Gastric Bypass

João Ettinger • Euler Ázaro
Rudolf Weiner • Kelvin D. Higa
Manoel Galvão Neto
Andre Fernandes Teixeira
Muhammad Jawad
Editors

Gastric Bypass

Bariatric and Metabolic Surgery Perspectives

Springer

Editors
João Ettinger
UNIME School of Medicine
Salvador
Bahia
Brazil

Euler Ázaro
Bahia School of Medicine and
Public Health
Salvador
Bahia
Brazil

Rudolf Weiner
Johann Wolfgang Goethe University
Frankfurt
Hessen
Germany

Kelvin D. Higa
Ste 460
Fresno, CA
USA

Manoel Galvão Neto
Gastro Obeso Center Clinic
São Paulo
São Paulo
Brazil

Andre Fernandes Teixeira
Orlando Health
Orlando, FL
USA

Muhammad Jawad
Orlando Health
Orlando, FL
USA

ISBN 978-3-030-28802-0 ISBN 978-3-030-28803-7 (eBook)
https://doi.org/10.1007/978-3-030-28803-7

This Springer imprint is published by the registered company Springer Nature Switzerland AG
The registered company address is: Gewerbestrasse 11, 6330 Cham, Switzerland

Contents

1 **History of the Gastric Bypass** 1
Arthur Belarmino Garrido Jr., Alexandre Amado Elias, Marcelo Roque de Oliveira, Renato Massaru Ito, and Henrique Yoshio Shirozaki

2 **Gastric Bypass: Mechanisms of Functioning** 7
Carel W. le Roux and Piriyah Sinclair

3 **Morbid Obesity** 23
Minna Ferrari Schleu and Karyne Freitas Barbosa

4 **Obesity and Related Diseases** 31
Mariana Freitas Ferreira Lopes

5 **Preparing for Gastric Bypass** 41
Joseph Sujka, Rena Moon, Muhammad Jawad, and Andre Fernandes Teixeira

6 **Preoperative Weight Loss in Gastric Bypass** 47
Gustavo Peixoto Soares Miguel, Paulo Henrique Oliveira de Souza, Luize Giuri Palaoro, Caroline Gravel, and Kassio Covre

7 **Preoperative Testing and Counseling** 53
Abraham Fridman

8 **Patient Selection for Metabolic Surgery** 61
Jose Guido Correa de Araujo Jr., Josemberg Marins Campos, Renata Paiva Barbosa, Maira Danielle Gomes, and Álvaro Antônio Bandeira Ferraz

9 **Psychiatric Issues During the Postoperative Period of Bariatric Surgery** 67
Adriano Segal and Debora Kinoshita Kussunoki

10 **Sleep-Disordered Breathing and Bariatric Surgery** 75
Michael V. J. Braganza and Stephen K. Field

11 **The Superobese Patient** 91
Michel Suter

12 **Airway Evaluation and Management** 99
Adriano Teixeira Fernandes, Macius Pontes Cerqueira, and Guilherme Oliveira Campos

13 Positioning the Bariatric Surgical Patient 111
Jay B. Brodsky

14 Developing the Laparoscopic Gastric Bypass 117
Cássio Renato Montenegro de Lima

15 Systemic Inflammation in the Morbidly Obese Patient 125
Antonio Jamel Coelho

16 Banded Gastric Bypass by Fobi Ring: Technique and Results. . . . 133
Mohit Bhandari, Hemant Kumar Nautiyal, Winni Mathur, and Susmit Kosta

17 Mini-Gastric Bypass and One-Anastomosis Gastric Bypass: Rationale 137
Mervyn Deitel, Cesare Peraglie, and David Hargroder

18 Simplified Gastric Bypass: The Brazilian Technique 145
Almino Cardoso Ramos and Eduardo Lemos de Souza Bastos

19 Roux-en-Y Gastric Bypass in the Elderly Patient 151
Denis Pajecki, Andre Morrell, and Marco Aurelio Santo

20 Gastric Bypass Reoperation for Weight Regain. 159
Gustavo Peixoto Soares Miguel, Paulo Henrique Oliveira de Souza, Isaac Walker de Abreu, Luize Giuri Palaoro, and Thales Ribeiro dos Santos Vecci

21 Conversion from Sleeve to Bypass. 171
Alcides José Branco Filho and André Thá Nassif

22 Gastrojejunostomy Testing. 177
Amador García Ruiz de Gordejuela and Jordi Pujol Gebelli

23 Closing the Mesenteric Defects 181
Mariano Palermo, Pablo A. Acquafresca, and Edgardo Serra

24 Preventing Complications 187
Felipe de la Cruz Vigo, José Luis de la Cruz Vigo, Elías Rodríguez Cuéllar, Pilar Gómez Rodríguez, and José María Canga Presa

25 Laparoscopic Gastric Bypass: Tricks and Tips 205
Fábio Almeida, Juliana Moura, and Antonio Alves Jr.

26 Psychiatric Assistance in Bariatric Surgery. 215
Adriano Segal and Debora Kinoshita Kussunoki

27 Perioperative Complications 221
Juliana Henrique, Luis Felipe Okida, Rene Aleman, Emanuele Lo Menzo, Samuel Szomstein, and Raul J. Rosenthal

28 Abdominal Pain After Gastric Bypass 235
Alexander Charles Morrell, André Luiz Gioia Morrell, Alexander Charles Morrell Jr., and Allan Gioia Morrell

29 Marginal Ulceration After (Laparoscopic) Roux-en-Y Gastric Bypass: Pathophysiology, Diagnostics, Treatment, and Prevention 247
U. K. Coblijn, B. A. van Wagensveld, S. M. Lagarde, and S. M. M. de Castro

30 Rhabdomyolysis 255
João Ettinger, Paulo Vicente Filho, Euler Ázaro, and Paulo Benigno

31 Depressive Disorders, Alcohol Use Disorders, and Suicidality in Bariatric Surgery 265
Adriano Segal

32 Nutritional Complications 273
Silvia Leite Faria, Orlando Pereira Faria, and Marina Kiyomi Ito

33 Eating Disorders 287
Debora Kinoshita Kussunoki

34 Gallbladder Stones and Choledocholitiasis 295
Pablo A. Acquafresca, Mariano Palermo, and Mariano E. Giménez

35 Hypoglycemia After Gastric Bypass 307
Glauco da Costa Alvarez

36 Dumping Syndrome 315
Christine Stier, Koschker Ann-Cathrin, and Sonja Chiappetta

37 Endoscopic Treatment of Roux-en-Y Gastric Bypass Complications 329
Lyz Bezerra Silva, Gabriel Tavares Xavier Simplicio, and Josemberg Marins Campos

38 Endoscopic Treatment of Weight Regain After Gastric Bypass 337
Luiz Gustavo de Quadros, Manoel Galvão Neto, Eduardo Grecco, Thiago Ferreira de Souza, Idiberto José Zotarelli Filho, and Andre Fernandes Teixeira

39 Laparoscopic Bariatric Surgery Training and the Credentialing Process 347
Kais A. Rona, Angela S. Volk, James R. Pellechi, Daniel H. Shin, and Christopher G. DuCoin

40 Training and Credentialing the Robotic Bariatric Surgeon 355
Kais A. Rona, Matthew N. Marturano, Leland P. Chan, and Christopher G. DuCoin

41 **Mechanisms of Control of Type 2 Diabetes with Gastric Bypass** ... 359
Manuel F. Landecho, Carlota Tuero, Víctor Valentí, Rafael Moncada, and Gema Frühbeck

42 **The Gut and Type 2 Diabetes Mellitus** ... 375
Stephen Boyce

43 **Shifts in the Intestinal Microbiota After Gastric Bypass** ... 395
Meera Nair, Carel W. le Roux, and Neil G. Docherty

44 **Infection: Diagnosis and Treatment** ... 403
Álvaro Antônio Bandeira Ferraz and Luciana Teixeira de Siqueira

45 **Gastric Bypass in Patients with Metabolic Syndrome** ... 411
Mariano Palermo, Maria del Pilar Quevedo, Edgardo Serra, and Marianela Aguirre Ackermann

46 **Gastric Bypass for Type 2 Diabetes Mellitus on BMI >35** ... 421
Jad Khoraki, Matthew G. Browning, Bernardo M. Pessoa, and Guilherme M. Campos

47 **Gastric Bypass for Type 2 Diabetes Mellitus on BMI < 35** ... 453
Admar Concon-Filho, Andre Fernandes Teixeira, Eduardo Grecco, Luiz Gustavo de Quadros, Manoel Galvão Neto, and Thiago Ferreira de Souza

48 **Postoperative Care** ... 459
Amador García Ruiz de Gordejuela and Jordi Pujol Gebelli

49 **Mini Gastric Bypass: Why It Is Better than Gastric Bypass in India** ... 465
Mohit Bhandari, Manoj Kumar Reddy, Winni Mathur, and Susmit Kosta

50 **Can Bariatric Surgery Improve the Microvascular Complications of Type 2 Diabetes?** ... 469
Loai A. Shakerdi, Carel W. le Roux, and Neil G. Docherty

Index ... 479

Contributors

Isaac Walker de Abreu Department of Surgical Clinics, Hospital Universitário Cassiano Antônio de Moraes – HUCAM/UFES, Vitória, ES, Brazil

Marianela Aguirre Ackermann Division of Bariatric Surgery Centro CIEN – DIAGNOMED, Institution to the University of Buenos Aires, Buenos Aires, Argentina

Pablo A. Acquafresca Division of Bariatric Surgery Centro CIEN – DIAGNOMED, Affiliated Institution to the University of Buenos Aires and DAICIM Foundation, Buenos Aires, Argentina

Rene Aleman Department of General Surgery and The Bariatric and Metabolic Institute, Cleveland Clinic Florida, Weston, FL, USA

Fábio Almeida SIGO – Serviço Integrado de Gastroenterologia e Obesidade and Unit of Bariatric Surgery of University Hospital of Universidade Federal de Sergipe, Aracaju, Sergipe, Brazil

Glauco da Costa Alvarez Department of Surgery, Federal University of Santa Maria, Santa Maria, Brazil

Antonio Alves Jr. SIGO – Serviço Integrado de Gastroenterologia e Obesidade and Unit of Bariatric Surgery of University Hospital of Universidade Federal de Sergipe, Aracaju, Sergipe, Brazil

Koschker Ann-Cathrin Department of Endocrinology, University Hospital Wuerzburg, Wuerzburg, Germany

Jose Guido Correa de Araujo Jr. Surgery Department, University Hospital, Pernambuco Federal University, Recife, Brazil

Euler Ázaro Bahia School of Medicine and Public Health, Salvador, Bahia, Brazil

Karyne Freitas Barbosa Endocrinology Division, São Rafael, Salvador, Bahia, Brazil

Renata Paiva Barbosa Esperança D'Or Hospital, Recife, Brazil

Eduardo Lemos de Souza Bastos International Federation for the Surgery of Obesity and Metabolic Disorders (IFSO), Naples, Italy

Gastro-Obeso-Center – Advanced Institute for Metabolic Optimization, São Paulo, Brazil

Division of Gastrointestinal Surgery, Marilia School of Medicine, São Paulo, Brazil

Brazilian Society of Bariatric and Metabolic Surgery (SBCBM), São Paulo, Brazil

Paulo Benigno Bahia School of Medicine and Public Health, Salvador, Bahia, Brazil

Mohit Bhandari Department of Surgery, Mohak Bariatrics and Robotics Surgical Center, Indore, India

Stephen Boyce Department of Surgery, Turkey Creek Medical Center, Knoxville, TN, USA

Michael V. J. Braganza Division of Respirology, Department of Medicine, Cumming School of Medicine, University of Calgary, Calgary, AB, Canada

Alcides José Branco Filho Department of Bariatric Surgery, Curitiba, Brazil

Jay B. Brodsky Department of Anesthesia, Perioperative and Pain Medicine, Stanford University School of Medicine, Stanford, CA, USA

Matthew G. Browning Division of Bariatric and Gastrointestinal Surgery, Department of Surgery, Virginia Commonwealth University, Richmond, VA, USA

Guilherme M. Campos Division of Bariatric and Gastrointestinal Surgery, Department of Surgery, Virginia Commonwealth University, Richmond, VA, USA

Guilherme Oliveira Campos Department of Anesthesiology, São Rafael Hospital, Salvador, Brazil

Josemberg Marins Campos Surgery Department, University Hospital, Pernambuco Federal University, Recife, Brazil

S. M. M. de Castro Department of Surgery, Onze Lieve Vrouwe Gasthuis, Amsterdam, The Netherlands

Macius Pontes Cerqueira Department of Anesthesiology, São Rafael Hospital, Salvador, Brazil

Leland P. Chan Department of Surgery, Tulane University School of Medicine, New Orleans, LA, USA

Sonja Chiappetta Ospedale Evangelico Betania, Naples, Italy

U. K. Coblijn Department of Surgery, Vrije Universiteit Medical Center, Amsterdam, The Netherlands

Antonio Jamel Coelho Department of Emergency, Hospital Barra D'Or, Rio de Janeiro, Brazil

Admar Concon-Filho Faculty of Medicine of ABC – FMABC, Santo André, Brazil

Concon Clinic, Valinhos, Brazil

Galileo Hospital and Maternity, Valinhos, Brazil

Kassio Covre Department of Surgical Clinics, Hospital Universitário Cassiano Antônio de Moraes – HUCAM/UFES, Vitória, ES, Brazil

Elías Rodríguez Cuéllar General, Digestive and Transplantation Surgery Department, 12 de Octubre University Hospital, Madrid, Spain

Mervyn Deitel Mini-Gastric Bypass–One Anastomosis Gastric Bypass Club, Toronto, ON, Canada

Neil G. Docherty Diabetes Complications Research Centre, Conway Institute, School of Medicine, University College Dublin, Dublin, Ireland

Christopher G. DuCoin Department of Surgery, University of South Florida, Tampa, FL, USA

Alexandre Amado Elias Bariatric Surgery, Instituto Garrido, São Paulo, SP, Brazil

João Ettinger, (Deceased) Bahia School of Medicine and Public Health, Salvador, Bahia, Brazil

Orlando Pereira Faria Bariatric and Metabolic Surgery, Gastrocirurgia de Brasília, Brasília, DF, Brazil

Silvia Leite Faria Gastrocirurgia de Brasília & University of Brasília, Brasília, DF, Brazil

Adriano Teixeira Fernandes Department of Anesthesiology, São Rafael Hospital, Salvador, Brazil

Álvaro Antônio Bandeira Ferraz Federal University of Pernambuco, Department of Surgery, Recife, Brazil

Stephen K. Field Division of Respirology, Department of Medicine, Cumming School of Medicine, University of Calgary, Calgary, AB, Canada

Abraham Fridman Griffin Hospital, Derby, CT, USA

Gema Frühbeck Metabolic Research Laboratory, University of Navarra, Pamplona, Spain

CIBER Fisiopatología de la Obesidad y Nutrición (CIBEROBN), Instituto de Salud Carlos III, Pamplona, Spain

Obesity & Adipobiology Group, Instituto de Investigaciones Sanitarias de Navarra (IdiSNA), Clínica Universidad de Navarra, Pamplona, Spain

Department of Endocrinology and Nutrition, Clínica Universidad de Navarra, Pamplona, Spain

Manoel Galvão Neto Faculty of Medicine of ABC – FMABC, Santo André, Brazil

Florida International University – FIU, Miami, FL, USA

EndoVitta Institute, São Paulo, Brazil

Arthur Belarmino Garrido Jr. Digestive Surgery, Hospital das Clínicas – University of São Paulo Medical School, São Paulo, SP, Brazil

Jordi Pujol Gebelli Bariatric Surgery Unit, General Surgery Department, Bellvitge University Hospital, Barcelona, Spain

Mariano E. Giménez Division of Bariatric Surgery Centro CIEN – DIAGNOMED, Affiliated Institution to the University of Buenos Aires and DAICIM Foundation, Buenos Aires, Argentina

Maira Danielle Gomes Surgery Department, University Hospital, Pernambuco Federal University, Recife, Brazil

Amador García Ruiz de Gordejuela Bariatric Surgery Unit, General Surgery Department, Bellvitge University Hospital, Barcelona, Spain

Caroline Gravel Department of Surgical Clinics, Hospital Universitário Cassiano Antônio de Moraes – HUCAM/UFES, Vitória, ES, Brazil

Eduardo Grecco ABC Medical School (FMABC), São Paulo, Brazil

David Hargroder Department of Surgery, Mercy Hospitals, Joplin, MO, USA

Juliana Henrique Department of General Surgery and The Bariatric and Metabolic Institute, Cleveland Clinic Florida, Weston, FL, USA

Marina Kiyomi Ito Department of Nutrition, University of Brasília, Brasília, DF, Brazil

Renato Massaru Ito Bariatric Surgery, Instituto Garrido, São Paulo, SP, Brazil

Muhammad Jawad Bariatric and Laparoscopy Center, Orlando Health, Orlando, FL, USA

Jad Khoraki Division of Bariatric and Gastrointestinal Surgery, Department of Surgery, Virginia Commonwealth University, Richmond, VA, USA

Susmit Kosta Department of Surgery, Mohak Bariatrics and Robotics Surgical Center, Indore, India

Debora Kinoshita Kussunoki Obesity and Diabetes Center, German Hospital Oswaldo Cruz, São Paulo, Brazil

Obesity and Metabolic Syndrome Outpatient Clinic, Service of Endocrinology and Metabolism-HCFMUSP/SP, São Paulo, Brazil

Brazilian Society of Bariatric and Metabolic Surgery, São Paulo, Brazil

Brazilian Association for the Study of Obesity and Metabolic Syndrome, São Paulo, Brazil

Segal Clinic, São Paulo, Brazil

S. M. Lagarde Department of Surgery, Erasmus Medical Center, Rotterdam, The Netherlands

Manuel F. Landecho General Health Check-Up Unit, Internal Medicine Department, Clinica Universidad de Navarra, Pamplona, Spain

Carel W. le Roux Diabetes Complications Research Centre, Conway Institute, School of Medicine, University College Dublin, Dublin, Ireland

Cássio Renato Montenegro de Lima Secretary of Health of Santa Catarina State, Florianópolis, Brazil

Mariana Freitas Ferreira Lopes Endocrinology Division, Department of Obesity, São Rafael Hospital (HSR), Salvador, Bahia, Brazil

Matthew N. Marturano Department of Surgery, Tulane University School of Medicine, New Orleans, LA, USA

Winni Mathur Department of Surgery, Mohak Bariatrics and Robotics Surgical Center, Indore, India

Emanuele Lo Menzo Department of General Surgery and The Bariatric and Metabolic Institute, Cleveland Clinic Florida, Weston, FL, USA

Gustavo Peixoto Soares Miguel Department of Surgical Clinics, Hospital Universitário Cassiano Antônio de Moraes – HUCAM/UFES, Vitória, ES, Brazil

Rafael Moncada CIBER Fisiopatología de la Obesidad y Nutrición (CIBEROBN), Instituto de Salud Carlos III, Pamplona, Spain

Obesity & Adipobiology Group, Instituto de Investigaciones Sanitarias de Navarra (IdiSNA), Clínica Universidad de Navarra, Pamplona, Spain

Department of Anesthesiology, Clínica Universidad de Navarra, Pamplona, Spain

Rena Moon Bariatric and Laparoscopy Center, Orlando Health, Orlando, FL, USA

Alexander Charles Morrell General Surgery/Bariatric and Metabolic Surgery/Robotic Surgery, Sociedade Beneficente Israelita Brasileira Hospital Albert Einstein, São Paulo, SP, Brazil

Allan Gioia Morrell General Surgery/Bariatric and Metabolic Surgery, Sociedade Beneficente Israelita Brasileira Hospital Albert Einstein, São Paulo, SP, Brazil

Andre Morrell Bariatric and Metabolic Surgery Unit – Gastroenterology Department – Surgical Division, Hospital das Clínicas – University of São Paulo, São Paulo, Brazil

André Luiz Gioia Morrell General Surgery/Bariatric and Metabolic Surgery, Sociedade Beneficente Israelita Brasileira Hospital Albert Einstein, São Paulo, SP, Brazil

Alexander Charles Morrell Jr. General Surgery/Bariatric and Metabolic Surgery, Sociedade Beneficente Israelita Brasileira Hospital Albert Einstein, São Paulo, SP, Brazil

Juliana Moura SIGO – Serviço Integrado de Gastroenterologia e Obesidade and Unit of Bariatric Surgery of University Hospital of Universidade Federal de Sergipe, Aracaju, Sergipe, Brazil

Meera Nair Diabetes Complications Research Centre, Conway Institute, School of Medicine, University College Dublin, Dublin, Ireland

André Thá Nassif Department of Bariatric Surgery, Curitiba, Brazil

Hemant Kumar Nautiyal Department of Surgery, Mohak Bariatrics and Robotics Surgical Center, Indore, India

Luis Felipe Okida Department of General Surgery and The Bariatric and Metabolic Institute, Cleveland Clinic Florida, Weston, FL, USA

Marcelo Roque de Oliveira Bariatric Surgery, Instituto Garrido, São Paulo, SP, Brazil

Denis Pajecki Bariatric and Metabolic Surgery Unit – Gastroenterology Department – Surgical Division, Hospital das Clínicas – University of São Paulo, São Paulo, Brazil

Luize Giuri Palaoro Department of Surgical Clinics, Hospital Universitário Cassiano Antônio de Moraes – HUCAM/UFES, Vitória, ES, Brazil

Mariano Palermo Division of Bariatric Surgery Centro CIEN – DIAGNOMED, Affiliated Institution to the University of Buenos Aires and DAICIM Foundation, Buenos Aires, Argentina

James R. Pellechi School of Medicine, Tulane Medical Center, New Orleans, LA, USA

Cesare Peraglie Department of Surgery, Heart of Florida Regional Medical Center, Davenport, FL, USA

Bernardo M. Pessoa Division of Bariatric and Gastrointestinal Surgery, Department of Surgery, Virginia Commonwealth University, Richmond, VA, USA

José María Canga Presa Laparoscopic Surgery Department, San Francisco Hospital, León, Spain

Luiz Gustavo de Quadros Department of Bariatric Endoscopy, Kaiser Day Hospital, São José do Rio Preto, Brazil

Maria del Pilar Quevedo Division of Bariatric Surgery Centro CIEN – DIAGNOMED, Institution to the University of Buenos Aires, Buenos Aires, Argentina

Almino Cardoso Ramos International Federation for the Surgery of Obesity and Metabolic Disorders (IFSO), Naples, Italy

Gastro-Obeso-Center – Advanced Institute for Metabolic Optimization, São Paulo, Brazil

Brazilian Society of Bariatric and Metabolic Surgery (SBCBM), São Paulo, Brazil

Manoj Kumar Reddy Department of Surgery, Mohak Bariatrics and Robotics Surgical Center, Indore, India

Pilar Gómez Rodríguez General, Digestive and Transplantation Surgery Department, 12 de Octubre University Hospital, Madrid, Spain

Kais A. Rona Department of Surgery, Tulane Medical Center, New Orleans, LA, USA

Raul J. Rosenthal Department of General Surgery and The Bariatric and Metabolic Institute, Cleveland Clinic Florida, Weston, FL, USA

Marco Aurelio Santo Bariatric and Metabolic Surgery Unit – Gastroenterology Department – Surgical Division, Hospital das Clínicas – University of São Paulo, São Paulo, Brazil

Minna Ferrari Schleu Endocrinology, Clínica Metta, Salvador, Bahia, Brazil

Adriano Segal Obesity and Diabetes Center, German Hospital Oswaldo Cruz, São Paulo, Brazil

Obesity and Metabolic Syndrome Outpatient Clinic, Service of Endocrinology and Metabolism-HCFMUSP/SP, São Paulo, Brazil

Brazilian Society of Bariatric and Metabolic Surgery, São Paulo, Brazil

Brazilian Association for the Study of Obesity and Metabolic Syndrome, São Paulo, Brazil

Segal Clinic, São Paulo, Brazil

Edgardo Serra Division of Bariatric Surgery Centro CIEN – DIAGNOMED, Affiliated Institution to the University of Buenos Aires and DAICIM Foundation, Buenos Aires, Argentina

Loai A. Shakerdi Clinical Research Centre, St. Vincent's University Hospital, Dublin, Ireland

Daniel H. Shin Tulane School of Medicine, New Orleans, LA, USA

Henrique Yoshio Shirozaki Bariatric Surgery, Instituto Garrido, São Paulo, SP, Brazil

Lyz Bezerra Silva Department of Surgery, Federal University of Pernambuco, Recife, Brazil

Gabriel Tavares Xavier Simplicio Department of Surgery, Federal University of Pernambuco, Recife, Brazil

Piriyah Sinclair Diabetes Complications Research Centre, University College Dublin, Dublin, Ireland

Luciana Teixeira de Siqueira Federal University of Pernambuco, Recife, Brazil

General Surgery Residence Program at the Federal University of Pernambuco Clinical Hospital, Recife, Brazil

Paulo Henrique Oliveira de Souza Department of Surgical Clinics, Hospital Universitário Cassiano Antônio de Moraes – HUCAM/UFES, Vitória, ES, Brazil

Thiago Ferreira de Souza ABC Medical School (FMABC), São Paulo, Brazil

Faculty of Medicine of ABC – FMABC, Santo André, Brazil

EndoVitta Institute, São Paulo, Brazil

University of São Paulo – USP, São Paulo, Brazil

Christine Stier Department of Surgical Endoscopy and Endocrinology, University Hospital Wuerzburg, Wuerzburg, Germany

Joseph Sujka Orlando Regional Medical Center, Department of Surgery, Orlando, FL, USA

Michel Suter Department of Surgery, Riviera-Chablais Hospital, Aigle-Monthey, Switzerland

Department of Visceral Surgery, University Hospital Lausanne, Lausanne, Switzerland

Samuel Szomstein Department of General Surgery and The Bariatric and Metabolic Institute, Cleveland Clinic Florida, Weston, FL, USA

Andre Fernandes Teixeira Bariatric and Laparoscopy Center, Orlando Health, Orlando, FL, USA

Carlota Tuero Department of General Surgery, Clínica Universidad de Navarra, Pamplona, Spain

Víctor Valentí Department of General Surgery, Clínica Universidad de Navarra, Pamplona, Spain

CIBER Fisiopatología de la Obesidad y Nutrición (CIBEROBN), Instituto de Salud Carlos III, Pamplona, Spain

Obesity & Adipobiology Group, Instituto de Investigaciones Sanitarias de Navarra (IdiSNA), Clínica Universidad de Navarra, Pamplona, Spain

Thales Ribeiro dos Santos Vecci Department of Surgical Clinics, Hospital Universitário Cassiano Antônio de Moraes – HUCAM/UFES, Vitória, ES, Brazil

Paulo Vicente Filho Bahia School of Medicine and Public Health, Salvador, Bahia, Brazil

Felipe de la Cruz Vigo General, Digestive and Transplantation Surgery Department, 12 de Octubre University Hospital, Madrid, Spain

José Luis de la Cruz Vigo Laparoscopic Surgery Department, San Francisco Hospital, León, Spain

Angela S. Volk Department of Surgery, Tulane Medical Center, New Orleans, LA, USA

B. A. van Wagensveld Department of Surgery, Onze Lieve Vrouwe Gasthuis, Amsterdam, The Netherlands

Idiberto José Zotarelli Filho São José do Rio Preto, Brazil

History of the Gastric Bypass

1

Arthur Belarmino Garrido Jr., Alexandre Amado Elias, Marcelo Roque de Oliveira, Renato Massaru Ito, and Henrique Yoshio Shirozaki

During the second half of the twentieth century, obesity of high degrees became frequent, affecting physical, psychological, and social health and increasing mortality rate. The current clinical therapies could not efficiently solve that situation. The first surgical attempts of treatment consisted of resection or bypass of large extensions of the small intestine, which caused malabsorption of nutrients and weight loss. But they provoked also intense undesirable side effects and were abandoned after about one decade [1, 2].

In 1966, Edward Mason [3] introduced to the bariatric surgery a different approach, based not in malabsorption but in restriction to the ingestion of food by the reduction of gastric capacity. He was inspired by the observation that the subtotal gastrectomies, then widely used in the treatment of peptic ulcers, often resulted in weight loss. The initial gastric bypass procedures consisted of horizontal section of the upper stomach, leaving a functioning pouch of 10% of its volume, and anastomosis to a proximal jejunal loop, excluding 90% of the gastric reservoir from the alimentary transit (Fig. 1.1).

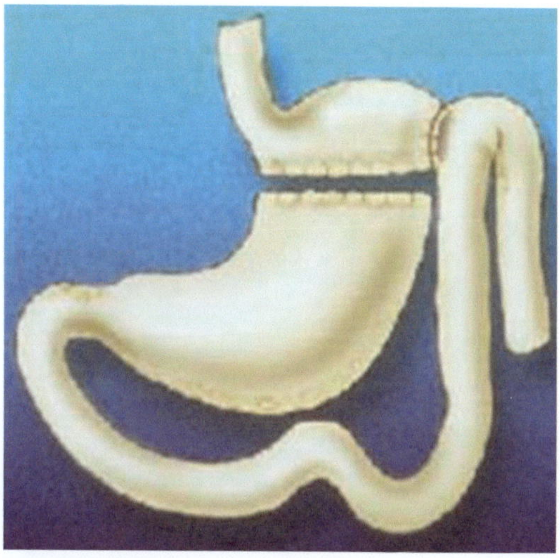

Fig. 1.1 MASON – 1st gastric bypass

The procedure was reluctantly accepted because vomiting, distress, and midterm recurrence of obesity were not rare, because of the large and distensible proximal pouch, the wide gastrojejunostomy, and the biliopancreatic reflux. With time, Mason and other surgeons improved the method by:

(a) Reducing the proximal pouch [4–6]
(b) Using surgical staplers to build the pouch [7, 8]
(c) Adopting Roux Y gastrojejunal anastomosis to prevent biliopancreatic reflux [9] (Fig. 1.2)
(d) Dividing the stapled stomach to facilitate the anastomosis and prevent rupture of the staple line [10]

A. B. Garrido Jr. (✉)
Digestive Surgery, Hospital das Clínicas – University of São Paulo Medical School, São Paulo, SP, Brazil

A. A. Elias · M. R. de Oliveira · R. M. Ito
H. Y. Shirozaki
Bariatric Surgery, Instituto Garrido, São Paulo, SP, Brazil

J. Ettinger et al. (eds.), *Gastric Bypass*, https://doi.org/10.1007/978-3-030-28803-7_1

(e) Encircling the gastrojejunostomy with a band of abdominal fascia as a ring of 11 mm diameter in order to prevent dilation of the outlet [11]
(f) Locating the proximal pouch near the small curvature, thicker, to prevent pouch dilation [12] (Fig. 1.3)

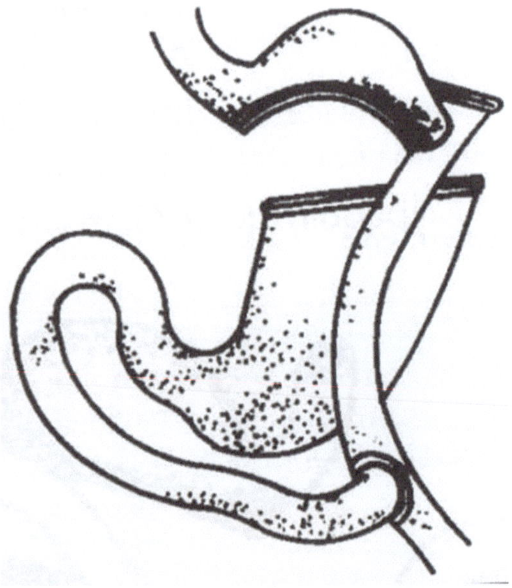

Fig. 1.2 GRIFFEN – RYGBP

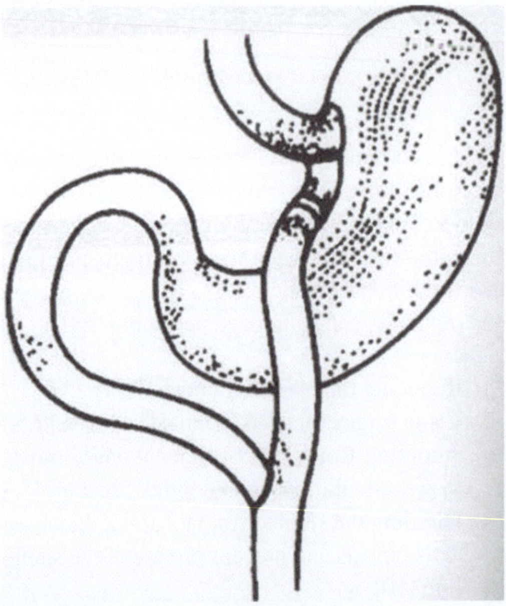

Fig. 1.3 TORRES – small curvature pouch

(g) Increasing the malabsorptive component using a gastroileal anastomosis Roux-en-Y (distal bypass), to correct obesity recurrence after regular bypass [13]
(h) Vertical division of the pouch near the small curvature with a silicone ring above the gastrojejunal anastomosis and interposition of a jejunal segment between the two parts of the stomach to prevent gastrogastric fistula [14–17]

In 1993, we started gastric bypass in Brazil at the University of São Paulo Medical School – Hospital das Clínicas [18]. We followed the technique learned from Raphael Capella:

- Upper midline incision
- Vertical pouch of about 20 ml divided by linear staplers (Fig. 1.4)
- Silicone ring of 6.5 cm circumference
- Retrocolic and retrogastric Roux-en-Y gastrojejunostomy: biliopancreatic limb 30–50 cm from the ligament of Treitz and alimentary limb 100 cm with 10 cm proximal jejunum interposed between the separated parts of the stomach (Fig. 1.5)

As proposed by Mathias Fobi, we employed routine upper abdominal drainage and gastrostomy (Fig. 1.6).

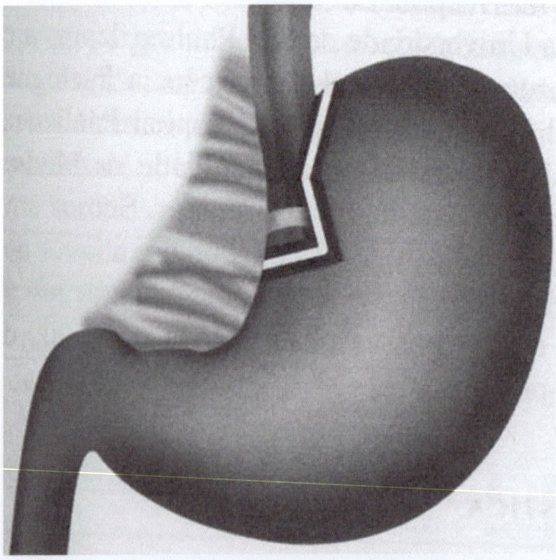

Fig. 1.4 CAPELLA – vertical pouch with silicone ring

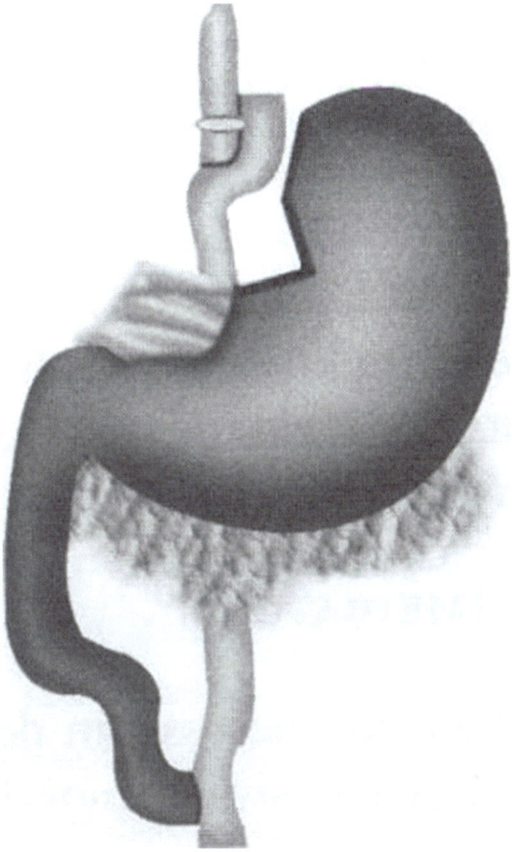

Fig. 1.5 CAPELLA – RYGBP with interposed loop

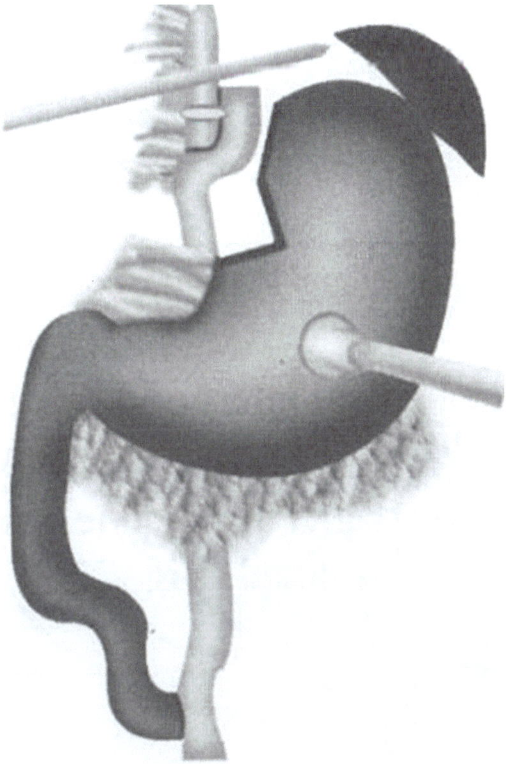

Fig. 1.6 FOBI – RYGBP with drainage and gastrostomy

This procedure was adopted by most Brazilian bariatric surgeons for over 10 years, and we performed 6000 surgeries of this procedure up to 2006. Average excess weight loss was about 65–70% after 5 years with near or over 50% weight regain rate of 10–15%. Improvement of associated diseases was outstanding. Most threatening immediate postoperative complications were staple line leaks (2%) and respiratory failure due to bronchopneumonia or pulmonary thromboembolism (1%). Mortality rate is 0.5%. Late complications mainly malnutrition, like anemia and hypoalbuminemia, needed careful follow-up control and were clearly related to the obstacle to protein ingestion caused by the silicone ring. From 2006, we abandoned the use of silicone ring (Fig. 1.7).

In 1995, Wittgrove and Clark [19] established a standard technique for laparoscopic gastric bypass. They helped us to learn it, and we progressively adapted to this new technology until quitting open gastric bypass for the last 10 years. Our group of surgeons in private practice performed over 15,000 laparoscopic Roux-en-Y gastric bypass (LRYGBP) surgeries without a ring (Fig. 1.8). Better exposure, advanced instruments, and surgeons' cumulated experience resulted in extraordinary reduction of surgical complications (less than 0.2% leaks and less than 0.01% of respiratory failures). Surgical mortality in the last 3 years was absent.

Similar progressive improvement in the results of LRYGBP is reported in most large series around the world [20–23].

The use of robotics in RYGBP started with the new millennium, the first reports of series dating from 2001 [24–26]. Tridimensional visualization and more accurate instrumental handling were emphasized. In São Paulo, Abdalla (2012) published an initial experience with robotic bariatric procedures like gastric band, vertical banded gastroplasty, and gastric bypass [27]. Under the supervision of Keith Kim from the Celebration

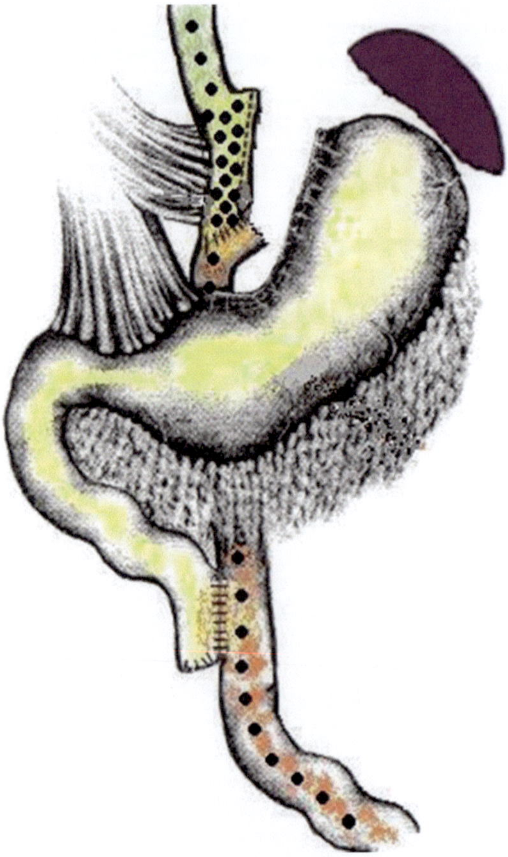

Fig. 1.7 Gastric bypass without ring

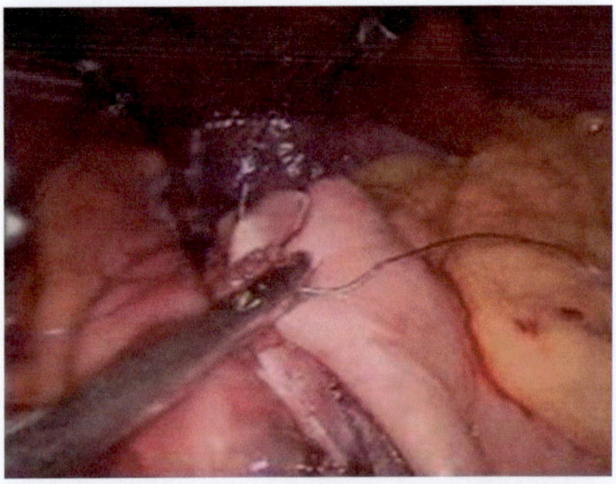

Fig. 1.8 LRYGBP – precision of robotic-assisted suture

(FL-USA) Robotic Center, Alexandre Amado Elias, in our group, started robotic RYGBP in 2010, counting presently 30 of those procedures performed (Figs. 1.8 and 1.9). The potential advantages of the method are becoming more

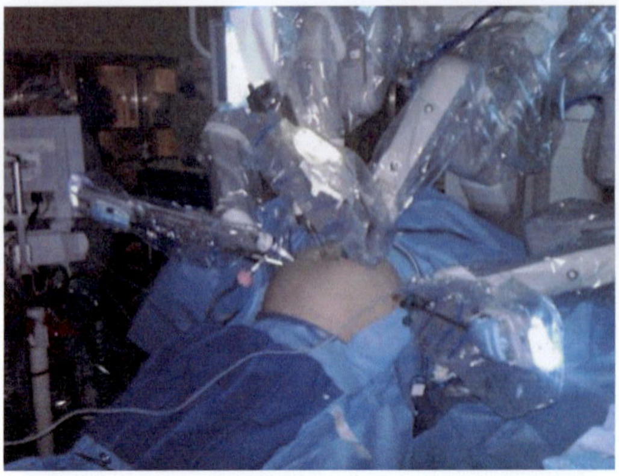

Fig. 1.9 Robotics in bariatric surgery – the robot in action

and more evident, especially in difficult cases, when precision is important. An example is the performance of RYGBP after previous gastric fundoplication.

Gastric bypass after 50 years of existence keeps representing a main tendency in surgical treatment of obesity and its comorbidities. The procedure is continuously benefiting from the progress of technology and better understanding of the obese patients and their needs and characteristics.

References

1. Kremen NA, Linner JH, Nelson CH. Experimental evaluation of the nutritional importance of proximal and distal small intestine. Ann Surg. 1954;140:439.
2. Buckwald H, Rucker RDJ. A history of morbid obesity. In: Najarian JS, Delaney JP, editors. Advances in gastrointestinal surgery. Chicago: Year Book Medical Publishers; 1984. p. 235.
3. Mason EE, Ito C. Gastric bypass in obesity. Surg Clin North Am. 1967;47:1345–52.
4. Mason EE, Printe KJ, Hartford C. Optimizing results of gastric bypass. Ann Surg. 1975;182:405–13.
5. Mason EE, Ito C. Graded gastric bypass. World J Surg. 1978;2:341–9.
6. Mason EE, Printen KJ, Blommers TJ. Gastric bypass and morbid obesity. Am J Clin Nutr (Suppl). 1980;33:395–405.
7. Alden JF. Gastric and jejuno-ileal bypass: a comparison in the treatment of morbid obesity. Arch Surg. 1977;112:799–806.
8. Griffen WO Jr, Bivins BA, Bell RM. Gastric bypass for morbid obesity. World J Surg. 1981;5:817–22.

9. Griffen WO Jr, Young VL, Stevenson CC. A prospective comparison of gastric and jejunoileal bypass procedures for morbid obesity. Ann Surg. 1977;186:500–9.
10. Miller DK, Goodman GN. Gastric bypass procedures. In: Deitel M, editor. Surgery for the morbidly obese patient. Philadelphia: Lea & Febiger; 1989. p. 113.
11. Linner JH, Drew RL. Roux-Y gastric bypass for morbid obesity. Scientific Exhibit, American College of Surgeons 73rd Clinical Congress, San Francisco, October 11–16, 1987.
12. Torres JC, Oca CF, Garrison RN. Gastric bypass: Roux-en-Y gastrojejunostomy from the lesser curvature. South Med J. 1983;76:1217–21.
13. Torres JC, Oca C. Gastric bypass lesser curvature with distal Roux-en-Y. Bariatric Surgery. 1987;5:10–5.
14. Fobi MAL, Lee H, Fleming A. The surgical technique of the banded Roux-en-Y gastric bypass. J Obesity Weight Reg. 1989;8:99–102.
15. Fobi MAL, Lee H, Felahy B, Che K, Ako P, Fobi N. Choosing an operation for weight control, and the transected banded gastric bypass. Obes Surg. 2005;15(1):114–21.
16. Capella RF, Capella J, Mandac H, Nath P. Vertical banded gastroplasty – gastric bypass. Obes Surg. 1991;1:219, Abstract.
17. Capella RF. Vertical banded gastroplasty – gastric bypass. Obes Surg. 1993;3:95, Abstract.
18. Garrido AB Jr, editor. Cirurgia da obesidade. São Paulo: Atheneu; 2002.
19. Wittgrove AC, Clark W, Schubert KR. Laparoscopic gastric bypass, Rou-en-Y: technique and results in 75 patients with 3–30 month follow-up. Obes Surg. 1996;6:500–4.
20. Weiss AC, Parina R, Horgan S, Talamini M. Quality and safety in obesity surgery – 15 years of Roux-en-Y gastric bypass outcomes from a longitudinal database. Surg Obes Relat Diseases. 2016;12(1):33–41.
21. Varban OA, Cassidy RB, Sheetz KH, Cain-Nielsen A, Carlin AM, et al. Technique or technology? Evaluating leaks after gastric bypass. Surg Obes Relat Diseases. 2016;12(2):264–73.
22. Nguyen NT, Wilson SE. Complications of anti-obesity surgery. Clin Pract Gastroenterol Hepatol. 2007;4:138–47.
23. Maciejewski ML, Livingston EH, Smith VA, Kavee AL, Kahwati LC, Henderson WG, et al. Survival among high-risk patients after bariatric surgery. JAMA. 2011;305(23):2419–26.
24. Artuso D, Wayne M, Grossi R. Use of robotics during laparoscopic gastric bypass for morbid obesity. JSLS. 2005;9:266–8.
25. Jacobsen G, Berger R, Horgan S. The role of robotic surgery in morbid obesity. Journal of laparoendoscopic & advanced surgical techniques. 2003;13(4):279–83.
26. Mohr CJ, Nadzam GS, Alami RS, Sanchez BR, Curet MJ. Totally robotic laparoscopic Roux-en-Y gastric bypass: results from 75 patients. Obes Surg. 2006;16(6):690–6.
27. Abdalla RZ, Garcia RB, De Luca CRP, Costa RID, Cozer CO. Experiência brasileira inicial em cirurgia da obesidade robô – assistida. ABCD. 2012;25(1) São Paulo.

Gastric Bypass: Mechanisms of Functioning

2

Carel W. le Roux and Piriyah Sinclair

Introduction

This chapter focusses on the underlying mechanisms of functioning of the Roux-en-Y gastric bypass (RYGB) – from its benefits (weight loss and comorbidity improvement) through to its complications. RYGB is no longer considered a purely mechanically restrictive and malabsorptive procedure but a metabolic procedure most likely to involve complex gut-brain signalling and physiological changes. It is likely that the gut has endocrine and metabolic functions that regulate appetite, satiety, weight and glucose metabolism. The full extent of these mechanisms is still not fully understood. Here we explore the current body of evidence.

The Benefits

Weight Loss

RYGB can result in up to 25% total body weight loss (68.2% excess weight loss) [1] which is maintained in the long term [2]. Traditionally, weight loss post RYGB was attributed to the mechanical effects of consuming a smaller volume and bypassing the small bowel. However, it is likely that there is a complex interplay of physiological mechanisms including:

1. Food intake
2. Food preferences
3. Calorie restriction
4. Energy Expenditure

C. W. le Roux (✉)
Diabetes Complications Research Centre, Conway Institute, School of Medicine, University College Dublin, Dublin, Ireland
e-mail: carel.leroux@ucd.ie

P. Sinclair
Diabetes Complications Research Centre, University College Dublin, Dublin, Ireland

Food Intake

Observations suggest that although dietary restriction with a low-calorie diet can initiate weight loss, randomized controlled trials (RCT) demonstrate poor maintenance of this weight loss [3, 4] Additionally, low-calorie diets result in increased hunger, decreased satiety, and fixation on energy-dense foods [5, 6]. This may be part of a normal physiological response to overcome the volume restriction and not due to lack of motivation [7].

Although RYGB has historically been considered a mechanically restrictive procedure resulting in caloric restriction, high-pressure manometry studies have revealed contrary findings after RYGB with normal pressures in the oesophagus, low pressures in the gastric pouch proximal to the anastomosis and higher pressures distal to the anastomosis [8]. Despite overall lower food intake, patients report decreased premeal hunger and increased satiety [9, 10]. Additionally, the fixation on energy-dense sweet

J. Ettinger et al. (eds.), *Gastric Bypass*, https://doi.org/10.1007/978-3-030-28803-7_2

and fatty foods is not reported unlike with caloric restriction [11, 12]. These changes in eating behaviour were first reported in the 1970s, where structured interviews were used to identify that patients reached satiety earlier post RYGB, commonly due to a “lack of desire” to eat more [13]. The reduction in calorie intake after RYGB is usually due to reduced meal size, reduced liquid intake, slower eating rate, and reduced calorie content of the actual foods eaten, compensated only partially by increased meal frequency [14, 15]. These findings may be explained by changes in the feedback signals from the GI tract to the brain after RYGB [15].

Further evidence that mechanical restriction does not have a significant role to play in gastric bypass mechanistically includes the fact that patients decrease their liquid intake, with no attempt to overcome mechanical restraint with food dilution, and blocking the hormone response in RYGB patients with a somatostatin analogue (keeping the pouch and stoma size constant) can double food intake [16].

After RYGB there is initially a decrease in daily energy intake to 600–700 kcal [17, 18]. This increases from the first month after surgery and continues to increase to 1000–1800 kcal during the first year [7, 17, 19, 20]. On average a reduction in intake of 1800 kcal per day compared to presurgery can be sustained for several years [19, 21]. Fat and carbohydrate intake decreases during the first post-operative year but returns to preoperative levels after the first year [17], although many patients increase their intake of lower glycaemic index carbohydrates over the longer term and have a compensatory reduction in intake of high glycaemic index carbohydrates and fatty foods [7]. Recommended protein intake is at least 1.5 g/kg/day. However, during the first year post-surgery, protein intake often falls to 0.5 g/kg [20]. We remain uncertain regarding the processes underlying this, but it may be explained by a temporary intolerance to the higher fat contents of meats and dairy foods [17, 18, 20]. The pattern of behaviour is suggestive of conditioned avoidance and not conditioned aversion.

There are several potential mechanisms for these noted observations in food intake, which include the following.

Mechanical Factors: Increased Transit of Food Through the Gastric Pouch into the Midgut

The technique of Roux-en-Y gastric bypass (RYGB) involves fashioning a small 15–30 ml gastric pouch, which is divided from the gastric remnant and anastomosed to the distal jejunum – forming a gastrojejunostomy. A Roux-en-Y jejuno-jejunostomy is then fashioned by anastomosing the alimentary or Roux limb with the excluded biliopancreatic limb (BPL).

The effect of the size of the gastric pouch and gastrojejunal anastomosis (stoma) in RYGB surgery on food intake and weight loss is controversial. Some studies suggest that the larger the pouch and stoma diameter, the less the weight loss [22–24]; others show no correlation between these variables [25, 26]. Initially restriction with a small stoma was thought to reduce transit of food from the oesophagus into the jejunum, but the current aim is rapid transit into the jejunum to reduce meal size [27]. As time from surgery progresses, the stoma becomes more “compliant,” allowing food to transit more easily from the pouch into the alimentary limb. However, food may also become stored in the pouch and not empty as rapidly as desired. Due to these varying factors, the initial size of the stoma may not affect weight loss in the long term [28].

Change in Gut Morphology

RYGB results in specific changes in the morphology of intestinal mucosa of animal models, including segmental hypertrophy of the small intestine [29–31]. In particular the muscular and mucosal layers are thicker in the Roux limb after RYGB, with increases in mucosal crypt depth and villi height. Similar changes may also be seen in the common channel, but not in the BPL. The mechanisms for this are unclear but may be a combination of increased release of GLP-2 from intestinal L cells [32] and stimulation of the intestine by nutrients and other factors. Post RYGB the hormonal secretory capacity of the small bowel increases, along with the L cell density (releasing GLP 1, GLP2 and PYY) and other enteroendocrine cells (e.g. cholecystokinin immunoreactive cells) [15].

Hormonal

Ghrelin was the first hormone to be studied with respect to weight loss after RYGB. Ghrelin affects glucose regulation, gut motility and gastric emptying. Initial studies suggested that ghrelin levels decreased post RYGB, and it was postulated that this led to reduced hunger after RYGB [7]. However, subsequent studies showed variability in fasting and postprandial ghrelin levels, with some showing an increase in fasting levels [7]. Overall there appears to be a comparative ghrelin deficiency post RYGB compared to the normal increases after diet-induced weight loss [33, 34]. However, it is unclear if the changes in circulating ghrelin affect weight loss or eating behaviours. In one study, ghrelin-deficient mice showed comparable food intake, body weight, dietary fat preference and glucose tolerance to wild-type mice post VSG [35].

Excluding ghrelin, the endogenous gut hormone response to a meal increases post RYGB, including glucagon-like peptide-1 (GLP-1), peptide YY (PYY), amylin and CCK (cholecystokinin). Two days post RYGB, the response has been shown to increase [16] and may remain increased for over a decade after RYGB [36]. It is postulated that the alteration in nutrient concentrations (higher in the distal segments) post RYGB gives stimulus to enteroendocrine cells to release these "satiety" hormones, and the increased secretion is thought to contribute to increased satiety, reduced food intake and sustained weight loss after RYGB. Other postulated mechanisms include the possibility of undiluted nutrients in the alimentary limb leading to increased levels of GLP-1, PYY and possibly CCK, as well as undiluted bile acids in the common limb stimulating L cell secretion.

The evidence for the effect of these hormones exists, but it is unclear whether they have a directly causal role in weight loss post RYGB. It is important to realize that this lack of clarity with respect to causality may be due to the fact that most studies look at single aspects and not the cumulative changes of all the hormones in parallel – the true effects mediating satiation after a meal are likely to be synergistic. Patients with the highest postprandial levels of satiety hormones lost the most weight post RYGB [37, 38]. Blocking satiety hormone release with the somatostatin analogue, octreotide increased food intake in rats and patients with RYGB, but not in sham-operated rats [39] or patients post adjustable gastric banding (AGB) surgery [9].

After RYGB PYY-knockout mice had lower weight loss compared to wild-type mice [40]. Pretreatment with exogenous PYY-specific antiserum revealed the usual effect of reduction in food intake in rats after bypass-type procedures [9]. PYY may also delay gastric emptying and orocaecal transit time but is unlikely to increase energy expenditure [41]. GLP-1 shows similar responses to PYY post RYGB but has also been associated with increases in secretion of insulin, which is usually considered fat storing [42, 43]. Studies looking at blocking the GLP-1 receptor and CCK receptor have been inconsistent [15], calling into question the significance of their role as single peptides in sustained weight loss post RYGB.

Leptin is an adipokine hormone produced mainly in adipose tissue as well as gastric mucosa. Leptin is known to be an appetite suppressant and affects energy expenditure and long-term weight loss. Obese patients have high leptin levels but also have leptin resistance. The leptin levels decrease post RYGB, but this correlates to weight loss. A study looking at leptin-deficient mice showed high rates of weight regain in the longer term [44].

Several areas in this field need further investigation, including the role of bile acids on hormone actions and how postprandial amylin secretion is triggered, as well as its effects on food intake and eating behaviour.

Neural

RYGB has been shown to influence neural responses [45], including a reduction in consumption of calorie-dense foods [13, 46–48], and has probable effects on energy expenditure. Several potential neural mechanisms have been postulated.

1. Vagus
Vagal afferent fibres in the gastric and proximal small bowel mucosa are sensitive to mechanical touch and can be activated by the volume of ingested food and degree of tension in the wall of the gastric pouch, which can in turn influence signals to the brain [49]. Sensory terminals known as intra-ganglionic laminar endings (IGLEs) may be activated in response to the stretch of the gastric wall, leading to reduced food intake [50]. During RYGB both the ventral and dorsal gastric branches are transected whilst fashioning the gastric pouch, which may play a role in satiation [51] and reduction in signalling of gut hormones such as ghrelin [52]. There is evidence that after RYGB, afferents in the vagal coeliac branches may become more sensitive to gut hormones [53]. This combined with the stretch-sensitive IGLEs in the pouch and Roux limb may explain the reduction in meal size, food preferences and reduced hunger.
2. Sympathetics
The sympathetic fibres in the distal stomach are also denervated during transection of the stomach. Gastric bypass has been associated with significantly reduced sympathetic contribution to resting energy expenditure and reduced resting sympathetic activity [54]. This may contribute to weight gain after gastric bypass surgery. Conversely, the coeliac plexus is associated with inhibition of peristalsis. Thus denervation should stimulate gut motility.
3. CNS centres for appetite regulation
Vagal afferents from the gut communicate centrally with hypothalamic centres associated with satiety, appetite regulation and hunger. They are hypothalamic groups of neurons, which act in antagonism. The melanocortin system, where melanocyte-stimulating hormone acts via the melanocortin-4 receptors to affect body weight, reduces food intake and increases energy expenditure and insulin sensitivity (although the latter may be due to weight loss) [55]. The second group of neurons synthesizing neuropeptide Y, agouti-related protein and gamma-aminobutyric acid reduce EE and increase food intake by inhibiting proopiomelanocortin [56]. These both need further study with respect to RYGB.
4. Other areas that require further investigation are changes within the enteric nervous system and the gastric electrical activity post RYGB.

Gut Microbiota

Gut flora is known to help modulate whole-body metabolism [57], including carbohydrate and energy metabolism, with fermentation of polysaccharides into short-chain fatty acids. Obese patients have altered gut flora, with increased *Firmicutes* and decreased *Bacteroidetes* species in animal [58] and human studies [59–61]. 'Obese microbiota' have an increased ability to harvest energy from the diet [62], and Germ-free mice colonized with an 'obese microbiota' had significantly greater total body fat [62]. This could be evidence for a significant role of gut flora in the pathophysiology of obesity.

Studies have shown that post RYGB, there is altered composition of endogenous gut microbiota, which is likely due to alterations in the acidity of the alimentary and biliopancreatic limbs with decreased *Firmicutes* and increased *Bacteroidetes* [63] and *Proteobacteria* (*Gammaproteobacteria*), in particular *Enterobacter hormaechei* [64], as well as *E coli*. In one study, RYGB increased *Escherichia* species and *Akkermansia* species independent of weight alteration and caloric restriction. When this gut flora was transferred to germ-free mice, they decreased body fat and body weight [65]. This could be explained, at least in part, by the increase in microbial production of short-chain fatty acids [65].

Weight loss in obese patients is associated with a low-grade inflammatory state [66]. The improvement of weight, inflammation and metabolic status after surgery has been associated with increased bacterial variety.

Bile Acids

Total plasma bile acids are increased post RYGB [67] for 3–4 years post-surgery, which could play a role in intestinal hypertrophy, anorexigenic hormone secretion and changes in gut flora and consequently weight loss. The increased bile acids may also increase energy expenditure by signalling via the cAMP-dependent thyroid hormone triggering enzyme type 2 iodothyronine deiodinase [68].

After RYGB bile flows down the BPL cells without mixing with food. These undiluted bile acids in the distal gut may stimulate the cell-membrane G protein coupled receptors (TGR5 receptors) on L cells [69], resulting in the changes in gut hormone response described above (e.g. increased GLP-1 and PYY). Bile acids also bind the farnesoid X receptor (FXR) in the jejunum, [70] which regulates lipid and glucose metabolism. FXR has been shown to regulate fibroblast growth factor 19 (FGF 19), which is released from the ileum, through the FGFR4 cell-surface receptor tyrosine kinase. FGF19 may contribute to the increased metabolic rate (with a role in mitochondrial activity and protein synthesis) and decreased adiposity seen post RYGB [71].

Food Preferences

Obese patients have a preference for energy-dense palatable food, a phenomenon termed 'hedonic hunger' [75]. However, this craving for sweet and high-fat foods decreases post RYGB even a year after surgery, and patients increase their intake of fruit, vegetables, protein, and low-fat food [76, 77]. Patients appear to have a heightened ability to detect sweet foods [78] but lose the desire for them. Initially, it was thought that dumping syndrome leads to a Pavlovian response of avoiding calorific foods [79]. However, the previously described changes are seen in patients who do not experience dumping [76, 80], and patients with severe dumping report continuing to like the taste of sweet foods.

It is still unclear which of the three processes involved in gustation have a predominant role in food preference: stimulus identification (sensory signals from taste stimuli), ingestive motivation (hedonic, palatability and reward) and digestive preparation (physiological reflexes that aid digestion and facilitate homeostasis) [81]. Alterations in taste sensitivity and palatability need further study. Studies using functional MRI (fMRI) have demonstrated reduced brain hedonic responses to high-calorie food (i.e. reduced activation of brain food-reward cognitive systems) post RYGB compared to matched weight loss post adjustable gastric banding [82], which may be mediated via gut hormones. There may also be an altered insulin/pancreatico-biliary homeostatic response to taste stimulation by sweet and fatty foods

The contribution of changes in food preferences to the RYGB effects on body weight is also not clear, with studies both describing no association [83] and others attributing decreased calorie intake and weight loss after RYGB to changes in food preferences [84]. Taken together the data reduction in preference for fatty foods may be a major contributor to reduced calorie intake in rodents and possibly in humans, again favouring conditioned avoidance as a mechanistic explanation.

Calorie Malabsorption

RYGB was originally intended to result in calorie malabsorption. However, the exclusion of the approximately 50 cm–150 cm of BPL (stomach, duodenum, proximal jejunum) after RYGB with an alimentary limb of 100–150 cm does not lead to calorie malabsorption, as the small bowel's total surface area capable of digestion and absorption is enough to prevent this. Furthermore there is hypertrophy of the small bowel in the alimentary limb and common channel, which are still in contact with nutrients [29–31]. RYGB may result in minor fat malabsorption by affecting pancreatic exocrine function – although this is unlikely to have any major impact on weight loss [72–74]. Most patients after RYGB report constipation, and as such significant calorie malabsorption is not possible.

Energy Expenditure

Changes in energy expenditure are likely to also be a minor but potentially important factor in weight loss maintenance post RYGB. The 'starvation response' [85] of reducing energy expenditure (EE) usually occurs during food restriction. However, total 24-hour EE has been shown to increase post RYGB in rodent models [85]; although this has not been shown consistently in human studies (which may be due to heterogeneity compared to laboratory animals [15]). A prevention of the expected decreased in EE could however contribute to the long-term maintenance of weight loss.

The mechanisms underlying the increase in EE are poorly understood, but areas that have been studied include:

- Higher-diet-induced thermogenesis appears the most consistent finding in both rodents and humans [7, 77] which may relate to gut hypertrophy after RYGB.
- Increased levels of postprandial GLP-1 may not contribute significantly as neither stimulation nor blockade has been shown to influence EE [15].
- Small bowel hypertrophy resulting in higher intestinal oxygen consumption and higher energy requirement [15].
- Increased metabolic rate of the small bowel, with increased carbohydrate consumption [73].
- Increased bile acid levels may also affect energy expenditure via the FXR receptor [15].

Reduced resting energy expenditure (REE) or basal metabolic rate post RYGB may predispose to weight regain [86], and it is important to increase REE by increasing physical activity and lean body mass (e.g. with increased protein intake).

Comorbidity Improvement/Resolution

As well as weight loss, RYGB results in obesity-related comorbidity improvement or resolution. Historically it was believed that most of the comorbidities that have been studied improve or resolve purely secondary to the surgery-induced weight loss. However, we now understand that complex metabolic mechanisms exist independent to weight loss. Type 2 diabetes mellitus (T2DM) and dyslipidaemia are two comorbidities that have been studied extensively after RYGB.

Comorbidities: Improvement/Resolution

- *Type 2 diabetes mellitus*
- *Dyslipidaemia*
- *Hypertension*
- *Obstructive sleep apnoea*
- *Musculoskeletal pain and function*
- *Gastroesophageal reflux disease (GORD)*
- *Non-alcoholic fatty liver disease*
- *PCOS symptoms*
- *Improved fertility*
- *Urinary incontinence*
- *Possible oncological risk reduction*
- *Psychosocial functioning*

Possible Mechanisms of T2DM Resolution

In one RCT, comparing RYGB with BPD and medical therapy, 75% of patients undergoing RYGB developed partial remission of diabetes at 2 years [87]. However, at 5 years 53% in the RYGB group went on to develop recurrent diabetes, and none of the patients were in complete remission of diabetes as judged by the American Diabetes Association criteria. Approximately 40% of obese patients with type 2 diabetes go into remission within days or weeks after RYGB [88], which suggests that the mechanisms underlying this are likely to be independent to weight loss.

Postulated mechanisms include:

- Gut hormones
- Bile acid kinetics
- Caloric restriction
- Weight loss

The main hormone that has been shown to contribute to improved glycaemic control is GLP-1. It has been associated with increased insulin secretion, increased insulin synthesis with beta cell proliferation [89] and improved beta cell function [90] (use of GLP-1 receptor antagonists results in relapse of impaired glucose tolerance), as well as inhibition of glucagon release [91]. A foregut and hindgut hypothesis has also been put forward [92]. The foregut hypothesis suggests that proximal jejunal and duodenal exclusion results in a signal that would otherwise lead to insulin resistance being inhibited, whilst the hindgut hypothesis suggests that accelerated delivery of concentrated nutrients to the distal intestine increases secretion of a signal that leads to improved glucose control. Further experiments [93] supporting the foregut hypothesis showed that bypassing a short segment of proximal intestine directly ameliorated type 2 diabetes, independently of effects on food intake, body weight, malabsorption or nutrient delivery to the hindgut.

In obese patients adipokines secreted from adipose tissue are known to induce a low-grade inflammatory state associated with insulin resistance; RYGB may induce some reduction in systemic inflammation, with evidence of reduced CRP levels post RYGB, potenitally improving whole-body insulin sensitivity [94]. Leptin may also play a role. When nutrients enter the jejunum, they are sensed by receptors that release leptin, which has been shown to reduce glucose levels [95].

Earlier we discussed the role of bile acids in stimulating GLP-1 secretion, which is one mechanism by which they exert an effect on glucose homeostasis and satiety. Bile acids may also directly affect insulin resistance by increasing energy expenditure in BAT (brown adipose tissue) via cAMP-dependent thyroid hormone-activating enzyme type 2 iodothyronine deiodinase and TGR5 [68]. Bile acids may also inhibit hepatic gluconeogenesis via FGF19 [96].

Caloric restriction results in reduced liver fat and improved hepatic insulin sensitivity [90], whilst weight loss leads to improved peripheral insulin sensitivity. The biliopancreatic limb post RYGB is usually around 50 cm. However, operations such as biliopancreatic diversion have a much longer BPL and greater reduction in insulin resistance, suggesting that the length of the BPL could be another influencing factor [97]. The melanocortin system may also be involved, as one population of MC4 receptors has been shown to mediate insulin sensitivity [55]. Clearly, there is an interplay of several mechanisms that lead to improved glucose control and T2DM resolution post RYGB.

Possible Mechanisms of Dyslipidaemia Resolution

Several studies post RYGB have shown reduction in total cholesterol, triglycerides, low-density lipoprotein cholesterol, very-low-density lipoprotein cholesterol and use/need for lipid-lowering medications, as well as increased high-density lipoprotein cholesterol (HDL-C) [98]. The effects on lipid profile are much greater post RYGB than other bariatric interventions [1, 99].

Mechanisms underlying this may include:

- Changes in food preferences (less fat intake)
- Reduction in cholesterol absorption
- Bile acids
- Reduction in hyperinsulinaemia

Higher turnover and plasma levels of bile salts, in particular cholic acid within bile, have been shown to reduce VLDL secretion and hepatic triglyceride accumulation [100]. This could be mediated via reduced expression of microsomal transfer protein, an essential enzyme for hepatic VLDL secretion [101]. Cholic acid's effect on reducing triglycerides may be mediated by reduced hepatic expression of SREBP-1c, which is involved in the fatty acid synthesis pathway [100]. Additionally, insulin is known to be fat storing and stimulate fatty acid synthesis in adipose tissue and the liver, as well as lead to the storage of triglycerides in adipose tissue and the liver. Reduction in hyperinsulinaemia may also play a role. The increase in circulating HDL-C has been attributed to fast gastric emptying with passage of nutrients directly into the jejunum stimulating ApoA4 secretion, which stabilizes HDL-C and induces increased plasma concentrations [102]. It would also be interesting to study whether length of the alimentary limb affects cholesterol absorption, as well as the enzymes involved in lipid metabolism.

The Complications

Complication rates after RYGB have decreased significantly with improved and more standardized techniques and improved training to increase surgeon experience quickly. 4% of patients have early complications including bleeding, perforation or leakage requiring return to theatre [99]. 15–20% have late complications including small bowel obstruction, abdominal pain or marginal ulceration requiring either surgical or endoscopic intervention [103]. The mechanistic aspects of these complications are discussed below.

Vitamin Deficiencies

- Vitamin B12
- Iron
- Folate
- Calcium and vitamin D

Vitamin B12 Deficiency

Up to 70% of patients have vitamin B12 deficiency post RYGB [104, 105]. The mechanisms underlying this may include:

- Achlorhydria reduces absorption of vitamin B12
- Reduced intake of meat
- Reduced production of intrinsic factor after surgery [106]

Iron Deficiency

Up to 49% of patients have iron deficiency post RYGB [107]. The mechanisms underlying this may include:

- Reduced iron absorption in the pouch secondary to less acid production [108]
- Reduced intake of red meat and iron rich foods

Folic Acid Deficiency

Up to 35% of patients have vitamin B12 deficiency post RYGB. The mechanisms underlying this may include:

- Folate absorption takes place in the proximal third of the small bowel, which is 'bypassed'.
- Vitamin B12 acts as a coenzyme and is often deficient.
- Less folate may be consumed.
- Acid is required for its absorption and is reduced.

Hypocalcaemia and Vitamin D Deficiency

Up to 10% of patients have calcium and 50% vitamin D deficiencies post RYGB [109]. The mechanisms underlying this may include:

- Calcium is predominantly absorbed in the proximal small bowel which is bypassed.
- Calcium can be lost from the bone, with higher bone turnover and reduced bone mass post RYGB [110, 111].
- Patients may become intolerant to foods rich in calcium, e.g. milk.

Hair Loss

Most patients have varying degrees of hair loss. Aetiological mechanisms include:

- Nutritional deficiencies (vitamin B, iron, calcium, zinc, etc.)
- Response to weight loss

Dental Problems

Dental problems can be due to:

- Vitamin deficiencies
- Malabsorption
- Reflux or vomiting post-surgery
- Salivary pH levels after surgery

Unexplained Abdominal Pain

Up to 95% of patients have some form of mild abdominal pain post RYGB [112–115], and up to 10% have chronic unexplained abdominal pain [112, 116]. This may be due to pain from internal hernias that spontaneously reduce, and jejuno-jejunal anastomosis may also contribute to chronic pain. Often patients undergo laparoscopy for diagnosis and treatment, as imaging often fails to elucidate the correct pathology. Pain accompanied by nausea and vomiting is usually pathological and may indicate obstruction, volvulus and/or ischaemia of herniated bowel and requires immediate attention [112, 117].

Change in Bowel Habits

Up to 46% of patients may have loose stool, diarrhoea or increased flatus post RYGB [118]. This may be secondary to bypassing a length of the small bowel, nutrient deficiencies and change in food intake. Patients may also have steatorrhoea post RYGB if they consume excessive fats. Many patients however have chronic constipation after RYGB which also needs active management.

(Early) Dumping Syndrome

Early dumping occurs 10–30 minutes after eating and is an outcome of rapid emptying of food into the jejunum due to the lack of a pylorus presumably causing neural activation in the proximal alimentary limb [119]. The food entering the jejunum is more undigested than usual and hyperosmolar, resulting in compensatory fluid shifts. Symptoms include bloating, sweating, nausea, abdominal pain, facial flushing, palpitations, dizziness and diarrhoea. Management involves dietary modification (patients should be advised to eat little and often, meals low in carbohydrate and fat, avoiding simple sugars and drinking fluids between meals and not with their food).

Postprandial Hypoglycaemia (Late Dumping)

Late dumping, or 'postprandial hypoglycaemia', happens 1–3 hours after ingesting a meal, even in patients without a previous history of diabetes, and is a result of the exaggerated insulin response to carbohydrates in the meal [120, 121]. Symptoms can include palpitations, sweating, confusion, fatigue, aggression, tremors and fainting. The proposed mechanisms involve increase β-cell mass, improve β-cell function and non-β-cell mechanisms, which may include a lack of ghrelin (a counter-regulatory measure to hypoglycaemia) [122, 123]. In addition the sustained weight loss can reduce insulin resistance which renders the previous insulin responses needed presurgery to suddenly become excessive. The aetiology of hypoglycaemia is likely to be different for individual patients and is also probably a mixture of the anatomic, hormonal and metabolic changes after RYGB [124]. Although treatment of this complication can be difficult, pancreatectomies are no longer advised [125], but rather a multimodal medical approach is favoured which aims to reduce insulin secretion from the pancreas or increasing insulin resistance at tissue level [126].

Loss of Bone Density

Loss of bone density [127] at central and peripheral sites continues 24 months post RYGB despite stabilization of weight loss. Mechanisms underlying this may include:

- Reduced mechanical load related to weight loss.
- Hyperparathyroidism secondary to:
  - Reduced calcium intake
  - Malabsorption of calcium and vitamin D
- Humoral factors from adipose tissue (oestradiol, leptin, adiponectin), the pancreas (e.g. insulin, amylin) or the gut (ghrelin, glucagon-like peptide-2, glucose-dependent insulinotropic peptide) may also play a role [128].

Kidney Stones

Calcium oxalate stones and oxalate nephropathy have been described post RYGB [129], and causative mechanisms include hyperoxaluria, low urine volume and hypocitraturia [130], with the latter two factors increasing calcium oxalate supersaturation.

Gallstones

Rapid weight loss and consequent changes in the composition of bile have been shown to increase gallstone formation [131]. In one study within 6 months post RYGB, gallstones had developed in 36% of patients and gallbladder sludge in 13% of patients [132]. A daily dose of 600 mg ursodeoxycholic acid for approximately 6 months has been shown to be effective prophylaxis against gallstone formation after RYGB [133] and is often prescribed in the post-operative phase. Some surgeons will undertake elective cholecystectomy at the time of RYGB if the patient has symptomatic gallstones, and although this has been shown to be safe and feasible without altering port placement, it has also been shown to significantly increase operative time and hospital stay [134]. Therefore, concomitant cholecystectomy and RYGB are not routinely performed for asymptomatic gallstones. Pancreatitis also appears to be increased after gastric bypass surgery and may be related to the increase in gallstone [135].

Gastric Remnant Distension

This is a rare complication of gastric bypass that can lead to perforation, peritonitis and subsequent death. Aetiological factors include:

- Distal obstruction
  - Mechanical
  - Paralytic ileus
- Injury to vagal fibres on the lesser curve of the stomach reducing gastric emptying

Management includes decompression with nasogastric tube on free drainage, percutaneous gastrostomy or surgical decompression if the above two methods have failed.

Stomal Stenosis

Patients with anastomotic stenosis may present with dysphagia, vomiting or reflux. The mainstay of treatment is endoscopic balloon dilatation, which may need to be repeated [136]. Revisional surgery is only used in patients who have failed endoscopic management.

Marginal Ulcers

Marginal ulcers occur in the gastric pouch and have several risk factors and associations:

Causes of marginal ulcers include:

- Poor tissue perfusion
  - Tissue tension or ischaemia at the anastomosis
  - Smoking
- Excess acid in the gastric pouch
  - Gastrogastric fistulas
- Nonsteroidal anti-inflammatories
- *Helicobacter pylori* infection [137]

The mainstay of management is acid suppression and treating the cause (e.g. stop smoking, stop NSAIDS, treat *H. pylori*, surgically manage gastrogastric fistula). Occasionally, surgical revision of the gastrojejunostomy and truncal vagotomy is required. Routine proton-pump therapy post RYGB to prevent this complication has been advocated [138].

Conclusion

The initial suggestion that it was based solely on mechanical restriction and calorie malabsorption is now obsolete. A complex symbiosis of gut hormones, bile acids, neural mechanisms, gut microbiota, food preferences and changes in energy expenditure is required to achieve the positive outcomes observed post gastric bypass. All operations have complications, and in the case of the Roux-en-Y gastric bypass, much work has been done to pre-empt these and manage them appropriately. As we learn more about the mechanisms of functioning of the Roux-en-Y gastric bypass, we realize that there is still so much more to learn. We must continue to study this fascinating operation to continue the journey of discovery.

References

1. Buchwald H, Avidor Y, Braunwald E, Jensen MD, Pories W, Fahrbach K, Schoelles K. Bariatric surgery: a systematic review and meta-analysis. JAMA. 2004;292(14):1724–37.
2. Olbers T, Gronowitz E, Werling M, Marlid S, Flodmark CE, Peltonen M, et al. Two-year outcome of laparoscopic Roux-en-Y gastric bypass in adolescents with severe obesity: results from a Swedish Nationwide Study (AMOS). Int J Obes. 2012;36(11):1388–95.
3. Sorensen TIA. Weight loss causes increased mortality: pros. Obes Rev. 2003;4(1):3–7.
4. Gerstein HC. Do lifestyle changes reduce serious outcomes in diabetes? N Engl J Med. 2013;369(2):189–90.
5. Sumithran P, Prendergast LA, Delbridge E, Purcell K, Shulkes A, Kriketos A, et al. Long-term persistence of hormonal adaptations to weight loss. N Engl J Med. 2011;365(17):1597–604.
6. Hofmann W, van Koningsbruggen GM, Stroebe W, Ramanathan S, Aarts H. As pleasure unfolds. Hedonic responses to tempting food. Psychol Sci. 2010;21(12):1863–70.
7. Abdeen G, Le Roux CW. Mechanism underlying the weight loss and complications of Roux-en-Y gastric bypass. Review Obes Surg. 2016;26:410–21.
8. Fandriks L. The role of the smaller stomach. 31-8-2011. Postgraduate course B, XVI World Congress of the International Federation for the Surgery of Obesity and Metabolic Disorders, Hamburg, Germany. Ref Type: Report.
9. Le Roux CW, et al. Gut hormone profiles following bariatric surgery favor an anorectic state, facilitate weight loss, and improve metabolic parameters. Ann Surg. 2006;243:108–14.
10. Dixon AF, Dixon JB, O'Brien PE. Laparoscopic adjustable gastric banding induces prolonged satiety: a randomized blind crossover study. J Clin Endocrinol Metab. 2005;90:813–9.
11. Miras AD, et al. Gastric bypass surgery for obesity decreases the reward value of a sweetfat stimulus as assessed in a progressive ratio task. Am J Clin Nutr. 2012;96:467–73.
12. Wilson-Perez HE, et al. The effect of vertical sleeve gastrectomy on food choice in rats. Int J Obes. 2012;37:288–2.
13. Halmi KA, Mason E, Falk JR, Stunkard A. Appetitive behavior after gastric bypass for obesity. Int J Obes. 1981;5(5):457–64.
14. Zheng H, Shin AC, Lenard NR, Townsend RL, Patterson LM, Sigalet DL, et al. Meal patterns, satiety, and food choice in a rat model of Roux-en-Y gastric bypass surgery. Am J Physiol Regul Integr Comp Physiol. 2009;297(5):R1273–82.
15. Lutz TA, Bueter M. Physiological mechanisms behind Roux-en-Y gastric bypass surgery. Dig Surg. 2014;31(1):13–24.
16. Le Roux CW, Welbourn R, Werling M, et al. Gut hormones as mediators of appetite and weight loss after Roux-en-Y gastric bypass. Ann Surg. 2007;246:780–5.
17. Miller GD, Norris A, Fernandez A. Changes in nutrients and food groups intake following laparoscopic Roux-en-Y gastric bypass (RYGB). Obes Surg. 2014;24(11):1926–32. 1–7. 23.
18. Xanthakos SA. Nutritional deficiencies in obesity and after bariatric surgery. Pediatr Clin N Am. 2009;56:1105–21.
19. Flancbaum L, Choban P, Bradley LR, BURGE JC. Changes in measured resting energy expenditure after Roux-en-Y gastric bypass for clinically severe obesity. Surgery. 1997;122:943–9.
20. Moize V, Geliebter A, Gluck ME, et al. Obese patients have inadequate protein intake related to protein intolerance up to 1 year following Roux-en-Y gastric bypass. Obes Surg. 2003;13:23–8.
21. Warde-Kamar J, Rogers M, Flancbaum L, Laferrère B. Calorie intake and meal patterns up to 4 years after Roux-en-Y gastric bypass surgery. Obes Surg. 2004;14:1070–9.
22. Heneghan HM, Yimcharoen P, Brethauer SA, Kroh M, Chand B. Influence of pouch and stoma size on weight loss after gastric bypass. Surg Obes Relat Dis. 2012;8(4):408–15.
23. Bueter M, Lowenstein C, Ashrafian H, Hillebrand J, Bloom S, Olbers T, et al. Vagal sparing surgical technique but not stoma size affects body weight loss in rodent model of gastric bypass. Obes Surg. 2010;20(5):616–22.
24. Campos GM, Rabl C, Mulligan K. FActors associated with weight loss after gastric bypass. Arch Surg. 2008;143(9):877–84.
25. Topart P, Becouarn G, Ritz P. Pouch size after gastric bypass does not correlate with weight loss outcome. Obes Surg. 2011;21(9):1350–4.
26. Madan A, Tichansky D, Phillips J. Does pouch size matter? Obes Surg. 2007;17(3):317–20.
27. Laurenius A, Larsson I, Bueter M, Melanson KJ, Bosaeus I, Forslund HB, et al. Changes in eating behaviour and meal pattern following Roux-en-Y gastric bypass. Int J Obes. 2012;36(3):348–55.
28. Gould J, Garren M, Boll V, Starling J. The impact of circular stapler diameter on the incidence of gastrojejunostomy stenosis and weight loss following laparoscopic Roux-en-Y gastric bypass. Surg Endosc. 2006;20(7):1017–20.
29. Bueter M, Lowenstein C, Olbers T, et al. Gastric bypass increases energy expenditure in rats. Gastroenterology. 2010;138:1845–53.
30. Mumphrey MB, Patterson LM, Zheng H, Berthoud HR. Roux-en-Y gastric bypass surgery increases number but not density of CCK-, GLP-1-, 5-HT-, and neurotensin-expressing enteroendocrine cells in rats. Neurogastroenterol Motil. 2013;25:e70–9.
31. Taqi E, Wallace LE, de Heuvel E, et al. The influence of nutrients, biliary-pancreatic secretions, and systemic trophic hormones on intestinal adaptation

in a Roux-en-Y bypass model. J Pediatr Surg. 2010;45:987–95.
32. le Roux CW, Borg C, Wallis K, et al. Gut hypertrophy after gastric bypass is associated with increased glucagon-like peptide 2 and intestinal crypt cell proliferation. Ann Surg. 2010;252:50–6.
33. Pournaras DJ, le Roux CW. Ghrelin and metabolic surgery. Int J Pept. 2010;2010:733–43.
34. Berthoud HR, Shin AC, Zheng H. Obesity surgery and gut-brain communication. Physiol Behav. 2011;105(1):106–19.
35. Chambers AP, Kirchner H, Wilson-Perez HE, et al. The effects of vertical sleeve gastrectomy in rodents are ghrelin independent. Gastroenterology. 2013;144:50–2. e55.
36. Dar MS, Chapman WH III, Pender JR, Drake AJ III, O'Brien K, Tanenberg RJ, et al. GLP-1 response to a mixed meal: what happens 10 years after Roux-en-Y gastric bypass (RYGB)? Obes Surg. 2012;22(7):1077–83.
37. Meguid MM, Glade MJ, Middleton FA. Weight regain after Roux-en-Y: a significant 20% complication related to PYY. Nutrition. 2008;24(9):832–42.
38. Dirksen C, Jorgensen NB, Bojsen-Moller KN, Kielgast U, Jacobsen SH, Clausen TR, et al. Gut hormones, early dumping and resting energy expenditure in patients with good and poor weight loss response after Roux-en-Y gastric bypass. Int J Obes. 2013 Nov;37(11):1452–9.
39. Batterham RL, Cohen MA, Ellis SM, le Roux CW, Withers DJ, Frost GS, et al. Inhibition of food intake in obese subjects by peptide YY3-36. N Engl J Med. 2003;349(10):941–8.
40. Chandarana K, Gelegen C, Karra E, Choudhury AI, Drew ME, Fauveau V, et al. Diet and gastrointestinal bypass-Induced weight loss the roles of ghrelin and peptide YY. Diabetes. 2011;60(3):810–8.
41. Sloth B, Holst JJ, Flint A, Gregersen NT, Astrup A. Effects of PYY1-36 and PYY3-36 on appetite, energy intake, energy expenditure, glucose and fat metabolism in obese and lean subjects. Am J Physiol Endocrinol Metab. 2007;292(4):E1062–8.
42. Troy S, Soty M, Ribeiro L, Laval L, Migrenne S, Fioramonti X, et al. Intestinal gluconeogenesis is a key factor for early metabolic changes after gastric bypass but not after gastric lap-band in mice. Cell Metab. 2008;8(3):201–11.
43. Peterli R, Wölnerhanssen B, Peters T, Devaux NÑ, Kern B, Christoffel-Court C, et al. Improvement in glucose metabolism after bariatric surgery: comparison of laparoscopic Roux-en-Y gastric bypass and laparoscopic sleeve gastrectomy: a prospective randomized trial. Ann Surg. 2009;250(2):234–41.
44. Hao Z, et al. Leptin deficient ob/ob mice and diet-induced obese miceresponded differently to Roux-en-Y bypass surgery. Int J Obes (Lond). 2015;39(5): 798–805.
45. Ochner CN, Kwok Y, Conceicao E, Pantazatos SP, Puma LM, Carnell S, et al. Selective reduction in neural responses to high calorie foods following gastric bypass surgery. Ann Surg. 2011;253(3):502–7.
46. Forman EM, Hoffman KL, McGrath KB, Herbert JD, Brandsma LL, Lowe MR. A comparison of acceptance- and control-based strategies for coping with food cravings: an analog study. Behav Res Ther. 2007;45(10):2372–86.
47. Lowe MR, van Steenburgh J, Ochner CN. Individual differences in brain activation in relation to ingestive behavior and obesity. Physiol Behav. 2009;5:561–71.
48. Lowe MR, Butryn ML, Didie ER, Annunziato RA, Thomas JG, Crerand CE, et al. The power of food scale. A new measure of the psychological influence of the food environment. Appetite. 2009;53(1):114–8.
49. Berthoud HR. Vagal and hormonal gut-brain communication: from satiation to satisfaction. Neurogastroenterol Motil. 2008;20(Suppl 1):64–72.
50. Zagorodnyuk VP, Chen BN, Brookes SJH. Intraganglioinic laminar endings are mechanotransduction sites of vagal tension receptors in the Guinea-pig stomach. J Physiol. 2001;534:255–68.
51. Berthoud HR. The vagus nerve, food intake and obesity. Regul Pept. 2008;149(13):15–25.
52. Le Roux CW, Neary NM, Halsey TJ, Small CJ, Martinez-Isla AM, Ghatei MA, Theodorou NA, Bloom SR. Ghrelin does not stimulate food intake in patients with surgical procedures involving vagotomy. J Clin Endocrinol Metab. 2005;90(8):4521–4.
53. Berthoud HR, Kressel M, Raybould HE, Neuhuber WL. Vagal sensors in the rat duodenal mucosa: distribution and structure as revealed by in vivo DiI-tracing. Anat Embryol (Berl). 1995;191(3):203–12.
54. Curry TB, Somaraju M, Hines CN, Groenewalk CB, Miles JM, Joyner MJ, Charkoudian N. Sympathetic support of energy expenditure and sympathetic nervous system activity after gastric bypass surgery. Obesity (Silver Spring). 2013;21(3):480–5.
55. Zechner JF, Mirshahi UL, Satapati S, et al. Weight-independent effects of roux-en-Y gastric bypass on glucose homeostasis via melanocortin-4 receptors in mice and humans. Gastroenterology. 2013;144:580–90. e58.
56. Miras AD, Le Roux CW. Mechanisms underlying weight loss after bariatric surgery. Nat Rev Gastroenterol Hepatol. 2013;10(10):575–84.
57. De La Serre CB, Ellis CL, Lee J, Hartman AL, Rutledge JC, Raybould HE. Propensity to high-fat diet-induced obesity in rats is associated with changes in the gut microbiota and gut inflammation. Am J Physiol Gastrointest Liver Physiol. 2010;299:G440–8.
58. Clarke SF, Murphy EF, Nilaweera K, Ross PR, Shanahan F, O Toole PW, et al. The gut microbiota and its relationship to diet and obesity: new insights. Gut Microbes. 2012;3(3):186–202.
59. Armougom F, Henry M, Vialettes B, Raccah D, Raoult D. Monitoring bacterial community of human gut microbiota reveals an increase in Lactobacillus in

obese patients and methanogens in anorexic patients. PLoS One. 2009;4(9):e7125.
60. Ley RE, Turnbaugh PJ, Klein S, Gordon JI. Microbial ecology: human gut microbes associated with obesity. Nature. 2006;444(7122):1022–3.
61. Turnbaugh PJ, Hamady M, Yatsunenko T, Cantarel BL, Duncan A, Ley RE, et al. A core gut microbiome in obese and lean twins. Nature. 2009;457(7228):480–4.
62. Turnbaugh PJ, Ley RE, Mahowald MA, Magrini V, Mardis ER, Gordon JI. An obesity-associated gut microbiome with increased capacity for energy harvest. Nature. 2006;444(7122):1027–131.
63. Sweeney TE, Morton JM. The human gut microbiome: a review of the effect of obesity and surgically induced weight loss. JAMA Surg. 2013;148(6):563–9.
64. Zhang H, DiBaise JK, Zuccolo A, Kudrna D, Braidotti M, Yu Y, et al. Human gut microbiota in obesity and after gastric bypass. Proc Natl Acad Sci. 2009;106(7):2365–70.
65. Liou AP, Paziuk M, Luevano JM, Machineni S, Turnbaugh PJ, Kaplan LM. Conserved shifts in the gut microbiota due to gastric bypass reduce host weight and adiposity. Sci Transl Med. 2013;5(178):178ra41.
66. Furet JP, Kong LC, Tap J, et al. Differential adaptation of human gut microbiota to bariatric surgery-induced weight loss: links with metabolic and low-grade inflammation markers. Diabetes. 2010;59:3049–57.
67. Pournaras DJ, Glicksman C, Vincent RP, Kuganolipava S, Alaghband-Zadeh J, Mahon D, et al. The role of bile after Roux-en-Y gastric bypass in promoting weight loss and improving glycaemic control. Endocrinology. 2012;153(8):3613–9.
68. Watanabe M, Houten SM, Mataki C, Christoffolete MA, Kim BW, Sato H, et al. Bile acids induce energy expenditure by promoting intracellular thyroid hormone activation. Nature. 2006;439(7075):484–9.
69. Katsuma S, Hirasawa A, Tsujimoto G. Bile acids promote glucagon-like peptide-1 secretion through TGR5 in a murine enteroendocrine cell line STC-1. Biochem Biophys Res Commun. 2005;329(1):386–9.
70. Kreymann B, Ghatei MA, Williams G, Bloom SR. Glucagon-like peptide-1. A physiological incretin in man. Lancet. 1987;330(8571):1300–4.
71. Holt JA, Luo G, Billin AN, Bisi J, McNeill YY, Kozarsky KF, et al. Definition of a novel growth factor-dependent signal cascade for the suppression of bile acid biosynthesis. Genes Dev. 2003;17(13):1581–91.
72. Kumar R, Lieske JC, Collazo-Clavell ML, Sarr MG, Olson ER, Vrtiska TJ, et al. Fat malabsorption and increased intestinal oxalate absorption are common after Roux-en-Y gastric bypass surgery. Surgery. 2011;149(5):654–61.
73. Odstrcil EA, Martinez JG, Santa Ana CA, Xue B, Schneider RE, Steffer KJ, et al. The contribution of malabsorption to the reduction in net energy absorption after long-limb Roux-en-Y gastric bypass. Am J Clin Nutr. 2010;92(4):704–13.
74. Carswell KA, Vincent RP, Belgaumkar AP, Sherwood RA, Amiel SA, Patel AG, et al. The effect of bariatric surgery on intestinal absorption and transit time. Obes Surg. 2014;24(5):796–805.
75. Lowe MR, Butryn ML. Hedonic hunger: a new dimension of appetite? Physiol Behav. 2007;91(4):432–9.
76. Ernst B, Thurnheer M, Wilms B, Schultes B. Differential changes in dietary habits after gastric bypass versus gastric banding operations. Obes Surg. 2009;19(3):274–80.
77. Olbers T, Bjorkman S, Lindroos A, Maleckas A, Lonn L, Sjostrom L, et al. Body composition, dietary intake, and energy expenditure after laparoscopic Roux-en-Y gastric bypass and laparoscopic vertical banded gastroplasty: a randomized clinical trial. Ann Surg. 2006;244(5):715–22.
78. Bueter M, Miras AD, Chichger H, Fenske W, Ghatei MA, Bloom SR, et al. Alterations of sucrose preference after Roux-en-Y gastric bypass. Physiol Behav. 2011;104(5):709–21.
79. Deitel M. The change in the dumping syndrome concept. Obes Surg. 2008;18(12):1622–4.
80. Thomas JR, Gizis F, Marcus E. Food selections of Roux-en-Y gastric bypass patients up to 2.5 years postsurgery. J Am Diet Assoc. 2010;110(4):608–12.
81. Spector AC, Glendinning JI. Linking peripheral taste processes to behavior. Curr Opin Neurobiol. 2009;19(4):370–7.
82. Scholtz S, Miras AD, Chhina N, Prechtl CG, Sleeth ML, Daud NM, et al. Obese patients after gastric bypass surgery have lower brain-hedonic responses to food than after gastric banding. Gut. 2014;63(6):891–902.
83. Laurenius A, Larsson I, Melanson KJ, Lindroos AK, Lonroth H, Bosaeus I, et al. Decreased energy density and changes in food selection following Roux-en-Y gastric bypass. Eur J Clin Nutr. 2013;67(2):168–73.
84. Kenler HA, Brolin RE, Cody RP. Changes in eating behavior after horizontal gastroplasty and Roux-en-Y gastric bypass. Am J Clin Nutr. 1990;52(1):87–92.
85. Nestoridi E, Kvas S, Kucharczyk J, Stylopoulos N. Resting energy expenditure and energetic cost of feeding are augmented after Roux-en-Y gastric bypass in obese mice. Endocrinology. 2012;153(5):2234–44.
86. Faria S, Kelly E, Faria O. Energy expenditure and weight regain in patients submitted to Roux-en-Y gastric bypass. Obes Surg. 2009;19(7):856–9.
87. Mingrone G, Panunzi S, De Gaetano A, et al. Bariatric-metabolic surgery versus conventional medical treatment in obese patients with type 2 diabetes: 5 year follow-up of an open-label, single-centre, randomised controlled trial. Lancet. 2015;386:964.
88. Pournaras DJ, Osborne A, Hawkins SC, Vincent RP, Mahon D, Ewings P, et al. Remission of type 2 diabetes after gastric bypass and banding: mechanisms and 2 year outcomes. Ann Surg. 2010;252(6):966–71.

89. Pournaras DJ, Le Roux CW. The effect of bariatric surgery on gut hormones that alter appetite. Diabetes Metab. 2009;35(6 Pt 2):508–12.
90. Svane MS, Bojsen-Møller KN, Madsbad S, Holst JJ. Updates in weight loss surgery and gastrointestinal peptides. Curr Opin Endocrinol Diabetes Obes. 2015;22(1):21–8.
91. Tang-Christensen M, Vrang N, Larsen PJ. Glucagon-like peptide containing pathways in the regulation of feeding behaviour. Int J Obes Relat Metab Disord. 2001;25(Suppl 5):S42–7.
92. Rubino F. Bariatric surgery: effects on glucose homeostasis. Curr Opin Clin Nutr Metab Care. 2006;9(4):497–507.
93. Rubino F, Forgione A, Cummings DE, Vix M, Gnuli D, Mingrone G, Castagneto M, Marescaux J. The mechanism of diabetes control after gastrointestinal bypass surgery reveals a role of the proximal small intestine in the pathophysiology of type 2 diabetes. Ann Surg. 2006;244(5):741–9.
94. Pournaras DJ, Nygren J, Hagström-Toft E, Arner P, le Roux CW, Thorell A. Improved glucose metabolism after gastric bypass: evolution of the paradigm. Surg Obes Relat Dis. 2016;12:1457–65. pii: S1550-7289(16)00110-6.
95. Rasmussen BA, et al. Jejunal leptin-P13K signaling lowers glucose production. Cell Metab. 2014;19(1):155–61.
96. Potthoff MJ, Boney-Montoya J, Choi M, He T, Sunny NE, Satapati S, Suino-Powell K, Xu HE, Gerard RD, Finck BN, Burgess SC, Mangelsdorf DJ, Kliewer SA. FGF15/19 regulates hepatic glucose metabolism by inhibiting the CREB-PGC-1α pathway. Cell Metab. 2011;13:729–38.
97. Nora M, Guimarães M, Almeida R, Martins P, Gonçalves G, MJÑ F, et al. Metabolic laparoscopic gastric bypass for obese patients with type 2 diabetes. Obes Surg. 2011;21(11):1643–9.
98. Nguyen NT, Varela E, Sabio A, et al. Resolution of hyperlipidemia after laparoscopic Roux-en-Y gastric bypass. J Am Coll Surg. 2006;203:24.
99. Sjostrom L, Lindroos AK, Peltonen M, Torgerson J, Bouchard C, Carlsson B, et al. Lifestyle, diabetes, and cardiovascular risk factors 10 years after bariatric surgery. N Engl J Med. 2004;351(26):2683–93.
100. Watanabe M, Houten SM, Wang L, et al. Bile acids lower triglyceride levels via a pathway involving FXR, SHP, and SREBP-1c. J Clin Invest. 2004;113:1408–141.
101. Hirokane H, Nakahara M, Tachibana S, Shimizu M, Sato R. Bile acid reduces the secretion of very low density lipoprotein by repressing microsomal triglyceride transfer protein gene expression mediated by hepatocyte nuclear factor-4. J Biol Chem. 2004;279:45685–92.
102. Raffaelli M, et al. Effect of gastric bypass versus diet on cardiovascular risk factors. Ann Surg. 2014;259:694–9.
103. Franco J, Ruiz P, Palermo M, Gagner M. A review of studies comparing three laparoscopic procedures in bariatric surgery: sleeve gastrectomy, Roux-en-Y gastric bypass and adjustable gastric banding. Obes Surg. 2011;21(9):1458–68.
104. Rhode BM, Arseneau P, Cooper BA, Katz M, Gilfix BM, MacLean LD. Vitamin B-12 deficiency after gastric surgery for obesity. Am J Clin Nutr. 1996;63(1):103–9.
105. LJ Bradley MS RD. Are vitamin B12 and folate deficiency clinically important after roux-en-Y gastric bypass? J Gastrointest Surg. 1998;2(5):436–42.
106. Decker GA, Swain JM, Crowell MD, Scolapio JS. Gastrointestinal and nutritional complications after bariatric surgery. Am J Gastroenterol. 2007;102(11):2571–80.
107. Halverson JD. Micronutrient deficiencies after gastric bypass for morbid obesity. Am Surg. 1986 Nov;52(11):594–8.
108. Smith CD, Herkes SB, Behrns KE, et al. Gastric acid secretion and vitamin B12 absorption after vertical Roux-gastric-Y bypass for morbid obesity. Ann Surg. 1993;218:91–6.
109. Brolin RE, LaMarca LB, Kenler HA, Cody RP. Malabsorptive gastric bypass in patients with superobesity. J Gastrointest Surg. 2002;6(2):195–205.
110. Coates PS, Fernstrom JD, Fernstrom MH, Schauer PR, Greenspan SL. Gastric bypass surgery for morbid obesity leads to an increase in bone turnover and a decrease in bone mass. J Clin Endocrinol Metab. 2004;89(3):1061–5.
111. Von Mach MA, Stoeckli R, Bilz S, Kraenzlin M, Langer I, Keller U. Changes in bone mineral content after surgical treatment of morbid obesity. Metabolism. 2004;53(7):918–21.
112. Comeau E, Gagner M, Inabnet WB, Herron DM, Quinn TM, Pomp A. Symptomatic internal hernias after laparoscopic bariatric surgery. Surg Endosc. 2005;19(1):34–9.
113. Garza E Jr, Kuhn J, Arnold D, Nicholson W, Reddy S, McCarty T. Internal hernias after laparoscopic Roux-en-Y gastric bypass. Am J Surg. 2004;188(6):796–800.
114. Cho M, Carrodeguas L, Pinto D, Lascano C, Soto F, Whipple O, et al. Diagnosis and management of partial small bowel obstruction after laparoscopic antecolic antegastric Roux-en-Y gastric bypass for morbid obesity. J Am Coll Surg. 2006;202(2):262–8.
115. Filip JE, Mattar SG, Bowers SP, Smith CD. Internal hernia formation after laparoscopic Roux-en-Y gastric bypass for morbid obesity. Am Surg. 2002;68(7):640–3.
116. Husain S, Ahmed AR, Johnson J, Boss T, O'Malley W. Small-bowel obstruction after laparoscopic Roux-en-Y gastric bypass: etiology, diagnosis, and management. Arch Surg. 2007;142(10):988.
117. Reddy SA, Yang C, McGinnis LA, Seggerman RE, Garza E, Ford KL III. Diagnosis of transmesocolic internal hernia as a complication of retrocolic gas-

tric bypass: CT imaging criteria. Am J Roentgenol. 2007;189(1):52–5.

118. Potoczna N, Harfmann S, Steffen R, et al. Bowel habits after bariatric surgery. Obes Surg. 2008;18:1287.
119. Mathews DH, Lawrence W, Poppell JW, Vanamee P, Randall HT. Change in effective circulating volume during experimental dumping syndrome. Surgery. 1960;48:185–94.
120. Tack J, Arts J, Caenepeel P, De Wulf D, Bisschops R. Pathophysiology, diagnosis and management of postoperative dumping syndrome. Nat Rev Gastroenterol Hepatol. 2009;6(10):583–90.
121. Ukleja A. Dumping syndrome: pathophysiology and treatment. Nutr Clin Pract. 2005;20(5):517–25.
122. Cummings DE, Weigle DS, Frayo RS, Breen PA, Ma MK, Dellinger EP, et al. Plasma ghrelin levels after diet-induced weight loss or gastric bypass surgery. N Engl J Med. 2002;346(21):1623–30.
123. Cummings DE, Foster-Schubert KE, Overduin J. Ghrelin and energy balance: focus on current controversies. Curr Drug Targets. 2005;6(2):153–69.
124. Kapoor RR, James C, Hussain K. Advances in the diagnosis and management of hyperinsulinemic hypoglycemia. Nat Clin Pract Endocrinol Metab. 2009;5(2):101–12.
125. Service GJ, Thompson GB, Service FJ, Andrews JC, Collazo-Clavell ML, Lloyd RV. Hyperinsulinemic hypoglycemia with nesidioblastosis after gastric-bypass surgery. N Engl J Med. 2005;353(3):249–54.
126. Patti ME, Goldfine AB. Hypoglycemia after gastric bypass: the dark side of GLP-1. Gastroenterology. 2014;146(3):605–8.
127. Yu EW, Bouxsein ML, Putman MS, Monis EL, Roy AE, Pratt JS, Butsch WS, Finkelstein JS. Two-year changes in bone density after Roux-en-Y gastric bypass surgery. J Clin Endocrinol Metab. 2015;100(4):1452–9.
128. Reid IR. Relationships among body mass, its components, and bone. Bone. 2002;31(5):547–55.
129. Nelson WK, Houghton SG, Milliner DS, et al. Enteric hyperoxaluria, nephrolithiasis, and oxalate nephropathy: potentially serious and unappreciated complications of Roux-en-Y gastric bypass. Surg Obes Relat Dis. 2005;1:481–5.
130. Canales BK, Gonzalez RD. Kidney stone risk following Roux-en-Y gastric bypass surgery. Transl Androl Urol. 2014;3(3):242–9.
131. Shiffman ML, Sugerman HJ, Kellum JM, Moore EW. Changes in gallbladder bile composition following gallstone formation and weight reduction. Gastroenterology. 1992;103:214.
132. Shiffman ML, Sugerman HJ, Kellum JM, et al. Gallstone formation after rapid weight loss: a prospective study in patients undergoing gastric bypass surgery for treatment of morbid obesity. Am J Gastroenterol. 1991;86:1000.
133. Sugerman HJ, Brewer WH, Shiffman ML, et al. A multicenter, placebo-controlled, randomized, double-blind, prospective trial of prophylactic ursodiol for the prevention of gallstone formation following gastric-bypass-induced rapid weight loss. Am J Surg. 1995;169:91.
134. Hamad GG, Ikramuddin S, Gourash WF, Schauer PR. Elective cholecystectomy during laparoscopic Roux-en-Y gastric bypass: is it worth the wait? Obes Surg. 2003;13:76.
135. Kumaravel A, Zelisko A, Schauer P, Lopez R, Kroh M, Stevens T. Acute pancreatitis in patients after bariatric surgery: incidence, outcomes, and risk factors. Obes Surg. 2014 Dec;24(12):2025–30.
136. Go MR, Muscarella P 2nd, Needleman BJ, et al. Endoscopic management of stomal stenosis after Roux-en-Y gastric bypass. Surg Endosc. 2004;18:56.
137. Rasmussen JJ, Fuller W, Ali MR. Marginal ulceration after laparoscopic gastric bypass: an analysis of predisposing factors in 260 patients. Surg Endosc. 2007;21:1090.
138. Gumbs AA, Duffy AJ, Bell RL. Incidence and management of marginal ulceration after laparoscopic Roux-Y gastric bypass. Surg Obes Relat Dis. 2006;2:460.

Morbid Obesity

3

Minna Ferrari Schleu and Karyne Freitas Barbosa

Obesity is a chronic disease with an increasing prevalence all over the world. Associated with the growth of global mortality and high risk of development of several systemic diseases, it has been noticed as a public health problem [1–3]. The number of obese patients in the world rose from 921 million in 1980 to 2.1 billion in 2013, with a prevalence of overweight over 50% in adults in certain areas of the globe [4]. Morbid obesity is defined as a BMI (body mass index) above 40 kg/m^2 [5]. It is known that the higher the BMI, the greater the associated risk [5] [6]. The prevalence of BMI above 40 increased in 70% between 2000 and 2010 [7]. This is a population that deserves special attention and care, and treatment should be stipulated for weight loss and control of associated comorbidities [8].

Morbidly Obese Patient Assessment

The patient with morbid obesity should be carefully evaluated to look for etiology, taking into account the genetic influences and environmental factors. Modern life habits play a fundamental role in this context, where we experience a decrease in physical activity levels and an increase in caloric intake [9]. In a morbidly obese patient, besides the evaluation of his lifestyle habits, it is important to evaluate the genetic influence, usually polygenic [10, 11]. The family history of obesity provides important information, as well as the time of the beginning of weight gain. The risk of obesity increases from 9% when only one parent is obese to 50% when both parents are. The earlier the onset of weight gain – childhood and adolescence – the greater the genetic influence on pathology [12].

Investigation for medications that lead to weight gain should be performed, the main ones being glucocorticoids, tricyclic antidepressants, antiepileptic, and antipsychotics [8].

The hormonal disorder most associated with morbid obesity is hypercortisolism. Signs and symptoms should be evaluated during medical history and physical examination, looking for buffalo hump, facial rounding and plethora, gross obesity of the trunk with wasting of the limbs, hirsutism, frontal balding, muscle weakness, spontaneous bruising, and acne. Hypercortisolism should be ruled out, even in patients without the classic findings of the syndrome. Thyroid evaluation should be performed knowing that hypothyroidism may contribute to obesity but never represents the only etiology for morbid obesity.

In morbid obesity, the genetic syndromes associated with overweight are more prevalent when compared to other degrees of obesity. Therefore they should always be evaluated [13].

M. F. Schleu (✉)
Endocrinology, Clínica Metta, Salvador, Bahia, Brazil

K. F. Barbosa
Endocrinology Division, São Rafael, Salvador, Bahia, Brazil

J. Ettinger et al. (eds.), *Gastric Bypass*, https://doi.org/10.1007/978-3-030-28803-7_3

The two major genetic syndromes associated with obesity are Prader-Willi syndrome and Bardet-Biedl syndrome, both monogenic. The predominant autosomal Prader-Willi syndrome has a prevalence of 1:25,000 live births and is characterized by hypogonadotropic hypogonadism, mental retardation, and binge eating, with onset of obesity in childhood and often associated with diabetes mellitus, dyslipidemia, and atheromatosis. Additional findings are childhood hypotonia, short stature, and behavioral abnormalities [14]. Bardet-Biedl syndrome, autosomal recessive, is characterized by early obesity, in the first years of life, pigmented retinopathy, polydactyl, mental retardation, male hypogonadism, and renal changes [15].

The major monogenic mutations are in the leptin gene, leptin receptor, proopiomelanocortin (POMC), and melanocortin (MC4R) receptor gene.

Mutation at the melanocortin receptor is the main cause of monogenic obesity, being prevalent in 1–6% of obese individuals, with a higher prevalence in the morbidly obese. These patients also present an increase in lean mass, bone mineral density, accelerated growth, and hyperinsulinemia [16]. Proopiomelanocortin deficiency (POMC) is characterized by hyperplasia with severe obesity onset in childhood, adrenal insufficiency with low levels of ACTH, cutaneous hypopigmentation, and reddish hair [17]. Leptin gene and receptor mutations manifest as hypogonadotropic hypogonadism, hyperphagia, and severe childhood obesity and represent 1–3% of cases of morbid obesity in obese individuals from consanguineous families [18, 19].

Associated Complications

The relative risk of death associated with overweight begins to increase with a BMI between 25 and 29 kg/m^2. Individuals with morbid obesity present a relative risk of death of two when compared to individuals of normal weight [20]. As with mortality, the risk of complications is also related to BMI. Morbidly obese patients have the highest risk rates among obese patients [20, 21].

Individuals with morbid obesity and BMI above 40 kg/m^2 have a 64% increased risk of developing DM 2, a 54% increased risk of hypertension, an additional 17% risk of developing asthma, a 34% increased risk of arthritis, and a 9% increased risk for hypercholesterolemia when compared to normal eutrophic adults [22].

The risk of arterial systemic hypertension becomes greater as the BMI increases, even after adjusting for other factors such as age and smoking. According to the Framingham Offspring Cohort, there is a linear positive correlation between BMI and LDL and triglyceride values and a negative correlation between BMI and HDL in nonsmokers [23].

Complications involving the liver may be present, ranging from elevated liver enzymes to cirrhosis, hepatic failure, and hepatocellular carcinoma. The prevalence of nonalcoholic fatty liver disease is even higher in morbidly obese individuals. Studies in this subgroup reveal rates that exceed 90% at the time of submission to bariatric surgery. And 5% of these patients may have undiagnosed cirrhosis [24, 25].

The risk of gallstones shows a positive correlation with BMI, which is more pronounced when it is above 30 kg/m^2 [26, 27]. Notably, in the morbid population, this risk is more pronounced, reaching seven times higher in women with BMI above 45 when compared to women with BMI <24 [27].

Male infertility is associated with obesity, especially among the morbidly obese [28]. Contributing factors are the reduction of testosterone levels due to its greater aromatization in estrogen in adipose tissue and the increase in SHBG levels [29–32]. Associated with hormonal disturbances, the increased testicle temperature due to the greater proximity of the surrounding tissues contributes to a higher rate of semen changes [28]. Similarly, female infertility is associated to BMI, being more frequent the higher the BMI, therefore more frequent in morbidly obese women. Chronic anovulation presents as the main cause [28].

The risk of depression and anxiety correlates positively with BMI and is more frequent in morbidly obese individuals when compared to other degrees of obesity [33, 34].

Obesity and overweight are associated with a higher incidence, morbidity, and mortality of several types of cancer. About 20% of cancers are associated with overweight. The higher the BMI, the greater the risk of cancers of the endometrium, breast, colorectal, kidneys, esophagus, and stomach [35–38].

The prevalence of respiratory function impairment in morbidly obese individuals is striking, even when compared with obese patients but with a lower BMI. Obstructive sleep apnea has a prevalence of 55–100% of morbidly obese subjects undergoing bariatric surgery [39, 40]. Higher mechanical pressure on the chest cavity, with consequent diaphragm compression, leads to a decrease in total lung capacity, expiratory reserve volume, and functional residual capacity, and thus from forced expiratory volume in the first second (FEV1) [41–44]. Studies have shown an inverse relationship between BMI and FEV1, the latter being an independent risk factor for cardiovascular diseases and stroke, as well as an independent predictor of death from all causes [44, 45].

Treatment of Severely Obese Patients

The cornerstone for treatment of obese patients is a multicomponent lifestyle intervention, and the same strategies are used to treat the morbid ones. It is based on behavioral changes with adherence to physical activity and a healthy diet. Pharmacological treatment and surgical treatment are reserved for those patients who do not respond to this approach. Some guidelines have been published to guide physicians [46–50].

The Look AHEAD trial brought us some evidence of efficacy of lifestyle intervention in severely obese individuals. In this trial, the most severely obese lost more weight than patients who were less obese. After 1 year, the severely obese lost 9.04% of initial body weight, while the overweight lost 7.43%. They also had comparable improvements in fitness, lipid levels, blood pressure, fasting glucose, and HbA1c [51, 52].

The great challenge is to bring these results to real life.

Very low-calorie diets (200 800 kcal/day) have been used occasionally in some centers, in severely obese patients, when rapid weight loss is necessary. Usually patients are maintained for up to 26 weeks on a high-quality protein diet in combination with electrolytes, vitamins, and trace elements. These can produce weight loss of around 2 kg/week (more in the first week as glycogen-bound fluid is lost). After 1 year, however, the weight change is not much different from other approaches [53].

US Food and Drug Administration (FDA) approved pharmacotherapy can be considered as an adjunct to lifestyle intervention in individuals with a BMI $\geq$ 30 or $\geq$ 27 kg/m^2 with at least one obesity-associated comorbidity. The AHA/ACC/TOS recommend an initial weight loss target of 5–10% of baseline weight within 6 months. These recommendations are based on that, even small changes in body weight, result in better control of associated morbidities and long-term health benefits [47].

Phentermine is a sympathomimetic amine anorectic approved, as monotherapy, for short-term treatment only in the USA. Topiramate is an antiepileptic drug associated with weight loss. Since both drugs, when used in monotherapy, can cause troublesome adverse events, they are now approved in a lower dose association for obesity management to minimize these side effects. Two studies, EQUIP and CONQUEST, and an extension study (SEQUEL) showed that the association of PHEN/TPM was effective in reducing body weight compared with placebo. An analysis of weight loss according to baseline BMI category was performed. PHEN/TPM was effective in all BMI categories. However, there was a significant treatment effect by baseline BMI category. The 15/92 mg group dose showed significantly greater percentage weight loss in the most severely obese subjects (baseline BMI 40 and 45) compared with 7.5/46 mg [54–56].

Lorcaserin, a 5-hydroxytriptamine (serotonin; 5-HT)2C receptor agonist, is also approved for weight management in the USA. It is used 10 mg twice daily and is effective compared with placebo after 1 and 2 years of treatment. In the BLOSSOM study, lorcaserin was associated with a decrease in the concomitant use of medications to treat dyslipidemia and hypertension and improved glycemic control. It is especially useful in those patients with cardiac arrhythmias or hypertension, as it is not associated with increases in blood pressure or pulse. Differences in weight loss as a function of baseline BMI have not been reported. Significant weight loss occurred in men and women across all BMI subgroups [57–59, 61, 62].

Naltrexone-bupropion is a sustained-release combination of an opioid receptor antagonist and a catecholamine reuptake inhibitor. It was approved by FDA and EMA for weight loss in people with overweight or obesity. Naltrexone and bupropion synergistically stimulate central melanocortin pathways and antagonize inhibitory feedback loops that limit weight reduction leading to improved energy expenditure and reduced appetite. A group of clinical trials also included morbidly obese subjects, but there are no reports of differences in weight loss across BMI subgroups [57, 60–62].

Orlistat is a reversible gastric and pancreatic lipase inhibitor that reduces fat absorption by ~30% when used 120 mg three times daily. In the XENDOS clinical trial, it produced significantly greater weight loss compared with placebo after 4 years. Orlistat therapy was accompanied by a ~50% risk reduction in progression to type 2 diabetes in those with impaired glucose tolerance. It was also associated with improvement of lipid profile, waist circumference, and blood pressure [63].

In terms of weight loss, it is less potent than other drugs approved for obesity treatment, with less impact in the management of the morbid patient, whose greater weight loss is desirable. The use of this drug, however, must be encouraged in those patients who cannot tolerate other drugs or in those that association of drugs is imperative to potentiate weight loss or to obtain metabolic benefits. There is no report of differences of weight loss across all BMI [57].

Liraglutide is a glucagon-like peptide-1 analogue that has recently been approved for the treatment of obesity at one daily dose of 3.0 mg, injected subcutaneously. Weight loss is mediated by appetite suppression and reduced energy intake. At the end of the SCALE trial, patients in the liraglutide group had lost an average of 8.4 ± 7.3 kg of body weight vs 2.8 ± 6.5 kg in the placebo group. The prevalence of prediabetes and development of type 2 diabetes were lower in the liraglutide group. Blood pressure and lipid levels also decreased. The most frequent adverse events were nausea and diarrhea. Titration of the dose is imperative to minimize these side effects.

Although it is a drug with a good safety profile, liraglutide seems to be less effective in patients with a mean BMI of 40 or higher than in patients with a lower BMI.

The FDA recommends that the drug should be discontinued after a 16-week period if 4% loss of baseline weight is not attained. The EMA recommends its discontinuation if 5% of weight loss is not reached after 12 weeks [61, 64].

The intragastric balloon became an interesting therapeutic option as it may confer a satisfactory weight loss in high-risk patients to improve the comorbidities and make a possible surgical procedure with a lower risk. Even in patients that are not submitted to surgery, studies show some weight loss in long-term follow-up. A study of 500 patients with BMI average 43 kg/m^2 showed loss average of 23.9 kg using a balloon filled with saline and methylene blue for 6 months. After 5 years, 41% of patients were reassessed and were still less obese, about 7 kg on average. A meta-analysis found 11.3% (8.2–14.4%) of total weight loss at 12 months after balloon placement [65].

AspireAssist is a percutaneous device of endoscopic gastrostomy designed to aspirate gastric contents. The device is implanted in a fashion similar to a conventional PEG tube. Approximately 20 min after meals, water is infused into the stomach, and gastric contents are drained. The device was recently approved by the FDA. The PATHWAY trial randomized subjects to AspireAssist with lifestyle counseling, or lifestyle counseling alone. The BMI of the AspireAssist group was 42.0 ± 5.1 kg/m^2, and the lifestyle counseling group had BMI of 40.9 ± 3.9 kg/m^2. At 52 weeks, an analysis showed 37.2% ± 27.5% weight loss in the AspireAssist group vs 13.0% ± 17.6% in the lifestyle counseling group. The most frequently reported adverse events were perioperative abdominal pain and postoperative granulation tissue and peristomal irritation. Additional studies for long-term outcomes are necessary [66].

Bariatric surgery is the most efficacious strategy and should be encouraged in those individuals in which the combination of pharmacological and non-pharmacological treatment was not effective. The percentage of weight loss will vary depending on the type of procedure performed. When comparing with the nonsurgical methods, bariatric surgery is associated with greater weight loss, higher percentage of improvement or remission of comorbidities, and improvement of quality of life. This option will be discussed in other chapters.

References

1. Stevens GA, Singh GM, Lu Y, Danaei G, Lin JK, Finucane MM, et al. National, regional, and global trends in adult overweight and obesity prevalences. Popul Health Metr [Internet]. 2012;10(1):22. Available from: http://www.ncbi.nlm.nih.gov/pubmed/23167948.
2. Finucane MM, Stevens GA, Cowan MJ, Danaei G, Lin JK, Paciorek CJ, et al. National, regional, and global trends in body-mass index since 1980: systematic analysis of health examination surveys and epidemiological studies with 960 country-years and 9??1 million participants. Lancet. 2011;377(9765):557–67.
3. Haslam DW, James WP. Obesity. Lancet. 2005;366:1197–209
4. Europe PMC Funders Group. Global, regional and national prevalence of overweight and obesity in children and adults 1980–2013: a systematic analysis. Lancet. 2014;384(9945):766–81.
5. National Institutes of Health. Weight management techniques. Pract Guid Identification, Eval Treat Overweight Obes Adults [Internet]. 2000;26–7. Available from: http://www.who.int/nutrition/topics/FFA_summary_rec_conclusion.pdf.
6. Manson J, Willett W, Stampfer M, Colditz G, Hunter DW, Hankinson S, et al. Body weight and mortality among women. N Engl J Med. 1995;333(11):677–85.
7. Sturm R, Ph D, Economist S. Morbid Obesity Rates Continue to Rise Rapidly in the US. Int J Obes. 2013;37(6):889–91.
8. Abeso. Obesidade: Diagnóstico e Tratamento de Crianças e Adolescentes. Diretrizes Brasileiras de Obesidade 2009/2010/ABESO. 2009. 63–70 p.
9. WHO. Obesity: preventing and managing the global epidemic. Report of a WHO consultation. World Health Organ Tech Rep Ser [Internet]. 2000;894:i–xii, 1–253. Available from: http://www.ncbi.nlm.nih.gov/pubmed/11234459.
10. Rodrigues AM, Suplicy HL, Radominski RB, Endocrinologia SS De. Implicações na Gênese da Obesidade. 47(Imc).
11. Coutinho W. Etiologia da obesidade. Abeso [Internet]. 2007;7(30):14. Available from: http://www.abeso.org.br/pdf/EtiologiaeFisiopatologia-Walmir Coutinho.pdf.
12. van den Bree MBM, Eaves LJ, Dwyer JT. Genetic and environmental influences on eating patterns of twins aged greater than or equals to 50 y. Am J Clin Nutr [Internet]. 1999;70(4):456–65. Available from: http://search.ebscohost.com/login.aspx?direct=true&AuthType=ip,shib&db=jlh&AN=2000000362&site=ehost-live.
13. Xia Q, Grant SFA. The genetics of human obesity. Ann N Y Acad Sci. 2013;1281(1):178–90.
14. Cassidy SB, Driscoll DJ. Prader-Willi syndrome. Eur J Hum Genet [Internet]. 2009;17(1):3–13. Available from: https://doi.org/10.1038/ejhg.2008.165
15. Forsythe E, Beales PL. Bardet-Biedl syndrome. Eur J Hum Genet [Internet]. 2013;21(1):8–13. Available from: http://www.nature.com/ejhg/journal/v21/n1/full/ejhg2012115a.html#bib39.
16. Farooqi IS, Keogh JM, Yeo GS, Lank EJ, Cheetham T, O'Rahilly S. Clinical spectrum of obesity and mutations in the melanocortin 4 receptor gene. N Engl J Med [Internet]. 2003;348:1085–95. Available from: internal-pdf://3543829267/MR4GENE.pdf\n http://www.ncbi.nlm.nih.gov/pubmed/12646665.
17. Krude H, Biebermann H, Luck W, Horn R, Brabant G, Grüters A. Severe early-onset obesity, adrenal insufficiency and red hair pigmentation caused by POMC mutations in humans. Nat Genet. 1998;19(2):155–7.
18. Farooqi S, Rau H, Whitehead J, O'Rahilly S. Ob gene mutations and human obesity. Proc Nutr Soc. 1998;57(3):471–5.
19. Farooqi IS, Wangensteen T, Collins S, Kimber W, Matarese G, Keogh JM, et al. Clinical and molecular genetic spectrum of congenital deficiency of the leptin receptor. N Engl J Med. 2007;356(3):237–47.
20. Calle EE, Thun MJ, Petrelli JM, Rodriguez C, Heath CW. Body-mass index and mortality in a prospective cohort of U.S. adults. N Engl J Med. 1999;341(15):1097–105.
21. Pi-Sunyer X. The medical risks of obesity. Postgrad Med. 2009;121(6):21–33.
22. Mokdad AH, Ford ES, Bowman BA, Dietz WH, Vinicor F, Bales VS, et al. Prevalence of obesity, diabetes, and obesity-related health risk factors, 2001. JAMA. 2003;289(1):76–9.
23. Barton M. Childhood obesity: a life-long health risk. Acta Pharmacol Sin. 2012;33(2):189–93.
24. Beymer C, Kowdley KV, Larson A, Edmonson P, Dellinger EP, Flum DR. Prevalence and predictors of asymptomatic liver disease in patients

undergoing gastric bypass surgery. Arch Surg. 2003;138(11):1240–4.
25. Machado M, Marques-Vidal P, Cortez-Pinto H. Hepatic histology in obese patients undergoing bariatric surgery. J Hepatol. 2006;45(4):600–6.
26. Field AE, Coakley EH, Must A, Spadano JL, Laird N, Dietz WH, et al. Impact of overweight on the risk of developing common chronic diseases during a 10-year period. Arch Intern Med. 2001;161(13):1581–6.
27. Stampfer MJ, Maclure KM, Colditz GA, Manson JE, Willett WC. Risk of symptomatic gallstones in women with severe obesity. Am J Clin Nutr. 1992;55(3):652–8.
28. Michalakis K, Mintziori G, Kaprara A, Tarlatzis BC, Goulis DG. The complex interaction between obesity, metabolic syndrome and reproductive axis: a narrative review. Metab Clin Exp. 2013;62:457–78.
29. Haffner SM. Sex hormones, obesity, fat distribution, type 2 diabetes and insulin resistance: epidemiological and clinical correlation. Int J Obes Relat Metab Disord. 2000;24(Suppl 2(2)):S56–8.
30. Weaver JU, Holly JM, Kopelman PG, Noonan K, Giadom CG, White N, et al. Decreased sex hormone binding globulin (SHBG) and insulin-like growth factor binding protein (IGFBP-1) in extreme obesity. Clin Endocrinol. 1990;33(3):415–22.
31. Lash MM, Armstrong A. Impact of obesity on women's health. Fertil Steril. 2009;91(5):1712–6.
32. Metwally M, Li TC, Ledger WL. The impact of obesity on female reproductive function. Obes Rev. 2007;8(6):515–23.
33. Gariepy G, Nitka D, Schmitz N. The association between obesity and anxiety disorders in the population: a systematic review and meta-analysis. Int J Obes. 2010;34(3):407–19.
34. Zhao G, Ford ES, Dhingra S, Li C, Strine TW, Mokdad AH. Depression and anxiety among US adults: associations with body mass index. Int J Obes. 2009;33(2):257–66.
35. Wolin KY, Carson K, Colditz GA. Obesity and cancer. Oncologist. 2010;15(6):556–65.
36. Gallagher EJ, LeRoith D. Epidemiology and molecular mechanisms tying obesity, diabetes, and the metabolic syndrome with cancer. Diabetes Care. 2013;36(SUPPL.2):233–9.
37. Calle EE, Teras LR, Thun MJ. Obesity and mortality. N Engl J Med. 2005;353:2197–9.
38. Reeves GK, Pirie K, Beral V, Green J, Spencer E, Bull D, et al. Cancer incidence and mortality in relation to body mass index in the Million Women Study: cohort study. BMJ. 2007;335(7630):1134.
39. Romero-Corral A, Caples SM, Lopez-Jimenez F, Somers VK. Interactions between obesity and obstructive sleep apnea: implications for treatment. Chest. 2010;137:711–9.
40. Frey WC, Pilcher J. Obstructive sleep-related breathing disorders in patients evaluated for bariatric surgery. Obes Surg. 2003;13(5):676–83.
41. McClean KM, Kee F, Young IS, Elborn JS. Obesity and the lung: 1. Epidemiology 1. Thorax. 2008;63(1468–3296 (Electronic)):649–54.
42. Parameswaran K, Todd DC, Soth M. Altered respiratory physiology in obesity. Can Respir J. 2006;13:203–10.
43. Sebastian JC. Respiratory physiology and pulmonary complications in obesity. Best Pract Res Clin Endocrinol Metab. 2013;27:157–61.
44. Salome CM, King GG, Berend N. Physiology of obesity and effects on lung function 2. J Appl Physiol. 2010;108(1522–1601 (Electronic)):206–11.
45. Schunemann HJ, Dorn J, Grant BJB, Winkelstein WJ, Trevisan M. Pulmonary function is a long-term predictor of mortality in the general population: 29-Year follow-up of the Buffalo Health Study. Chest. 2000;118(3):656–64.
46. Yumuk V, Frühbeck G, Oppert JM, Woodward E, Toplak H. An EASO position statement on multidisciplinary obesity management in adults. Obes Facts. 2014;7(2):96–101.
47. Eckel RH, Jakicic JM, Ard JD, de Jesus JM, Miller NH, Hubbard VS, et al. 2013 AHA/ACC guideline on lifestyle management to reduce cardiovascular risk. Circulation. 2014;129(25 suppl 2):S76–99.
48. Apovian CM, Aronne LJ, Bessesen DH, McDonnell ME, Murad MH, Pagotto U, et al. Pharmacological management of obesity: an endocrine society clinical practice guideline. J Clin Endocrinol Metab. 2015;100(2):342–62.
49. Jensen MD, Ryan DH, Apovian CM, Loria CM, Ard JD, Millen BE, et al. 2013 AHA/ACC/TOS guideline for the management of overweight and obesity in adults. J Am Coll Cardiol. 2013;1:1–70.
50. (UK) NCGC. Obesity: identification, assessment and management of overweight and obesity in children, young people and adults: partial update of CG43. National Institute for Health and Clinical Excellence: Guidance. 2014.
51. Wadden TA. Eight-year weight losses with an intensive lifestyle intervention: The look AHEAD study. Obesity. 2014;22(1):5–13.
52. Unick JL, Beavers D, Jakicic JM, Kitabchi AE, Knowler WC, Wadden TA, et al. Effectiveness of lifestyle interventions for individuals with severe obesity and type 2 diabetes: results from the look AHEAD trial. Diabetes Care. 2011;34(10):2152–7.
53. Gilden Tsai A, Wadden TA. The evolution of very-low-calorie diets: an update and meta-analysis. Obesity. 2006;14(8):1283–93.
54. Allison DB, Gadde KM, Timothy Garvey W, Peterson CA, Schwiers ML, Najarian T, et al. Controlled-release phentermine/topiramate in severely obese adults: a randomized controlled trial (EQUIP). Obes (SilverSping, Md). 2012;20(2):330–42.
55. Gadde KM, Allison DB, Ryan DH, Peterson CA, Troupin B, Schwiers ML, et al. Effects of low-dose, controlled-release, phentermine plus topiramate combination on weight and associated comorbidities in overweight and obese adults (CONQUER): a randomised, placebo-controlled, phase 3 trial. Lancet. 2011;377(9774):1341–52.
56. Garvey WT, Ryan DH, Look M, Gadde KM, Allison DB, Peterson CA, Schwiers M, Day WW, Bowden

C. Two-year sustained weight loss and metabolic benefits with controlled release phentermine. Am J Clin Nutr. 2012;95(2):297–308.

57. Macdaniels JS, Schwartz TL. Effectiveness, tolerability and practical application of the newer generation anti-obesity medications. Drugs Context. 2016;5:11.
58. BELVIQ® Prescribing Information. 2012. Available from URL: http://www.accessdata.fda.gov/drugsatfda_docs/label/2012/022529lbl.pdf.
59. Smith SR, Weissman NJ, Anderson CM, Sanchez M, Chuang E, Stubbe S, et al. Multicenter, placebo-controlled trial of lorcaserin for weight management. N Engl J Med [Internet]. 2010;363(3):245–56. Available from: http://www.nejm.org/doi/abs/10.1056/NEJMoa0909809\npapers2://publication/doi/10.1056/NEJMoa0909809.
60. Apovian CM, Aronne L, Rubino D, Still C, Wyatt H, Burns C, et al. A randomized, phase 3 trial of naltrexone SR/bupropion SR on weight and obesity-related risk factors (COR-II). Obesity. 2013;21(5):935–43.
61. Bray GA, Frühbeck G, Ryan DH, Wilding JPH. Management of obesity. Lancet [Internet]. 2016;6736(16):1–10. Available from: https://doi.org/10.1016/S0140-6736(16)00271-3.
62. Fujioka K. Current and emerging medications for overweight or obesity in people with comorbidities. Diabetes Obes Metab. 2015;17:1021–32.
63. Jarl S, Mark N. Xenical in the prevention of diabetes in obese subjects (XENDOS) study. Diabetes Care. 2004;27(1):155–61.
64. Pi-Sunyer X, Astrup A, Fujioka K, Greenway F, Halpern A, Krempf M, et al. A randomized, controlled trial of 3.0 mg of liraglutide in weight management. N Engl J Med [Internet]. 2015;373(1):11–22. Available from: http://www.ncbi.nlm.nih.gov/pubmed/26132939.
65. Kim SH, Chun HJ, Choi HS, Kim ES, Keum B, Jeen YT. Current status of intragastric balloon for obesity treatment. World J Gastroenterol. 2016;22:5495–504.
66. Kumar N. Weight loss endoscopy: Development, applications, and current status. World J Gastroenterol. 2016;22(31):7069–79.

Obesity and Related Diseases

4

Mariana Freitas Ferreira Lopes

Obesity is a significant risk factor for and contributor to increased morbidity and mortality, most importantly from cardiovascular disease (CVD) and diabetes but also from cancer and chronic diseases, including osteoarthritis, liver and kidney disease, sleep apnea, and depression. The prevalence of obesity has increased steadily over the past five decades, and obesity may have a significant impact on quality-adjusted life years. Obesity is also strongly associated with an increased risk of all-cause mortality as well as cardiovascular and cancer mortality. Despite the substantial effects of obesity, weight loss can result in a significant reduction in risk for the majority of these comorbid conditions [1, 2].

This chapter will review significant associations of obesity with comorbidities and some of the potential mechanisms involved.

Obesity and Comorbidity

Diabetes

The condition most strongly influenced by body weight is type 2 diabetes. In the Nurses' Health Study, which followed 114.281 middle-age women for 14 years, the risk of developing diabetes was 93 times higher among women who had a body mass index (BMI) of 35 or higher at the start of the study, compared with women with BMIs lower than 22 [3]. Weight gain during adulthood also increased diabetes risk, even among women with BMIs in the healthy range. The Health Professionals Follow-Up Study found a similar association in men [4].

More recently, investigators conducted a systematic review of 89 studies on weight-related diseases and then did a statistical summary, or meta-analysis, of the data. Of the 18 weight-related diseases they studied, diabetes was at the top of the risk list: Compared with men and women in the normal weight range (BMI lower than 25), men with BMIs of 30 or higher had a 7-fold higher risk of developing type 2 diabetes, and women with BMIs of 30 or higher had a 12-fold higher risk [5].

Fat cells, especially those stored around the waist, secrete hormones and other substances that fire inflammation. Plasma leptin, interleukin-6 (IL-6), tumor necrosis factor-α (TNF-α), and non-esterified fatty acid levels are all elevated in obesity.

Recent studies have identified "links" between obesity and type 2 diabetes involving proinflammatory cytokines (TNF-α, IL-6), deranged fatty acid metabolism, and cellular processes such as mitochondrial dysfunction and endoplasmic reticulum stress. Although inflammation is an essential component of the immune system and part of the healing process, inappropriate inflammation causes a variety of health problems [6].

M. F. F. Lopes (✉)
Endocrinology Division, Department of Obesity, São Rafael Hospital (HSR), Salvador, Bahia, Brazil

J. Ettinger et al. (eds.), *Gastric Bypass*, https://doi.org/10.1007/978-3-030-28803-7_4

Two mechanisms might be involved in the pathogenesis of inflammation. Firstly, glucose and macronutrient intake causes oxidative stress and inflammatory changes. Chronic obesity might thus be a proinflammatory state with oxidative stress. Secondly, the increased concentrations of TNF-α and IL-6, associated with obesity and type 2 diabetes, might interfere with insulin action by suppressing insulin signal transduction. This might interfere with the anti-inflammatory effect of insulin [7].

Therefore distinct mechanisms have been proposed to link obesity to insulin resistance and predispose to type 2 diabetes:

1. Increased production of adipokines/cytokines, including tumor necrosis factor-α, interleukin-6 (IL-6), resistin, and retinol-binding protein 4, that contribute to insulin resistance as well as reduced levels of adiponectin [8]
2. Ectopic fat deposition, particularly in the liver and perhaps also in skeletal muscle, and the dysmetabolic sequelae [8]
3. Mitochondrial dysfunction, evident by decreased mitochondrial mass and/or function. Mitochondrial dysfunction could be one of many important underlying defects linking obesity to diabetes, both by decreasing insulin sensitivity and by compromising β-cell function [7, 8]

Several large trials have shown that moderate weight loss can prevent or delay the start of diabetes in people who are at high risk [9–11].

Cardiovascular Disease (CVD)

Body weight is directly associated with various cardiovascular risk factors. As BMI increases, so do blood pressure, low-density lipoprotein (LDL) cholesterol, triglycerides, blood sugar, and inflammation. These changes translate into increased risk for coronary heart disease, stroke, and cardiovascular death:

- *Coronary Artery Disease*. Numerous studies have demonstrated a direct association between excess body weight and coronary artery disease (CAD). The BMI-CAD Collaboration Investigators conducted a meta-analysis of 21 long-term studies that followed more than 300,000 participants for an average of 16 years. Study participants who were overweight had a 32% higher risk of developing CAD, compared with participants who were at a normal weight; those who were obese had an 81% higher risk [12]. Although adjustment for blood pressure and cholesterol levels slightly lowered the risk estimates, they remained highly significant for obesity. The investigators estimated that the effect of excess weight on blood pressure and blood cholesterol accounts for only about half of the obesity-related increased risk of coronary heart disease. The higher incidence of CAD events in obese patients seems to be related to endothelial dysfunction and subclinical inflammation in addition to the worsening of CVD risk factors.

  Excess abdominal visceral adipose tissue, irrespective of the BMI, has been associated with a constellation of atherogenic abnormalities such as insulin resistance, increased triglycerides and apolipoprotein B levels, low high-density lipoprotein cholesterol, and an increased proportion of small dense low-density lipoprotein (LDL) and high-density lipoprotein (HDL) particles, the latter lipid abnormalities being generally described as the atherogenic dyslipidemia. Imaging cardiometabolic studies recently conducted in large cohort studies (Framingham Heart Study and the Jackson Heart Study) have shown that excess visceral adiposity accompanied by excess ectopic fat deposition such as excess heart, liver, and intrathoracic fat was significantly associated with cardiac and metabolic abnormalities.

  Obesity also induces a variety of structural adaptations/alterations in cardiovascular (CV) structure/function [13]. Chronic excessive accumulation of body fat causes adaptations of the CV system aiming at maintaining whole-body homeostasis. Increased cardiac output and a decrease in peripheral resistance are of importance in this adaptive state. Over the long term, such an increase in cardiac burden induces ventricular remodeling with enlargement of the cardiac cavities and increased wall tension which may eventually lead to left ventricular (LV) hypertrophy (LVH). In the heart itself, many additional alterations are observed along with increased adiposity. In healthy individuals, epicardial fat depot is distributed on the heart surface, close to the coronary arteries. With obesity, outside of the intracellular accumulation of fat, a higher amount of extracellular fat deposition builds up in the epicardium. The proximity of epicardial fat and coronary arteries might be associated with the atherosclerosis burden [14, 15]. Also, epicardial fat deposition is correlated with the amount of visceral fat which seems to produce potential proinflammatory adipokines/cytokines and macrophage signals that may be involved in the development of coronary artery disease. For instance, in visceral obesity, epicardial fat could influence blood vessels by its action as a paracrine organ while secreting locally pro-atherosclerotic molecules (such as interleukin or IL-1β, IL-6, or tumor necrotic factor-α) and less adiponectin compared to subcutaneous fat. Fat infiltration within the heart may cause direct damage that may lead to heart failure [16, 17].

Indeed, among the 5881 participants followed for 14 years in the Framingham Heart Study, 496 subjects developed CAD. Obese subjects were two times more at risk of developing CAD than normal weight individuals. An increased risk of 5% for men and 7% for women for every unit increase in BMI was observed after adjustment for established risk factors 42 suggesting a direct link between excess body fat and cardiac dysfunction.

- *Stroke*. Ischemic (clot-caused) stroke and coronary artery disease share many of the same disease processes and risk factors. A meta-analysis of 25 prospective cohort studies with 2.3 million participants demonstrated a direct, graded association between excess weight and stroke risk. Overweight increased the risk of ischemic stroke by 22%, and obesity increased it by 64%. There was no significant relationship between overweight or obesity and hemorrhagic (bleeding-caused) stroke, however [18]. A repeat analysis that statistically accounted for blood pressure, cholesterol, and diabetes weakened the associations, suggesting that these factors mediate the effect of obesity on stroke.
- *Cardiovascular Death*. In a meta-analysis of 26 observational studies that included 390,000 men and women, several racial and ethnic groups, and samples from the United States and other countries, obesity was significantly associated with death from CAD and cardiovascular disease. Women with BMIs of 30 or higher had a 62% greater risk of dying early from CAD and also had a 53% higher risk of dying early from any type of cardiovascular disease, compared with women who had BMIs in the normal range (18.5–24.9). Men with BMIs of 30 or higher had similarly elevated risks [19].

Cancer

Epidemiological studies have associated obesity with a range of cancer types, although the mechanisms by which obesity induces or promotes tumorigenesis vary by cancer site.

In an exhaustive review of the data, released in 2007, an expert panel assembled by the World Cancer Research Fund and the American Institute for Cancer Research concluded that there was convincing evidence of an association between obesity and cancers of the esophagus, pancreas, colon and rectum, breast, endometrium, and kidney and a probable association between obesity and gallbladder cancer [20]. Abdominal obesity and weight gain during adulthood were also linked with several cancers. A later systematic review and meta-analysis confirmed direct associations between obesity and cancers. Obese subjects have an approximately 1·5–3·5-fold increased risk of developing these cancers (colon and rectum, endometrium, esophagus, kidney, ovary, and pancreas) compared with normal weight subjects, and it has been estimated that between 15% and 45% of these cancers can be attributed to overweight (BMI 25·0–29·9 kg/m2) and obesity [21, 22].

Several possible mechanisms have been suggested to explain the association of obesity with increased risk of certain cancers:

Fat tissue produces excess amounts of estrogen, high levels of which have been associated with the risk of breast, endometrial, and some other cancers. Obese people often have increased levels of insulin and insulin-like growth factor-1 (IGF-1) in their blood, which may promote the development of certain tumors [23].

Fat cells produce hormones (adipokines) that may stimulate or inhibit cell growth. For example, leptin, which is more abundant in obese people, seems to promote cell proliferation, whereas adiponectin, which is less abundant in obese people, may have antiproliferative effects. Fat cells may also have direct and indirect effects on other tumor growth regulators, including mammalian target of rapamycin (mTOR) and AMP-activated protein kinase. Obese people often have chronic low-level, or "subacute," inflammation, which has been associated with increased cancer risk. Other possible mechanisms include altered immune responses, effects on the nuclear factor kappa beta system, and oxidative stress. All these factors may act directly or indirectly on the tumor microenvironment to drive tumor progression via the stimulation of cell survival/antiapoptosis, cell proliferation, angiogenesis, and invasion/metastasis of cancer cells [23–25].

Depression

Association between obesity and depression has repeatedly been established. An analysis of 17 cross-sectional studies found that people who were obese were more likely to have depression than people with healthy weights [26]. Since the studies included in the analysis assessed weight and mood only at one point in time, the investigators could not say whether obesity increases the risk of depression or depression increases the risk of obesity. New evidence confirms that the relationship between obesity and depression may be a two-way street: A meta-analysis of 15 long-term studies that followed 58,000 participants for up to 28 years found that people who were obese at the start of the study had a 55% higher risk of developing depression by the end of the follow-up period and people who had depression at the start of the study had a 58% higher risk of becoming obese [27].

Level of obesity appears to be an independent risk factor for common mental health disorders. Several reviewers have suggested that severe obesity puts individuals at greater risk of depression [28, 29].

Extremely obese people who seek bariatric surgery have been found to have lower self-esteem and higher depression scores than less obese individuals who seek pharmacological and behavioral weight loss interventions [30]. One study found that almost two-thirds of morbidly obese patients presenting for bariatric surgery had a psychiatric diagnosis, with major depression being the most common. Most patients were depressed about the negative effects of obesity in every aspect of their life, for example, health, social life, finances, mobility, and functioning [31].

The exact mechanism how obesity increases the risk for depression has not yet been definitively identified. Possible mechanisms include activation of inflammation, dysregulation of oxidant/antioxidant system balance, changes in the hypothalamic-pituitary-adrenal axis, insulin resistance, leptin resistance, altered plasma glucose, reduced neuronal brain-derived neurotrophic factor (BDNF), and decreased serotonergic neurotransmission in various regions of the brain and also social or cultural factors.

Reproduction

Obesity can influence various aspects of reproduction, from sexual activity to conception. Among women, the association between obesity and infertility, primarily ovulatory infertility, is represented by a classic U-shaped curve. In the Nurses' Health Study, infertility was lowest in women with BMIs between 20 and 24 and increased with lower and higher BMIs [32]. This study suggests that 25% of ovulatory infertility in the United States may be attributable to obesity. During pregnancy, obesity increases the risk of early and late miscarriage, gestational diabetes, preeclampsia, and complications during labor and delivery [33]. It also slightly increases the chances of bearing a child with congenital anomalies [34]. One small randomized trial suggests that modest weight loss improves fertility in obese women [35].

Strong evidence shows that insulin resistance is an integral part of polycystic ovarian syndrome, especially in obese women. In most women with the syndrome, hyperinsulinemia – driven or revealed by excess weight gain – promotes ovarian androgen secretion and abnormal follicular development, leading to dysfunctional ovarian and menstrual activity. Androgens are carried in the circulation bound to sex hormone-binding globulin (SHBG). Conditions of high androgen and insulin concentrations are associated with lower levels of SHBG, resulting in high free androgen activity. Thus, clinical manifestations of polycystic ovarian syndrome are associated with androgen activity and include hirsutism, acne, and alopecia, as well as oligomenorrhea and ovulation failure [36].

The impact of obesity on male fertility is less clear. In a study by Hammoud and colleagues, the incidence of low sperm count (oligospermia) and poor sperm motility (asthenospermia) increased with BMI, from 5.3% and 4.5%, respectively, in normal weight men to 15.6 and 13.3% in obese men [37]. In contrast, a study by Chavarro and colleagues found little effect of body weight on semen quality except at the highest BMIs (above 35), despite major differences in reproductive hormone levels with increasing weight [38]. Hypogonadism is an important comorbidity of obesity that is often overlooked. Hypogonadism, defined as the presence of low testosterone level measured on at least two occasions along with signs or symptoms that are owing to low testosterone, has been shown to be strongly correlated with obesity. In fact, it has been reported that obesity is probably the single most common cause of testosterone deficiency in the developed world, with approximately 52.4% of all obese men having testosterone levels below 300 ng/dL [39].

Sexual function may also be affected by obesity. Data from the Health Professionals Follow-Up Study [40], the National Health and Nutrition Examination Survey (NHANES) [41], and the Massachusetts Male Aging Study [42] indicate that the odds of developing erectile dysfunction increase with increasing BMI. Of note, weight loss appears to be mildly helpful in maintaining erectile function [43].

Respiratory Diseases

Excess weight impairs respiratory function via mechanical and metabolic pathways. The accumulation of abdominal fat, for example, may limit the descent of the diaphragm and, in turn, lung expansion, while the accumulation of visceral fat can reduce the flexibility of the chest wall, sap respiratory muscle strength, and narrow airways in the lungs [44]. Cytokines generated by the low-grade inflammatory state that accompanies obesity may also impede lung function.

Of these respiratory diseases, it has already been well established that obesity can lead to obstructive sleep apnea (OSA) and obesity hypoventilation syndrome (OHS).

In a meta-analysis of seven prospective studies that included 333,000 subjects, obesity increased the risk of developing asthma in both men and women by 50% [45]. More recent data suggest that the prevalence of wheezing and bronchial hyper-responsiveness, two symptoms often associated with asthma, is increased in overweight and obese individual. Indeed, epidemiological studies have reported that obesity is a risk factor for the development of asthma [46].

Obesity is also a major contributor to obstructive sleep apnea (OSA), which is estimated to affect approximately 1 in 5 adults; 1 in 15 adults has moderate or severe obstructive sleep apnea. This condition is associated with daytime sleepiness, accidents, hypertension, cardiovascular disease, and premature mortality. Between 50% and 75% of individuals with OSA are obese. Clinical trials suggest that modest weight loss can be helpful when treating sleep apnea [47, 48].

Furthermore, a number of studies indicate that obesity is also associated with a higher risk of developing deep vein thrombi, pulmonary emboli, pulmonary hypertension, and pneumonia.

Finally, weight reduction has been shown to be effective in improving the symptoms and severity of several respiratory diseases, including OSA and asthma.

Cognitive Function

Numerous studies have demonstrated that both obesity and metabolic disorders are associated with poorer cognitive performance, cognitive decline, and dementia. Body weight is a potentially modifiable risk factor for Alzheimer's disease and dementia. When we consider the growing population of overweight and obese people worldwide, along with an increasingly aging population, understanding the pathophysiology of obesity on the central nervous system is essential.

A meta-analysis of 10 prospective cohort studies that included almost 42,000 subjects followed for 3–36 years demonstrated a U-shaped association between BMI and Alzheimer's disease. Compared with being in the normal weight range, being underweight was associated with a 36% higher risk of Alzheimer's disease, while being obese was associated with a 42% higher risk [49]. The associations were stronger in studies with longer follow-up. A more recent meta-analysis demonstrated a similarly strong association between obesity and Alzheimer's disease [50].

It is evident that there is a deleterious effect of obesity/high fat feeding on cognitive performance. In human clinical studies, obesity has been shown to increase the risk of the development of mild cognitive impairment, in the form of short-term memory and executive function deficits, as well as dementia and Alzheimer's disease. The exact mechanisms or mediators that underlie the connections between obesity and the risk of cognitive impairment are still unknown, but potential avenues of further research include brain atrophy, disruption in cerebrovascular function, development of Alzheimer's disease-related pathology, and systemic and central inflammation. Increased adiposity has been correlated with reduced volume in a number of brain regions.

Amyloid plaques and neurofibrillary tangles containing tau protein are the pathological markers of Alzheimer's disease, accompanied by microglia activation and astrogliosis. Higher levels of amyloid-beta (Aβ, the main component of amyloid plaques) precursor protein (APP) and tau expression have been reported in hippocampal sections from morbidly obese patients without cognitive impairment, compared to a cohort of nonobese controls. Indeed increased levels of plasma amyloid proteins have been found in a number of studies of obese individuals suggesting a possible mechanism linking midlife obesity with the later development of Alzheimer's disease [50, 51].

Systemic inflammation can contribute to cognitive decline and dementia. Cytokines, such as IL-1β and IL-6, have been shown to disrupt neural circuits involved in cognition and memory. A recent meta-analysis identified that increased plasma levels of C-reactive protein and IL-6 is associated with an increase of dementia.

Moreover, increasing evidence suggests that the vascular effects of obesity have a key role in the development of vascular cognitive impairment in aged people by promotion of atherosclerosis in large cerebral arteries and alterations at the level of the cerebral microcirculation.

Musculoskeletal Disorders

Excess weight places mechanical and metabolic strains on bones, muscles, and joints. Osteoarthritis of the knee and hip are both positively associated with obesity, and obese patients account for one-third of all joint replacement operations [52].

Obesity has been implicated in the development or progression of a wide variety of musculoskeletal conditions:

- Osteoarthritis (knee, hip, hand)
- Low back pain (degenerative disc disease of the lumbar spine, spinal canal stenosis, and zygapophyseal joint disease)
- Diffuse idiopathic skeletal hyperostosis
- Gait disturbance
- Soft tissue conditions (e.g., carpal tunnel syndrome, plantar fasciitis)
- Gout
- Fibromyalgia
- Connective tissue disorders (rheumatoid arthritis)

There is a significant positive association between musculoskeletal disorders and the level of obesity. The Centers for Disease Control and Prevention [53] recently reported that in the United States, more than 31% of obese adults reported a doctor diagnosis of arthritis compared to only 16% of nonobese people.

Osteoarthritis (OA) is the most common form of arthritis and the leading cause of chronic disability among older people. Large longitudinal studies have demonstrated that obesity is a significant risk factor for both the development and progression of tibiofemoral knee OA (both symptomatic and radiographic) [52]. An association, though modest, has also been demonstrated between obesity and OA at other sites such as the hip, hand, and patellofemoral joint, suggesting that both mechanical and metabolic factors may be responsible for the link between OA and obesity.

Gout is the most common form of crystal-induced arthritis and in the United States affects more than 1% of adults [53]. It results from the deposition of monosodium urate crystals. Obesity is a well-known modifiable risk factor in the pathogenesis of gout, and serum uric acid is positively associated with BMI. The size of the visceral fat area is the strongest contributor to elevated serum uric acid concentration, decreased uric acid clearance, and increased urinary uric acid/creatinine ratio. Weight loss is advocated in the overall management of gout.

Fibromyalgia is a complex disorder resulting in pain, disturbed sleep, and altered mood. A number of risk factors are associated with this condition, and obesity also plays a role. In a pilot study of overweight and obese women with fibromyalgia, the relationship between BMI and fibromyalgia symptoms were assessed after a 20-week behavioral weight loss treatment [54]. Participants lost, on average, 4.4% of their initial weight, and weight loss predicted a reduction in fibromyalgia symptoms, pain interference, body satisfaction, and quality of life. In a study of obese subjects undergoing bariatric surgery, there was a significant reduction in fibromyalgia syndrome at follow-up 6–12 months later [55].

Obese patients were more likely to have radicular pain and neurologic signs [56]. Obesity was a significant, independent determinant of chronicity in a prospective cohort study in workers claiming compensation for lower-back pain [57]. In morbidly obese subjects with lower-back pain undergoing bariatric surgery, weight loss significantly improved the degree of functional disability and resulted in less frequent lower-back pain and the use of reduced doses of medications [58].

Nonalcoholic Fatty Liver Disease

Obesity is associated with an increased risk of nonalcoholic fatty liver disease (NAFLD). Steatosis, the hallmark feature of NAFLD, occurs when the rate of hepatic fatty acid uptake from plasma and de novo fatty acid synthesis is greater than the rate of fatty acid oxidation and export (as triglyceride within very low-density lipoprotein). Therefore, an excessive amount of intrahepatic triglyceride (IHTG) represents an imbalance between complex interactions of metabolic events. The presence of steatosis is associated with a constellation of adverse alterations in glucose, fatty acid, and lipoprotein metabolism. It is likely that abnormalities in fatty acid metabolism, in conjunction with adipose tissue, hepatic, and systemic inflammation, are key factors involved in the development of insulin resistance, dyslipidemia, and other cardiometabolic risk factors associated with NAFLD [59].

The prevalence rate of NAFLD increases with increasing BMI. An analysis of liver histology [60] obtained from liver donors, automobile crash victims, autopsy findings, and clinical liver biopsies suggests that the prevalence rates of steatosis and steatohepatitis are approximately 15% and 3%, respectively, in nonobese persons; 65% and 20%, respectively, in persons with class I and II obesity (BMI 30.0–39.9 kg/m^2); and 85% and 40%, respectively, in extremely obese patients (BMI ≥40 kg/m^2). The relationship between BMI and NAFLD is influenced by racial/ethnic background and genetic variation in specific genes.

Other Conditions

A number of additional health outcomes have been linked to excess weight. These include the development of gallstones in men and women [61], chronic kidney disease [62], and acute pancreatitis [63].

Obesity harms virtually every aspect of health, from shortening life and contributing to chronic conditions such as diabetes and cardiovascular disease to interfering with sexual function, breathing, mood, and social interactions. Obesity isn't necessarily a permanent condition. Diet, exercise, medications, and even surgery can lead to weight loss. Prevention of obesity could vastly improve individual and public health, reduce suffering, and save billions of dollars each year in healthcare costs.

References

1. Grundy SM. Obesity, metabolic syndrome, and cardiovascular disease. J Clin Endocrinol Metabol. 2004;89:2595–600.
2. Haslam DW, James WP. Obesity. Lancet. 2005;366(9492):1197–209.
3. Colditz GA, Willett WC, Rotnitzky A, Manson JE. Weight gain as a risk factor for clinical diabetes mellitus in women. Ann Intern Med. 1995;122:4816.
4. Koh-Banerjee P, Wang Y, Hu FB, Spiegelman D, Willett WC, Rimm EB. Changes in body weight and body fat distribution as risk factors for clinical diabetes in US men. Am J Epidemiol. 2004;159:11509.
5. Guh DP, Zhang W, Bansback N, Amarsi Z, Birmingham CL, Anis AH. The incidence of co-morbidities related to obesity and overweight: a systematic review and meta-analysis. BMC Public Health. 2009;9:88.
6. Rocha VZ, Libby P. Obesity, inflammation, and atherosclerosis. Nat Rev Cardiol. 2009;6:399409.
7. Dandona P, Aljada A, Bandyopadhyay A. Inflammation: the link between insulin resistance, obesity and diabetes. Trends Immunol. 2004;25:4–7.
8. Rabe K, et al. Adipokines and insulin resistance. Mol Med. 2008;14:741.
9. Knowler WC, Barrett-Connor E, Fowler SE, et al. Reduction in the incidence of type 2 diabetes with lifestyle intervention or metformin. N Engl J Med. 2002;346:393403.
10. Li G, Zhang P, Wang J, et al. The long-term effect of lifestyle interventions to prevent diabetes in the China Da Qing diabetes prevention study: a 20-year follow-up study. Lancet. 2008;371:17839.
11. Tuomilehto J, Lindstrom J, Eriksson JG, et al. Prevention of type 2 diabetes mellitus by changes in lifestyle among subjects with impaired glucose tolerance. N Engl J Med. 2001;344:134350.
12. Bogers RP, Bemelmans WJ, Hoogenveen RT, et al. Association of overweight with increased risk of coronary heart disease partly independent of blood pressure and cholesterol levels: a meta-analysis of 21 cohort studies including more than 300,000 persons. Arch Intern Med. 2007;167:17208.
13. Poirier P, Martin J, Marceau P, Biron S, Marceau S. Impact of bariatric surgery on cardiac structure, function and clinical manifestations in morbid obesity. Expert Rev Cardiovasc Ther. 2004;2:193–201.
14. Shimabukuro M, Hirata Y, Tabata M, et al. Epicardial adipose tissue volume and adipocytokine imbalance are strongly linked to human coronary atherosclerosis. Arterioscler Thromb Vasc Biol. 2013;33:1077–84.
15. Vela D, Buja LM, Madjid M, et al. The role of periadventitial fat in atherosclerosis. Arch Pathol Lab Med. 2007;131:481–7.
16. Iacobellis G, Sharma AM. Epicardial adipose tissue as new cardio-metabolic risk marker and potential therapeutic target in the metabolic syndrome. Curr Pharm Des. 2007;13:2180–4.
17. Baker AR, Silva NF, Quinn DW, et al. Human epicardial adipose tissue expresses a pathogenic profile of adipocytokines in patients with cardiovascular disease. Cardiovasc Diabetol. 2006;5:1.
18. Strazzullo P, DElia L, Cairella G, Garbagnati F, Cappuccio FP, Scalfi L. Excess body weight and incidence of stroke: meta-analysis of prospective studies with 2 million participants. Stroke. 2010;41:e41826.
19. McGee DL. Body mass index and mortality: a meta-analysis based on person-level data from twenty-six observational studies. Ann Epidemiol. 2005;15:8797.
20. American Institute for Cancer Research, World Cancer Research Fund. Food, nutrition, physical activity and the prevention of cancer. Washington, DC: American Institute for Cancer Research; 2007.
21. Polednak AP. Estimating the number of U.S. incident cancers attributable to obesity and the impact on temporal trends in incidence rates for obesity-related cancers. Cancer Detect Prev. 2008;32(3):190–9.

22. Ballard-Barbash R, Berrigan D, Potischman N, Dowling E. Obesity and cancer epidemiology. In: Berger NA, editor. Cancer and energy balance, epidemiology and overview. New York: Springer-Verlag New York, LLC; 2010.
23. Roberts DL, Dive C, Renehan AG. Biological mechanisms linking obesity and cancer risk: new perspectives. Annu Rev Med. 2010;61:301–16.
24. Grivennikov SI, Greten FR, Karin M. Immunity, inflammation, and cancer. Cell. 2010;140(6):883–99.
25. Wolin KY, Carson K, Colditz GA. Obesity and cancer. Oncologist. 2010;15(6):556–65.
26. de Wit L, Luppino F, van Straten A, Penninx B, Zitman F, Cuijpers P. Depression and obesity: a meta-analysis of community-based studies. Psychiatry Res. 2010;178:2305.
27. Luppino FS, de Wit LM, Bouvy PF, et al. Overweight, obesity, and depression: a systematic review and meta-analysis of longitudinal studies. Arch Gen Psychiatry. 2010;67:2209.
28. Markowitz S, Friedman MA, Arent SM. Understanding the relation between obesity and depression: causal mechanisms and implications for treatment. Clin Psychol Sci Pract. 2008;15(1):1–20.
29. Scott KM, Bruffaerts R, Simon GE, Alonso J, Angermeyer M, de Girolamo G, et al. Obesity and mental disorders in the general population: results from the world mental health surveys. Int J Obes. 2008;32(1):192–200.
30. Gundersen C, Mahatmya D, Garasky S, Lohman B. Linking psychosocial stressors and childhood obesity. Obes Rev. 2010;3:10.
31. Vaidya V. Psychosocial aspects of obesity. Adv Psychosom Med. 2006;27:73–85.
32. Rich-Edwards JW, Spiegelman D, Garland M, et al. Physical activity, body mass index, and ovulatory disorder infertility. Epidemiology. 2002;13:18490.
33. Huda SS, Brodie LE, Sattar N. Obesity in pregnancy: prevalence and metabolic consequences. Semin Fetal Neonatal Med. 2010;15:706.
34. Stothard KJ, Tennant PW, Bell R, Rankin J. Maternal overweight and obesity and the risk of congenital anomalies: a systematic review and meta-analysis. JAMA. 2009;301:63650.
35. Clark AM, Ledger W, Galletly C, et al. Weight loss results in significant improvement in pregnancy and ovulation rates in anovulatory obese women. Hum Reprod. 1995;10:270512.
36. Ramsay JE, Greer I, Sattar N. Obesity and reproduction. Br Med J. 2006;333:1159.
37. Hammoud AO, Wilde N, Gibson M, Parks A, Carrell DT, Meikle AW. Male obesity and alteration in sperm parameters. Fertil Steril. 2008;90:22225.
38. Chavarro JE, Toth TL, Wright DL, Meeker JD, Hauser R. Body mass index in relation to semen quality, sperm DNA integrity, and serum reproductive hormone levels among men attending an infertility clinic. Fertil Steril. 2010;93:222231.
39. Lamm S, Chidakel A, Bansal R, et al. Urologic Clinics of North America. 2016;43:239–45.
40. Bacon CG, Mittleman MA, Kawachi I, Giovannucci E, Glasser DB, Rimm EB. A prospective study of risk factors for erectile dysfunction. J Urol. 2006;176:21721.
41. Saigal CS, Wessells H, Pace J, Schonlau M, Wilt TJ. Predictors and prevalence of erectile dysfunction in a racially diverse population. Arch Intern Med. 2006;166:20712.
42. Johannes CB, Araujo AB, Feldman HA, Derby CA, Kleinman KP, McKinlay JB. Incidence of erectile dysfunction in men 40 to 69 years old: longitudinal results from the Massachusetts male aging study. J Urol. 2000;163:4603.
43. Wing RR, Rosen RC, Fava JL, et al. Effects of weight loss intervention on erectile function in older men with type 2 diabetes in the look AHEAD trial. J Sex Med. 2010;7:15665.
44. McClean KM, Kee F, Young IS, Elborn JS. Obesity and the lung: 1. Epidemiology. Thorax. 2008;63:64954.
45. Beuther DA, Sutherland ER. Overweight, obesity, and incident asthma: a meta-analysis of prospective epidemiologic studies. Am J Respir Crit Care Med. 2007;175:6616.
46. Murugan AT, Sharma G. Obesity and respiratory diseases. Chron Respir Dis. 2008;5:233–42.
47. Nerfeldt P, Nilsson BY, Mayor L, Udden J, Friberg D. A two-year weight reduction program in obese sleep apnea patients. J Clin Sleep Med. 2010;6:47986.
48. Tuomilehto HP, Seppa JM, Partinen MM, et al. Lifestyle intervention with weight reduction: first-line treatment in mild obstructive sleep apnea. Am J Respir Crit Care Med. 2009;179:3207.
49. Beydoun MA, Beydoun HA, Wang Y. Obesity and central obesity as risk factors for incident dementia and its subtypes: a systematic review and meta-analysis. Obes Rev. 2008;9:204–18.
50. Profenno LA, Porsteinsson AP, Faraone SV. Meta-analysis of Alzheimers disease risk with obesity, diabetes, and related disorders. Biol Psychiatry. 2010;67:50512.
51. Craft S. Insulin resistance syndrome and Alzheimer's disease: age-and obesity-related effects on memory, amyloid, and inflammation. Neurobiol Aging. 2005;26:65–9.
52. National Center for Chronic Disease Prevention and Health Promotion. Arthritis related statistics 2006. Division of Adult and Community Health, Health Care and Aging Studies Branch 2006.
53. Saag KG, Choi H. Epidemiology, risk factors, and lifestyle modifications for gout. Arthritis Res Ther. 2006;8(Suppl 1):S2.
54. Shapiro JR, Anderson DA, Danoff-Burg S. A pilot study of the effects of behavioral weight loss treatment on fibromyalgia symptoms. J Psychosom Res. 2005;59:275–82.
55. Hooper MM, Stellato TA, Hallowell PT, Seitz BA, Moskowitz RW. Musculoskeletal findings in obese subjects before and after weight loss following bariatric surgery. Int J Obes. 2007;31:114–20.

56. Fanuele JC, Abdu WA, Hanscom B, Weinstein JN. Association between obesity and functional status in patients with spine disease. Spine. 2002;27:306–12.
57. Fransen M, Woodward M, Norton R, Coggan C, Dawe M, Sheridan N. Risk factors associated with the transition from acute to chronic occupational back pain. Spine. 2002;27:92–8.
58. Melissas J, Kontakis G, Volakakis E, Tsepetis T, Alegakis A, Hadjipavlou A. The effect of surgical weight reduction on functional status in morbidly obese patients with low back pain. Obes Surg. 2005;15:378–81.
59. Tsuneto A, Hida A, Sera N, et al. Fatty liver incidence and predictive variables. Hypertens Res. 2010;33:63843.
60. Wanless IR, Lentz JS. Fatty liver hepatitis (steatohepatitis) and obesity: an autopsy study with analysis of risk factors. Hepatology. 1990;12:1106–10.
61. Tsai CJ, Leitzmann MF, Willett WC, Giovannucci EL. Prospective study of abdominal adiposity and gallstone disease in US men. Am J Clin Nutr. 2004;80:3844.
62. Kopple JD. Obesity and chronic kidney disease. J Ren Nutr. 2010;20:S2930.
63. Martinez J, et al. Obesity is a definitive risk factor of severity and mortality in acute pancreatitis: an updated meta-analysis. Pancreatology. 2006;6:206–9.

Preparing for Gastric Bypass

5

Joseph Sujka, Rena Moon, Muhammad Jawad, and Andre Fernandes Teixeira

Bariatric surgery is a commonly performed surgical procedure for control of morbid obesity. Its use has continued to grow with a total of 196,000 bariatric surgery procedures performed in 2015, a significant increase from 158,000 in 2011 [1]. Gastric bypass, including Roux-en-Y and duodenal switch, are some of the most common forms of bariatric surgery. To optimize weight loss after bypass, patients should undergo careful selection, teaching, biochemical testing, psychiatric evaluation, nutritional assessment, and diet changes.

Patient Selection

Medical management can be initially attempted for control of severe obesity, but failure rates remain high. As a result, many patients are evaluated for surgery once medical management has failed. In 1991 the NIH set out the following guidelines for patients looking to undergo bariatric surgery (NIH):

- They have a low likelihood of responding to nonsurgical techniques.
- They are motivated and informed about operative risks.
- BMI > 40 kg/m^2 or body weight greater than 100 lbs above ideal body weight.
- BMI between 35 and 40, if they have one high-risk comorbid condition or body weight greater than 80 lbs above ideal body weight with a comorbidity.

The Society of American Gastrointestinal Endoscopic Surgeons (SAGES) has similar recommendations stating that patients who have a body mass index greater than 40 kg/m^2 or BMI greater than 35 kg/m^2 with significant comorbidities who can show that dietary attempts at weight control are ineffective should be considered for surgery [2]. Utilizing these guidelines patients are able to be appropriately triaged for surgical intervention and started on the process of becoming ready for their chosen operative intervention.

Teaching

There are a variety of bariatric procedures that can be utilized to control morbid obesity including bypass; these include banding, sleeve gastrectomy, intragastric balloons, and others. Patients seeking bariatric surgery should first undergo education about the various options available to them for control of morbid obesity.

J. Sujka
Orlando Regional Medical Center, Department of Surgery, Orlando, FL, USA
e-mail: joseph.sujka@orlandohealth.com

R. Moon · M. Jawad · A. F. Teixeira (✉)
Bariatric and Laparoscopy Center, Orlando Health, Orlando, FL, USA
e-mail: reena.moon@orlandohealth.com; Muhammad.jawad@orlandohealth.com; andre.teixeira@orlandohealth.com

J. Ettinger et al. (eds.), *Gastric Bypass*, https://doi.org/10.1007/978-3-030-28803-7_5

A study evaluating 297 consecutive patients undergoing preoperative teaching found it affected patient surgical decision-making. The patients underwent teaching about types of operations including banding, bypass, or other procedures, through 3 weekly interactive 2 hour sessions. The study found that after education, 45 patients (15%) decided to change their surgical option and 27 (9%) declined surgery [3]. We encourage patients to not only attend classes related to bypass surgery but also to read and explore the topic through books and videos. Once the patient has decided on a procedure, we discuss this with them in more depth and begin operative clearance and planning.

Biochemical Testing

All patients preparing to undergo bariatric surgery should have basic laboratory evaluation including CBC, CMP, and a nutritional workup. Key nutritional elements to evaluate include prealbumin, albumin, thiamine, folate, 25-OH vitamin D, iron, and ferritin. Additional elements to consider testing are calcium and parathyroid hormone (if vitamin D is a concern), prothrombin time (if vitamin K is a concern), B_{12}, vitamin A, zinc, selenium, niacin, biotin, and copper. Nutritional assessment by a registered dietician is essential in this process [2].

Nutritional Assessment

We require that every patient undergo evaluation by a registered dietitian prior to undergoing surgery. Their ongoing involvement throughout the patient's care is essential to a good outcome. Preoperatively they talk about weight loss prior to surgery and behavioral changes, test patients for nutritional deficiencies, and discuss postoperative weight loss goals and eating strategies. After surgery dietitians are essential in the ongoing monitoring of the patient and should continue to be involved in the patient's weight loss process.

Behavioral Changes

One of the most important changes to make for a patient preoperatively is eating habits. It is important to identify behaviors preoperatively that may result in weight loss, results that are less than optimal. Specifically, identifying binge eating and snacking has had a discernible effect on a patient's bariatric surgery outcome. Carbohydrate addiction has also been evaluated but was not shown to have any effect on surgical outcomes.

Binge eating disorder is defined in the DSM-5 as recurrent episodes of eating more food in a short period than most people would under the same circumstances. This includes eating quickly and eating when not feeling hungry. This results in feeling of guilt, embarrassment, disgust, and psychological distress [4]. A prospective study analyzed 216 obese patients and classified them into 3 subgroups: no binge eating, sub-threshold binge eating, and binge eating disorder. These patients were followed up 3 years after surgery. The study found that patients with no history of binge eating had a greater percent excess BMI loss than those with sub-threshold or binge eating disorder [5]. This suggests that identification and correction of binge eating could lead to better outcomes after bypass surgery.

Snacking is another behavior that has been found to affect the weight loss of a patient who undergoes bypass surgery. A study of 75 patients evaluated the weight loss difference between patients who snack regularly, eat a large amount of sweets, and those with a normal eating pattern. They found a significant difference (p = 0.04) between normal eaters and snackers, finding that patients who snacked had a higher caloric intact, highest number of daily meals, and least excess weight loss of the groups examined. In light of these findings, the examiners recommended that patients receive additional screening to target these patients for additional behavioral therapy [6].

Carbohydrate addiction is the idea that patients may be addicted to specific food groups and that this may affect postoperative bypass surgery weight gains. A study evaluating 104 consecutive patients in a single program evaluated patients on a 0–60 scale to determine their level of carbohydrate craving. They compared the level of carbohydrate craving to successful excess weight loss following surgery. They defined success as percent excess weight loss greater than 50%. They found no statistically significant difference in the level of preoperative carbohydrate craving between successful and unsuccessful patients postoperatively. This indicates that carbohydrate craving does not seem to affect postoperative weight loss success. This, however, does not rule out other cravings affecting postoperative weight loss success [7].

Preoperative Weight Loss

The effect of weight loss prior to bariatric surgery is a heavily debated topic. Some debate that weight loss preoperatively has positive short-term effects on difficulty of surgery and resulting morbidities and that in the long-term patients are more successful with their overall weight loss. No study has elucidated an optimal amount of weight loss and what effects this has on bariatric surgery outcomes, but some have suggested the positive benefits.

A 2005 single institution study of 90 subjects found a positive correlation between weight lost and postoperative excess weight loss and a negative correlation between BMI and excess weight loss after 1 year. For every 1% initial weight loss, an increase of 1.8% of postoperative excess weight loss was seen, and for every 1 unit of BMI increase, there was a decrease of 1.34% excess weight loss. This suggests that those with weight loss prior to surgery have an increased benefit on total loss and those unable to lose weight may be less able to lose weight postoperatively [8].

A 2008 single institution study evaluated 150 patients to see if preoperative total body weight correlated with 3–4 year weight loss outcomes. Ninety-five patients were followed up for 4 years, and the author found that excess body weight loss preoperatively correlated positively with maintaining weight loss outcomes postoperatively. This may be due to a variety of factors but most likely underscores that those who are motivated to lose weight preoperatively develop improved habits and eating behaviors resulting in a more durable weight loss after surgery [9].

A recently published study in 2013 attempted to determine what effects specific percent of weight loss preoperatively correlated with operative outcomes, morbidity, and weight loss at 1 year. The study was a retrospective review of prospective single institution data. It included 548 patients who underwent laparoscopic Roux-en-Y gastric bypass surgery. These patients were divided into three groups depending on the amount of weight lost after surgery. Group A was <5%, B 5–10%, and C > 10%. Comparing these three groups, they found that there were significant differences in operative time, length of hospital stay, morbidity rate, and mean excess weight lost. Those patients with greater preoperative weight loss benefited in all these categories [10].

Most patients attempt to lose weight preoperatively through traditional means such as diet and exercise, but there has been some interest in utilizing adjuncts such as intragastric balloon for patients with massive obesity unable to lose weight through traditional means. One study found that super obese patients can lose up to 10% of excess weight in 3 months through utilization of an intragastric balloon. Going forward adjuncts may be utilized to help decrease patient's weight to further improve bariatric surgical outcomes [11].

Psychiatric Evaluation

Psychiatric evaluation remains an important part of an obese patient's preoperative workup. Some go as far to say that it is as important to the patient as nutritional counseling and preoperative clearance. Patients commonly do not grasp the severity of their problem, and many use food as a comfort mechanism. It is important that these habits are brought to the surface, so they do not interfere with weight loss after surgery. By dealing with these issues prior to surgery, the outcome of bariatric surgery can be improved.

Psychiatrists have various tools to evaluate patients that include, but aren't limited to, the Symptom Checklist 90, Wahler Physical Symptoms Inventory, and Personality Assessment screen. These tools are utilized in the setting of a formal interview where the psychiatrist can delve more deeply into issues relating to the patient's obesity. Psychiatrists commonly discuss personal trauma, (abuse, etc.), emotional dysfunction, (such as suicidal ideation), depression, substance abuse, and support systems after surgery. Patients need to be ready with supportive friends and family postoperatively and have dealt with all these factors to optimize their surgical result. This will help prevent patients from falling back into self-destructive behavior that may worsen their surgical outcomes.

The concept of psychiatry playing a strong role in bariatric surgery has become better accepted, but there are those who do not believe it plays a strong role as nutritional counseling and other support systems surrounding bariatric surgery. A 2014 single institution study evaluated 485 patients who underwent laparoscopic Roux-en-Y gastric bypass surgery. These patients were evaluated by a psychiatrist preoperatively and given green (453) or yellow light evaluations (19). Those with yellow light evaluations were recommended for additional psychiatric therapy. The study compared percent excess weight loss (%EWL) and percent body mass index change through a 3-year follow-up after surgery. They found that there was no statistically significant difference in %EWL or percent body mass index over the 3-year follow-up. Given the small number of yellow evaluation patients, there is not enough power to detect a difference in the groups, but it does give an interesting counterargument to the value of psychiatric evaluation [12].

Endoscopy

Preoperative EGD is routine in some centers. However, there is debate on whether or not it should be and whether the risks outweigh the benefits. Several studies have been performed in the last several years to examine this, and the results have been mixed. One study evaluated 169 patients and had no complications relating to the EGD. They found that only 33.3% of patients had negative EGDs; however, only 2 had changes to their operative plan [13]. Another study evaluated 468 patients with abnormal findings in 147 (46%) patients. In this study the surgical management was only changed in 4% of patients [14]. The most recent study, 2013, examined 412 patients with a negative EGD in 191 (55.8%) of patients. None of the findings changed the surgical management of these patients and were all determined to be benign [15]. Based on these and other findings, EGD is a relatively safe method for preoperative evaluation of the bypass patient but does not need to be routinely utilized as a screening method prior to bypass surgery.

Conclusion

The preparation of the patient for bariatric surgery is multifaceted. It requires multiple teams and specialties working in tandem for the best possible outcomes. This continued multidisciplinary perspective continues to push the field of bariatric surgery forward and improves the weight loss seen by patients.

References

1. American Society for Metabolic and Bariatric Surgery. [Online].; 2016 [cited 2016 August 14. Available from: https://asmbs.org/resources/estimate-of-bariatric-surgery-numbers
2. Nguyen N. The SAGES manual: a practical guide to bariatric surgery. 2008th ed. New York: Springer; 2008.
3. Giusti V, De Lucia A. Impact of preoperative teaching on surgical option of patients qualifying for bariatric surgery. Obes Surg. 2004;14:1241–6.
4. Association AP. Diagnostic and statistical manual of mental disorders. 5th ed. Washington, DC: American Psychiatric Association; 2013.
5. Sallet P, Sallet J. Eating behavior as a prognostic factor for weight loss after gastric bypass. Obes Surg. 2007;17:445–51.
6. Faria S, Kelly E. Snack-eating patients experience lesser weight loss after Roux-en-Y gastric bypass surgery. Obes Surg. 2008;19:1293–6.

7. Madan A, Orth W. Preoperative carbohydrate "addiction" does not predict weight loss after laparoscopic gastric bypass. Obes Surg. 2006;16:879–82.
8. Alvarado R, Alami R. The impact of preoperative weight loss in patients undergoing laparoscopic Roux-en-Y gastric bypass. Obes Surg. 2005;15:1282–6.
9. Alger-Mayer S, Polimeni J. Preoperative weight loss as a predictor of long-term success following Roux-en-Y gastric bypass. Obes Surg. 2008;18:772–5.
10. Giordano S, Victorzon M. The impact of preoperative weight loss before laparoscopic gastric bypass. Obes Surg. 2014;24:669–74.
11. Alfalah H, Philippe B. Intragastric balloon for preoperative weight reduction in candidates for laparoscopic gastric bypass with massive obesity. Obes Surg. 2006;16:147–50.
12. Won E, Tran T. A comparative study of three-year weight loss and outcomes after laparoscopic gastric bypass in patients with "yellow light" psychological clearance. Obes Surg. 2014;24:1117–9.
13. Zeni T, Frantzides C. Value of preoperative upper endoscopy in patients undergoing laparoscopic gastric bypass. Obes Surg. 2006;16:142–6.
14. Azagury D, Dumonceau J. Preoperative work-up in asymptomatic patients undergoing Roux-en-Y gastric bypass: is endoscopy mandatory. Obes Surg. 2006;16:1304–11.
15. Peromaa-Haavisto P, Victorzon M. Is routine preoperative upper GI endoscopy needed prior to gastric bypass. Obes Surg. 2013;23:736–9.

Preoperative Weight Loss in Gastric Bypass

6

Gustavo Peixoto Soares Miguel,
Paulo Henrique Oliveira de Souza,
Luize Giuri Palaoro, Caroline Gravel,
and Kassio Covre

Introduction

Bariatric surgery has been widely performed, and gastric bypass still represents one of the most performed procedures throughout the world [1]. Roux-en-Y gastric bypass (RYGB) has good results in terms of weight loss and can achieve a mean of 51–72% excess of weight loss (%EWL) [2]; however, the increasingly number of procedures leads to a necessity to improve patient selection and get optimized results in terms of weight loss and minimize postoperative complications.

In this context, preoperative weight loss may be an adjunct to achieve better results, and some centers recommend it [3, 4]. Preoperative weight loss can be undertaken by individual patients to evaluate the ability to adhere to dietary changes and to comply with the treatment, to potentially decrease operating time and intraoperative complications, to reduce the size of the liver and visceral load, and to influence postoperative weight loss and other complications [5]. A significant weight loss (>10% EWL) before bariatric surgery also ensures a better health status of obese patients with and without comorbidities [6].

Impact of Preoperative Weight Loss in Surgical Outcomes

Success in bariatric surgery is multifactorial, and besides preoperative body mass index (BMI), psychosocial disorders, and technical issues, preoperative weight loss can be one of the contributors [7]. Nevertheless, there are conflicting data in the literature as to the true effect of a preoperative weight loss regimen on various aspects of clinical outcome after bariatric surgery, including postoperative weight loss and surgical complications. Also, the large majority of the available studies regarding preoperative weight loss are observational and uncontrolled [5].

Impact in Postoperative Weight Loss

In one of the few randomized controlled trials (RCT) assessing the role of preoperative weight loss, Alami et al. (2007) randomized 100 patients undergoing laparoscopic RYGB (LRYGB) in two groups. In one group, patients should demonstrate a 10% weight loss before their scheduled surgery, and patients in the control group completed their routine preoperative workup. There was a higher %EWL up to 3-month follow-up,

G. P. S. Miguel (✉) · P. H. O. de Souza
L. G. Palaoro · C. Gravel · K. Covre
Department of Surgical Clinics, Hospital Universitário Cassiano Antônio de Moraes – HUCAM/UFES, Vitória, ES, Brazil

J. Ettinger et al. (eds.), *Gastric Bypass*, https://doi.org/10.1007/978-3-030-28803-7_6

however, not sustained to the 6-month period. A new study has evaluated the same sample of patients at a 1-year follow-up, and data were then analyzed with consideration of patients who had lost a minimum of 5% of their excess weight preoperatively. Weight loss group had a lower BMI and a higher percentage of excess body weight loss at 1-year postoperatively [8].

In the other published RCT, 294 patients were randomized to preoperative very low-calorie diet (VLCD) and to control group. The distribution between the groups was 136 patients in the control group and 137 in the VLCD group, and after a 30-day follow-up, the authors reported no difference in BMI and BMI loss. However, besides the short follow-up period, this study protocol was not primarily designed to evaluate any potential increased weight reduction [9].

There are some observational studies with a wide variation between them (sample size, study design, degree of preoperative weight loss, duration of follow-up) in which a positive relation has been reported in some, while no relation could be confirmed in others and even negative correlation was reported [5, 7].

A large Swedish cohort of patients who underwent RYGB had a median preoperative weight loss of −4.5%, and it was observed that the improvement in postoperative weight loss was related to the amount of weight loss before surgery, what indicates that there seems to be a positive "dose-response" relationship between pre- and postoperative weight loss [3]. A similar correlation was observed by Alvarado et al. (2010) in a 90-patient retrospective analysis with a 7.25% mean preoperative weight loss with a 1-year follow-up. In another prospective study with a longer follow-up, there was a significant positive correlation between preoperative weight loss and weight loss at 3 and 4 years after gastric bypass surgery [10]. There is also a trend in which patients with a higher preoperative weight loss sustained also a higher postoperative weight loss [11]. Other findings suggest that benefit from preoperative weight loss may be limited to male patients, but different procedures were analyzed, and only a minimum of 2% of weight loss was required [12].

Nevertheless, some studies report no association between preoperative and postoperative weight loss. A retrospective analysis of 300 patients who have gained or lost weight preoperatively has shown that there was no association between preoperative percent excess weight change and weight loss outcomes in 2 years after LRYGB [13]. A 2-year follow-up negative correlation was also found in a nonrandomized, single center, prospective study, even with marginal statistical significance [14]. Riess et al. (2008) concluded that patients who underwent LRYGB and presented more than 4.54 kg lost preoperatively had a worst outcome in terms of %EWL after 1-year follow-up [15]. This finding, however, is questionable, due to a significant heterogeneity between the groups.

Impact in Complications and Other Outcomes

One of the other advocated reasons to stimulate preoperatively weight loss is the potential of this strategy in reducing perioperative complications. It has been speculated that preoperative weight loss treatment may induce a catabolic state, contributing to an elevated risk of complications. However, there are some proposed mechanisms in which patients may benefit, and one possible explanation might be that patients exposed to preoperative weight loss could be expected to have a better glucose control in the postoperative period. A period of hypocaloric nutrition in obese, insulin-resistant subjects will improve insulin sensitivity, mainly due to depletion of glycogen stores and increased glucose uptake. Therefore, patients with improved insulin sensitivity before operation are likely to have better glucose control postoperatively, which has been convincingly shown to be associated with improved outcome after surgery [5]. Besides metabolic issues, preoperative weight loss can facilitate surgical technique, improving surgery duration and minimizing technical problems.

Many of the studies addressed this issue, but there is no homogeneity between them about the definition and reported types of complications.

The categories included bleeding, wound infection, anastomotic leak, need for reoperation during the initial hospitalization, and thromboembolic complications. Some studies also included late complications such as incisional hernia and marginal ulcers.

There are controversial results, and even the few RCTs had no consistent results. Alami et al. (2007) found a greater total operating room time in the non-weight loss group, but there was no difference in estimated blood loss, hospital length of stay, and intraoperative or postoperative complication rates, between the groups. This finding was maintained after reassessment of the same population after 1 year [8]. In a 30-day follow-up analysis, Van Nieuwenhove et al. (2011) showed a significantly higher number of complications in control group, compared to preoperative weight loss group.

A Scandinavian study of a large population-based cohort (22,327 patients) with a median preoperative weight loss of 4.7% analyzed the relation between weight loss before surgery and postoperative complications. When comparing patients in the 75th to the 25th percentile of preoperative weight loss, the risk of any complication was reduced by 13%. For specific complications, the corresponding risks were reduced for anastomotic leakage by 24%, deep infection/abscess by 37%, and minor wound complications by 54% [16]. Giordano et al. (2014) showed a higher overall early postoperative complications, with a lower incidence in the group with >10% preoperative weight loss [17]. In a recent retrospective paper, although no statistical significance in postoperative complications, a higher rate of complications in patients with preoperative weight gain compared to those with weight loss was observed [13]. Another study, despite no difference in postoperative weight loss, observed a trend to lower rate of postoperative complications [15]. Another study showed no difference in terms of surgical complications [18, 19].

The lower incidence of complications and shorter operative time can be related to technical aspects during the surgical procedure. The loss of weight can result in decrease of liver volume and intra-abdominal fat that leads to a better visualization of gastroesophageal junction and makes the division of the small gastric pouch and the gastrojejunostomy easier. Furthermore, traction to a fatty liver may cause trauma with increased risk for bleeding.

RCTs have different findings regarding LRYGB operative time comparing groups with preoperative weight loss and control groups. In fact, one of them compared operating room time, what can also take into account the anesthetic time, while the other refers to operating time [4, 9].

In a nonrandomized prospective evaluation, Edholm et al. (2011) compared liver volume and laparoscopic visibility after a 4-week low-calorie diet. The intrahepatic fat content, as assessed by magnetic resonance technique, decreased by 40%, and the liver volume decreased by 12%. Also, low-calorie group had better score regarding the laparoscopic size of the left liver lobe, sharpness of the liver edge, and exposure of the hiatal region as compared to the controls [18]. In another prospective analysis, a very low-calorie diet was given during 12 weeks; liver volume, visceral, and subcutaneous tissue were measured by both CT scan and MRI. BMI had a 10.6% decrease, liver volume reduced in 18.7%, and both subcutaneous and visceral adipose tissues reduced around 17%. Interestingly, the authors observed that most of the liver volume reduction occurred in the first 2 weeks of weight loss, whereas visceral adipose tissue and body weight decreased at a uniform rate over the 12-week study period [20]. A RCT also found that median perceived visual analog scale of difficulty encountered by the surgeon during the operation was significantly higher in the control group compared with the group that received a VLCD preoperatively [9] (Fig. 6.1).

Superobesity is a well-known risk factor for complications and obesity recidivism. An optimized and thorough preoperative evaluation should be performed in this group of patients, in which a preoperative weight loss can benefit even more. Some studies, therefore, analyzed outcomes after preoperative weight loss achieved by

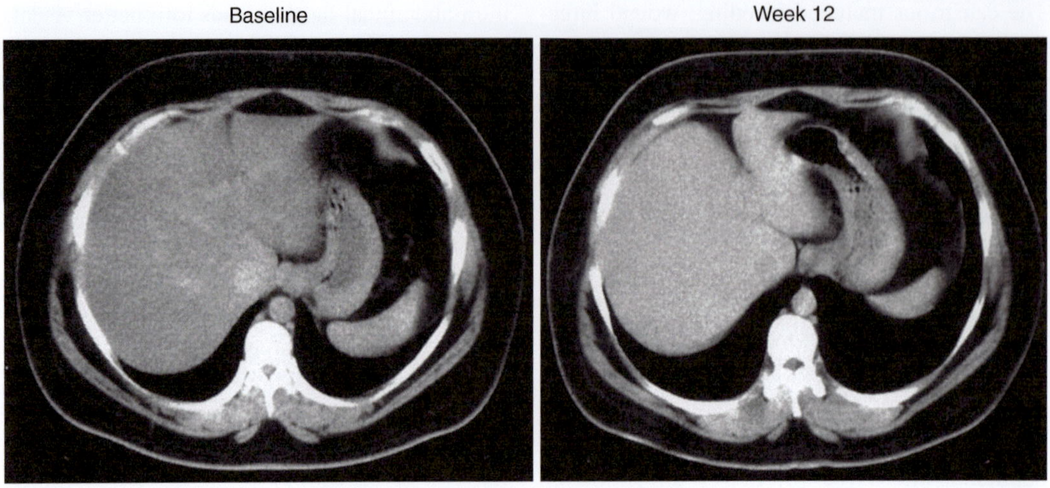

Fig. 6.1 Single cross-sectional images of the liver performed by computed tomography at baseline and week 12 of a very low-energy diet. The images, taken from within a series of contiguous 8-mm slices used to calculate total liver volume, illustrate the extent of the change in liver volume with weight loss in a 35-year-old man with an initial liver volume of 3.7 L and a final liver volume of 2.4 L. A 35% reduction in liver size and a weight loss of 18 kg were observed. (From: Colles et al. [20])

different methods in this group of patients. A retrospective, case-control study compared the records of 60 super-super obese patients with preoperative intragastric balloon (23 cases) or without (37 cases). The case group reached an 11.2% preoperative weight loss, and follow-up analysis revealed a more important weight loss for the case group only at 1 month after surgery; after this period, a similar and constant weight loss is observed in both groups. Moreover, a shorter operative time and less postoperative complications were observed in the intragastric balloon (IGB) group [21]. In a series of 20 super-obese patients, there was observed a mean of 19.7% preoperative weight loss, due to a hospitalization and multidisciplinary program, and no postoperative major complications were observed, highlighting a tendency toward a positive effect in this special group of patients [22].

Methods of Preoperative Weight Loss

There are a lot of ways in how weight loss was achieved preoperatively in the various published studies (informal vs. formal nutrition consult, liquid diet, low-calorie diet, very low-calorie diet). The components of a successful program, which will likely include both exercises and nutritional counseling, as well as the most effective dietary plan to achieve a significant amount of preoperative rapid weight loss, are unknown. The multidisciplinary team should try to identify the most feasible plan, according to the patient. Some predictive factors for compliance of preoperative weight loss recommendations are known, such as a high weight loss goal and a frequent self-weighing [23].

Although numerous preoperative weight loss strategies have been proposed, most of the available studies did not define or detail the specific utilized diet. Based on medical weight loss data, very low-calorie diets (VLCD) defined as 800 or less kcal/day and low-calorie diets (LCD) defined as 800–1200 kcal/day are possible to be prescribed and are generally associated with the greatest absolute losses in the shortest periods.

Protein shakes or meal replacement shakes are options to accomplish a VLCD. A recent review showed 15 studies regarding its use. Duration of the intervention was variable (median 4 weeks), and there are significant variations to standard protocols. Despite the majority of studies were assessed as weak methodological quality, 10 out of the 14 studies that reported on weight loss achieved greater than 5% total weight loss compared to baseline weight. Seven of these studies achieved greater than 10% [24].

An option used in superobesity with a BMI ≥50 kg/m^2 is IGB. Alfalah et al. (2006) showed that preoperative placement of an IGB can reduce the excess weight by 10% within 3 months, but extending this period failed to improve these results further [25]. This lack of long-term effectiveness is showed by other studies, although IGB can be considered a safe method, with around 3% of morbidity [26, 27]. Most of the patients return to their initial weight at 12 months after balloon removal [28], the reason why the IGB is recommended mainly as a "bridge" therapy, improving preoperative conditions. Zerrweck et al. (2012) show that IGB prior to LRYGB in super-super obese patients significantly reduced excess BMI. It was associated with a shorter operative time and a lower overall risk of significant adverse outcomes [21].

Ultimately, various treatment modalities are appropriate for each patient, and multidisciplinary team must use their judgment in selecting from among the different feasible treatment options.

Conclusion

Then, bariatric surgery programs should be free to recommend preoperative weight loss according to the specific needs and circumstances of the patient. This strategy, despite no evidence that strongly support its benefits, must be encouraged due to its potential in reducing surgical complications and improving postoperative weight loss.

References

1. Angrisani L, Santonicola A, Iovino P, Formisano G, Buchwald H, Scopinaro N. Bariatric surgery worldwide 2013. Obes Surg. 2015;25(10):1822–32.
2. Puzziferri N, Roshek TB, Mayo HG, Gallagher R, Belle SH, Livingston EH. Long term follow-up after bariatric surgery. JAMA. 2014;312(9):934–42.
3. Gerber P, Anderin C, Gustafsson UO, Thorell A. Weight loss before gastric bypass and postoperative weight change: data from the Scandinavian Obesity Registry (SOReg). Surg Obes Relat Dis. 2016;12(3):556–62.
4. Alami RS, Morton JM, Schuster R, Lie J, Sanchez BR, Peters A, et al. Is there a benefit to preoperative weight loss in gastric bypass patients? A prospective randomized trial. Surg Obes Relat Dis. 2007;3(2):141–5.
5. Gerber P, Anderin C, Thorell A. Weight loss prior to bariatric surgery: an updated review of the literature. Scand J Surg. 2014;104:33–9.
6. Sepu E, Ve LGA. Prospective study of the clinical, anthropometrical, and biochemical improvement following a mandatory weight loss of > 10% before bariatric. Surgery. 2016;11(2):1–6.
7. Livhits M, Mercado C, Yermilov I, Parikh JA, Dutson E, Mehran A, et al. Preoperative predictors of weight loss following bariatric surgery: systematic review. Obes Surg. 2012;22(1):70–89.
8. Solomon H, Liu GY, Alami R, Morton J, Curet MJ. Benefits to patients choosing preoperative weight loss in gastric bypass surgery: new results of a randomized trial. J Am Coll Surg. 2009;208(2):241–5.
9. Van Nieuwenhove Y, Dambrauskas Z, Campillo-Soto a, van Dielen F, Wiezer R, Janssen I, et al. Preoperative very low-calorie diet and operative outcome after laparoscopic gastric bypass: a randomized multicenter study. Arch Surg. 2011;146(11):1300–5.
10. Alvarado R, Alami RS, Hsu G, Safadi BY, Sanchez BR, Morton MJ, Curet MJ. The impact of preoperative weight loss in patients undergoing laparoscopic Roux-en-Y gastric bypass. Obes Surg. 2005;15:1282–6.
11. Alger-Mayer S, Polimeni JM, Malone M. Preoperative weight loss as a predictor of long-term success following Roux-en-Y gastric bypass. Obes Surg. 2008;18(7):772–5.
12. Mrad BA, Johnson Stoklossa C, Birch DW. Does preoperative weight loss predict success following surgery for morbid obesity? Am J Surg. 2008;195(5):570–4.
13. Blackledge C, Graham LA, Gullick AA, Richman J, Stahl R, Grams J. Outcomes associated with preoperative weight loss after laparoscopic Roux-en-Y gastric bypass. Surg Endosc. 2016;30(11):5077–83.
14. Pekkarinen T, Mustonen H, Sane T, Jaser N, Juuti A, Leivonen M. Long-term effect of gastric bypass and sleeve gastrectomy on severe obesity: do preoperative weight loss and binge eating behavior predict the outcome of bariatric surgery? Obes Surg. 2016;26(9):2161–7.
15. Riess KP, Baker MT, Lambert PJ, Mathiason MA, Kothari SN. Effect of preoperative weight loss on laparoscopic gastric bypass outcomes. Surg Obes Relat Dis. 2008;4(6):704–8.
16. Anderin C, Gustafsson UO, Heijbel N, Thorell A. Weight loss before bariatric surgery and postoperative complications: data from the Scandinavian Obesity Registry (SOReg). Ann Surg. 2015;261(5):909–13.

17. Giordano S, Victorzon M. The impact of preoperative weight loss before laparoscopic gastric bypass. Obes Surg. 2014;24(5):669–74.
18. Edholm D, Kullberg J, Haenni A, Hedberg J, Ahlström H, Sundbom M. Preoperative 4-week low-calorie diet reduces liver volume and intrahepatic fat, and facilitates laparoscopic gastric bypass in morbidly obese. Obes Surg. 2011;21:345–50.
19. Huerta S, Dredar S, Hayden E, Siddiqui AA, Anthony T, Asolati M, et al. Preoperative weight loss decreases the operative time of gastric bypass at a veterans administration hospital. Obes Surg. 2008;18(5):508–12.
20. Colles SL, Dixon JB, Marks P, Strauss BJ, O'Brien PE. Preoperative weight loss with a very-low-energy diet: quantitation of changes in liver and abdominal fat by serial imaging. Am J Clin Nutr. 2006;84(2):304–11.
21. Zerrweck C, Maunoury V, Caiazzo R, Branche J, Dezfoulian G, Bulois P, et al. Preoperative weight loss with intragastric balloon decreases the risk of significant adverse outcomes of laparoscopic gastric bypass in super-super obese patients. Obes Surg. 2012;22(5):777–82.
22. Santo MA, Riccioppo D, Pajecki D, De CR, Kawamoto F, Cecconello I. Preoperative weight loss in super-obese patients: study of the rate of weight loss and its effects on surgical morbidity. Clin (São Paulo, Brazil). 2014;69(12):828–34.
23. Bergh I, Kvalem IL, Risstad H, Cameron LD, Sniehotta FF. Predictors of preoperative weight loss in morbidly obese adults waiting for bariatric surgery: a prospective cohort study. Obes Surg. 2015;25(9):1610–7.
24. Ross LJ, Wallin S, Osland EJ, Memon MA. Commercial very low energy meal replacements for preoperative weight loss in obese patients: a systematic review. Obes Surg. 2016;26(6):1343–51.
25. Alfalah H, Philippe B, Ghazal F, et al. Intragastric balloon for preoperative weight reduction in candidates for laparoscopic gastric bypass with massive obesity. Obes Surg. 2006;16:147–50.
26. Imaz I, Martinez-Cervell C, Garcia-Alvarez EE, et al. Safety and effectiveness of the intragastric balloon for obesity. A meta-analysis. Obes Surg. 2008;18:841–6.
27. Fernandes M, Atallah AN, Soares BG, et al. Intragastric balloon for obesity. Cochrane Database Syst Rev. 2007;1:CD004931.
28. Angrisani L, Lorenzo M, Borrelli V, et al. Is bariatric surgery necessary after intragastric balloon treatment? Obes Surg. 2006;16:1135–7.

Preoperative Testing and Counseling

7

Abraham Fridman

Introduction

A laparoscopic gastric bypass (LGBP) was first described in 1994 and has since been used worldwide for the treatment of morbid obesity [1]. To properly identify patients who will be successful in the long term, a thorough preoperative work-up is recommended. In this chapter a proper preoperative work-up will be described and explained to decrease complications and increase compliance in all patients who end up undergoing a LGBP.

History

All patients interested in a LGBP should undergo an extensive preoperative evaluation for obesity-related comorbidities and causes of obesity. This evaluation should include a comprehensive medical history, psychosocial history, and physical examination.

A complete preoperative history and physical should be obtained on every patient prior to bariatric surgery. Obesity-related comorbidities should be identified at this time, including but not limited to diabetes, cardiac disease, gastroesophageal reflux disease (GERD), and obstructive sleep apnea (OSA). The physician should identify any potential medical, environmental, or social causes of morbid obesity in each patient. Weight loss history, commitment to the planned procedure, and any potential exclusions related to surgical risk should be identified at this time. A thorough physical exam should be performed on all patients to assess for any potential medical or surgical contraindications to the planned bariatric procedure. Medications and medical history should be reviewed in detail. Any mobility limitations should be evaluated and documented as these patients are more likely to have perioperative complications [2].

Data supports the association of smoking cigarettes with an increased risk of marginal ulceration and postoperative pneumonia [3]. Smoking cessation is recommended at least 6 weeks prior to LGBP [4]. This timing of smoking cessation has not been supported by other studies, and therefore cessation should be recommended at any time prior to surgery.

Candidates for LGBP should be counseled to avoid pregnancy preoperatively and for 12–18 months postoperatively. Estrogen therapy should be discontinued before LGBP (one cycle for oral contraceptives in premenopausal women; 3 weeks of hormone replacement therapy in postmenopausal women) to reduce the risk for postoperative thromboembolic phenomena [2].

A. Fridman (✉)
Griffin Hospital, Derby, CT, USA

J. Ettinger et al. (eds.), *Gastric Bypass*, https://doi.org/10.1007/978-3-030-28803-7_7

Laboratory Testing

All patients should undergo routine laboratory screening prior to undergoing a gastric bypass. Routine testing should include a complete blood count, chemistry, coagulation profile, kidney function, urine analysis, liver function testing, lipid panel, and fasting blood glucose. Routine screening for primary hypothyroidism simply due to the presence of an obese state is not recommended [5]. However, many insurance companies require TSH testing before bariatric surgery.

Lipid profile and preoperative triglyceride levels positively correlate with nonalcoholic steatohepatitis, and high-density lipoprotein levels negatively correlate with nonalcoholic fatty liver disease. This data supports the utility of preoperative lipid profiling [6]. All patients should undergo an appropriate nutritional evaluation, including micronutrient measurements, before any bariatric surgical procedure. Malabsorptive procedures require a more extensive evaluation [7, 8]. Patients should be screened with iron studies, B12 and folic acid, B1, and Vitamin D.

Psychosocial and Nutritional Evaluation

Psychosocial factors have significant potential to affect long-term outcomes of bariatric surgery. Thus, it is recommended that bariatric behavioral health clinicians with specialized knowledge and experience be involved in the evaluation and care of patients before and after surgery. Their main role is to identify factors that may pose challenges to optimal surgical outcome and to provide recommendations to the patient and the bariatric team on how to address these issues [9]. Presurgical psychosocial evaluation has been adopted by most third-party payers and most bariatric surgery programs [10].

The primary objective for the psychosocial evaluation for bariatric surgery is to provide screening and identification of risk factors or potential postoperative challenges that may contribute to a poor postoperative outcome [11]. Obtaining a comprehensive history of the patient's weight trajectory over time, including past weight loss attempts, is an essential component of the evaluation [12]. It clarifies the various environmental and physiologic contributors that have affected the patient's weight [13]. Clinical experience and expert opinion, as well as most published sets of practice guidelines, suggest that it remains important to carefully assess past and current eating disorder symptoms [14, 15]. Binge eating disorder, night eating syndrome, self-induced vomiting/purging, and anorexia nervosa should be carefully screened for. Other eating behaviors like skipping meals, eating in the absence of hunger, consuming large portions, obtaining meals outside the home, and grazing can all compromise weight loss outcomes.

Patients with severe obesity tend to exhibit more psychopathology than healthy weight individuals or those with less severe obesity [16]. Psychological disorders like depression, bipolar disorder, anxiety, and schizophrenia should all be identified and treated prior to undergoing surgery. Clark et al. found that patients who had undergone past treatment for psychiatric or substance abuse disorders demonstrated better weight loss 2 years after surgery [17]. Patients should be well-informed, motivated, and willing to engage in the necessary postoperative dietary and behavioral changes.

GI Evaluation

There is controversy among different centers and studies whether upper endoscopy (EGD) or radiographic study like an upper gastrointestinal series (UGI) should be routinely or selectively used. The European Association for Endoscopic Surgery recommends performing either an UGI or an EGD for all patients undergoing bariatric procedures [18]. Loewen et al. found the positive EGD findings led to a change in medical treatment in 18% of patients out of a group of 447 [19]. In another study, out of 536 patients, 4.9% had changed or altered operative procedures due to endoscopic findings [20]. However, there are multiple other studies in the literature that do not show a benefit to doing routine preoperative GI evaluations [21, 22].

In operations that exclude anatomy, like the LGBP, it is acceptable to perform a preoperative EGD or UGI, because up to 80% of patients with pathological findings can be asymptomatic [23]. EGD is a better modality due to its ability to visualize and biopsy lesions. Proper cancer screening with colonoscopy should be performed prior to LGBP if clinically warranted.

Prevalence of *Helicobacter pylori* (*H. pylori*) varies from 8.7% anywhere up to 85.5% in different populations [23, 24]. There is evidence that supports screening, which reduced incidence of perforation postoperatively and potentially reduced marginal ulcers from 6.8% to 2.4% with preoperative diagnosis and treatment [20]. However, other studies conclude that gastric ulcers are related to surgical procedures and not *H. pylori* infection [25]. Evidence overall does not support routine screening, but in high prevalence areas, routine screening is recommended.

Venous Thromboembolic Events (VTE/DVT)

History of VTE or pulmonary embolism (PE) should be obtained in all patients. Based on the BOLD database, overall risk of VTE was 0.42%, with most events occurring after discharge and within 30 days. Risk of VTE was found to be greater in patients undergoing a LGBP than a lap band [26]. Appropriate diagnostic evaluation for DVT (ultrasound) should be obtained in patients with history of thromboembolism. Prophylactic use of IVC filters prior to LGBP does not prevent PE and may lead to additional complications [27]. A longer duration of chemoprophylaxis is recommended for patients at high risk for postoperative VTE.

Cholelithiasis/Abdominal Ultrasound

The incidence of gallstones and or cholecystectomy in autopsy populations is up to 45% in females as reported in a Danish study [28]. The Swedish obesity study showed that obese patients have a significantly higher prevalence of cholelithiasis, cholecystitis, cholecystectomies, and pancreatitis as compared with the reference population. Obesity surgery significantly increased the incidence of cholelithiasis, cholecystitis, and cholecystectomies in men. In both genders, weight loss was related to an increased incidence of biliary disease [29]. Transabdominal ultrasonography (US) remains an effective diagnostic tool to assess for cholelithiasis with sensitivity and specificity greater than 87–96% (may have a limited sensitivity in the obese patient) [30]. It is a noninvasive test, with minimal to no radiation exposure, which has a very high yield.

It is well established, as mentioned before, that obesity is a significant risk factor for stone formation and that the presence of gallstones is proportionate to the degree that the individual is overweight. It has also been shown that rapid weight loss from any cause is strongly associated with stone formation [29]. Approximately 30% of post-bariatric surgery patients newly develop gallstones within 12–18 months after LGBP, and about 1/3 of these patients are symptomatic [31]. Different effects of surgery have been explained as the cause of increased biliary disease after LGBP. Some suggest that it is the altered anatomy and the diversion of food from the distal stomach or duodenum decreases gallbladder contractility [32]. Other data supports that it is the metabolic and neuronal alterations that play a greater role than an alteration of anatomy [33].

Prophylactic cholecystectomy in all patients continues to be advocated by some, but it is performed far less often now. A selective approach to cholecystectomy can be undertaken and is guided with either preoperative or intraoperative assessment of the gallbladder. Patients who are symptomatic and have signs of gallbladder disease should undergo an US and have a cholecystectomy if abnormalities are diagnosed on preoperative US. Tucker et al. found 12% incidence of gallbladder pathology, with 65% of those patients undergoing a concomitant cholecystectomy at the same time as the LGBP. 17.6% of the patients who did not undergo a cholecystectomy required a subsequent operation. They concluded that cholecystectomy for US confirmed pathology is feasible and safe and reduces future gallbladder-related morbidity [34]. On the other hand, Papasavas et al. suggest that the gallbladder does not need to be evaluated in patients without symptomatic disease due to lack of significant gallbladder disease postoperatively [35]. However, a case can be made that since the access to the biliary tree after a LGBP is more difficult, a preoperative or concomitant cholecystectomy should be performed to minimize the risk for a more complicated procedure in the future. Although there is controversy regarding preoperative gallbladder evaluation prior to LGBP, data supports preoperative gallbladder evaluation with an US and a subsequent cholecystectomy if abnormalities are detected.

Medical Subspecialty Evaluation

Pulmonary

In patients considered for LGBP, a chest radiograph and standardized screening for obstructive sleep apnea (OSA) (with confirmatory polysomnography if screening tests are positive) should be considered. OSA is prevalent before bariatric surgery in up to 94% of patients, 38% being undiagnosed [36]. Predictive models lack sufficient sensitivity and specificity. Moderate to severe OSA is associated with increased mortality and adverse outcomes in the bariatric surgery group [37]. Routine screening preoperatively should be considered, with further diagnostic testing and treatment of appropriate at-risk patients. Standard preoperative management of OSA with continuous positive airway pressure is recommended.

Patients seeking bariatric surgery also commonly suffer from other pulmonary ailments like asthma, dyspnea, chronic pulmonary obstructive disease (COPD), and obesity hypoventilation syndrome (OHS). Some of these patients suffer from more severe hypoxemia than OSA patients. If severe disease is confirmed, patients should have preoperative arterial blood gas measurements and pulmonary function tests [38].

Cardiology

Increase in BMI has steadily shown to predict increased cardiovascular mortality, and that increase can be two to four times higher than normal weight individuals [39]. Patients with a known heart disease may require a formal cardiology consultation before bariatric surgery. Noninvasive cardiac testing beyond an electrocardiogram is determined on the basis of the individual risk factors and findings on history and physical examination. Patients at risk for heart disease should undergo evaluation for perioperative beta-adrenergic blockade. In a cohort comprised of many bariatric surgery patients, the continuation of beta-blockers was associated with fewer cardiac events and improved 90-day mortality rates [40].

Endocrinology

Type 2 diabetes mellitus (T2D) is one of the risk factors contributing to postoperative complications and death after LGBP. Preoperative glycemic control should be optimized using a diabetes comprehensive plan (diet, physical activity, pharmacotherapy, etc.). Reasonable targets for preoperative glycemic control include a Hgb A1C <6.5–7%., fasting blood glucose <110, and a 2-hour postprandial blood glucose of <140 mg/dL [41]. A shorter duration and better glycemic control preoperatively is associated with a higher rate of T2D remission after surgery [42]. In a study of 468 patients undergoing LGBP, elevated preoperative hemoglobin A1C was associated with elevated postoperative hyperglycemia. Postoperative hyperglycemia is independently associated with wound infections, acute renal failure, and reduced T2D remission rates [43].

Informed Consent

Completely informed consent requires both the physician and the patient to be informed with all of the information. Informed consent for bariatric surgery is a dynamic process of education and patient comprehension which begins at the initial consultation and does not end till the time of the actual surgery. Disclosure of the risks and benefits plays a vital role as well. Educational objectives, active teaching (and learning), and assessments are recommended. These should be communicated clearly and presented at a 6th–8th grade level [44]. Multimedia, social media, and other interactive tools have shown promise in improving patient comprehension and understanding of the proposed procedure. Informational seminars that have been adopted by many programs are vital in the beginning of the patient experience, but education should be ongoing throughout the work-up. Promotion of realistic expectations is recommended, and the benefits of the procedure should not be overstated [45]. Thorough discussion for the need of long-term follow-up, vitamin supplementation, and the cost required for both is vital to postoperative success. Consent should include the experience of the surgeon within the specific procedure offered and whether the hospital is an accredited institution or not.

While many statistics can be given to the patient, care must be taken to not just highlight the positive ones. An objective assessment of patient's individual risks, outcomes, and expectations should be provided. If there is a significant variance between individual and national statistics, these should be clearly highlighted to the patient [46]. Patients often forget significant elements of their preoperative teaching and education, including risks of serious complications. Therefore this discussion should be held again immediately prior to the proposed operation. There have also been legal precedents that perhaps individual facility and surgeons' specific complication rates be included in the consent process [47]. The ultimate consent privilege lies with the patient alone. Therefore, it is prudent and safer to have a well-educated and truly informed patient prior to the procedure.

Conclusion

Preoperative work-up for LGBP is very important in the subsequent success and happiness of the patient. It is essential to set up practice standards such that each patient can be approached in a standardized and evidence-based fashion preoperatively to optimize care. Standardized preoperative protocols will limit errors of omission and inappropriate offerings of surgery. They will ensure no patient gets left behind or falls through the cracks while increasing efficiency and avoiding unnecessary testing [46].

References

1. Wittgrove AC, Clark GW, Tremblay LJ. Laparoscopic gastric bypass, Roux-en-Y: preliminary report of five cases. Obes Surg. 1994;4(4):353–7.
2. Mechanik JL, Youdim A, Jones DB, Garvey WT, Hurley DL, McMahon MM. Clinical practice guidelines for the perioperative nutritional, metabolic, and nonsurgical support of the bariatric surgery patient-2013 update: cosponsored by American Association of Clinical Endocrinologists, The Obesity Society, and American Society for Metabolic & Bariatric Surgery. Surg Obes Relat Dis. 2013;9:159–91.
3. Felix EL, Kettelle J, Mobley E, Swartz D. Perforated marginal ulcers after laparoscopic gastric bypass. Surg Endosc. 2008;22:2128–32.
4. Schumann R, Jones SB, Cooper B, Kelley SD, Bosch MV, Ortiz VE, et al. Update on best practice recommendations for anesthetic perioperative care and pain management in weight loss surgery. Obesity (Silver Spring). 2009;17:889–94.
5. Garber J, Cobin RH, Gharib H, Hennessey JV, Klein I, Mechanik JI, et al. Clinical practice guidelines for hypothyroidism in adults: cosponsored by American Association of Clinical Endocrinologists and the American Thyroid Association. Endocr Pract. 2012;11:1–207.
6. Kashyap SR, Diab DL, Baker AR, Yerian L, Bajaj H, Gray-McGuire C, et al. Triglyceride levels and not adipokine concentrations are closely related to severity of non-alcoholic fatty liver disease in an obesity surgery cohort. Obesity. 2009;17:1696–701.
7. Toh SY, Zarshenas N, Jorgensen J. Prevalence of nutrient deficiencies in bariatric patients. Nutrition. 2009;25:1150–6.
8. Aasheim ET, Bjorkman S, Sovik TT, Engstrom M, Hanvold SE, Mala T, et al. Vitamin status after bariatric surgery: a randomized study of gastric bypass and duodenal switch. Am J Clin Nutr. 2009;90:15–22. Erratum in: Am J Clin Nutr 2010;91:239–40.
9. Sogg S, Lauretti J, West-Smith L. Recommendations for the presurgical psychosocial evaluation of bariatric surgery patients. Surg Obes Relat Dis. 2016;12:731–49.
10. Bauchowitz AU, Gonder-Freederick LA, Olbrisch ME, Azarbad L, Ryee MY, Woodson M, et al.

Psychosocial evaluation of bariatric surgery candidates: a survey of present practices. Psychosom Med. 2005;67:825–32.
11. Lanyon R, Maxwell B. Predictors of outcomes after gastric bypass surgery. Obes Surg. 2007;17(3):321–8.
12. Gould J, Ellsmere J, Fanelli R, Hutter M, Jones S, Pratt J, et al. Panel report: best practices for the surgical treatment of obesity. Surg Endoosc. 2011;25(6):1730–40.
13. Ashton D, Favretti F, Segato G. Preoperative psychological testing: another form of prejudice. Obes Surg. 2008;18(10):1330–7.
14. Wadden TA, Sarwer DB. Behavioral assessment of candidates for bariatric surgery: a patient oriented approach. Obesity. 2006;14(Suppl 2):53S–62S.
15. Sogg S, Mori DL. Revising the Boston interview: incorporating new knowledge and experience. Surg Obes Relat Dis. 2008;4(3):455–63.
16. Malik S, Mitchell JE, Engel S, Crosby R, Wonderlich S. Psychopathology in bariatric surgery candidates: a review of studies using structured diagnostic interviews. Compr Psychiatry. 2014;55(2):248–59.
17. Clark MM, Balsiger BM, Sletten CD, Dahlman KL, Ames G, Williams DE, et al. Psychosocial factors and 2 year outcome following bariatric surgery for weight loss. Obes Surg. 2003;13(5):739–45.
18. Sauerland S, Angrisani L, Belachew M, Chevallier JM, Favretti F, Finer N, European Association of Endoscopic Surgery, et al. Obesity surgery: evidence based guidelines of the European Association of Endoscopic Surgery (EAES). Surg Endosc. 2005;19(2):200–21.
19. Loewen M, Giovanni J, Barba C. Screening endoscopy before bariatric surgery: a series of 448 patients. Surg Obes Relat Dis. 2008;4(6):709–12.
20. Schirmer B, Erenoglu C, Miller A. Flexible endoscopy in the management of patients undergoing Roux-en-Y gastric bypass. Obes Surg. 2002;12:634–8.
21. Korenkov M, Sauerland S, Shah S, Junginger T. Is routine preoperative upper endoscopy in gastric banding patients really necessary? Obes Surg. 2006;16(1):45–7.
22. Ghassemian AJ, Macdonald KG, Cunningham PG, Swanson M, Brown BM, Morris PG, et al. The work-up for bariatric surgery does not require a routine upper gastrointestinal series. Obes Surg. 1997;7(1):16–8.
23. Kuper MA, Kratt T, Kramer KM, Zdichavsky M, Schneider JH, Glatzle J, et al. Effort, safety, and findings of routine preoperative endoscopic evaluation of morbidly obese patients undergoing bariatric surgery. Surg Endosc. 2010;24(8):1996–2001.
24. Al-Akwaa AM. Prevalence of Helicobacter pylori infection in a group of morbidly obese Saudi patients undergoing bariatric surgery: a preliminary report. Saudi J Gastroenterol. 2010;16:264–7.
25. Yang CS, Lee WJ, Wang HH, Huang SP, Lin JT, Wu MS. The influence of Helicobacter pylori infection on the development of gastric ulcer in symptomatic patients after bariatric surgery. Obes Surg. 2006;16:735–9.
26. Winegar DA, Sherif B, Pate V, Demaria EJ. Venous thromboembolism after bariatric surgery performed by Bariatric Surgery Center of Excellence Participants: analysis of the Bariatric Outcomes Longitudinal Database. Surg Obes Relat Dis. 2011;7:181–8.
27. Birkmeyer NJ, Share D, Baser O, Carlin AM, Finks JF, Pesta CM, et al. Preoperative placement of inferior vena cava filters and outcomes after gastric bypass surgery. Ann Surg. 2010;252:313–8.
28. Teilum D. The prevalence of gallstones in autopsies from Danish urban area. Frederiksberg 1914–1955. Acta Chir Scand. 1989;155(2):103–6. Available at: http://www.ncbi.nlm.nih.gov/pubmed/2787087. Accessed 30 Sept 2016.
29. Torgerson JS, Lindroos AK, Naslund I, Peltonen M. Gallstones, gallbladder disease, and pancreatitis: cross-sectional and 2 year data from the Swedish obese subjects (SOS) and SOS reference studies. Am J Gastroenterol. 2003;98:1032–41.
30. Birtwhistle RV, Sauerbrei EE. Ultrasonography in the diagnosis of gallbladder disease. Can Fam Physician. 1983;29:1621–5. Available at: http://www.pubmedcentral.nih.gov/articlerender.fcgi?artid=2153898&tool=pmcentrez&rendertype=abstract. Accessed 30 Sept 2016.
31. Miller K, Hell E, Lang B, Lengauer E. Gallstone formation prophylaxis after gastric restrictive procedures for weight loss: a randomized double-blind placebo-controlled trial. Ann Surg. 2003;238(5):697–702.
32. Erlinger S. Gallstones in obesity and weight loss. Eur J Gastroenterol Hepatol. 2000;12(12):1347–52.
33. Bastouly M, Arasake CH, Ferreira JB, Zanoto A, Borges FGHP, Del Grande JC. Early changes in post-prandial gallbladder emptying in morbidly obese patients undergoing Roux-en-Y gastric bypass: correlation with the occurrence of biliary sludge and gallstones. Obes Surg. 2009;19(1):22–8.
34. Tucker ON, Fajnwaks P, Szomstein S, Rosenthal RJ. Is concomitant cholecystectomy necessary in obese patients undergoing laparoscopic gastric bypass surgery. Surg Endosc. 2008;22(11):2450–4.
35. Papasavas PK, Gagne DJ, Ceppa FA, Caushaj PF. Routine gallbladder screening is not necessary in patients undergoing laparoscopic Roux-en-Y gastric bypass. Surg Obes Relat Dis. 2006;2(1):41–6.
36. Rasmussen JJ, Fuller WD, Ali MR. Sleep apnea syndrome is significantly underdiagnosed in bariatric surgical patients. Surg Obes Relat Dis. 2012;8(5):569–73.
37. Flum DR, Belle SH, King WC, Wahed AS, Beck P, Chapman W, et al. Perioperative safety in the longitudinal assessment of bariatric surgery. N Engl J Med. 2009;361:445–54.
38. Piper AJ, Grunstein RR. Obesity hypoventilation syndrome: mechanisms and management. Am J Respir Crit Care Med. 2011;183:292–8.
39. Litwin SE. Which measures of obesity best predict cardiovascular risks? J Am Coll Cardiol. 2008;52:616–9.
40. Kwon S, Thompson R, Florence M, Maier R, McIntyre L, Rogers T, et al. B-blocker continuation after noncardiac surgery: a report from the surgical

care and outcomes assessment program. Arch Surg. 2012;147:467–73.
41. Handelsman Y, Mechanick JY, Blonde L, et al. American Association of Clinical Endocrinologists Medical Guidelines for clinical practice for developing a diabetes mellitus comprehensive care plan. Endoc Practice. 2011;17(Suppl 2):1–52.
42. Hall TC, Pellen MGC, Sedman PC, Jain PK. Preoperative factors predicting remission of type 2 diabetes mellitus after Roux-en-Y gastric bypass surgery for obesity. Obes Surg. 2010;20:1245–50.
43. Pena M, Romagnuolo J, Morgan K, Byrne TK, Baker M. Preoperative hemoglobin A1c and postoperative glucose control in outcomes after gastric bypass for obesity. Surg Obes Relat Dis. 2012;8(6):685–90.
44. Raper SE, Sarwer DB. Informed consent issues in the conduct of bariatric surgery. Surg Obes Relat Dis. 2008;4:60.
45. Heinberg LJ, Keting K, Simonelli L. Discrepancy between ideal and realistic goal weights in three bariatric procedures: who is likely to be unrealistic? Obes Surg. 2010;20:148–53.
46. Tichansky DS, Sudan R. Preoperative care of the bariatric patient. In: Nguyen NT, Blackstone RP, Morton JM, Ponce J, Rosenthal RJ, editors. The ASMBS textbook of bariatric surgery. New York: Springer Science + Business Media; 2015. p. 77–84.
47. Plerhoples TA, Lau JN. Informed consent. In: Tichansky DS, Morton J, Jones DB, editors. The SAGES manual of quality, outcomes, and patient safety. New York: Springer Science + Business Media; 2012. p. 521–8.

Patient Selection for Metabolic Surgery

8

Jose Guido Correa de Araujo Jr., Josemberg Marins Campos, Renata Paiva Barbosa, Maira Danielle Gomes, and Álvaro Antônio Bandeira Ferraz

The global prevalence of T2DM has increased significantly on the past decades. WHO reports an increase from 30 million individuals in 1985 to 177 million individuals in 2000, and with maintained progress on incidence, it is expected over 500 million diabetic individuals by 2030 [1]. Important to state that a significant group of the diabetic population is unaware of the condition and, therefore, chronically exposed to continued hyperglycaemia and consequently high morbidity and mortality due to the lack of treatment. On 2014, the United States National Institutes of Health (NIH) Centres for Disease Control related a 9.3% (29.1 million) prevalence of diabetes on the American population, stressing that approximately 30% (8.1 million) of this population are nondiagnosed diabetic patients [2].

Diabetes is responsible for three million deaths annually, ranging 1.7–5.2% of all reported death causes, remaining a fifth death cause worldwide, and several papers suggest there is under notification of diabetes-related deaths [3–5].

J. G. C. de Araujo Jr. (✉)
J. M. Campos · M. D. Gomes
Surgery Department, University Hospital, Pernambuco Federal University, Recife, Brazil

R. P. Barbosa
Esperança D'Or Hospital, Recife, Brazil

Á. A. B. Ferraz
Federal University of Pernambuco, Department of Surgery, Recife, Brazil

Great attention is driven to the Asiatic population, wherein ethnic distinctive physiology of body fat storage and its influence in metabolic arrangements pose an increased risk for metabolic syndrome with less body mass index (BMI) when compared to the occidental population. In China in 2010, diabetes prevalence was 11.6%, and prediabetes was as high as 51% [6]. The Asiatic population is at risk for a high prevalence of the so-called metabolically obese phenotype, wherein early-onset increased abdominal adiposity can coexist with normal body weight or low BMI [7]. Impairment of insulin sensitivity and β cell function induced by free fatty acids derived from abdominal adipose tissue leads to T2DM and metabolic syndrome even with low BMIs.

Although long-term glycaemic control can delay or ameliorate the evolution of diabetes to cardiovascular risk and chronic complications, barely half of the diabetic population can achieve adequate glycaemic control relying solely on medical treatment and behavioural changes [8, 9]. Longitudinal studies such as UKPDS demonstrated the limited results on long-term glycaemic control in this population, suggesting that novel therapies be used to improve diabetes control and prevent chronic complications of the disease [10, 11].

On the other hand, the past decades have witnessed great enthusiasm with the results of bariatric surgeries, mainly gastric bypass but also other procedures, on treating diabetes in T2DM patients. Bariatric procedures were widely

J. Ettinger et al. (eds.), *Gastric Bypass*, https://doi.org/10.1007/978-3-030-28803-7_8

accepted as a treatment for T2DM particularly after significant data with strong evidence reporting complete diabetes remission in 78.1% and improvement (remission + amelioration) in 86.6% of the patients treated with gastric bypass [12, 13]. Bariatric surgery has been reported to improve glycaemic control and other metabolic targets, providing a cost-effective alternative approach to treat T2DM patients. Considering cardiometabolic risk reduction and glycaemic control, bariatric surgery has been indicated currently to treat obesity patients who cannot achieve good control with medical treatment [14].

The effectiveness of bariatric surgery in diabetes remission with mechanisms not entirely related to weight loss raised the question on how nonobese or mild obesity diabetics would respond to surgical treatment. In 2006, Cohen et al. [15] published a series of 37 diabetic patients with BMI < 35 kg/m^2 with severe comorbidities, submitted to laparoscopic gastric bypass with a 4-year follow-up. Thirty patients had comorbidities remission, and mean excess weight loss was 81%. De Sá et al. [16] analysed 27 patients with BMI < 35 kg/m^2 submitted to Roux-en-Y gastric bypass (RYGB) to treat uncontrolled T2DM, with a mean follow-up of 20 months. On the postoperative follow-up, an excess weight loss of 94% was achieved, and 74% of the patients completely discontinued medications, whereas 48% achieved complete diabetes remission. Preoperative BMI or drug scheme did not influence glycaemic control or diabetes remission, whereas long-standing diabetes was associated with inferior results.

Several randomized trials are currently evaluating metabolic surgery for T2DM in patients with BMI < 35 kg/m^2. Shimizu et al. [17] evaluated 18 studies, with a total of 477 patients. Remission rate of 64% was achieved, considered as a patient with discontinued medications, plus fasting plasma glucose (FPG) <126 mg/dl and HgbA1c <6.5%. Schauer et al. [18] presented a randomized trial of bariatric surgery vs intensive medical therapy for obese patients with diabetes, wherein 34% of the population studied had a BMI lower than 35 kg/m^2. Diabetes remission rate for the bypass group at 1 year was 42% vs 12% for medical treatment.

The Diabetes Surgery Study randomized clinical trial [19] performed a comprehensive review of the available literature and compared gastric bypass to intensive medical therapy in 120 patients with a 12-month follow-up, with target on ADA criteria for metabolic syndrome control: HgbA1c < 7%, systolic blood pressure < 130 mmHg and LDL <100 mg/dL. Most patients in both groups were obese with BMI < 35 kg/m^2. At 1 year follow-up, 75% of the bypass group had met the criteria for diabetes remission, compared to only 32% of the medical treatment group.

Recently, elucidation of the complex physiopathology on energy storage and expenditure has raised novel targets on the preoperative evaluation of patients who can benefit from metabolic surgery. BMI remains important, but strong evidence suggest that visceral fat, more than BMI itself, has the potential adverse influence on glycaemic control through impairing insulin resistance and β-cell function. Therefore, anatomical rearrangement of the gastrointestinal tract and its well-known effect on entero-hormonal changes in fact benefits a great number of patients regardless of weight loss. Current recognized strong predictors of good postoperative metabolic results of bariatric surgery include recently diagnosed diabetes and preserved β-cell function as measured by C-peptide levels [20].

Surgery is evaluated to T2DM patients considering patient ability to tolerate surgical procedures and always with a tailored approach to risk-benefit relations on an individual basis. Bariatric surgeries have repeatedly been reported as a low-morbidity and safe procedure, with overall mortality rates ranging from 0.1% to 0.2% and a major complication rate of 2.5% [21, 22]. Despite low morbidity and mortality, a complete comprehensive preoperative workup with multidisciplinary evaluation is warranted in standards of care required to all bariatric and metabolic interventions, as it is routine for all elective operations. Surgery is better avoided in patients with high surgical risk for adverse cardiovascular events or other critical medical conditions, which can preclude surgery as a treatment for T2DM and metabolic syndrome. Accessing the specific type of diabetes, screening for chronic complications of the disease and measurement of β-cell function and the grade of pancreatic endocrine insufficiency are of special value to help predict chances of diabetes recurrence and exclude unrecognized type 1 diabetes.

Bariatric surgery in patients who present moderate or severe obesity has long been established as a gold standard to treat T2DM alongside with obesity [13]. In the past decade, bariatric surgery has gained wide acceptation also in patients with T2DM and metabolic syndrome who present mild obesity and even overweight patients, who present poor glycaemic and metabolic control with medical treatment. The key to success with the surgical treatment relies on adequate selection of the patient for metabolic surgery to treat T2DM. Given that metabolic syndrome is closely related to the obesity phenotype – with patients who present central obesity posing an increased risk – several papers have addressed the value of BMI as a sensible parameter to select obese patients for metabolic surgery [23, 24]. Panuzi et al. [25] published meta-analysis of all studies to date on diabetes remission in patients with T2DM and found no significant differences in diabetes remission when studies with preoperative BMI < 35 kg/m^2 (remission rate 72%) were compared to preoperative BMI ≥ 35 kg/m^2 (remission rate 71%).

In the Asiatic population, studies have addressed the need to identify other parameters rather than BMI who would correlate better with the risk of T2DM.

Yu et al. [26] published a retrospective review of prospectively collected data of 68 ethnic Chinese with mean BMI of 31.5 kg/m^2 submitted to RYGB, evaluated for metabolic outcomes. Of note, preoperative visceral fat area (VFA) was evaluated with magnetic resonance imaging. Diabetes remission was defined as no medications and HbgA1c < 6.5% at 1 year following surgery. The authors found that remission was achieved in 73.5% of the patients. When the remission group was compared to non-remission patients, BMI and waist circumference did not differ, whereas remission patients had a shorter duration of diabetes, lower preoperative HgbA1c levels, higher C-peptide levels and more visceral fat area, suggesting that those patients who present more visceral adiposity can significantly benefit from RYGB, and VFA might be of great value in the preoperative decision making.

The selection of a patient for metabolic surgery should be based therefore in the presence of metabolic syndrome with a poor control of diabetes, with a specific approach to diabetes and metabolic syndrome. The evaluation of diabetic patients should include a cutoff point of HgbA1c of 7% as preconized by American Diabetes Association (ADA). In addition, better results will be achieved in individuals with diabetes with short (<5 years) duration and C-peptide >2.9 ng/dL, who represent better residual β-cell function [27].

Because of such amount of evidence, an international consensus conference was held in Rome-IT in 2007. The first Diabetes Surgery Summit (DSS-I) [28] encouraged randomized clinical trials to evaluate bariatric surgery as a valid treatment for T2DM in comparison to intensive lifestyle changes and medical treatment. The RCTs published on the sequence of DSS-I are repeatedly corroborating the findings that metabolic surgery is superior to medical interventions in reducing cardiovascular risk factors and achieving better glycaemic control in the range of obesity patients.

Again, because of the great number of studies addressing the topic of bariatric surgery as a treatment for T2DM in mildly obese patients, the International Diabetes Federation also positioned and published in 2011 a Position Statement considering bariatric surgery as an acceptable treatment modality for T2DM in patients with a BMI < 35 kg/m^2 and poor control with medical treatment [29].

Based on the accumulated level 1 and 1A evidence of good short- and long-term results with metabolic surgery in grade I obese diabetics, comparable to grade II and III obese diabetics, with low morbidity and mortality of RYGB, Campos et al. [30] published, on behalf of the Brazilian Bariatric and Metabolic Surgery Society, a Position Statement on metabolic surgery in which a "Metabolic Risk Score" is proposed to select patients for metabolic surgery (Table 8.1). The score consists of obligatory and complementary criteria. On the complementary

Table 8.1 Metabolic risk score for metabolic surgery

Metabolic risk score	
Obligatory criteria	Type 2 diabetes mellitus
	Age 30–65
	BMI ≥ 30 kg/m²
	Baseline C-peptide >1 ng/dL and negative Anti-GAD
	HgbA1c 2 points above reference regardless of medical treatment
	Surgical indication corroborated by endocrinologist
Complementary criteria	BMI: 30–30,9 kg/m²: 0 points 31–31.9 kg/m²: +1 point 32–32.9 kg/m²: +2 points 33–33.9 kg/m²: +3 points 34–34.9 kg/m²: +4 points
	Albuminuria >30 mg/g creatinine: +1 point
	C-peptide >50% baseline after mixed meal test: +1 point
	Hypertension: +1 point
	Dyslipidaemia: +1 point
	Macrovascular disease: +1 point
	NASH: +1 point
	Sleep apnoea: +1 point
	Diabetes time: 2–5 years: +2 points 5–10 years: +1 point >10 years: −1 point >15 anos: −2 points
	Insulin use >5 years: −1 point

From Campos et al. [30]

field, patients are attributed positive scores (+1) to criteria which are supposed to influence positively on postoperative outcomes and negative scores (−1) for criteria which are supposed to negatively influence postoperative outcomes. Metabolic surgery will be indicated when patients meet all obligatory criteria and score 7 points or more on the complementary criteria field.

In 2016, Rubino et al. [31] published the results of the Diabetes Surgery Summit II (DSS-II), which represents the most complete evidence to date, thus definitely introducing bariatric surgery in the treatment algorithm of diabetes in obese subjects, including mild obesity with poor medical control, establishing new guidelines that recommend bariatric surgery as an option, alongside with medical and lifestyle interventions, to treat T2DM. These guidelines were supported by more than 40 international societies representing various clinical and surgical societies worldwide. The guidelines are described on the sequence, and its use should be encouraged as a reference for the use of bariatric surgery as a recommended treatment of T2DM in obese patients. The algorithm for the selection of patients for metabolic surgery suggested in DSS-II is represented in Table 8.2.

Table 8.2 Patients with type 2 diabetes

Nonobese (BMI < 30 kg/m² or 27.5 for Asians)
Nonsurgical treatment
Obese (BMI ≥ 30 kg/m² or ≥ 27.5 kg/m² for Asians)
Class I obese (BMI 30.0–39.4 kg/m² or 27.5–32.4 kg/m² for Asians)
Optimal lifestyle and medical treatment
Adequate glycaemic control – nonsurgical treatment
Poor glycaemic control – consider metabolic surgery
Class II obese (BMI 35.0–39.9 kg/m² or 32.5—37.4 for Asians)
Optimal lifestyle and medical treatment
Adequate glycaemic control – consider metabolic surgery
Poor glycaemic control – recommend metabolic surgery
Class III obese (BMI ≥ 40 kg/m² or ≥ 37.5 for Asians)
Preoperative assessment – recommend metabolic surgery

Algorithm for the treatment of T2DM, as recommended by DSS-II voting delegates (From Rubino et al. [31]) Indications consider that patients are clinically able to tolerate surgery)

In conclusion, the current options for medical treatment of T2DM are insufficient to achieve adequate glycaemic control in most obese diabetic patients, particularly in the long-term follow-up. Metabolic surgery in diabetic patients with a BMI < 35 kg/m² is safe and effective and appears to have similar results as in patients with BMI greater than 35 kg/m², improving diabetes control when compared to lifestyle and medical interventions alone. The indication for metabolic surgery must be made in a tailored approach considering risk-benefit relations and after a complete and thorough preoperative assessment by a committed multidisciplinary team in a certified institution for the surgical treatment of obesity and metabolic syndrome patients. Worldwide, surgical societies for the treatment of obesity and metabolic syndrome strongly encourage the development of randomized clinical trials to answer questions related to cost-effectiveness and long-term follow-up of surgery in diabetic patients with mild obesity and to determine more adequate parameters than BMI alone to achieve more precise selection of the ideal patients for surgery.

References

1. Wild S, Roglic G, Green A, Sicree R, King H. Global prevalence of diabetes: estimates for the year 2000 and projections for 2030. Diabetes Care. 2004;27:1047–53.
2. National Institutes of Health. National Institute of Diabetes and Digestive and Kidney Diseases: National Diabetes Statistics, 2014. http://www.cdc.gov/diabetes/pubs/statsreport14/national-diabetes-report-wcb.pdf
3. Conway B, Miller RG, Costacou T, Fried L, Kelsey S, Evans RW, Orchard TJ. Adiposity and mortality in type 1 diabetes. Int J Obes. 2009;33(7):796–805.
4. Idris I, Thomson GA, Sharma JC. Diabetes mellitus and stroke. Int J Clin Pract. 2006;60(1):48–56.
5. Cugnet-Anceau C, Bauduceau B. Glycaemic control and cardiovascular morbid-mortality: the contribution of the 2008 studies. Ann Endocrinol. 2009;70(1):48–54.
6. Xu Y, Wang L, He J, Bi Y, Li M, Wang T, Wang L, Jiang Y, Dai M, Lu J, Xu M, Li Y, Hu N, Li J, Mi S, Chen CS, Li G, Mu Y, Zhao J, Kong L, Chen J, Lai S, Wang W, Zhao W, Ning G. Prevalence and control of diabetes in Chinese adults. JAMA. 2013;310:948–59.
7. Chan JC, Malik V, Jia W, Kadowaski T, Yajnik CS, Yoon KH, Hu FB. Diabetes in Asia: epidemiology, risk factors and pathophysiology. JAMA. 2009;301:2129–40.
8. Liebl A, Mata M, Eschwege E. Evaluation of risk factors for development of complications in type II diabetes in Europe. Diabetologia. 2002;45:S23–8.
9. Resnick HE, Foster GL, Bardsley J, Ratner RE. Achievement of American Diabetes Association clinical practice recommendations among US adults with diabetes, 1999–2002: the National Health and Nutrition Examination Survey. Diabetes Care. 2006;29:531–7.
10. Koro CE, Bowlin SJ, Bourgeois N, Fedder DO. Glycemic control from 1988 to 2000 among US adults diagnosed with type 2 diabetes: a preliminary report. Diabetes Care. 2004;27:17–20.
11. UK Prospective Diabetes Study Group (UKPDS). Intensive blood-glucose control with sulphonylureas or insulin compared with conventional treatment and risk of complications in patients with type 2 diabetes (UKPDS 33). Lancet. 1998;352:837–53.
12. Buchwald H, Avidor Y, Braunwald E, Jensen MD, Pories W, Fahrbach K, Schoelles K. Bariatric Surgery. A systematic review and meta-analysis. JAMA. 2004;292:1724–37.
13. Buchwald H, Estok R, Fahrbach K, Banel D, Jensen MD, Pories WJ, Bantle JP, Sledge I. Weight and type 2 diabetes after bariatric surgery: systematic review and meta-analysis. Am J Med. 2009;122:248–56.
14. Cummings DE, Cohen RV. Bariatric/Metabolic surgery to treat type 2 diabetes in patients with a BMI < 35kg/m2. Diabetes Care. 2016;39:924–33.
15. Cohen R, Pinheiro JS, Correa JL, Schiavon CA. Laparoscopic Roux-en-Y gastric bypass for BMI < 35m2: a tailored approach. Surg Obes Relat Dis. 2006;2:401–4.
16. De Sá VC, Ferraz AA, Campos JM, Ramos AC, Araujo JG, Ferraz EM. Gastric bypass in the treatment of type 2 diabetes in patients with a BMI of 30–35Kg/m2. Obes Surg. 2011;21:283–7.
17. Shimizu H, Timratana P, Schauer PR. Review of metabolic surgery for type 2 diabetes and body mass index less than 35%. J Obes. 2012;2012:147256.
18. Schauer PR, Kashyap SR, Wolski K, et al. Bariatric surgery vs. intensive medical therapy in obese patients with diabetes. N Engl J Med. 2012;366(17):1567–76.
19. Ikramuddin S, Korner J, Lee W, Connet J. Roux-en-Y gastric bypass vs intensive medical management for the control of type 2 diabetes, hypertension and hyperlipidemia. The Diabetes Surgery Study Randomized clinical trial. JAMA. 2013;309(21):2240–9.
20. Pok EH, Lee WJ. Gastrointestinal metabolic surgery for the treatment of type 2 diabetes mellitus. World J Gastroenterol. 2014;20(39):14315–28.
21. Birkmeyer NJ, Dimick JB, Share D. Hospital complication rates with bariatric surgery in Michigan. JAMA. 2010;304(4):435–42.
22. Nguyen NT, Masoomi H, Magno CP, et al. Trends in use of bariatric surgery, 2003–2008. J Am Coll Surg. 2011;213(2):261–6.
23. Sjöström L, Peltonen M, Jacobson P, et al. Association of bariatric surgery with long-term remission of type 2 diabetes and with microvascular and macrovascular complications. JAMA. 2014;311:2297–304.
24. Mingrone G, Panuzi S, de Gaetano A, et al. Bariatric-metabolic surgery versus conventional medical treatment in obese patients with type 2 diabetes: a 5 year follow-up of an open-label, single-centre, randomised controlled trial. Lancet. 2015;386:964–73.
25. Panuzi S, De Gaetano A, Carnicelli A, Mingrone G. Predictors of remission of diabetes mellitus in severely obese individuals undergoing bariatric surgery: do BMI or procedure choice matter? A meta-analysis. Ann Surg. 2015;261:559–467.
26. Yu H, Di J, Bao Y, Zhang P, Zhang L, Tu Y, Han X, Jia W. Visceral fat area as a new predictor of short-term diabetes remission after Roux-en-Y Gastric bypass surgery in Chinese patients with a body mass

index less than 35Kg/m2. Surg Obes Relat Dis. 2015;11(1):6–11.
27. Dixon JB, Chuang LM, Chong K, Chen SC, Lambert GW, Straznicky NE, Lambert EA, Lee WJ. Predicting the glycemic response to gastric bypass surgery in patients with type 2 diabetes. Diabetes Care. 2013;36:20–6.
28. Rubino F, Kaplan LM, Schauer PR, Cummings DE. The Diabetes Surgery Summit consensus conference: recommendations for the evaluation and use of gastrointestinal surgery to treat type 2 diabetes mellitus. Ann Surg. 2010;251:399–405.
29. Dixon JB, Zimmet P, Alberti KG, Mbanya JC, Rubino F. Bariatric surgery for diabetes: the International Diabetes Federation takes a position. J Diabetes. 2011;3(4):261–4.
30. Campos J, Ramos A, Szego T, Zilberstein B, Feitosa H, Cohen R. The role of metabolic surgery for patients with obesity grade I and type 2 diabetes not controlled clinically. Arq Bras Cir Dig. 2016;29:102–6.
31. Rubino F, Nathan DM, Eckel RH, et al.; 2nd Diabetes Surgery Summit. Metabolic surgery in the treatment algorithm for type 2 diabetes: a joint statement by the international diabetes organizations. Diabetes Care. 2016;39:861–877.

9 Psychiatric Issues During the Postoperative Period of Bariatric Surgery

Adriano Segal and Debora Kinoshita Kussunoki

Introduction

The most effective treatment for severe obesity in terms of weight loss and weight loss maintenance, in terms of positive impacts on many quality of life (QoL) and health markers – including mental health markers – and also in terms of overall mortality decrease is the surgical approach [1]. This is a well-known fact, as described and explained throughout this book. Regardless of that, there are many clinical and psychological concerns associated to the follow-up of bariatric surgeries (BS). These concerns are, in great part, justifiable and seem to result from, at least, two causes:

1. Although not always declared, there is also a generalized fear that there are some psychological and/or psychiatric complications resulting from the procedure, regardless of the care offered. It is our opinion that this fear is much more a consequence of prejudice against obesity – associated or not to psychosomatic unproven theories in relation to its etiology – than just scientifically based caution. This particular point is further discussed in our chapter on depression, suicide and drug abuse disorders.
2. BS obviously are not a panacea for obesity. They are not even "the easiest way" or "the last chance," as many patients, family members, and, unfortunately, some health professionals wish for despise and/or fear in a sometimes concurringly, confusingly, or counterproductively manner. Patients and health team must be aware that being submitted to this type of procedure equals taking on a lifelong commitment of collaboration (in the true sense of the word, i.e., a joint work) with the multiprofessional team, especially during the postoperative period (PO), and start acting accordingly. This attitude is probably the main way for achieving procedure success in the long run, not only in terms of weight and comorbidity reduction but also in terms of preventing adverse events and complications, which may sometimes become irreversible [2].

The prevalence of some psychiatric disorders (PD) in the BS candidates is higher than in the overall population [3]. However, at the same time, psychiatric improvement is expected in a large part of these patients [4], probably as a result of the removal of an important stressing factor, that is, severe obesity. This disease exerts stress not only through

A. Segal (✉) · D. K. Kussunoki
Obesity and Diabetes Center, German Hospital Oswaldo Cruz, São Paulo, Brazil

Obesity and Metabolic Syndrome Outpatient Clinic, Service of Endocrinology and Metabolism-HCFMUSP/SP, São Paulo, Brazil

Brazilian Society of Bariatric and Metabolic Surgery, São Paulo, Brazil

Brazilian Association for the Study of Obesity and Metabolic Syndrome, São Paulo, Brazil

Segal Clinic, São Paulo, Brazil

J. Ettinger et al. (eds.), *Gastric Bypass*, https://doi.org/10.1007/978-3-030-28803-7_9

the huge psychological burden that being obese represents – a lot was already said about the stigma of obesity in modern society – but also through somatic pathways such as biochemical, hormonal, inflammatory, clinical, and multidrug regimen side effects, among others. In this chapter, we will address part of these aspects.

Psychiatric Disorders Identified During the PO

For a significant part of the BS patients, PO will represent at least half of their lives, usually more. Therefore, it is reasonable to expect a higher chance of PD onset during the PO than on the preoperative period, without a true cause/effect relation. This can be simply an effect of the longer period of time patient is expected to live after the surgery, a point it is worth to be studied.

In fact, there is no cause/effect relation in great part of the cases, despite some contrary assumptions [4]. The cause/effect relation, which some attribute to BS or to weight loss, is far from consensual in the scientific community.

These new PDs may in fact *appear* in the PO (the patient never presented PD before surgery) or simply may *be diagnosed* in the PO (patient had a PD or history of PD, which remained unknown to the team for some reason). These PDs may or may not be related to bariatric surgery or weight loss.

Some candidate causes of PD onset during the PO are:

- *Age group*: the age group of great part of BS candidates is usually close to the age of the first psychiatric state. With the increasing number of adolescents submitted to these procedures, this will probably become a main reason [5].
- *Gender*: The majority of the BS candidates are female, and there is a higher prevalence of PD in females, notably mood, anxiety, and eating disorders [6, 7].
- *Eating disorders* (*not present during preoperative*) that may be caused by any of the PO changes. For instance, in 2004, we described a state characterized by important changes in the relationship with food combined with an intense and irrational fear of weight regain. Unlike in anorexia nervosa (AN), high-calorie foods – usually tastier and easier to swallow – are often chosen. Additionally, the core criteria for AN and bulimia nervosa (BN) are absent in the Postsurgical Eating Avoidance Disorder (PSEAD) [4].
- *Behavioral changes* resulting from specific malnutrition [8].
- *Pharmacokinetic changes of alcohol* in some techniques (especially in those techniques with the Roux Y), favoring a more effective alcohol absorption and faster damage to target organs (liver, pancreas, heart, and brain) [9, 10].
- *High levels of association* between eating disorders and substance abuse [11].
- *Reward deficiency syndrome* (RDS) [12].

We have chosen not to include the last three items under the concept of "compulsion change." Due to the fact there is no sufficient scientific evidence to support this concept, using it would only help to perpetuate prejudice in an area which it is already abundant enough.

On the other hand, some aspects can "produce" PDs in the PO. Actually those PDs already existed in the preoperative period. Those are [12, 13]:

- *Insufficient psychiatric anamnesis*: as many teams do not include a psychiatrist, psychiatric issues tend to be investigated by nonspecialist professionals. The inclusion of psychiatrists is recommended due to the higher than normal prevalence of PDs in that population. Their presence in the team tends to mitigate this kind of error.
- *Mood disorders* that can be mistaken as "expected" depressive reactions in the presence of morbid obesity or in the presence of food restriction secondary to most bariatric procedures.
- *Bipolar spectrum states* may take years to be diagnosed as such; thereby they can be mistreated as unipolar depression or general anxiety disorder, in the case of mixed states.

- *Intentional misinformation by the patient and/or family member* due to shame or with the aim of not being contraindicated for surgery. It is worth noting that this item can be a somehow iatrogenic consequence of health professionals' prejudice, of inadequate formation, or of denials of surgery approval in the presence of all PDs. Some teams still use the expression "postpone surgery" as an euphemism to contraindication, despite the fact that there are only few and well-defined cases in which this posture is justifiable. The cases in which surgeries are "postponed" are much more abundant than those cases mentioned.

Interference of PDs in the Outcome of BSs

Regardless the PD being pre-existing or appearing after the BS, it can interfere with the patient compliance to clinical and nutritional follow-up and, possibly, interfere in the global outcome. Therefore, each pathology must be detected and treated as early as possible in order to avoid negative impacts on weight loss, on the nutritional status and on the patient's QoL and global health [12].

It is important to emphasize that there is no need for normalization/complete remission of the majority of PDs before BS, at least from the evidence-based medicine point of view [12]. Exceptions of that stance are the states in which the patient cannot fully understand the surgical and nonsurgical procedures that will take place, their needs, limits, and consequences. In those conditions, the patient is temporarily or permanently incapable of reasoning and deciding, leading to the necessity of full treatment before the surgical decision is taken. Also, in the states in which there is a substance abuse disorder present (see specific chapter), the surgery should be postponed. The first group is comprised of active psychotic states at the time of preoperative procedures, acute mania, acute and severe depressions, and states with innate or acquired cognitive impairment, reversible or not. In the case of reversible states, when reverted, they do not constitute contraindication [4, 12–14].

Furthermore, for some authors [14], slow preoperative evaluations/preparations can be not only a type of prejudice, in face of the current means of scientific evidences, but also useless.

In the table below [6, 12], some PDs and their relations with BS PO are shown:

Disorder (DSM V)	Related symptoms	Others
Major depressive disorder	Changes in mobility and/or motor autonomy; increased appetite; weight gain and sleepiness (depressive episodes with atypical characteristics); gloominess; and pessimistic thoughts. Somatic symptoms bring patient back to the office with uncommon BS complaints Risk and/or suicidal behavior include not following nutritional scheme directions	Depressive episodes with atypical characteristics are more frequent in BD 1 and BD 2 and major depressive disorder recurring with a seasonal pattern. Mania episodes that present after BS may be preceded by atypical preoperative depression
Bipolar disorders (BD)	*Mania*: lack of impulse control (including eating in some cases). Poor compliance to treatment regimens. There is association of BD with absenteeism, school failure, divorces, and in more severe cases, violent behavior Marked irritability and mood instability Increased suicide risk in mixed states *Hypomania*: less severe presentations *Weight gain* with mood stabilizers and atypical antipsychotics must be observed BS may help in compliance to the posology scheme in specific cases Some obesity treatments may induce mania or hypomania episodes in these patients	Uncontrolled shopping, excessive spending, alcohol abuse, as well as other substances, unusual sexual behavior (for the patient), excessive involvement in highly enjoyable activities with a potential for harmful consequences Higher rates of diabetes mellitus type 2, even before psychopharmacological treatment

Disorder (DSM V)	Related symptoms	Others
Schizophrenia	*Patients with negative symptoms* show decrease in physical and social activities *Positive symptoms* must be treated prior to BS and patients must be followed up Change in mobility and/or autonomy Variable weight gain with different kinds of antipsychotics. In some cases, BS may help in compliance to the posology scheme	More visceral obesity and metabolic syndrome even before starting treatment with antipsychotics.
Anxiety disorders	*Choking phobia:* patient avoids solid foods or food that could get "stuck" *Agoraphobia*: possibly associated to greater use of delivery fast food and/or visiting 24-hour store at night	Higher cortisol levels
Obsessive compulsive disorder	Rituals and compulsions that make compliance to nutritional schemes or to clinical follow-up more difficult Prader-Willi syndrome: impulsive and compulsive behaviors, hyperphagia	Eating with symmetry rituals may lead to overeating
Substance use disorders	Non-compliance to clinical and nutritional follow-up Risky behaviors May be at an increased risk of becoming addicted to alcohol as result of changes in alcohol absorption and metabolism Malnutrition (*crack/cocaine*) or sometimes insufficient weight loss (*Cannabis*), case reports only	Search for psychiatric comorbidities. Treating an underlying PD makes it easier to treat the addiction
BN	Weight maintenance achieved through inappropriate compensatory behaviors (self-induced vomiting, laxatives and diuretics abuse, prolonged fasting, excessive exercise) Differentiate between bulimic symptoms and involuntary vomiting immediately after PO. Some of these may later evolve to provoked vomiting, be it to lose weight or as a response to gastric discomfort	The presence of inappropriate compensatory practices must be investigated, not only in preoperative period but especially in the PO
Binge eating disorder and night eating syndrome	Difficulty to keep with the proposed nutritional schemes and less weight loss	High comorbidity rate with mood and anxiety disorders
PSEAD (not in DSM V)	Higher and/or faster weight loss than expected and tests are not compatible with technique used Resistance to any type of dietary or medical approach Intense and irrational fear of going back to weight before BS	Differential diagnosis between AN and PSEAD must be done. In DSM V, PSEAD could be classified as Atypical AN

Interference of BSs on Present PDs

Possible Psychiatric Presentations Resulting from Nutritional Deficiencies [12]

Pellagra

Caused by deficiency of niacin and/or tryptophan, pellagra is usually associated to alcohol abuse, unbalanced vegetarian diets, and extreme malnutrition. It is classically described as the *Five Ds*: dermatitis, diarrhea, delirium, dementia, and death. Replacement promotes a fast recovery; however if the deficiency is maintained, recovery tends to be slower or permanent damage may arise.

Beriberi

Vitamin B1 (thiamine) deficiency is characterized by cardiovascular and neurological alterations and associated to Wernicke-Korsakoff syndrome. Symptoms include apathy, depression, irritability, nervousness, and concentration deficit. Long-lasting cases could cause severe and irreversible memory loss.

Wernicke-Korsakoff Syndrome (WKS)

WKS is a severe neuropsychiatric syndrome due to B1 deficiency commonly caused by alcohol abuse and/or poor nutrition.

Wernicke's encephalopathy symptoms are confusion, loss of motor coordination, tremors, ataxia, visual alterations, nystagmus, and palpebral ptosis.

Korsakoff's syndrome includes anterograde and retrograde amnesia, inventing stories (confabulation), and hallucinations.

Vitamin B12 Deficiency

Vitamin B12 – which needs the intrinsic factor produced by the gastric mucosa to be absorbed – deficiency is characterized by megaloblastic anemia, neurological manifestations resulting from nervous degenerations, and mental alterations.

Apathy, depression, and irritability are common. In some cases, acute confusional state (*delirium*), illusions, hallucinations, and dementia are observed.

Symptoms reversion is usually fast after early and continuous administration of vitamin B12.

Psychiatric Alterations as Result of Weight Loss [12, 13]

The idea that diets cause a negative psychological impact is widely disseminated among lay people and also among some health professionals. That is possibly a result of – or was reinforced by – the first trials carried out on this topic, from 1950 to 1970. These studies were not randomized controlled trials, and their results were mainly based on non-standardized clinical evaluations. Controlled trials, with standardized tools carried out as from 1969, have shown opposite results, with patients presenting improvement in mental health parameters. There is a consensus about the psychological and QoL improvement in successfully treated obese patients, proportional to the amount of weight loss and regardless of the method.

Eating disorders will be further discussed in a specific chapter.

Psychiatric Alterations as Result of the Surgical Procedures [12]

Here, we will mention the changes in the many different moments of PO. It is worth noting that part of them are common to any type of surgery similar to BS in terms of physiological impact and preparation, and the other part is associated to nutritional deficiencies.

Immediate PO (1st Day)

Delirium (acute confusional state)

- Postanesthesia
- Anesthetics and previously suspended long half-life drug interactions
- Others (embolism or strokes in the CNS, unbalanced electrolytes, other metabolic/physiological acute disturbances)
- Substance use or abstinence (licit or illicit)

Mediate (1st Month) and Late PO (from 2nd Month)

- Substance use or abstinence (licit or illicit)
- Reemerging psychiatric syndromes known in preoperative
- Reemerging of psychiatric syndromes unknown before the surgery (see above)
- States caused by dietary deficiencies (see above and other chapters of book)
- Use of licit or illicit substances leading to psychiatric states (via intoxication or triggering)
- Attempted suicide [15]

At Any Time in Any Surgery (Not Only BS)

Many psychiatric conditions may be present in the PO of any type of surgery, without a cause-effect relationship. These can include factitious disorder, Münchhausen syndrome, and simulation.

Factitious disorder is characterized by intentionally produced or simulated physical or psychological symptoms or syndromes with the purpose of playing the role of a sick person in the absence of external incentives or immediate gain. In general, an individual is not aware of the motivation. Münchhausen syndrome is the most chronic and severe variant of its presentation and seems to be most frequent in men.

Simulation presents with a clear direct gain such as indemnifications, running from the police, and finding a place to stay at night.

Somatization

This is a polysymptomatic state with onset before 30 years of age, which takes place for many years and is characterized by a combination of pain, gastrointestinal, sexual, and neurological symptoms. The symptoms are not intentionally produced.

Epilepsy with Psychiatric, Psychological, and/or Behavioral Symptoms

Epileptic fits present signs and symptoms that reflect the affected area of the brain. It can present motor, sensitive, sensory-perceptive, autonomic, and even psychological manifestations [12]. Epileptic fits in the temporal lobe often present automatism, including crying, laughing, shouting, walking, running, and kissing. The more common secondary reactions and feelings during these fits are fear, anxiety, depression, depersonalization, pleasure, and displeasure. Aura, when present, may involve feelings of fear or anxiety, changes in gastric motility, or a feeling of smelling strange things.

Psychopharmacological Treatment in the PO

Obviously there are few differences in treatments of PDs in the PO compared to other situations where they are used. The same psychotherapeutic, biological, psychopharmacological, and social approaches must be instituted.

However, some items must be observed, and only the last one is unique to BS:

1. Choosing the drug which is less associated to weight gain/metabolic alterations whenever possible
2. Be aware of drug and food interactions of psychoactive drugs
3. Be aware of pharmacokinetic and pharmacodynamic changes that could change the serum levels of the prescribed medication (s) [16–18]

Conclusion

There is a high association of PDs and obesity, notably in BS candidates.

This fact makes psychiatrist's presence on the multidisciplinary team strictly required. Psychologists with proper training may be able to diagnose some PDs (by means of clinical open, semistructured or structured interviews) but have no technical capacitation for thoroughly treating the majority of PDs.

On the other hand, BSs seem to have a positive effect on most pre-existing PDs, even though it shows no effect or even some negative effect on a minority of cases.

There are no evidences that suggest weight loss causes worsening of pre-existing states, provided the adequate psychiatric care is properly implemented.

Likewise, PDs with onset in the PO can be the result of many factors, alone or combined, and also may be more common in one surgical technique than in another (i.e., malnutrition, alcohol pharmacokinetics alterations). While a meaningful part of them can be addressed through prevention or specific treatment, only a minority is directly caused by BSs. In all cases, a comprehensive evaluation is granted.

One point worth being discussed is the apparently higher risk of suicide in BS PO, as mentioned above. For example, in a study cited above [15], there were higher suicide rates among surgical patients when compared to the overall population and paired according to gender and age. The study did not match for BMI nor the presence of previous psychiatric disorder and/or dietary disorders. The authors of that important study state that "suicides are not necessarily attributed to the bariatric surgery, but may be related to myriad factors." We agree that, although this outcome should be kept in mind as there is a substantial number of studies addressing this point, it should not be viewed as a well-proven cause-effect relationship.

Despite an enormous amount of literature, definite knowledge available is still insufficient, especially when the broadening of indications for BSs and the metabolic surgeries are considered. Specific, prospective, and adequately designed trials are still necessary. With the available data, BS are safe among psychiatric patients when proper care is taken.

Acknowledgment The authors would like to thank Rodrigo Rezende for his English revision.

References

1. Yumuk V, Tsigos C, Fried M, Schindler K, Busetto L, Micic D, et al. European guidelines for obesity management in adults. Obes Facts. 2015;8(6):402–24.
2. Segal A, Kussunoki D. Psychiatric disorders and postoperative follow-up. In: Rios B. Integrated health in bariatric surgery. 2015. ebook available at http://www.bariatric.today/
3. Duarte-Guerra L, Coêlho B, Santo M, Wang Y. Psychiatric disorders among obese patients seeking bariatric surgery: results of structured clinical interviews. Obes Surg. 2014;25(5):830–7.
4. Segal A, Kinoshita Kussunoki D, Aparecida Larino M. Post-surgical refusal to eat: anorexia nervosa, bulimia nervosa or a new eating disorder? A case series. Obes Surg. 2004;14(3):353–60.
5. Olbers T, Gronowitz E, Werling M, Mårlid S, Flodmark C, Peltonen M, et al. Two-year outcome of laparoscopic Roux-en-Y gastric bypass in adolescents with severe obesity: results from a Swedish Nationwide Study (AMOS). Int J Obes. 2012;36(11):1388–95.
6. American Psychiatric Association. Diagnostic and statistical manual of mental disorders. 5th ed. Arlington: American Psychiatric Association; 2013.
7. Buchwald H, Avidor Y, Braunwald E. Bariatric surgery. A systematic review and meta-analysis. ACC Curr J Rev. 2005;14(1):13.
8. Fujioka K. Follow-up of nutritional and metabolic problems after bariatric surgery. Diabetes Care. 2005;28(2):481–4.
9. Hagedorn J, Encarnacion B, Brat G, Morton J. Does gastric bypass alter alcohol metabolism? Surg Obes Relat Dis. 2007;3(5):543–8.
10. King W, Chen J, Mitchell J, Kalarchian M, Steffen K, Engel S, et al. Prevalence of alcohol use disorders before and after bariatric surgery. JAMA. 2012;307(23):2516.
11. Ross HIvis F. Binge eating and substance use among male and female adolescents. Int J Eat Disord. 1999;26(3):245–60.
12. Segal A, Kussunoki DK. Transtornos Psiquiátricos no Pós-Operatório. In: Pereira A, Freire CC, Godoy EP, Viegas F, Marchesini JCD, Zanela MT (Eds): Cirurgia Bariátrica e Metabólica - Abordagem Multiprofissional. Editora Rubio. Rio De Janeiro RJ, 2019. p 371–79.
13. Segal A. Obesidade e comorbidade psiquiátrica: caracterização e eficácia terapêutica de atendimento multidisciplinar na evolução de 34 pacientes. São Paulo, 1999. Thesis (Doutorate) – Faculdade de Medicina da Universidade de São Paulo.
14. Ashton D, Favretti F, Segato G. Preoperative psychological testing – another form of prejudice. Obes Surg. 2008;18(10):1330–7.
15. Tindle H, Omalu B, Courcoulas A, Marcus M, Hammers J, Kuller L. Risk of suicide after long-term follow-up from bariatric surgery. Am J Med. 2010;123(11):1036–42.
16. Hamad G, Helsel J, Perel J, Kozak G, McShea M, Hughes C, et al. The effect of gastric bypass on the pharmacokinetics of serotonin reuptake inhibitors. Am J Psychiatr. 2012;169(3):256–63.
17. Semion K, Dorsey J, Bourgeois J. Intravenous valproate use in bipolar II disorder after gastric bypass surgery. J Neuropsychiatry Clin Neurosci. 2005;17(3):427–a-429.
18. Padwal R, Brocks D, Sharma A. A systematic review of drug absorption following bariatric surgery and its theoretical implications. Obes Rev. 2010;11(1):41–50.

Sleep-Disordered Breathing and Bariatric Surgery

10

Michael V. J. Braganza and Stephen K. Field

Introduction

Obesity has become increasingly prevalent globally. According to WHO research, the number of obese individuals has *doubled* since 1980. It has been estimated that roughly 1/3 of North Americans are categorized as obese, defined as having a BMI > 30 [1]. Worldwide, it is estimated that roughly 10% of the population meets this definition [2, 3]. Obesity is a chronic disease with systemic consequences. The respiratory system is no exception.

There are variety of mechanisms by which obesity can impact respiratory function. Furthermore, there is emerging evidence that the prognosis and natural history of some disease processes, including asthma, COPD, and several kinds of cancer, are influenced by obesity [2]. It increases the risk for pulmonary embolism as well as for aspiration pneumonia. Obesity, in the absence of other conditions, can cause respiratory complications in the perioperative setting. Bag-mask ventilation, endotracheal intubation, and operative oxygenation can all be compromised by excess adiposity. The focus of this chapter will be on sleep-related complications in bariatric surgery. The reader should be aware that excess adipose tissue can have a variety of adverse effects beyond its deleterious effects on sleep.

M. V. J. Braganza · S. K. Field (✉)
Division of Respirology, Department of Medicine, Cumming School of Medicine, University of Calgary, Calgary, AB, Canada
e-mail: sfield@ucalgary.ca

Pulmonary Complications of Obesity

Several mechanical and physiologic alterations are present in the obese. Excess weight increases oxygen consumption and carbon dioxide production and mechanically disadvantages the respiratory system [4]. These changes can be slowly progressive and not perceived by the patient. Symptoms, when present, typically occur with exertion. In extreme cases, obesity heightens ventilatory demand, increases the work of breathing, mechanically disadvantages the respiratory muscles, and decreases the compliance (stiffens) the respiratory system [2].

Subdivisions of Lung Volumes and Pulmonary Function Tests

A grasp of pulmonary function testing, including spirometry, plethysmography, the determination of lung volumes, and the measurement of diffusion capacity, is essential to understanding the effects of obesity on respiration. Figure 10.1 demonstrates the subdivision of lung volumes. The abbreviations used for the various lung volumes and spirometric parameters are shown in Table 10.1.

J. Ettinger et al. (eds.), *Gastric Bypass*, https://doi.org/10.1007/978-3-030-28803-7_10

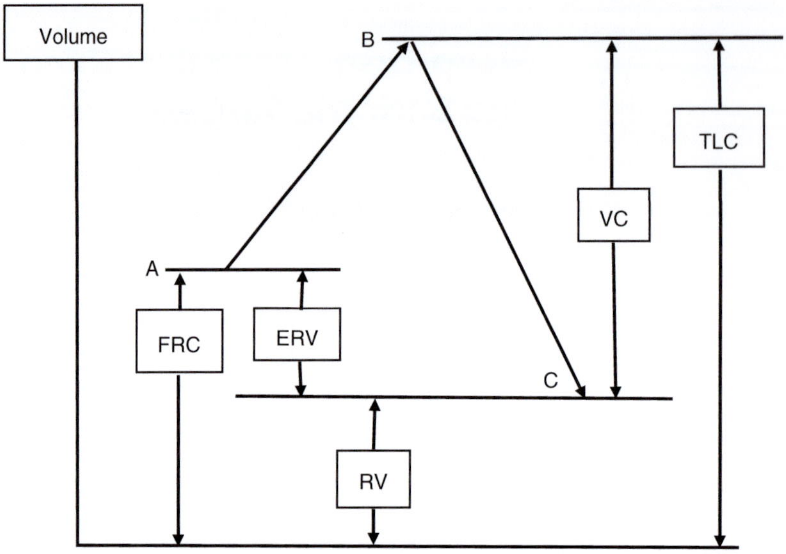

Fig. 10.1 Subdivision of lung volumes

Table 10.1 Common spirometric and subdivision of lung volume terms

FEV_1	Forced expiratory volume in 1 second
FVC	Forced vital capacity
FEV_1/FVC	Ratio of FEV_1 and FVC
TV	Tidal volume
FRC	Functional residual capacity
RV	Residual volume
ERV	Expiratory reserve volume
VC	Vital capacity
TLC	Total lung capacity

Functional residual capacity (FRC) (A) is the lung volume at the end of a passive expiration and is the point where the tendency of the lung to collapse is balanced by the equal and opposite recoil of the chest wall. If one makes a maximal inspiratory effort, the inspiratory limit is the total lung capacity (TLC) (B) or maximum lung volume. If one then makes a maximal expiratory effort, the expired volume is the vital capacity (VC), and the remaining air in the lungs is the residual volume (RV) (C). The volume difference between the FRC and the RV is called the expiratory reserve volume (ERV).

Obese patients will commonly have preserved total lung capacity [2, 4–6]. However, there are some changes that are considered typical for the obese patient. In obese patients, the increased weight compresses the chest wall reducing the lung volume where the recoil of the chest wall is balanced by the tendency of the lung to collapse reducing both FRC and ERV but RV remains relatively preserved. ERV decreases exponentially with increasing BMI (Fig. 10.2) [5, 7, 8]. The ERV may be reduced over 40% in those with a BMI of 30 kg/m^2–55 kg/m^2. In patients with a BMI $\geq$ 60 kg/m^2, the ERV can be reduced by 80%. Figure 10.3 demonstrates the effects of severe obesity on lung volumes.

Total lung capacity (TLC) is only minimally decreased, even in cases of morbid obesity [9–11] (Fig. 10.3). Any reductions in TLC are likely on the basis of increasing diaphragmatic impedance and intercostal adiposity. The chest wall, despite the increased load, is only minimally affected. Tidal volumes are generally (but not universally) reduced. The morbidly obese (BMI > 40 kg/m^2) may have an increased respiratory rate, as well as an increased minute ventilation [12].

Spirometry is the most frequently used test for assessing pulmonary function and measures vital capacity and expiratory flow rates (Fig. 10.4). The most commonly used flow rate is the FEV_1. Reductions in FEV_1 with relative preservation of FVC are seen in obstructive lung diseases including asthma and COPD. In restrictive diseases such as interstitial lung disease and chest wall disorders including morbid obesity, both FEV_1 and FVC are reduced in a similar proportion. There is an inverse relationship between weight and FEV_1 and FVC. These changes are particularly apparent

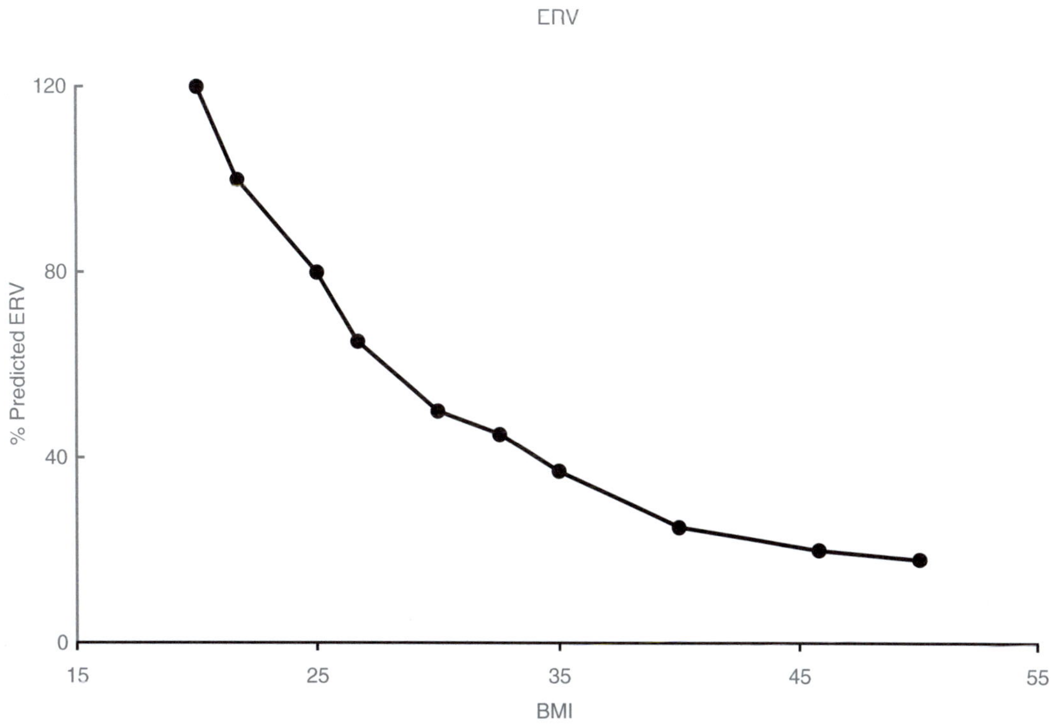

Fig. 10.2 Predicted ERV decreases exponentially with increasing BMI

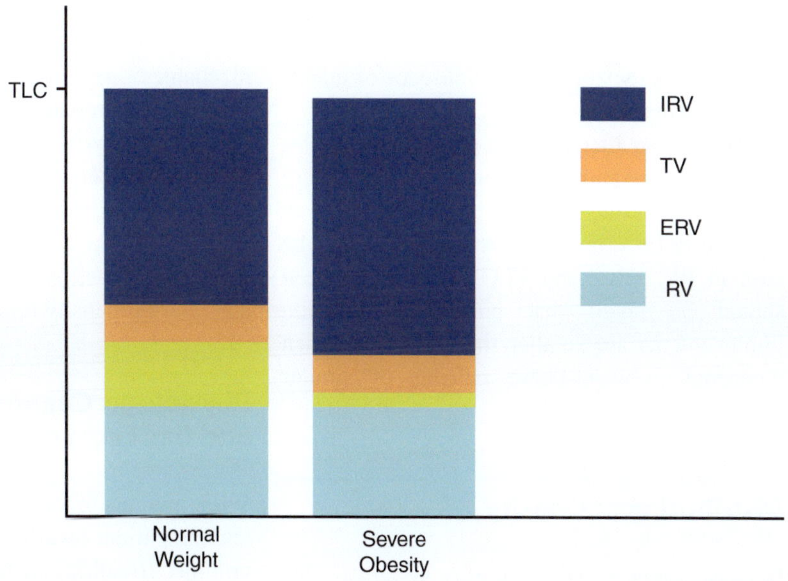

Fig. 10.3 The effect of severe obesity on lung volumes. The reduction in FRC is due to a decrease in ERV. The TLC is minimally affected

once the BMI exceeds 40 kg/m^2 [13]. A cross-sectional study of 1674 adults demonstrated that a 1 cm increase in waist circumference resulted in 13 ml/second and 11 ml average reductions in FEV_1 and FVC, respectively [6].

Diffusion capacity is a measure of the gas exchange ability of the lungs and is reduced in diseases of lung parenchyma such as emphysema and interstitial lung diseases. It is generally pre-

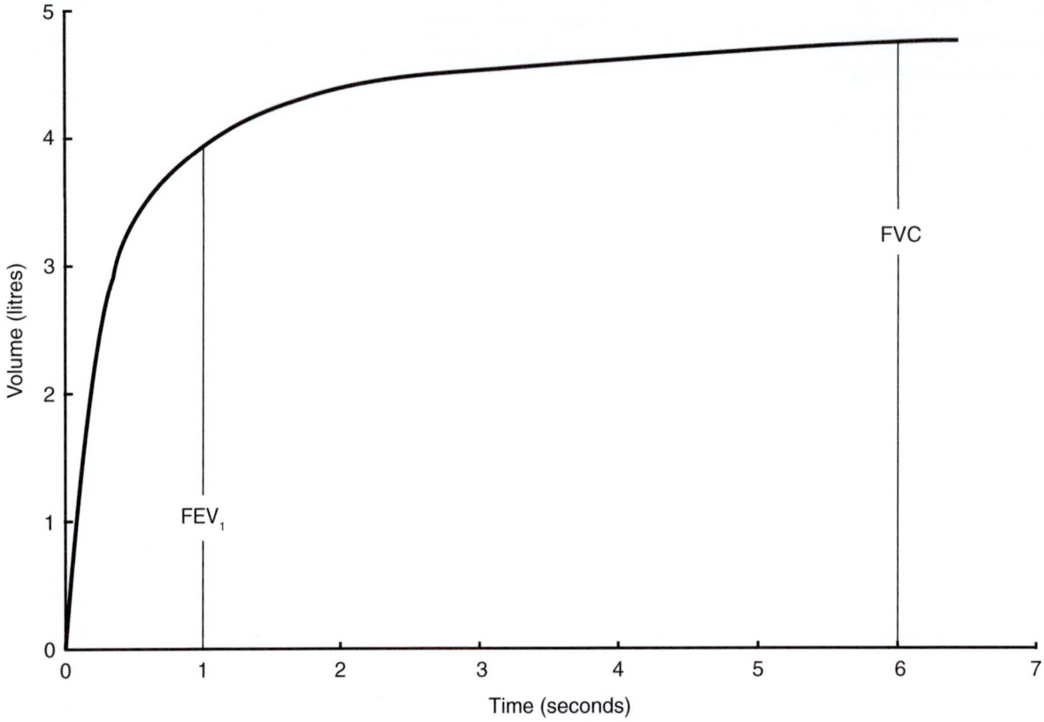

Fig. 10.4 The expiratory spirogram. The FEV1 is the volume of air forcefully expired in 1 second. The FVC is the total volume of air that can forcefully be expired. Though decreases in both are is seen in obesity, changes are most apparent when BMI exceeds 40 kg/m^2

served in obese patients in the absence of underlying lung disease.

Weight loss after bariatric surgery is the most effective intervention to improve pulmonary function. It is associated primarily with an increase in ERV, but improvements may also be seen in RV, FRC, and TLC [14]. However, it should be noted that pulmonary function improvements are smaller than expected when compared to never-obese patients of similar height and ethnicity [13].

Distribution of Obesity

In obese patients, the respiratory system is also affected by adipose tissue distribution. Fat distributed around the lower thorax and upper abdomen, both in subcutaneous tissue and around the viscera, impedes chest wall motion. This is referred to as central obesity. Peripheral obesity, where fat distribution is concentrated on the hips and extremities, has less of an effect on chest wall mechanics. An increased waist-to-hip ratio (WHR), a surrogate for central obesity, predicts this respiratory impairment better than BMI [2, 6]. Other markers of central obesity include waist circumference, abdominal height, and subscapular skinfold thickness [4]. Weight gain affects respiratory function more in men since they have a greater propensity for central obesity.

Physiologic Changes and Gas Exchange in Obesity

With increasing obesity, the ERV is reduced, and the patient breathes at a lower absolute lung volume. Breathing at lower lung volumes may cause airway closure. In turn, atelectasis may develop in the dependent lung zones. Total respiratory compliance may be reduced both by chest wall restriction and atelectasis [7]. The relative contributions of each are variable and likely patient specific [15–19]. These processes are exacerbated by abdominal pressure on the diaphragm in the supine position, a concern during abdominal surgery. In extreme obesity, tidal volumes (TV) are reduced with a compensatory increase in the respiratory rate that is particularly evident during exercise [4, 20].

Even in the absence of lung disease, gas exchange may be compromised in the morbidly obese. Airway closure and atelectasis will reduce ventilation to the dependent lung zones where perfusion is greatest. The resulting ventilation/perfusion mismatch may cause hypoxemia.

Effect of Obesity on Sleep

One of the major consequences of obesity on the respiratory system, sleep-disordered breathing (SDB), is often unnoticed and undiagnosed [21, 22]. SDB encompasses a variety of conditions, including upper airways resistance syndrome (UARS), obstructive sleep apnea (OSA), central sleep apnea (CSA), Cheyne-Stokes respiration, and obesity hypoventilation syndrome (OHS). These conditions are associated with a variety of adverse clinical outcomes, including poor neurocognitive performance, psychiatric disturbances, increased risk of motor vehicle accidents, and cardiovascular morbidities and hypertension, stroke, and coronary artery disease. SDB also represents a significant risk factor for perioperative complications, including cardiorespiratory failure and prolonged intubation. These conditions are associated with significant socioeconomic burden. Among these conditions, OSA is the most clinically relevant to the bariatric surgeon. The other disorders of breathing are briefly reviewed below.

Central Sleep Apnea and Cheyne-Stokes Respiration

CSA is characterized by the cessation of airflow and of ventilatory effort. The condition can be idiopathic or secondary to another process (i.e., Cheyne-Stokes respiration).

Cheyne-Stokes respiration is a cyclical breathing pattern characterized by apnea followed by rapid frequency crescendo-decrescendo tidal volumes terminating with another apnea. Cheyne-Stokes respiration is commonly associated with congestive heart failure, neurologic disease, and sedative medications. It is unrelated to obesity.

Obesity Hypoventilation Syndrome

OHS is a severe form of sleep-disordered breathing. It is defined by the presence of chronic daytime hypercarbia ($PaC0_2 > 45$ mmHg) not caused by other conditions such as severe lung disease, neurological disease, or sedative or narcotic medication, in patients with obesity (BMI > 30 kg/m^2). It is often referred to as obesity-related respiratory insufficiency in the literature. It often occurs in association with OSA; 80% of those with OHS have OSA. It is estimated that 10–20% of those with OSA have OHS, with higher prevalence among the morbidly obese [23]. The pathogenesis is incompletely understood. Several different proposed mechanisms, including mechanical impedance due to excessive adipose tissue, an impaired central response to hypercarbia and hypoxemia, as well as neurohormonal disturbances, are thought to play a role [23]. It has a similar clinical presentation to OSA but is often more severe. It is associated with cognitive deficits, pulmonary hypertension and consequent right heart failure, and endothelial dysfunction with resultant adverse cardiovascular effects. It is also a significant risk factor for perioperative complications. Bariatric surgery may be effective treating this condition [24]. A small study of 31 patients who underwent bariatric surgery demonstrated significant improvements in $Pa0_2$ and $PaC0_2$ 1 year after surgery. However, in 12 of these patients, both $Pa0_2$ and $PaC0_2$ had worsened 5 years later in the absence of weight gain [25]. This indicates that SDB, including OSA, can recur despite successful surgery. Patients with OHS have an increased risk of perioperative death due to higher rates of postoperative respiratory failure and venous thromboembolism [26]. All patients with OHS should undergo polysomnography prior to surgery. OHS should be optimized medically prior to surgery with continuous positive airway pressure (CPAP).

Obstructive Sleep Apnea

OSA is characterized by cyclical cessation or reduction of airflow due to upper airway obstruction that occurs during sleep [9]. Obesity is its major risk factor. For every 10 kg increase in body weight, the risk of OSA increases twofold. An increase in BMI of 6 kg/m^2, or an increase in abdominal/hip girth of 13–15 cm, is associated with a fourfold increase in the risk OSA [27]. Other risk factors include craniofacial abnormalities, acromegaly, hypothyroidism, and increased neck circumference [28]. When defined by an apnea-hypopnea index (AHI) of ≥5, its prevalence ranges from 15 to 30% in males and 5 to 15% in females in the North American population [27]. The vast majority of patients are both undiagnosed and untreated [29].

Pathophysiology

It is a common misconception that the pathogenesis of OSA is simply due to fat and soft tissue directly obstructing the airway. There are multiple mechanisms postulated to contribute to upper airway obstruction. Anatomical factors, including enlarged soft tissue structures such as the tongue, tonsils, soft palate, and uvula surrounding the airway, can reduce airway patency. In the recumbent position, diaphragm excursion is reduced in the obese resulting in decreased intrathoracic pressure and lung volumes. This reduces the "tug" on the trachea applied indirectly through traction from the mediastinal structures [9]. Thickening the walls of the lateral pharyngeal walls and narrowing the airway also play a role [9]. Airway edema due to cephalad displacement of fluid from the lower extremities occurs in patients with OSA while recumbent. Neurohormonal influences on the thalamus and peripheral inflammation may also contribute [9].

Even in extreme obesity, the airway itself is rarely compromised during wakefulness. This phenomenon, known as the "wakeful stimuli," highlights a key aspect of OSA's pathogenesis [9]. In the obese, nocturnal pharyngeal collapsibility directly contributes to OSA pathogenesis. More than 20 skeletal muscles, known as pharyngeal dilation muscles, ensure airway patency in humans. When an individual falls asleep, the activity of these pharyngeal dilator muscles declines, as has been demonstrated by electromyography (EMG). The decreased activity is proportionally greater in the pharyngeal muscles than the reductions in other respiratory muscles, including the diaphragm [30]. As sleep deepens, pharyngeal muscle activity progressively lessens, making the upper airway more compliant and vulnerable to collapse. When inspiration reduces intraluminal airway pressure below the tissue pressure (applied by pharyngeal muscles, submucosal fat, and edema), the compliant pharyngeal tube will obstruct. This effect is exaggerated when the patient enters rapid eye movement (REM) sleep, a state where the accessory respiratory and pharyngeal muscles are effectively paralyzed [9].

An apneic event occurs when the upper airway obstructs, resulting in hypoventilation. The resultant hypercarbia and hypoxemia cause an arousal, associated with an adrenergic surge that restores upper airway patency by lessening (or fragmenting) sleep with an associated increase in pharyngeal muscle tone. Catecholamines and other hormones are released. The cycle occurs repetitively with subsequent sleep fragmentation that is associated with daytime symptoms including (but are not limited to) excessive daytime sleepiness, unrefreshing sleep, and snoring [29, 31, 32]. Neurocognitive complaints, including memory impairment, decreased occupational performance, depression, anxiety, and decreased sexual drive, are commonly described [29]. The large negative intrapleural pressures generated during episodes of airway obstruction may result in gastroesophageal reflux [32]. Biochemical disturbances can become apparent. Hypoventilation and consequent hypercarbia may cause respiratory acidosis. The kidneys respond to the respiratory acidosis by increasing retention of bicarbonate ($HC0_3$). The result is a chronic metabolic alkalosis. Chronic hypoxemia stimulates renal production of erythropoietin, increasing bone marrow production of erythrocytes to increase oxygen-carrying capacity. This may manifest as (secondary) polycythemia, which may be associated with increased risk of venous thromboembolism [33]. Severe OSA is associated with insulin resistance and impaired glucose tolerance, conditions that are harbingers for diabetes. Additional hormonal effects include elevated serum leptin, which is associated with weight and satiety regulation, as well as respiratory control [9, 34]. OSA is associated with an increased risk of workplace accidents and motor vehicle collisions [35, 36]. Special attention should be paid to patients in high-risk occupations, particularly those in transportation or heavy industry, where accidents due to excessive sleepiness can have severe consequences both for the patient and public.

OSA has been linked with a variety of cardiovascular risk factors and endothelial dysfunction. It is associated with increased risks of congestive heart failure and cerebrovascular disease [37]. In severe cases, patients can develop cor pulmonale. There is a strong correlation between the severity of OSA and hypertension that is independent of obesity [38, 39]. An increase in the apnea-hypopnea index (AHI) (see definition below) by one event/hour increases the odds of hypertension by 1%. [38] OSA is associated with cardiac arrhythmias, particularly atrial fibrillation and supraventricular tachyarrhythmias [40–43]. Whether OSA is independently associated with ischemic heart disease remains controversial [44]. However, there is evidence that OSA, particularly when more severe, is associated with coronary artery disease and decreased survival (Fig. 10.5) [45–48].

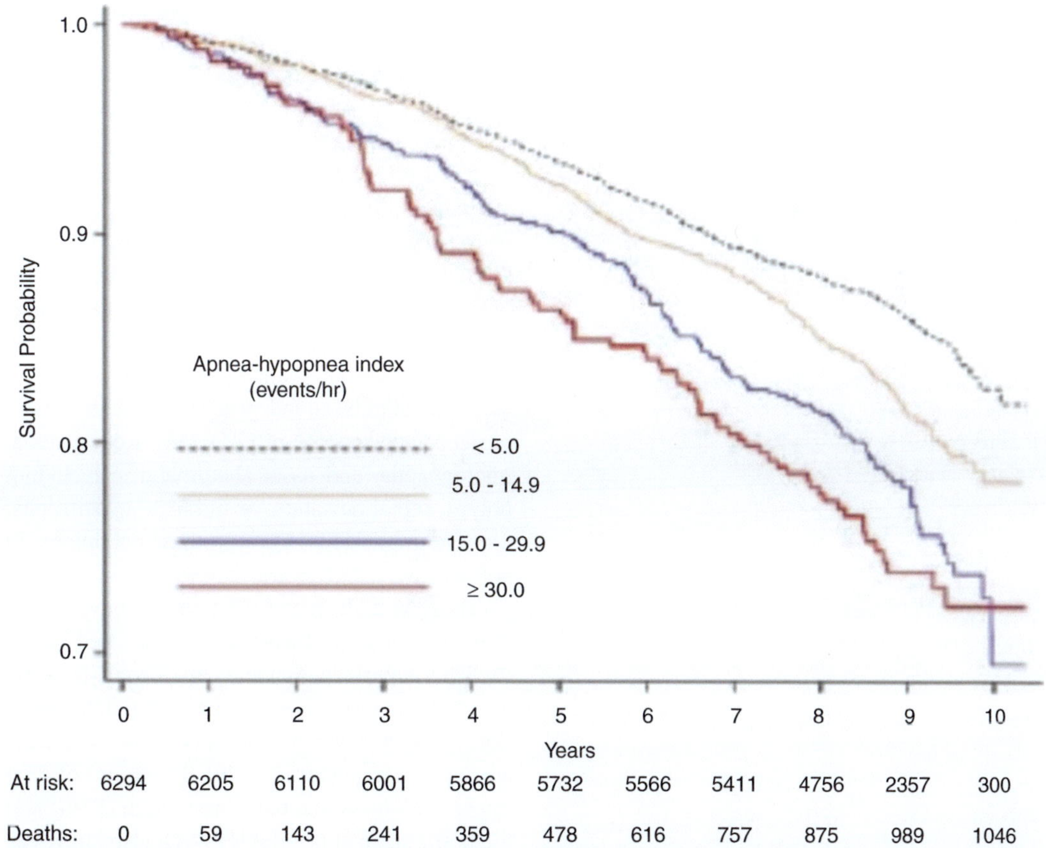

Fig. 10.5 Probability of survival in patients with different severities of OSA as measured by AHI. (Reproduced with permission from [48])

Diagnosis and Classification of OSA

The criterion for diagnosis and severity of OSA most often used is the AHI. An apnea is cessation (≥90% reduction) of airflow for a minimum of 10 seconds. An event is considered obstructive if there is continuing respiratory effort during the apnea. A hypopnea has variable definitions. This chapter will use the definition suggested by the American Academy of Sleep Medicine; a hypopnea is a decrease in airflow by 30% for ≥10 seconds associated with arterial oxygen desaturation of ≥3% measured by oximetry [49].

An AHI of ≥5 is considered abnormal. An AHI ≥ 5 associated with symptoms of obstructive sleep apnea is diagnostic of OSA (Table 10.2). Severe OSA is most often defined as an AHI >30 (Table 10.3); however there is some controversy surrounding this definition [50, 51]. The reader should be aware that other markers of severity include, but are not limited to, the nadir arterial oxygen saturation, as well as length and pattern of desaturations. The study of OSA is a rapidly changing field, and these definitions are likely to change as our understanding increases.

Numerous screening tools have been developed to predict OSA in individuals referred for evaluation of SDB. However, a diagnosis of SDB, particularly OSA, should be suspected in every patient referred for bariatric surgery. Several studies have demonstrated that the prevalence of OSA is between 70% and 80% in the bariatric surgery population [52–54].

Table 10.2 Symptoms of OSA

Symptoms of OSA
Excessive daytime sleepiness Choking or gasping during sleep
Unrefreshing sleep
Recurrent awakenings from sleep
Witnessed apneas
Daytime fatigue
Impaired concentration
Cognitive deficits
Depression/mood changes
GERD
Morning headaches

Table 10.3 Severity of OSA as determined by AHI

Severity of OSA	
Classification	AHI
Normal	<5
Mild	5–15
Moderate	16–30
Severe	>30

The evaluation for OSA should begin with a detailed clinical and sleep history. A patient should be interrogated about snoring, witnessed apneas, and nocturnal gasping. Often, it is helpful to ask the patient's bed partner these questions as many patients themselves may be unaware. Psychiatric and cognitive disturbances, such as depression and decreased ability to concentrate or remember, are classic symptoms of OSA. A comprehensive evaluation should include an estimate of total sleep time, questions about insomnia, and reasons for waking (e.g., nocturia). Daytime sleepiness should be quantified by a standardized tool, such as the Epworth Sleepiness Scale, seen below (Fig. 10.6) [29]. A score of 11 or more indicates abnormal daytime sleepiness. A history of conditions associated with OSA including hypertension, cerebrovascular disease, and motor vehicle accidents should be sought.

Physical examination is also important in the assessment. Increased neck circumference (≥16 inches in women, ≥17 inches in men) also increases the risk of OSA. Oropharyngeal crowding due to obesity, macroglossia, an oversized uvula, or tonsillar hypertrophy increases the risk of OSA. This is reflected in the Mallampati score, which has been shown to be an independent predictor of both presence and severity of OSA [55]. Retrognathia, micrognathia, and nasal abnormalities, including polyps, septal deviation, or turbinate hypertrophy, are also implicated. However, these conditions do not improve with bariatric surgery.

Those at high risk of OSA should have objective confirmation of disease presence and severity. The American Academy of Sleep Medicine (AASM) recommends that objective determination of OSA severity is necessary to determine appropriate management [29]. Two types of testing are endorsed: the polysomnogram (PSG) and the home sleep apnea test (HSAT), also known as the portable monitor (PM). The PSG is an in-laboratory, supervised overnight study where the

How Sleepy Are You?

How likely are you to doze off or fall asleep in the following situations? You should rate your chances of dozing off, not just feeling tired. Even if you have not done some of those things recently try to determine how they would have affected you. For each situation, decide whether or not you would have:

- No chance of dozing =0
- Slight chance of dozing =1
- Moderate chance of dozing =2
- High chance of dozing =3

Write down the number corresponding to your choice in the right hand column. Total your score below.

Situation	Chance of Dozing
Sitting and reading	•
Watching TV	•
Sitting inactive in a public place (e.g., a theater or a meeting)	•
As a passenger in a car for an hour without a break	•
Lying down to rest in the afternoon when circumstances permit	•
Sitting and talking to someone	•
Sitting quietly after a lunch without alcohol	•
In a car, while stopped for a few minutes in traffic	•

Total Score = ____________________

Fig. 10.6 Epworth sleepiness scale

subject is observed sleeping by a certified sleep technician. It is considered the gold standard for diagnosis [29, 56].

The attended PSG is a complex and costly test that monitors several physiologic and mechanical parameters throughout sleep. Electroencephalography (EEG), electrooculography (EOG), muscle activity, airflow, oxygen saturation, respiratory effort, and cardiac rate and rhythm are all simultaneously monitored under direct observation by a trained sleep technologist. It is recommended that the results are summarized and interpreted by a certified sleep physician. SDB is a common concern, and many areas have limited PSG capacity. Wait lists for diagnosis of OSA can be lengthy. A Canadian study demonstrated that OSA patients may wait up to 11.6 months and 16.2 months for initiation of medical or surgical treatment, respectively [57].

HSAT is a useful alternative to the PSG for the diagnosis of suspected OSA, particularly when there is a high pretest probability of moderate-to-severe disease [29, 56]. The HSAT records fewer physiologic variables. At a minimum, it should record airflow, respiratory effort, and oxygen saturation. Its accuracy is affected by comorbid sleep disorders or major comorbid medical disorders. Exclusion of significant cardiopulmonary, vascular, and neurological comorbidities is necessary. These tests do not measure EEG and cannot reliably determine when the patient is sleeping. Consequently, they generally underestimate the severity of SDB. They are not recommended for patients with moderate-to-severe pulmonary disease, neuromuscular disease, and congestive heart failure and those with a comorbid sleep disorder.

Treatment

OSA is a chronic disease and should be managed in a multidisciplinary manner. Therapy should always include behavioral and lifestyle modification. This includes diet, exercise, and weight loss. Patients should also be advised to avoid sedating medications and alcohol, particularly at nighttime. These interventions rarely lead to complete OSA remission but should always be promoted [58]. A systematic review and meta-analysis confirmed that lifestyle interventions are effective at reducing OSA severity as measured by AHI [59].

CPAP is considered the mainstay therapy for OSA. When used properly, CPAP can be curative. [29]. CPAP utilizes a pressurized hose and upper airway interface (facemask or nasal cannula) to pneumatically splint open and stabilize the airway throughout the respiratory cycle during sleep. Since CPAP became widely available in the 1980s, its major limitation has been patient compliance. A patient is considered to be compliant if they use their CPAP for ≥4 hours nightly for ≥70% of nights [60]. However, reality often falls far short of this goal. A review found that 29–83% do not use CPAP for 4 hours [61]. Twelve–25% of patients will entirely abandon CPAP within 3 years [62]. This has led to the development of alternative modalities of treatment. Alternatives and adjuncts include medications, positional therapies, exercise regimes to strengthen the upper airway, oral appliances, upper airway surgery, tracheostomy, and, sometimes as a last resort, bariatric surgery. Several experimental therapies are also in development, including a variety of upper airway muscle stimulators.

Bariatric surgery is an effective means to promote and maintain weight loss [63]. Consequently, it can be a very effective therapeutic option for the treatment of OSA. A 2004 meta-analysis of outcomes in bariatric surgery demonstrated that SDB is the most responsive obesity-related pathology [63]. Several reviews have demonstrated a marked reduction in nocturnal respiratory events following bariatric surgery [64, 65]. When compared to nonsurgical weight loss, bariatric surgery is more effective at reducing both BMI and AHI [66]. A systematic review of 13 900 patients with OSA who underwent various bariatric procedures demonstrated that 75% had an improvement in their AHI. However, only 4% had complete resolution of OSA (AHI < 5). For this reason, bariatric surgery is considered an *adjunctive* therapy [29]. Despite marked weight loss in patients following successful surgery, the body of evidence indicates that the majority have an elevated (but improved) AHI or RDI following recovery from bariatric surgery [63, 64]. A meta-analysis by Buchwald quotes resolution of OSA symptoms in 85.7% of bariatric surgery patients [63]. However, only the minority of studies included in this analysis objectively quantitated respiratory disturbances following surgery. PSG analysis following surgery demonstrates that 62% of patients have a residual AHI of ≥15, which would be characterized as moderately severe OSA. Although OSA may improve following surgery, patients should first be offered a noninvasive alternative. Most patients will still require CPAP following bariatric surgery [67]. This remains the case several years after surgery, despite the bariatric patient experiencing marked weight loss. A randomized controlled trial that compared conventional weight loss to bariatric surgery demonstrated that after 2 years, despite a significant sustained improvement in BMI in the surgical patients, the AHI were similar in two groups [68]. Another smaller trial had similar findings [69]. These studies highlight the importance of continuing conventional therapies for the management of OSA postoperatively, over the long term, regardless of weight loss. Following significant weight loss (≥10%), objective testing to determine OSA severity and for appropriateness of prescribed CPAP is necessary. The AASM recommends a follow-up sleep study be performed on any bariatric patient in whom moderate-to-severe OSA existed preoperatively. [29]

Perioperative Management of Sleep Apnea and Sleep-Disordered Breathing

Perioperative risk is higher in those with OSA compared to other subjects undergoing a wide range of surgical procedures [70–72]. The bariatrician's expectation should be that their patient has OSA of some severity. Screening tools for OSA, such as the Berlin Questionnaire, STOP-BANG score, and Sleep Apnea Clinical Score, were not validated in patient populations being evaluated for bariatric surgery [73–75]. Nonetheless, some experts suggest using them as a screening tool in bariatric populations [31]. There is a vigorous debate in which specific screening tests or specific preoperative care is necessary for SDB in patients referred for bariatric surgery.

Existing recommendations regarding perioperative care are largely based on expert opinion, which are variable. Some suggest that all patients being evaluated for bariatric surgery should be screened using an objective sleep study (PSG or HSAT) to determine presence and severity of OSA [76–81]. Others suggest the selective use of PSG only in circumstances where there is objective evidence of cardiac or pulmonary disease [82, 83]. Others disagree that every patient should be screened because of the relatively low perioperative complication rates seen in bariatric surgery in general. There is no evidence to suggest that preoperative PSG decreases the complication rate. A commonly seen complication, postoperative oxygen desaturation, may not be clinically significant [84]. What is not controversial is that those with significant comorbidities, such as right or left heart failure, pulmonary hypertension, and hypercapnia, should be studied with PSG preoperatively [31].

Patients with confirmed OSA awaiting bariatric surgery should have their SDB treatment optimized prior to surgery. Those with moderate-to-severe OSA are at highest risk for perioperative complications, especially if the patient is still symptomatic (daytime tiredness, hypercapnia) or if there has been excessive recent weight gain. Evaluation may include a repeat PSG, HSAT, or consultation with a sleep specialist. Patients should be screened for concomitant OHS, as daytime hypercapnia is associated with adverse perioperative outcomes. An arterial blood gas while awake can be used to screen for hypercarbia ($PaC0_2$ > 45 mmHg). A metabolic alkalosis ($HC0_3$ > 27 mmol) that is otherwise unexplained is also a relatively sensitive indicator of OHS [85].

The pathophysiology of OSA itself can be exacerbated at several stages during surgery. Medications, most notably sedatives, opioids, anesthetics, and paralytics, can reduce upper airway tone, increasing the likelihood and severity of apneic events. Furthermore, these agents depress central respiratory drive and may inhibit the protective arousal response. Complications from intubation, most notably laryngeal edema or tracheal stenosis, can further compromise an already tenuous airway. Positioning a patient supine, the position where OSA is worst, can also exacerbate OSA. Fluid administration during surgery can cause pharyngeal edema further compromising the upper airway. Lastly, many patients neglect to inform their clinicians that they have OSA and consequently forget to bring their therapeutic devices (CPAP, bi-level positive pressure, oral appliances) to hospital.

Surgical risk is also increased by conditions associated with OSA, such as pulmonary arterial hypertension, metabolic syndrome, arterial hypertension, and coronary artery disease. Hypoxemia due to OSA, particularly when untreated, can cause cardiac arrhythmias. A meta-analysis of 3942 patients showed that OSA patients are two to four times more likely to experience postoperative oxygen desaturations, respiratory failure, or adverse cardiac events or require ICU admission [70]. Not surprisingly, bariatric patients with OSA are at increased risk of prolonged hospitalization, with consequently increased healthcare costs [86]. They have an increased risk respiratory compromise during sedation. These concerns highlight why numerous experts continue to advocate for the need to screen bariatric patients to determine the severity of OSA. With respect to postoperative care, expert opinion advises continuous monitoring on a designated surgical or medium care unit, particularly when patients are known to have moderate or severe OSA. In the absence of complications, routine ICU admission is not necessary [31].

Bariatric surgery patients represent a high-risk surgical group. However, it is important to note that OSA does not confer additional risk above that of the bariatric patient without a formal diagnosis of SDB [76, 77, 87]. A meta-analysis of 13 studies with 98 935 patients compared perioperative outcomes in bariatric surgery patients with confirmed OSA to those without a formal diagnosis. Morbidity rates ranged from 0 to 25% but were similar in each group. There was no increased risk of cardiopulmonary morbidity, intensive care utilization, mortality, or length of stay after bariatric surgery for those with a history of OSA [77]. It is important to note that this study did not analyze preoperative care; those with diagnosed OSA may have received preoperative optimization of SDB prior to surgery.

There has been debate on whether CPAP should be administered following bariatric surgery. Concerns of anastomotic complications by positive airway pressure causing digestive tract distention have been reported [88]. However, several reviews of large patient cohorts, particularly those undergoing Roux-en-Y gastrectomy, suggest that it is safe and advisable [89, 90]. If positive pressure is omitted, early ambulation and incentive spirometry are critical [91].

Our understanding of obesity and its consequences for the respiratory system has increased substantially. It is clear that further research is of paramount importance given the global epidemic of obesity. Bariatric surgery is one of the most effective means of reversing the deleterious effects of excess fat on pulmonary function and OSA. The pathophysiology of OSA is complex, requiring an understanding of physiology, upper airway mechanics, and neurohormonal interplay. Perioperative identification and optimization of patients with OSA is important prior to bariatric surgery. Though usually not curative, OSA can improve considerably after bariatric surgery. As bariatric surgery rates increase, it will be important to monitor the outcomes in this interesting patient group.

References

1. Ogden CL, Carroll MD, Kit BK, Flegal KM. Prevalence of obesity among adults: United States, 2011–2012. NCHS Data Brief. 2013;131(131):1–8.
2. McClean KM, Kee F, Young IS, Elborn JS. Obesity and the lung: 1. Epidemiology. Thorax. 2008;63(7):649–54.
3. WHO. Obesity and overweight internet. http://www.who.int/mediacentre/factsheets/fs311/en/2016
4. Salome CM, King GG, Berend N. Physiology of obesity and effects on lung function. J Appl Physiol (1985). 2010;108(1):206–11.
5. Biring MS, Lewis MI, Liu JT, Mohsenifar Z. Pulmonary physiologic changes of morbid obesity. Am J Med Sci. 1999;318(5):293–7.
6. Chen Y, Rennie D, Cormier YF, Dosman J. Waist circumference is associated with pulmonary function in normal-weight, overweight, and obese subjects. Am J Clin Nutr. 2007;85(1):35–9.
7. Pelosi P, Croci M, Ravagnan I, Tredici S, Pedoto A, Lissoni A, et al. The effects of body mass on lung volumes, respiratory mechanics, and gas exchange during general anesthesia. Anesth Analg. 1998;87(3):654–60.
8. Sood A. Altered resting and exercise respiratory physiology in obesity. Clin Chest Med. 2009;30(3):445–54, vii.
9. Dempsey JA, Veasey SC, Morgan BJ, O'Donnell CP. Pathophysiology of sleep apnea. Physiol Rev. 2010;90(1):47–112.
10. Gifford AH, Leiter JC, Manning HL. Respiratory function in an obese patient with sleep-disordered breathing. Chest. 2010;138(3):704–15.
11. Jones RL, Nzekwu MM. The effects of body mass index on lung volumes. Chest. 2006;130(3):827–33.
12. Littleton SW. Impact of obesity on respiratory function. Respirology. 2012;17(1):43–9.
13. Parameswaran K, Todd DC, Soth M. Altered respiratory physiology in obesity. Can Respir J. 2006;13(4):203–10.
14. Thomas PS, Cowen ER, Hulands G, Milledge JS. Respiratory function in the morbidly obese before and after weight loss. Thorax. 1989;44(5):382–6.
15. Naimark A, Cherniack RM. Compliance of the respiratory system and its components in health and obesity. J Appl Physiol. 1960;15:377–82.
16. Sharp JT, Henry JP, Sweany SK, Meadows WR, Pietras RJ. The total work of breathing in normal and obese men. J Clin Invest. 1964;43:728–39.
17. Hedenstierna G, Santesson J. Breathing mechanics, dead space and gas exchange in the extremely obese, breathing spontaneously and during anaesthesia with intermittent positive pressure ventilation. Acta Anaesthesiol Scand. 1976;20(3):248–54.
18. Pelosi P, Croci M, Ravagnan I, Vicardi P, Gattinoni L. Total respiratory system, lung, and chest wall mechanics in sedated-paralyzed postoperative morbidly obese patients. Chest. 1996;109(1):144–51.

19. Suratt PM, Wilhoit SC, Hsiao HS, Atkinson RL, Rochester DF. Compliance of chest wall in obese subjects. J Appl Physiol Respir Environ Exerc Physiol. 1984;57(2):403–7.
20. Sampson MG, Grassino AE. Load compensation in obese patients during quiet tidal breathing. J Appl Physiol Respir Environ Exerc Physiol. 1983;55(4):1269–76.
21. Young T, Peppard PE, Gottlieb DJ. Epidemiology of obstructive sleep apnea: a population health perspective. Am J Respir Crit Care Med. 2002;165(9):1217–39.
22. Peppard PE, Young T, Barnet JH, Palta M, Hagen EW, Hla KM. Increased prevalence of sleep-disordered breathing in adults. Am J Epidemiol. 2013;177(9):1006–14.
23. Mokhlesi B, Kryger MH, Grunstein RR. Assessment and management of patients with obesity hypoventilation syndrome. Proc Am Thorac Soc. 2008;5(2):218–25.
24. Sugerman HJ, Fairman RP, Baron PL, Kwentus JA. Gastric surgery for respiratory insufficiency of obesity. Chest. 1986;90(1):81–6.
25. Mokhlesi B. Obesity hypoventilation syndrome: a state-of-the-art review. Respir Care. 2010;55(10):1347–62; discussion 63–5.
26. DeMaria EJ, Portenier D, Wolfe L. Obesity surgery mortality risk score: proposal for a clinically useful score to predict mortality risk in patients undergoing gastric bypass. Surg Obes Relat Dis. 2007;3(2):134–40.
27. Young T, Palta M, Dempsey J, Skatrud J, Weber S, Badr S. The occurrence of sleep-disordered breathing among middle-aged adults. N Engl J Med. 1993;328(17):1230–5.
28. Flemons WW. Clinical practice. Obstructive sleep apnea. N Engl J Med. 2002;347(7):498–504.
29. Epstein LJ, Kristo D, Strollo PJ Jr, Friedman N, Malhotra A, Patil SP, et al. Clinical guideline for the evaluation, management and long-term care of obstructive sleep apnea in adults. J Clin Sleep Med. 2009;5(3):263–76.
30. Orem J, Lovering AT, Dunin-Barkowski W, Vidruk EH. Tonic activity in the respiratory system in wakefulness, NREM and REM sleep. Sleep. 2002;25(5):488–96.
31. Riad W, Chung F. Preoperative screening for obstructive sleep apnea in morbidly obese patients. Int Anesthesiol Clin. 2013;51(3):13–25.
32. Fleetham J, Ayas N, Bradley D, Fitzpatrick M, Oliver TK, Morrison D, et al. Canadian Thoracic Society 2011 guideline update: diagnosis and treatment of sleep disordered breathing. Can Respir J. 2011;18(1):25–47.
33. Davis G, Patel JA, Gagne DJ. Pulmonary considerations in obesity and the bariatric surgical patient. Med Clin North Am. 2007;91(3):433–42, xi.
34. Gami AS, Caples SM, Somers VK. Obesity and obstructive sleep apnea. Endocrinol Metab Clin N Am. 2003;32(4):869–94.
35. Tregear S, Reston J, Schoelles K, Phillips B. Obstructive sleep apnea and risk of motor vehicle crash: systematic review and meta-analysis. J Clin Sleep Med. 2009;5(6):573–81.
36. Ayas N, Skomro R, Blackman A, Curren K, Fitzpatrick M, Fleetham J, et al. Obstructive sleep apnea and driving: a Canadian Thoracic Society and Canadian Sleep Society position paper. Can Respir J. 2014;21(2):114–23.
37. Somers VK, White DP, Amin R, Abraham WT, Costa F, Culebras A, et al. Sleep apnea and cardiovascular disease: an American Heart Association/American College of Cardiology Foundation Scientific Statement from the American Heart Association Council for High Blood Pressure Research Professional Education Committee, Council on Clinical Cardiology, Stroke Council, and Council on Cardiovascular Nursing. J Am Coll Cardiol. 2008;52(8):686–717.
38. Lavie P, Herer P, Hoffstein V. Obstructive sleep apnoea syndrome as a risk factor for hypertension: population study. BMJ. 2000;320(7233):479–82.
39. Nieto FJ, Young TB, Lind BK, Shahar E, Samet JM, Redline S, et al. Association of sleep-disordered breathing, sleep apnea, and hypertension in a large community-based study. Sleep Heart Health Study. JAMA. 2000;283(14):1829–36.
40. Mehra R, Benjamin EJ, Shahar E, Gottlieb DJ, Nawabit R, Kirchner HL, et al. Association of nocturnal arrhythmias with sleep-disordered breathing: The Sleep Heart Health Study. Am J Respir Crit Care Med. 2006;173(8):910–6.
41. Braga B, Poyares D, Cintra F, Guilleminault C, Cirenza C, Horbach S, et al. Sleep-disordered breathing and chronic atrial fibrillation. Sleep Med. 2009;10(2):212–6.
42. Needleman M, Calkins H. The role of obesity and sleep apnea in atrial fibrillation. Curr Opin Cardiol. 2011;26(1):40–5.
43. Harbison J, O'Reilly P, McNicholas WT. Cardiac rhythm disturbances in the obstructive sleep apnea syndrome: effects of nasal continuous positive airway pressure therapy. Chest. 2000;118(3):591–5.
44. McEvoy RD, Antic NA, Heeley E, Luo Y, Ou Q, Zhang X, et al. CPAP for prevention of cardiovascular events in obstructive sleep apnea. N Engl J Med. 2016;375(10):919–31.
45. Peker Y, Hedner J, Kraiczi H, Loth S. Respiratory disturbance index: an independent predictor of mortality in coronary artery disease. Am J Respir Crit Care Med. 2000;162(1):81–6.
46. Young T, Finn L, Peppard PE, Szklo-Coxe M, Austin D, Nieto FJ, et al. Sleep disordered breathing and mortality: eighteen-year follow-up of the Wisconsin sleep cohort. Sleep. 2008;31(8):1071–8.
47. Campos-Rodriguez F, Pena-Grinan N, Reyes-Nunez N, De la Cruz-Moron I, Perez-Ronchel J, De la Vega-Gallardo F, et al. Mortality in obstructive sleep apnea-hypopnea patients treated with positive airway pressure. Chest. 2005;128(2):624–33.

48. Punjabi NM, Caffo BS, Goodwin JL, Gottlieb DJ, Newman AB, O'Connor GT, et al. Sleep-disordered breathing and mortality: a prospective cohort study. PLoS Med. 2009;6(8):e1000132. https://doi.org/10.1371/journal.pmed.1000132.
49. Berry RB, Gamaldo CE, Harding SM, Brooks R, Lloyd RM, Vaughn BV, et al. AASM scoring manual version 2.2 updates: new chapters for scoring infant sleep staging and home sleep apnea testing. J Clin Sleep Med. 2015;11(11):1253–4.
50. Strohl K, Wheatley J, Young T, Douglas N, Levy P, McNicholas W, Fleetham J, et al. Sleep-related breathing disorders in adults: recommendations for syndrome definition and measurement techniques in clinical research. The Report of an American Academy of Sleep Medicine Task Force. Sleep. 1999;22(5):667–89.
51. Punjabi NM. COUNTERPOINT: is the apnea-hypopnea index the best way to quantify the severity of sleep-disordered breathing? No. Chest. 2016;149(1):16–9.
52. Frey WC, Pilcher J. Obstructive sleep-related breathing disorders in patients evaluated for bariatric surgery. Obes Surg. 2003;13(5):676–83.
53. Ravesloot MJ, van Maanen JP, Hilgevoord AA, van Wagensveld BA, de Vries N. Obstructive sleep apnea is underrecognized and underdiagnosed in patients undergoing bariatric surgery. Eur Arch Otorhinolaryngol. 2012;269(7):1865–71.
54. Khan A, King WC, Patterson EJ, Laut J, Raum W, Courcoulas AP, et al. Assessment of obstructive sleep apnea in adults undergoing bariatric surgery in the longitudinal assessment of bariatric surgery-2 (LABS-2) study. J Clin Sleep Med. 2013;9(1):21–9.
55. Nuckton TJ, Glidden DV, Browner WS, Claman DM. Physical examination: Mallampati score as an independent predictor of obstructive sleep apnea. Sleep. 2006;29(7):903–8.
56. Canadian Sleep S, Blackman A, McGregor C, Dales R, Driver HS, Dumov I, et al. Canadian Sleep Society/Canadian Thoracic Society position paper on the use of portable monitoring for the diagnosis of obstructive sleep apnea/hypopnea in adults. Can Respir J. 2010;17(5):229–32.
57. Rotenberg B, George C, Sullivan K, Wong E. Wait times for sleep apnea care in Ontario: a multidisciplinary assessment. Can Respir J. 2010;17(4):170–4.
58. Peppard PE, Young T, Palta M, Dempsey J, Skatrud J. Longitudinal study of moderate weight change and sleep-disordered breathing. JAMA. 2000;284(23):3015–21.
59. Araghi MH, Chen YF, Jagielski A, Choudhury S, Banerjee D, Hussain S, et al. Effectiveness of lifestyle interventions on obstructive sleep apnea (OSA): systematic review and meta-analysis. Sleep. 2013;36(10):1553–62, 62A–62E.
60. Kribbs NB, Pack AI, Kline LR, Smith PL, Schwartz AR, Schubert NM, et al. Objective measurement of patterns of nasal CPAP use by patients with obstructive sleep apnea. Am Rev Respir Dis. 1993;147(4):887–95.
61. Weaver TE, Grunstein RR. Adherence to continuous positive airway pressure therapy: the challenge to effective treatment. Proc Am Thorac Soc. 2008;5(2):173–8.
62. Engleman HM, Wild MR. Improving CPAP use by patients with the sleep apnoea/hypopnoea syndrome (SAHS). Sleep Med Rev. 2003;7(1):81–99.
63. Buchwald H, Avidor Y, Braunwald E, Jensen MD, Pories W, Fahrbach K, et al. Bariatric surgery: a systematic review and meta-analysis. JAMA. 2004;292(14):1724–37.
64. Greenburg DL, Lettieri CJ, Eliasson AH. Effects of surgical weight loss on measures of obstructive sleep apnea: a meta-analysis. Am J Med. 2009;122(6):535–42.
65. Sarkhosh K, Switzer NJ, El-Hadi M, Birch DW, Shi X, Karmali S. The impact of bariatric surgery on obstructive sleep apnea: a systematic review. Obes Surg. 2013;23(3):414–23.
66. Ashrafian H, Toma T, Rowland SP, Harling L, Tan A, Efthimiou E, et al. Bariatric surgery or non-surgical weight loss for obstructive sleep apnoea? a systematic review and comparison of meta-analyses. Obes Surg. 2015;25(7):1239–50.
67. Lettieri CJ, Eliasson AH, Greenburg DL. Persistence of obstructive sleep apnea after surgical weight loss. J Clin Sleep Med. 2008;4(4):333–8.
68. Dixon JB, Schachter LM, O'Brien PE, Jones K, Grima M, Lambert G, et al. Surgical vs conventional therapy for weight loss treatment of obstructive sleep apnea: a randomized controlled trial. JAMA. 2012;308(11):1142–9.
69. Pillar G, Peled R, Lavie P. Recurrence of sleep apnea without concomitant weight increase 7.5 years after weight reduction surgery. Chest. 1994;106(6):1702–4.
70. Kaw R, Chung F, Pasupuleti V, Mehta J, Gay PC, Hernandez AV. Meta-analysis of the association between obstructive sleep apnoea and postoperative outcome. Br J Anaesth. 2012;109(6):897–906.
71. Memtsoudis S, Liu SS, Ma Y, Chiu YL, Walz JM, Gaber-Baylis LK, et al. Perioperative pulmonary outcomes in patients with sleep apnea after noncardiac surgery. Anesth Analg. 2011;112(1):113–21.
72. Mokhlesi B, Hovda MD, Vekhter B, Arora VM, Chung F, Meltzer DO. Sleep-disordered breathing and postoperative outcomes after elective surgery: analysis of the nationwide inpatient sample. Chest. 2013;144(3):903–14.
73. Flemons WW, Whitelaw WA, Brant R, Remmers JE. Likelihood ratios for a sleep apnea clinical prediction rule. Am J Respir Crit Care Med. 1994;150(5 Pt 1):1279–85.
74. Netzer NC, Stoohs RA, Netzer CM, Clark K, Strohl KP. Using the Berlin Questionnaire to identify patients at risk for the sleep apnea syndrome. Ann Intern Med. 1999;131(7):485–91.
75. Chung F, Yegneswaran B, Liao P, Chung SA, Vairavanathan S, Islam S, et al. STOP questionnaire:

a tool to screen patients for obstructive sleep apnea. Anesthesiology. 2008;108(5):812–21.
76. Weingarten TN, Flores AS, McKenzie JA, Nguyen LT, Robinson WB, Kinney TM, et al. Obstructive sleep apnoea and perioperative complications in bariatric patients. Br J Anaesth. 2011;106(1):131–9.
77. de Raaff CA, Coblijn UK, de Vries N, van Wagensveld BA. Is fear for postoperative cardiopulmonary complications after bariatric surgery in patients with obstructive sleep apnea justified? A systematic review. Am J Surg. 2016;211(4):793–801.
78. Lopez PP, Stefan B, Schulman CI, Byers PM. Prevalence of sleep apnea in morbidly obese patients who presented for weight loss surgery evaluation: more evidence for routine screening for obstructive sleep apnea before weight loss surgery. Am Surg. 2008;74(9):834–8.
79. O'Keeffe T, Patterson EJ. Evidence supporting routine polysomnography before bariatric surgery. Obes Surg. 2004;14(1):23–6.
80. Rao A, Tey BH, Ramalingam G, Poh AG. Obstructive sleep apnoea (OSA) patterns in bariatric surgical practice and response of OSA to weight loss after laparoscopic adjustable gastric banding (LAGB). Ann Acad Med Singap. 2009;38(7):587–93.
81. Sareli AE, Cantor CR, Williams NN, Korus G, Raper SE, Pien G, et al. Obstructive sleep apnea in patients undergoing bariatric surgery – a tertiary center experience. Obes Surg. 2011;21(3):316–27.
82. Catheline JM, Bihan H, Le Quang T, Sadoun D, Charniot JC, Onnen I, et al. Preoperative cardiac and pulmonary assessment in bariatric surgery. Obes Surg. 2008;18(3):271–7.
83. Schumann R, Jones SB, Cooper B, Kelley SD, Bosch MV, Ortiz VE, et al. Update on best practice recommendations for anesthetic perioperative care and pain management in weight loss surgery, 2004–2007. Obesity (Silver Spring). 2009;17(5):889–94.
84. Kurrek MM, Cobourn C, Wojtasik Z, Kiss A, Dain SL. Morbidity in patients with or at high risk for obstructive sleep apnea after ambulatory laparoscopic gastric banding. Obes Surg. 2011;21(10):1494–8.
85. Macavei VM, Spurling KJ, Loft J, Makker HK. Diagnostic predictors of obesity-hypoventilation syndrome in patients suspected of having sleep disordered breathing. J Clin Sleep Med. 2013;9(9):879–84.
86. Memtsoudis SG, Stundner O, Rasul R, Chiu YL, Sun X, Ramachandran SK, et al. The impact of sleep apnea on postoperative utilization of resources and adverse outcomes. Anesth Analg. 2014;118(2):407–18.
87. Mokhlesi B, Hovda MD, Vekhter B, Arora VM, Chung F, Meltzer DO. Sleep-disordered breathing and postoperative outcomes after bariatric surgery: analysis of the nationwide inpatient sample. Obes Surg. 2013;23(11):1842–51.
88. Vasquez TL, Hoddinott K. A potential complication of bi-level positive airway pressure after gastric bypass surgery. Obes Surg. 2004;14(2):282–4.
89. Huerta S, DeShields S, Shpiner R, Li Z, Liu C, Sawicki M, et al. Safety and efficacy of postoperative continuous positive airway pressure to prevent pulmonary complications after Roux-en-Y gastric bypass. J Gastrointest Surg. 2002;6(3):354–8.
90. Ramirez A, Lalor PF, Szomstein S, Rosenthal RJ. Continuous positive airway pressure in immediate postoperative period after laparoscopic Roux-en-Y gastric bypass: is it safe? Surg Obes Relat Dis. 2009;5(5):544–6.
91. Jensen C, Tejirian T, Lewis C, Yadegar J, Dutson E, Mehran A. Postoperative CPAP and BiPAP use can be safely omitted after laparoscopic Roux-en-Y gastric bypass. Surg Obes Relat Dis. 2008;4(4):512–4.

The Superobese Patient

11

Michel Suter

Introduction and Definition

Like cancer and other chronic and progressive medical conditions, obesity has traditionally been divided into different stages according to the severity of the disease. Although the World Health Organization (WHO) recognizes that BMI may not always express similar degrees of fatness between individuals, this organization defines obesity as abnormal or excessive fat accumulation that may impair health, with a body mass index of 30 kg/m^2 as a threshold [1]. The risks associated with obesity are continuous and increase with disease severity. WHO recognizes three classes of obesity according to the body mass index (BMI). Class 1 obesity refers to patients with modest obesity and a BMI between 30 and 34.9 kg/m^2, class 2 includes patients with a BMI between 35 and 39.9 kg/m^2, and class 3 refers to patients with a BMI $\geq$ 40 kg/m^2. In the nonspecialized literature, the latter patients are offered referred to as massively obese, or extremely obese. In bariatric medicine, which essentially deals with patients in the WHO class 2 and 3 categories, it is useful to further divide morbid obesity into more classes. This may be helpful in selecting patients for various bariatric procedures, for specific surgical approaches, for preoperative patient preparation and/or weight loss, etc. It is also useful to have categories encompassing patient groups that can reasonably be compared between each other both regarding risks, results of surgery, morbidity and mortality, or any other specific issue. The superobese patient is defined arbitrarily has having a BMI $\geq$ 50 kg/m^2. Other terms are being used for even more severe sub-categories such as patients with BMI > 60 (super-super-obese) or above 70 (mega-obese).

M. Suter (✉)
Department of Surgery, Riviera-Chablais Hospital, Aigle-Monthey, Switzerland

Department of Visceral Surgery, University Hospital Lausanne, Lausanne, Switzerland
e-mail: michelsuter@netplus.ch

Clinical Characteristics of the Superobese Patient

As stated above, the BMI does not necessarily reflect the same amount of excess fat in different individuals, since BMI is related to total weight and not only fat mass. Defining the severity of obesity according to BMI classes in fact can be profoundly misleading. Indeed, some patients in the low BMI range are very sick, with severe metabolic syndrome, poorly controlled diabetes, coronary artery disease, and other severe comorbidities, while other superobese patients seem to be perfectly healthy apart from their massive overweight, with virtually no or only mild comorbid condition(s). As BMI increases, however, the proportion of fat mass in body composition increases as well. In general, the heavier an

J. Ettinger et al. (eds.), *Gastric Bypass*, https://doi.org/10.1007/978-3-030-28803-7_11

individual, especially in the higher extreme ranges, the more excess fat he/she has accumulated. As for every obese individual, excess fat may or may not be associated with a variety of conditions, and this depends among other factors from fat distribution. In general, central visceral fat is far more toxic than peripheral subcutaneous fat. Central, or visceral, obesity causes a chronic inflammatory state that can affect almost every organ system. Even in favorable cases, superobese patients have more visceral fat and therefore are at higher risk to develop severe obesity-related complications, especially of metabolic nature, such as dyslipidemia, type 2 diabetes, hypertension, fatty liver disease, and all components of the metabolic syndrome. Increasing obesity also affects the respiratory and cardiovascular systems. Massive obesity reduces both static and dynamic lung function parameters and promotes left ventricular concentric hypertrophy and dilatation. Indeed, it has been shown that superobese patients have higher left ventricular mass than less obese patients, with higher left ventricular and left atrial volumes, despite similar ejection fractions [2]. Insulin resistance is also higher in superobese patients [2], and type 2 diabetes is more prevalent [3]. Superobese patients more often present with the obesity-related hypoventilation syndrome and dyspnea [3, 4], and the sleep apnea syndrome is more common in these individuals. Studies have shown that the hypopnea/apnea index increases linearly with the BMI [5, 6]. Functional limitation related to osteoarthritis is more severe in superobese than in less obese patients [7]. Superobesity has been shown to increase obstetric risks. Preeclampsia and macrosomia are more prevalent during pregnancy, and there is an increased need for cesarean sections for delivery [8]. Superobesity has also been shown to increase risks and/or costs in various types of surgery, including joint replacement surgery [9, 10] and bariatric surgery, especially with an open approach [11, 12], although this role has been challenged in recent laparoscopic series [13–16]. Even if surgery-related morbidity is not increased per se in the superobese, complications in this group of patients are poorly tolerated due to very limited physiological reserves, which may lead to prolonged intensive care unit stay and longer time on mechanical ventilation [17].

Evaluation of the Superobese Patient Before Bariatric/Metabolic Surgery

Superobese patients are complex with often multiple etiological factors, including genetics, for their obesity. Any patient presenting or referred for possible bariatric surgery must be screened in details by a specialized multidisciplinary team, and this applies particularly to the superobese. Superobese patients have often been severely obese for many years. This long-standing condition, together with its greater severity, is likely to already have a significant impact on many organ systems. All possible obesity-related comorbidities must be looked for. Those that may affect operative and perioperative risks or the choice of a bariatric operation, like cardiovascular and respiratory status, or severe metabolic abnormalities, are of particular importance. The nutritional status must be assessed very carefully, since superobese patients paradoxically are particularly prone to multiple micronutrient deficiencies. Treatment for obesity-related comorbidities or any other medical condition that may affect surgical outcome must be optimized before surgery, and nutritional deficiencies must be corrected in order to minimize surgical risks.

Preoperative evaluation should also focus on all potential factors that play a role in the development/maintenance of extreme obesity and especially those that are deemed modifiable. The social and family environment needs to be assessed, and eating habits must be carefully evaluated. Identifying psychological issues related to extreme obesity, and possible issues that might result from massive weight loss, is important. These problems need to be addressed appropriately, and special needs for postoperative psychological support must be recognized. Identifying eating disorders (emotional eating, stress eating, night eating, etc.), and poor dietary choices, and addressing them aggressively with the help of dieticians and psychologists are of paramount importance before surgery. If left untreated, they will negatively impact the results of any bariatric procedure, especially in the long term. Patients must be made aware of the fact that Roux-en-Y gastric bypass (RYGB), while being extremely powerful, remains merely a tool that will help them eat less by reducing hunger, increasing satiety, and inducing some mechanical restriction. They must understand that RYGB by no way will prevent them from eating too much (more calories than they spend), or too often, or from making poor dietary choices and drinking high caloric beverages. Patients therefore must be carefully instructed about the type of diet they should follow after surgery and in the long term. Because they are more limited from a physical point of view, and often do very little physical activity, if any, superobese patients need to be instructed about the importance of progressively increasing their physical activity during the weight loss phase and the importance of maintaining a sufficient level of physical activity, and its role in weight maintenance thereafter. Superobese patients, like all bariatric individuals, must be instructed about the likely need for life-long nutritional supplementations, the absolute necessity of a specialized follow-up, and especially the reasons behind it. They need to be informed about the standard follow-up scheme and be made aware that deviations from the latter are possible according to postoperative evolution. They must realize the chronic character of their condition, the risks for weight regain and/or recurrence of comorbidities over time, and understand that they can seek help from members of the multidisciplinary team at anytime according to their needs.

As superobese individuals have very limited physiological reserves, preoperative evaluation from an anesthetist perspective is essential so that intra- or postoperative problems can be anticipated. This may require extensive cardiovascular of pulmonary work-up. C-PAP treatment must be initialized several weeks before surgery in patients with severe sleep apnea syndrome so that the machine can be fine-tuned according to the patient's needs and they can adjust to it. Severe obesity-related hypoventilation syndrome needs to be recognized, as this is likely to worsen during surgery in supine position, especially under the conditions of laparoscopy with pneumoperitoneum and increased intra-abdominal pressure. Evaluation by a cardiologist is sometimes required, even in asymptomatic patients, especially in patients with long-standing diabetes. Individuals with severe ventricular dysfunction may require special intraoperative monitoring. For patients with foreseeable difficulties, a critical care facility must be available for the immediate postoperative period.

Patients in the superobese category often have massive skin folds and not unusually present with intertrigo and chronic inflammation in various areas. This also causes difficulties with personal hygiene. Preoperative care of such areas is important to minimize the risks for postoperative infections. Also, since these patients are likely to develop massive, and sometimes really debilitating, skin folds after weight loss, they can benefit even before they undergo bariatric surgery from the expertise and counseling of a well-trained plastic surgeon.

Choice of Procedure

Although the topic of the present book is Roux-en-Y gastric bypass, a chapter dedicated to the superobese patient failing to at least discuss this issue would be out of scope. Indeed, it has been repeatedly shown that RYGB-associated weight loss, expressed as excess weight loss or excess BMI loss (with BMI = 25 accepted as ideal weight), is less in superobese patients compared with less obese individuals. If one considers the percentage of total body weight loss, however, results of the various procedures do not differ much between all obesity classes [15]. Weight regain over the years is another issue that can be a problem after every bariatric procedure and in all obesity classes. After RYGBP, weight regain has also been shown to be more important in more obese patients [18–20]. Altogether, insufficient weight loss or substantial weight regain may affect at least 40% of superobese patients after standard RYGBP. This has also been demonstrated, albeit to a lesser extent, after biliopancreatic diversion [21]. Finally, since RYGB is a relatively complex bariatric procedure, its risks are sometimes perceived as sky-scraping in high-risk patients such as superobese individuals. In fact, some surgeons argue that some superobese patients, if not all of them, could/should benefit from a two-stage approach. In the latter, the first stage consists of a sleeve gastrectomy, a procedure that many consider as relatively low-risk and simple, allowing for substantial initial weight loss and reduction of perioperative risk. During the second stage, a more efficient, but also more risky, procedure can then be performed to ensure optimal weight loss and maintenance.

Several studies, including one randomized controlled trial, have shown that biliopancreatic diversion with duodenal switch (BPD-DS) provides greater weight loss and better weight maintenance than RYGB in the superobese patient, at the expense of increased perioperative morbidity as well as long-term morbidity [19, 22, 23]. If weight loss and/or control of comorbidities are the main issue, all other factors being equal, it seems reasonable to prefer BPD-DS over RYGB. If on the contrary safety is essential, RYGB or sleeve gastrectomy (SG) seem preferable. In fact, many would currently argue that SG is the best option. The current literature, however, lacks long-term results of SG, both in general and in this particular group of patients, to support this view. Because of these potential differences in outcomes, the choice of surgical procedure must be discussed in details with the patient who should have his/her say in the decision process, unless there is a clear contraindication to one or the other options. Since malabsorptive surgery carries additional risks of nutritional deficiencies, including protein malnutrition, it seems appropriate, however, to offer the latter only to very compliant patients who accept the intensive follow-up program and the multiple long-term nutritional supplementations that this kind of procedure requires. Performing a SG first allows for prolonged observation of the patient and his/her overall behavior after the first operation. It also avoids performing procedures with a high risk of severe nutritional complications in poorly compliant patients.

Preoperative Preparation of the Patients

As already mentioned, treatment of comorbidities should be optimized before surgery, and nutritional deficiencies need to be corrected. Patients with massive obesity may benefit from preoperative weight loss in order to reduce operative difficulties as well as perioperative risks.

While many superobese patients can undergo surgery without specific difficulties, with reasonable risks and an operative morbidity similar to that observed in less obese patients, risk-reduction strategies can be necessary, and are sometimes mandatory, in patients with very high BMIs, or in patients with very severe cardiorespiratory comorbidities. The latter may benefit from preoperative weight loss in order to make them more easily transportable, to facilitate intraoperative management by the anesthetist as well as surgical exposure, and sometimes only to make surgery possible. In these extreme cases, though, a significant amount of preoperative weight loss is necessary, without which surgery carries prohibitive risks or is simply not possible. In many other patients, preoperative weight loss is helpful mostly for risk reduction. This may require prolonged supervised very low-calorie diet, or even inpatient low-calorie diet [24, 25]. Very low-calorie diet has been shown to help reducing perioperative morbidity after RYGB [26]. The use of a temporary intragastric balloon has also been demonstrated as effective in diminishing perioperative morbidity [27]. In a recent multicenter trial comparing intragastric balloon therapy with standard medical care in superobese patients before RYGB, however, there was no difference in perioperative outcomes between the two groups, despite the fact that mean weight loss was significantly greater in the balloon group [28]. Intragastric balloons can be followed by a variety of complications, and this risk must be balanced against the risks of the same surgical procedure performed in a slightly heavier patient. Preoperative weight loss strategies may imply a significant delay of several months since indication for surgery is confirmed and the procedure itself can be carried out. In order to ensure optimal compliance, patients need to be informed about why this is necessary.

Superobese patients very often have fatty liver disease. An extremely enlarged liver can occasionally make any type of surgery completely impracticable, but most often makes surgery more difficult and challenging. A large liver is difficult to retract efficiently and is prone to bleeding because of its fragile consistency. This results in poor visual exposure and consequently technical difficulties during surgery, especially RYGB, notably during creation of the gastric pouch and confection of the gastrojejunostomy. Short-term induced preoperative weight loss using low-calorie diet has been shown to improve surgical exposure due to a significant reduction of the liver volume. In a study using a 9-week low-calorie diet, Collins et al. have shown a significant reduction not only in weight but also in subcutaneous abdominal fat, in visceral adipose tissue, along with an 18% reduction in liver volume [29]. Sekino et al. have shown that the maximal effect on liver size is obtained after only 2–4 weeks [30]. We currently advise every bariatric patient to follow a very low-fat/low-carbohydrates diet during 2 weeks before surgery and 3 weeks in the superobese.

Special Requirements for the Superobese Patient

Facilities where superobese patients are treated must be equipped with appropriate furniture (beds, chairs, etc.) that accommodates these patients easily and safely, both on the regular ward and in the intensive care unit. Restrooms must be wide enough, with solid toilets, ideally floor-mounted, that can sustain the heaviest patients. Special equipment for patient transfer may be required.

The entire setting of the operating room must be friendly to the superobese patient. The operative table must be able to sustain weights up to 350 kg in all positions, included deep reverse Trendelenburg. It also needs to be wide enough. As superobese patients are also very thick, the operative field is higher than in less obese patients, especially in males with abdominal obesity. The operative table must therefore be adjustable in height to a very low position so that the surgeon can operate comfortably without the need to stand on a step. If a stool is required, it must be wide enough to accommodate not only the surgeon but also the pedals he might need to activate surgical instruments like electrocoagulation or suction. Special mattresses or gel cushions should be used to secure the patient on the operative table and to prevent pressure sores and rhabdomyolysis. Rhabdomyolysis is more common in superobese patients and can develop even after an operation of relatively short duration, typically less than 2 hours. The thickness of the subcutaneous fat layer in some superobese patients can interfere with the establishment of pneumoperitoneum and placement of trocars. It can cause increased torque during surgery and increased fatigue to the surgical team. Intraoperative exposure is often more difficult because of increased intra-abdominal fat and liver size. Furthermore, tissues are often very fragile and prone to oozing during manipulation. This requires extreme softness during tissue handling and may require special instrumentation, with longer trocars and surgical instruments. Additional trocars should be used liberally, as they can greatly facilitate movements, speed up the procedure, and improve safety. Additional 5 mm trocars are very well tolerated and leave scars that are barely visible in the long term. Insufflation can be a problem in the superobese, especially in patients with a massive abdominal apron that falls between the legs. This may require special support to the abdominal wall and possibly a second insufflator.

Aftercare in the Superobese Patient Population

Superobese patients require close follow-up by the multidisciplinary team just as any other bariatric patients. Dietary counseling and psychological support can be very important in this fragile group of individuals, notably during the rapid weight loss phase. Once they have stabilized their weight, they need to be referred to plastic surgery for consideration of body contouring and reconstructive surgery, since massive skin folds are often impairing functionality.

As mentioned earlier, superobese patients are more prone than less obese individuals to important weight regain. To prevent this, dietary support is essential, but increasing physical activity is even more important. These patients must be encouraged to exercise on a daily basis, and support by physiotherapist or other types of coaches may be beneficial. Group exercising is often of great help and can help with patient motivation.

Conclusions

Superobese patients often have more obesity-related comorbidities and are therefore at increased risk for bariatric/metabolic surgery. Furthermore, surgery in these individuals is often more difficult from a technical point of view, with difficulties establishing pneumoperitoneum, manipulating laparoscopic instruments, and getting adequate exposure during the procedure. Preoperative work-up is of paramount importance. Preoperative preparation of the patient according to its findings and preoperative weight loss are necessary steps to ensure optimal patient outcomes. From a logistical point of view, special equipment and adapted surgical instruments must be readily available. These procedures should only be performed by very experienced bariatric surgeons, and anesthesia must be conducted by experienced bariatric anesthetists. Postoperative care requires involvement of multiple specialists, including plastic surgery once weight has stabilized.

References

1. World health Organization. www.who.int/mediacentre/factsheets/fs311/en/. Accessed 13 Sept 2016.
2. Antonini-Canterin F, Mateescu AD, Vriz O, La Carrubba S, Di Bello V, Carerj S, Zito C, Sparacino L, Marzano B, Usurelu C, Ticulescu R, Ginghina C, Nicolosi GL, Popescu BA. Cardiac structure and function and insulin resistance in morbidly obese patients: does superobesity play an additional role? Cardiology. 2014;127:144–51.
3. Kakarla VR, Nandipati K, Lalla M, Castro A, Merola S. Are laparoscopic bariatric procedures safe in superobese (BMI $\geq$ 50 kg/m^2) patients? An NSQIP data analysis. Surg Obes Relat Dis. 2011;7:452–8.
4. Muñoz S, Nowzaradan Y, Varon J. Extreme obesity in the intensive care unit: the malignant obesity hypoventilation syndrome. J Intensive Care Med. 2013;28:134–5.
5. Matthew R, Castriotta RJ. High hypopnea/apnea ratio (HAR) in extreme obesity. J Clin Sleep Med. 2014;10:391–6.
6. Lopez PP, Stefan B, Schulman CI, Byers PM. Prevalence of sleep apnea in morbidly obese patients who presented for weight loss surgery evaluation: more evidence for routine screening for obstructive sleep apnea before weight loss surgery. Am Surg. 2008;74:834–8.
7. Fabris SM, Faintuch J, Brienze SL, Brito GB, Sitta IS, Mendes EL, Fonseca IC, Cecconello I. Are knee and foot orthopedic problems more disabling in the superobese? Obes Surg. 2013;23:201–4.
8. Marshall NE, Guild C, Cheng YW, Caughey AB, Halloran DR. Maternal superobesity and perinatal outcomes. Am J Obstet Gynecol. 2012;206:417.e1–6.
9. Werner BC, Burrus MT, Browne JA, Brockmeier SF. Superobesity (body-mass index > 50 kg/m^2) and complications after total shoulder arthroplasty: an incremental effect of increasing body mass index. J Shoulder Elb Surg. 2015;24:1868–75.
10. Meller MM, Toossi N, Johanson NA, Gonzalez MH, Son MS, Lau EC. Risk and cost of 90-day complications in morbidly and superobese patients after total knee arthroplasty. J Arthroplast. 2016;31:2091–8.
11. Livingston EH, Arterburn D, Schifftner TL, Henderson WG, DePalma RG. National surgical quality improvement program analysis of bariatric operations: modifiable risk factors contribute to bariatric surgical adverse outcomes. J Am Coll Surg. 2006;203:625–33.
12. Fernandez AZ, DeMaria EJ, Tichansky DS, Kellum JM, Wolfe LG, Meador J, Sugerman HJ. Multivariate analysis of risk factors for death following gastric bypass for treatment of morbid obesity. Ann Surg. 2004;239:698–702.
13. Fazylov RM, Savel RH, Horovitz JH, Pagal MK, Coppa GF, Nicastro J, Lazzaro RS, Macura JM. Association of super-obesity and male gender with elevated mortality in patients undergoing the duodenal switch procedure. Obes Surg. 2005;15:618–23.
14. Dresel A, Kuhn JA, McCarthy TM. Laparoscopic Roux-en-Y gastric bypass in morbidly obese and super morbidly obese patients. Am J Surg. 2004;187:230–2.
15. Dayer-Jankechova A, Fournier P, Allemann P, Suter M. Complications after laparoscopic Roux-en-Y gastric bypass in 1573 consecutive patients: are there predictors? Obes Surg. 2016;26:12–20.
16. Suter M, Calmes JM, Paroz A, Romy S, Giusti V. Results of Roux-en-Y gastric bypass in morbidly versus superobese patients: similar body weight loss,

correction of comorbidities, and improvement of quality of life. Arch Surg. 2009;144:312–8.
17. Marino JL, Stapleton RD, Wang M, Day AG, Cahill NE, Dixon AE, Suratt BT, Heyland DK. Extreme obesity and outcomes in critically ill patients. Chest. 2011;140:1198–206.
18. Magro DO, Geloneze B, Delfini R, Pareja BC, Callebas F, Pareja JC. Long-term weight regain after gastric bypass: a 5-year prospective study. Obes Surg. 2008;18:648–51.
19. Topart P, Becouarn G, Ritz P. Weight loss is more sustained after biliopancreatic diversion with duodenal switch than Roux-en-Y gastric bypass in superobese patients. Surg Obes Relat Dis. 2013;9:526–30.
20. Christou NV, Look D, MacLean LD. Weight gain after short-and long-limb gastric bypass in patients followed for longer than 10 years. Ann Surg. 2006;244:734–40.
21. Biron S, Hould FS, Lebel S, Marceau S, Lescelleur O, Simard S, Marceau P. Twenty years of biliopancreatic diversion. What is the goal of surgery? Obes Surg. 2004;14:160–4.
22. Sovik TT, Taha O, Aasheim ET, Engström M, Kristinsson J, Björkman S, Schou CF, Lönroth H, Mala T, Olbers T. Randomized clinical trial of laparoscopic gastric bypass versus laparoscopic duodenal switch for superobesity. Br J Surg. 2010;97:160–6.
23. Risstad H, Sovik TT, Engström M, Aasheim ET, Fagerland MW, Olsen MF, Kristinsson JA, LeRoux CW, Bohmer T, Birkeland KI, Mala T, Olbers T. Five-year outcomes after laparoscopic gastric bypass and laparoscopic duodenal switch in patients with body mass index of 50 to 60: a randomized clinical trial. JAMA Surg. 2015;150:352–61.
24. Huerta S, Li Z, Anthony T, Livingston EH. Feasibility of a supervised inpatient low-calorie diet program for massive weight loss prior to RYGB in superobese patients. Obes Surg. 2010;20:173–80.
25. Orlando G, Gervasi R, Luppino IM, Vitale M, Amato B, Silecchia G, Puzziello A. The role of a multidisciplinary approach in the choice of the best surgery approach in a super-super-obesity case. Int J Surg. 2014;12(suppl 1):S103–6.
26. Van Nieuwenhove Y, Dambrauskas Z, Campillo-Soto A, van Dielen F, Wiezer R, Janssen I, Kramer M, Thorell A. Preoperative very low-calorie diet and operative outcome after laparoscopic gastric bypass. A randomized multicenter study. Arch Surg. 2011;146:1300–5.
27. Zerrweck C, Maunoury V, Caiazzo R, Branche J, Dezfoulian G, Bulois P, Verkindt H, Pigeyre M, Arnalsteen L, Pattou F. Preoperative weight loss with intragastric balloon decreases the risk of significant adverse outcomes of laparoscopic gastric bypass in super-super obese patients. Obes Surg. 2012;22:777–82.
28. Coffin B, Maunoury V, Pattou F, Xébuterne X, Schneider S, Coupaye M, et al. Impact of intragastric balloon before laparoscopic gastric bypass on patients with superobesity: a randomized multicenter study. Obes Surg. 2016;27:902. https://doi.org/10.1007/s11695-016-2383-x.
29. Collins J, McCloskey C, Titchner R, Goodpaster B, Hoffman M, Hauser D, Wilson M, Eid G. Preoperative weight loss in high-risk superobese bariatric patients: a computed tomography-based analysis. Surg Obes Relat Dis. 2011;7:480–5.
30. Sekino Y, Imajo K, Sakai E, Uchiyama T, Iida H, Endo H, et al. Time-course of changes of visceral fat area, liver volume and liver fat area during intragastric balloon therapy in Japanese super-obese patients. Intern Med. 2011;50:2449–55.

Airway Evaluation and Management

12

Adriano Teixeira Fernandes, Macius Pontes Cerqueira, and Guilherme Oliveira Campos

Introduction

Proper handling of the airway and alveolar ventilation is essential for anesthesia in any patient population. In obese patients, ensuring airway patency is challenging and involves not only anesthesia induction time but also the entire process of anesthesia, including awakening and the post anesthetic recovery period. Obese patients are more susceptible to adverse ventilatory events during the entire perioperative period [1].

The advent of gastric bypass surgeries has caused anesthesia in obese patients to become more frequent, and numerous publications on the subject have emerged. This fact has led to a better understanding of the anatomical and physiological peculiarities of obese patients and their repercussions in the perioperative period. Improved knowledge about the pharmacokinetic and pharmacodynamic aspects of anesthetics and practical training for an obese population has permitted anesthesiologists to improve their clinical skills to overcome most difficulties in handling the airway and ventilation in this population.

The ASA Closed Claims 2005 [1] found that the airway-related and respiratory complications were more frequent in obese patients, especially during extubation. The 2011 NAP4 (National Audit Project of The Royal College of Anesthetists and The Difficult Airway Society) in the United Kingdom also found that complications related to supraglottic airway devices (SGD) were four times more frequent in obese patients [2].

The American Society of Anesthesiologists (ASA) defines a difficult airway (DA) as a clinical situation in which a conventionally trained anesthesiologist experiences difficulty with face-mask ventilation, difficulty with tracheal intubation, or both [3]. Difficulty with use of supraglottic airway devices (SGD), such as laryngeal masks, was also described in the same guideline. Considering this guideline of the ASA, many morbidly obese patients may have an airway management-related problem, as obesity is an independent risk factor for difficult ventilation.

Respiratory and Airway Changes in the Obese Population

The main respiratory obesity changes are due to the accumulation of adipose tissue in the chest wall, diaphragm, abdomen (visceral and abdominal wall), and in tissues adjacent to the upper airway, such as walls of the pharynx, tongue, uvula, tonsillar pillars, and tonsils [4–6].

Thoracic and abdominal fat accumulation are responsible for decreased thoracic compliance and consequent restrictive ventilatory disturbances, characterized in the obese by

A. T. Fernandes (✉) · M. P. Cerqueira
G. O. Campos
Department of Anesthesiology,
São Rafael Hospital, Salvador, Brazil

J. Ettinger et al. (eds.), *Gastric Bypass*, https://doi.org/10.1007/978-3-030-28803-7_12

decreased functional residual capacity (FRC). The residual volume (RV) usually remains normal in the obese, and decreased FRC is due to a decreased expiratory reserve volume. The sharp reduction in FRC when approaching the residual volume can trigger the early closure of distal airways in the dependent lung areas, with uncoupling of the ventilation-perfusion and hypoxemia [5].

The closure of distal airways resulting from decreased FRC, which mainly occurs in a supine position, can limit the expiratory flow and cause air trapping in dependent alveoli, and this causes the appearance of regional hyperinflation and positive pressure at the end of the expiration or intrinsic PEEP (PEEPi), which invariably increases respiratory work [7]. The use of CPAP may abolish PEEPi and thus decrease respiratory work.

Obese patients have higher oxygen consumption and increased carbon dioxide production compared to nonobese patients. This is due to increased basal metabolic activity caused by the large volume of adipose tissue, which promotes increased alveolar ventilation with the consequently increased work of breathing. Other factors contribute to increased work when breathing, such as reduction of the thoracic and abdominal compliance, and increased ventilatory drive by the presence of neurohumoral stimuli, such as leptin hormone, which is elevated in the obese [7].

Obesity can cause dynamic obstruction of the upper airway during sleep and obstructive sleep apnea (OSA). The prevalence of OSA is high in morbidly obese individuals, and the prevalence is even higher in morbidly obese men (in the United States, the prevalence ranges from 79.5% to 82.8% in men and 43.0% to 67.9% in women) [8]. In the nonobese population, the average prevalence is one-third of that found in obese patients. OSA is characterized by episodes of apnea and hypopnea (partial stoppage or a decrease in airflow despite respiratory efforts against a closed glottis) of 10 seconds or more, and these episodes occur repeatedly during sleep causing oxygen desaturation. The patency of the airway at the pharynx is dependent on transmural pressure. The continued opening of the oropharynx is guaranteed by the contraction of the palatine tensor muscle, genioglossus, and the muscles of the hyoid bone. The inspiratory diaphragmatic contraction promotes negative pressure in the oropharynx and contributes to its collapse. During sleep, and also under an anesthetic effect, the pharyngeal muscles are relaxed, and the great mass of peripharyngeal and subcutaneous fat encountered in the obese causes an increase in extraluminal pressure, which leads to occlusion of the upper airway and collapse of the pharynx. These airway changes explain why OSA is a disorder highly associated with obesity [4, 9].

Obesity and Perioperative Hypoxemia

The increase in oxygen consumption, decreased functional residual capacity, and ventilation-perfusion mismatch caused by atelectasis contribute to a higher incidence of perioperative hypoxemia, a shorter time to the onset of desaturation at the induction of anesthesia and shorter available time for airway handling or a shorter "safe apnea period" [10]. An increased susceptibility to postoperative hypoxemia with the use of opioid analgesics is also observed [4, 11].

Obesity and Risk of Gastric Contents Aspiration

Prophylaxis with H2 blockers and prokinetics has been proposed since pioneering publications that included recommendations for bariatric surgery, once obesity was considered a risk factor for regurgitation and gastric contents aspiration [12]. However, the literature is controversial on this issue. There are more recent trials that have not identified delayed emptying of the stomach or even found faster gastric emptying in the obese than in nonobese patients [13], and significant differences in the pH/gastric volume set were not observed in obese patients compared to nonobese patients [14].

Warner [15], in a retrospective study with over 172,000 patients, also found no increased risk of obesity-related aspiration of the gastric contents. Subsequently, Mahajan [16] identified lower pH and increased gastric volume, which was enough for greater risk of aspiration in the obese compared to nonobese patients undergoing surgery. A good response to prokinetics and H2 blockers was also identified. Prophylaxis for morbidly obese patients who were candidates for surgery or patients with a body mass index (BMI) above 35 with comorbidities was then considered as necessary. We believe that the prevention of aspiration with prokinetic and hydrochloric acid production blockers should always be considered for morbidly obese patients and for those with BMI >35 with comorbidities when undergoing surgery.

Obesity and Difficult Airway (DA)

A difficult airway is a broad term that includes difficult intubation of the trachea, difficult mask ventilation, and, more recently, difficulty in supraglottic device ventilation [17]. However, other factors, such as higher propensity to hypoxic phenomena with little tolerance to apnea and the possible risk of gastric contents aspiration, make the handling of difficult airways in this population a challenging task.

Dealing with airway-related problems comprises searching for the clinical predictors of a difficult airway and a strategic plan of actions to ensure safe and successful airway management. Some of these strategies have been published as algorithms. The first algorithm was published by the American Society of Anesthesiologists (ASA) in 1993. In 2005, a reduction in claims related to airway complications in the United States was observed [1], which was likely due to the publication of the ASA Difficult Airway Guidelines in 1993. The most recent algorithm by the ASA was delivered in 2013 [3]. Subsequently, other anesthesiology societies published recommendations for the management of difficult airways, and among them, the Difficult Airway Society – United Kingdom (DAS) is the most popular and most cited guideline [18]. The majority of airway guidelines is grounded in the consensus of the opinion of experts, since there are only a few controlled studies on the subject.

Airway Evaluation in the Obese

The assessment of the airway begins by anamnesis. The history of difficult intubation or ventilation is a major indicator of a difficult airway. Diseases related to the difficulty of cervical mobility, such as rheumatoid arthritis, ankylosing spondylitis, and diabetes mellitus, are associated with difficult laryngoscopy and intubation. Obstructive sleep apnea is a clinical condition that is an independent risk factor for difficulty with ventilation and intubation.

Although polysomnography is the final exam for the diagnosis of OSA, using the STOP-BANG questionnaire (Table 12.1) in the preanesthetic evaluation has high sensitivity and specificity, and as a simple tool, it is recommended in the preanesthetic evaluation of patients who have not had polysomnography performed [19, 20]. The presence of more than three criteria in the STOP-BANG questionnaire and OSA diagnosed by polysomnography is a predictor of difficult intubation, difficult mask ventilation (DMV), and complications during extubation and postanesthetic recovery [20–22].

Table 12.1 The STOP-BANG questionnaire for detecting a difficult airway

S	Snoring	More than three positive answers are associated with a difficult airway
T	Tiredness during the day	
O	Observed respiratory pause	
P	High blood pressure	
B	Body mass index kg/m^2 >35	
A	Age above 50	
N	Neck circumference >40 cm	
G	Gender – male sex	

Adapted from Toshniwal et al. [20]

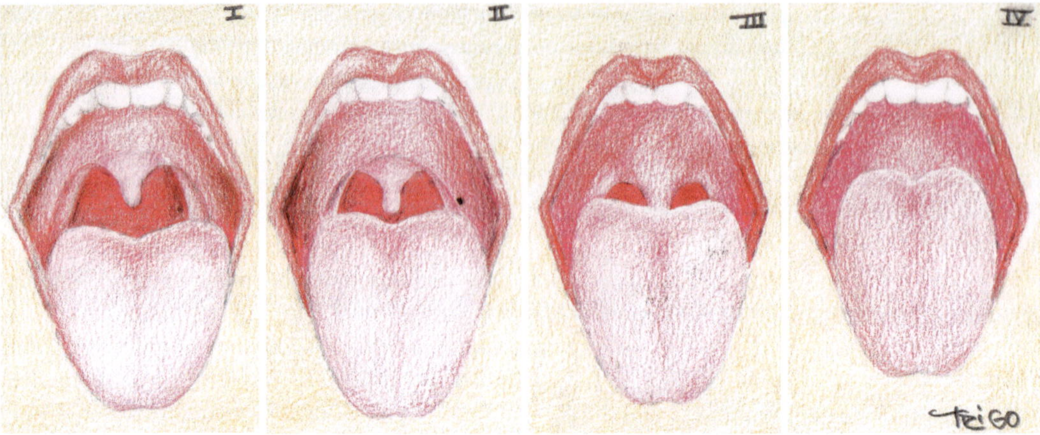

Fig. 12.1 Artistic interpretation of the Mallampati classification modified by Samsoon and Young, 1987. Class I, soft palate fauces, uvula, and pillars visible; class II, soft palate fauces and uvula visible; class III, soft palate and base of uvula visible; class IV, soft palate not visible at all

Body Mass Index (BMI)

Although described in some studies [23], the association of higher BMI and difficult intubation is quite controversial. In some studies, BMI was not an independent risk factor for difficult intubation (DI), especially those that used the Cormack-Lehane classification as a criteria for DI [24, 25]. If care was taken to establish good positioning, there was no more difficulty in intubating obese patients [25]. Nevertheless, when evaluating the difficulty of mask ventilation, the degree of obesity (higher BMI) is often considered a major risk factor. Anatomical issues that lead to an increase in airway resistance and lower thoracic compliance and diaphragmatic compression may explain this [21, 22, 26].

Mallampati Classification (MP)

Mallampati classification, modified by Samsoon and Young [27], evaluates the oropharyngeal structures by inspection with the patient in maximum mouth opening, and this can be graded from 1 to 4, as shown in Fig. 12.1. In obese population studies, patients with grade 3 or 4 MP have higher risk for DI [23, 25] and ventilation with a face mask [22].

Table 12.2 Difficult mask ventilation predictive factors [21, 22, 49, 50]

Age >48
Short neck
Neck circumference >40 cm
Limited jaw protrusion
Mallampati classification 3 or 4
Male gender
Facial hair
OSA/snoring history
Lack of teeth
BMI >34
History of difficult intubation
Neck radiation

Neck Circumference (NC)

The NC should be measured at the level of the thyroid cartilage. In obese patients, the NC is considered important criteria for DI according to several studies. It is estimated that a NC >40 cm means a 5% increase in the risk of the DI, while a NC >60 cm increases this risk by 35% [25, 28].

Other Predictors of a Difficult Airway

Other classic criteria, which are not only relevant to the obese population, should be considered in the preoperative evaluation of DA risk. Such widely cited criteria are shown in (Tables 12.2 and 12.3).

Table 12.3 Difficult intubation predictive factors [3, 20, 25]

Interincisor distance <3 cm
Relatively long upper incisors
Neck circumference >40 cm
Short neck
Limited jaw protrusion
Mallampati classification 3 or 4
Highly arched palate
OSA/STOP-BANG score >3
Neck extension limited
History of difficult intubation
Congenital or acquired deformities
Age >49 years

Difficult Supraglottic Device Ventilation Predictive Factors

Supraglottic devices, broadly represented by laryngeal masks, had their use established in the general population, and they have been proven to provide effective ventilation in elective situation as well as in the rescue of ventilation when ventilation by face mask turns impossible, especially in the obese. A failure rate of 3–5% can be anticipated in obese patients with SGD ventilation, even if second-generation devices, as the ProSeal® laryngeal mask, are used [29]. Recently, a proposal for a new scoring system to predict difficult ventilation through the SGD has been published (Table 12.4). Nevertheless, it was not a high sensitivity score, only 23%. Therefore, it can be used only as a screening aid to alert the anesthetist [30].

Table 12.4 The simplified scoring system to predict difficult ventilation through a SGD; 0–3 signified a low risk, and 4–7 signified a high risk of difficult ventilation through a SGD

Perioperative variables	Points
Male gender	1
Age >45 years	1
Short thyromental distance <5.5 cm	3
Limited neck movements	2

Adapted from Saito et al. [30]

Airway Management

During preparation for the induction of anesthesia in an obese patient, emphasis should be placed on maintaining adequate oxygenation. Strategies must be designed in accordance with the arsenal of devices and equipment available. Although the vast majority of obese patients does not represent greater difficulty in airway management compared to nonobese patients, independent of a difficult airway that has been diagnosed, some measures must be taken universally, particularly proper positioning and effective preoxygenation.

Positioning

Proper positioning is one of the most important measures for an effective direct laryngoscopy (DL). It allows the alignment of the oral and pharyngeal axis, which adds to the direct laryngoscopy maneuver and allows visualization of the laryngeal structures in most individuals. The best position described for the general population is the "sniffing position" (flexion of the lower neck to 35° using a cushion elevation and extension of the face plane to 15°) [31]. However, in obese individuals, the large fat mass can hinder the confluence of the oral and pharyngeal axis, making it a poor position for good visualization of the glottis and intubation in some patients. In the obese, "ramp" positioning, associated with elevation of the head above the chest, or the "HELP" position (head-elevated position laryngoscopy) [32] was superior to the traditional position, providing better visualization of the glottis [33]. In this postural setting, the goal is the horizontal alignment between the sternal notch and the external auditory meatus, (Fig. 12.2); thus, the necessary angle of elevation of the thorax is variable, depending on the anteroposterior distance of the chest of patients.

Once in a supine position, the obese patient will increase the volume of occlusion by decreasing the functional residual capacity, which will lead to worsening of ventilation, atelectasis, and decreased tissue oxygenation. Another advantage of ramp positioning is that it promotes significant improvement in preoxygenation and a significant increase in the safe apnea time [34] and facilitates ventilation with a face mask and use of supraglottic airway devices if necessary.

The HELP position can be achieved with use of specific devices developed by the medical industry [35], through the use of pillows and sheets, or by a specific setting of the surgical table with comparable efficacy [36], as shown in Figs. 12.2 and 12.3. Figure 12.4 shows an example of a commercial positioning device.

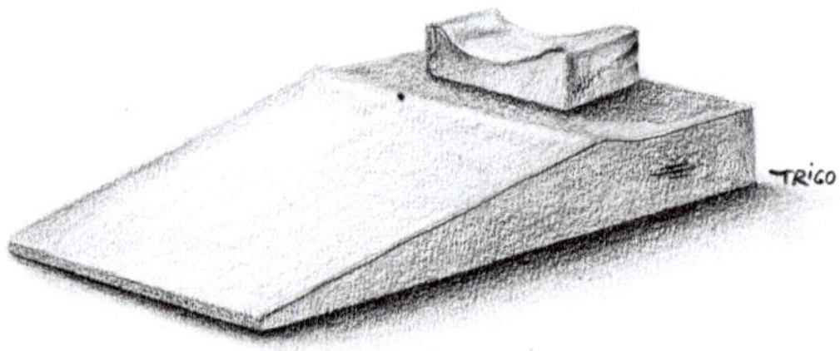

Fig. 12.2 Artistic interpretation of Troop ELEVATION pillow®, Mercury medical, a commercial device for positioning of obese patients

Preoxygenation

The use of 100% oxygen before induction of general anesthesia is formally recommended in most well-recognized airway guidelines [3, 18]. In obese patients, this practice is particularly impor-

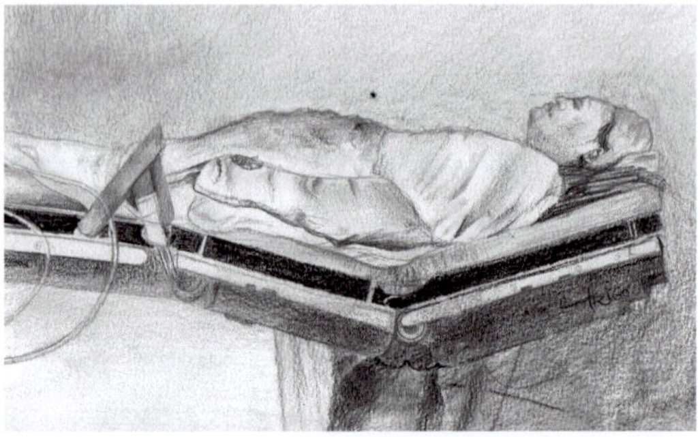

Fig. 12.4 Artistic interpretation of the correct positioning of the obese patient for airway management with the use of the surgical table setting

Fig. 12.3 Artistic interpretation of the uncorrect positioning (top) and correct positioning or HELP (bottom) of the obese patient for airway management with the use of Linens and blankets

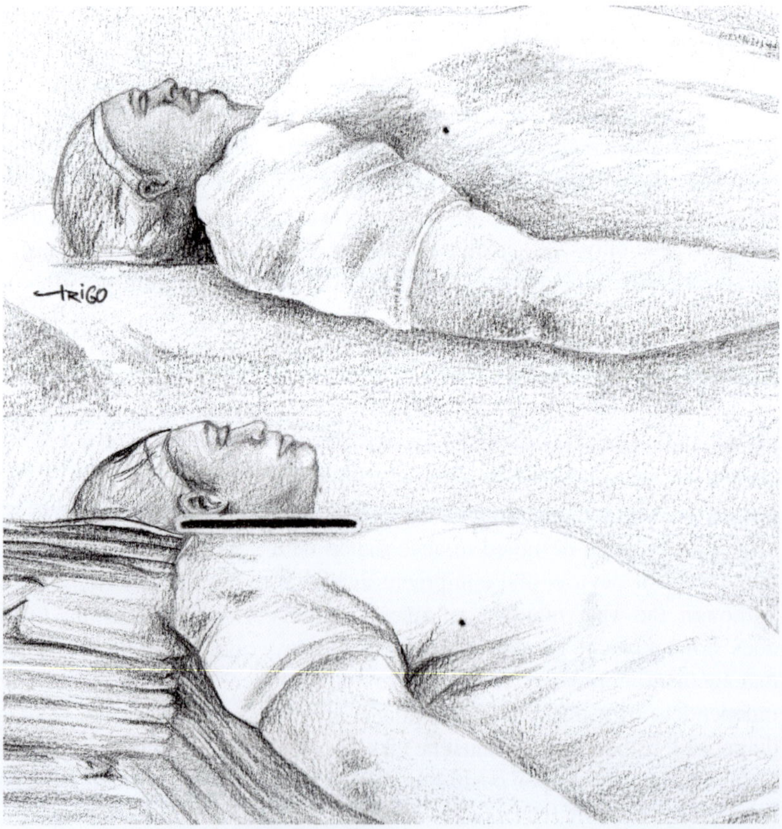

tant since this group of patients has a shorter safe apnea period due to reduced FRC. The preoxygenation with 100% oxygen lengthens the interval to onset of hypoxemia, adding precious extra time for airway management.

The use of CPAP during the induction period was effective in reducing atelectasis and increasing apnea safe time [37].

Anticipated Difficult Airway

Facing a suspected DA in an obese patient, a strategy must be developed considering the available equipment and devices as well as the technical skills of the anesthesiologist. An important part of this planning is the request for qualified help.

"Awake fiberoptic intubation" (AFI) is currently considered the gold standard for anticipated difficult airways. The use of this technique should be particularly preferred in cases where difficult mask ventilation is predicted because the spontaneous breathing of the patient will be preserved [3, 4, 38]. "Awake intubation" requires proper planning. The psychological preparation of patients, local anesthesia of the airway, and judicious and titrated use of analgesics such as fentanyl, remifentanil, dexmedetomidine, and ketamine are extremely important for the success of this procedure [39]. In obese patients, performing peripheral blocks is more time-consuming and risky due to anatomical characteristics; therefore, techniques such as topical or atomized 2% lidocaine are simpler and equally effective [40]. "Topicalization" may also be well achieved by the use of a 4% gel or 10% spray lidocaine. The positioning for AFI, either nasal or oral, may be achieved with the patient in a supine position with the head up at 45°, facing the anesthesiologist. The AFI is still the safest technique for cases of DA [3].

Another option for "awake intubation" is indirect laryngoscopy with the use of video laryngoscopes with specific blades for DA. These devices do not require optimal alignment of the oral and pharyngeal axis, allowing visualization of the glottis with less discomfort to the patient compared to conventional laryngoscopy with a Macintosh blade. The video laryngoscopes are superior to conventional laryngoscopes in obese patients [41].

Once a patient becomes uncooperative, it precludes awake techniques, and tracheal intubation of these patients can only be done after general anesthesia. In such cases, the use of video laryngoscopes can be a good option for an anticipated difficult airway as well as intubation through a laryngeal mask [42].

The emergence of supraglottic devices, especially laryngeal masks, provided excellent backup for ventilation in difficult mask ventilation patients both at the time of induction and after extubation, if airway rescue becomes necessary. Among the group of supraglottic devices, the second-generation laryngeal masks are preferred, since they have an esophageal channel that allows the placement of a gastric drainage tube; it also provides a better seal, allowing good ventilation in patients with reduced compliance and the use of PEEP. Another useful SGD for the obese is the intubating laryngeal mask (ILMA). It allows successful intubation in most obese patients while allowing ventilation [42]. The techniques that combine the use of a SGD, such as ILMA with a flexible fiberoptic for tracheal intubation, can increase the success rate of airway establishment [43].

Unanticipated Difficult Airway

Difficulty of intubation and ventilation that is not recognized in the preanesthetic evaluation is a potentially lethal situation.

The care of patients with difficult intubation and preserved ventilation aims to maintain adequate oxygenation until tracheal intubation is achieved or the patient is awakened. It is recommended that once the difficulty of intubation is identified, there is an immediate request for qualified help, and avoiding repeated attempts of laryngoscopies must be emphasized. Insistence on laryngoscopy can result in trauma to the airway, making it difficult or even completely impossible for ventilation or subsequent use of other devices.

Laryngoscopy attempts should be restricted to no more than three or four by optimizing the positioning of the head and neck, trying to change blades or use a video laryngoscope, externally manipulating the larynx, or using the elastic bougie as a guide for intubation. Some practical algorithms detail the strategies for handling this type of situation [3, 18].

The use of supraglottic airway devices takes place immediately after intubation failure to maintain ventilation. In addition to ventilation, SGD can be used as a secondary technique for intubation either by intubation laryngeal mask (ILMA) or by the use of a fiberoptic through the laryngeal mask. In the event that face mask ventilation is difficult or impossible, supraglottic devices are good choices, especially the second-generation laryngeal masks, which provide a better seal and allow gastric suctioning.

In extreme cases, when intubation or ventilation of a patient is impossible with the available techniques, even with the use of supraglottic devices, the only option is to perform emergency cricothyrotomy, a lifesaving procedure that has increased difficulty in obese patients due to the difficulty of identifying cervical structures in this group of patients [44–46].

It is important that the algorithms are adapted to local resources and that the anesthesia staff is conscious of the priorities in every typical scenario of airway management. Regular training in critical situations must be encouraged.

Planning Extubation

In 2005, the ASA Closed Claims Project noticed that the events that led to death and serious brain damage outcomes were mainly related to extubation and anesthesia recovery times, and they were more frequent in obese patients [1]. More recently, NAP4 observed that 30% of the adverse events associated with anesthesia occurred upon emergence from anesthesia and during recovery time and that obesity is the most common pathology, which was present in 45% of cases [2].

In 2011, the Difficult Airway Society published guidelines for extubation based on four fundamentals: planning, preparation, execution, and post extubation care [47]. Despite being based on the opinion of experts, as currently strong scientific evidence is unavailable, this report considers extubation as an important chapter in the management of airways. The general requirements for successful extubation are hemodynamic, metabolic and respiratory stability and normothermia (temperature >35.5 °C).

Obese patients have higher risk of airway obstruction, hypoxemia, and aspiration of gastric contents after extubation than nonobese patients. Therefore, they need proper planning for extubation to avoid major respiratory events. Airway obstruction is the most common cause of hypoxemia in obese patients during extubation and recovery from anesthesia. Airway obstruction can be caused by the loss of muscle tone, which is required for opening of the airway; laryngospasm due to the presence of secretions or blood in the airway; laryngeal edema caused by instrumental trauma during intubation; or even by a hypersensitivity reaction [2]. Failure of a neuromuscular blockade reversal has often been related to some of these postoperative events [48] as well as residual sedation by analgesics and anesthetics. The total reversal of anesthesia and neuromuscular blockade is then essential. The adequacy of spontaneous ventilation must be confirmed as well as eye-opening and the capacity to obey simple commands. Reversal of a neuromuscular blockade can be ensured if the T4/T1 train-of-four ratio is above 0.9 [48]. It is mandatory that the airway be free of blood and secretions through proper aspiration.

Instituting preoxygenation before extubation is recommended, especially if there was any difficulty in intubation or ventilation, as it ensures extra time for rescue ventilation and oxygenation if extubation failure occurs.

As suggested for induction of anesthesia, the resumption of the HELP position is also mandatory since this position enhances chest compliance and facilitates ventilation through the mask, the use of supraglottic devices, or reintubation if it becomes necessary.

Difficult airway patients should be considered high-risk patients for extubation, and placing an airway exchange catheter before extubation should be considered to serve as a reintubation guide in the case of extubation failure [4]. Patients with difficult ventilation criteria, mainly previous BiPAP/CPAP users, should maintain BiPAP/CPAP use in the post extubation period since this improves ventilation [11]. A laryngeal mask must also be available to serve as a ventilatory backup device for extubation of these patients [2]. In the remaining patients, only the "HELP" position plus oxygen supplementation through a nasal cannula, coupled with the basic measures above, is sufficient for uneventful extubation.

References

1. Peterson GN, Domino KB, Caplan RA, Posner KL, Lee LA, Cheney FW. Management of the difficult airway: a closed claims analysis. Anesthesiology [Internet]. 2005;103(1):33–9. Available from: http://www.scopus.com/inward/record.url?eid=2-s2.0-21744442282&partnerID=40&md5=83742e2a13adb7ada5e5de089e31bbe8\n, http://content.wkhealth.com/linkback/openurl?sid=WKPTLP:landingpage&an=00000542-200507000-00009
2. Cook TM, Woodall N, Frerk C, Project on behalf of the FNA. Major complications of airway management in the UK: results of the Fourth National Audit Project of the Royal College of Anaesthetists and the Difficult Airway Society. Part 1: Anaesthesia. Br J Anaesth [Internet]. Oxford University Press; 2011 May 1 [cited 2016 Aug 18];106(5):617–31. Available from: http://bja.oxfordjournals.org/lookup/doi/10.1093/bja/aer058.
3. Apfelbaum JL, Hagberg CA, Caplan RA, Blitt CD, Connis RT, Nickinovich DG, et al. Practice guidelines for management of the difficult airway: an updated report by the American Society of Anesthesiologists Task Force on Management of the Difficult Airway. Anesthesiology [Internet]. 2013;118(2):251–70. Available from: http://www.ncbi.nlm.nih.gov/pubmed/23364566
4. Aceto P, Perilli V, Modesti C, Ciocchetti P, Vitale F, Sollazzi L. Airway management in obese patients. Surg Obes Relat Dis [Internet]. 2013;9:809–15. Available from: http://ovidsp.ovid.com/ovidweb.cgi?T=JS&CSC=Y&NEWS=N&PAGE=fulltext&D=emed11&AN=2013627486, http://sfx.scholarsportal.info/uhn?sid=OVID:embase&id=pmid:&id=doi:10.1016/j.soard.2013.04.013&issn=1550-7289&isbn=&volume=9&issue=5&spage=809&pages=809-815&date=201
5. Salome CM, King GG, Berend N. Physiology of obesity and effects on lung function. J Appl Physiol. 2010;108(1):206–11.
6. Isono S. Obesity and obstructive sleep apnoea: mechanisms for increased collapsibility of the passive pharyngeal airway. Respirology. 2012;17:32–42.
7. Lin CK, Lin CC. Work of breathing and respiratory drive in obesity. Respirology. 2012;17(3):402–11.
8. Peppard PE, Young T, Barnet JH, Palta M, Hagen EW, Hla KM. Increased prevalence of sleep-disordered breathing in adults. Am J Epidemiol. 2013;177(9):1006–14.
9. Benumof JL. Obesity, sleep apnea, the airway and anesthesia. Curr Opin Anaesthesiol. 2004;17(1):21–30.
10. Jense HG, Dubin SA, Silverstein PI, O'Leary-Escolas U. Effect of obesity on safe duration of apnea in anesthetized humans. Anesth Analg [Internet]. 1991 Jan [cited 2016 Sep 7];72(1):89–93. Available from: http://www.ncbi.nlm.nih.gov/pubmed/1984382.
11. Schumann R. Anaesthesia for bariatric surgery. Best Pract Res Clin Anaesthesiol [Internet]. 2011 Mar [cited 2016 May 21];25(1):83–93. Available from: http://www.sciencedirect.com/science/article/pii/S1521689610000960.
12. Ogunnaike BO, Jones SB, Jones DB, Provost D, Whitten CW. Anesthetic considerations for bariatric surgery. Anesth Analg [Internet]. 2002;95(3):1793–805. Available from: http://www.anesthesia-analgesia.org/content/95/6/1793.short.
13. Buchholz V, Berkenstadt H, Goitein D, Dickman R, Bernstine H, Rubin M. Gastric emptying is not prolonged in obese patients. Surg Obes Relat Dis [Internet]. 2013 Sep;9(5):714–7. Available from: http://linkinghub.elsevier.com/retrieve/pii/S1550728912001013.
14. Harter RL, Kelly WB, Kramer MG, Perez CE, Dzwonczyk RR. A comparison of the volume and pH of gastric contents of obese and lean surgical patients. Anesth Analg. 1998;86:147–52.
15. Warner MA, Warner ME, Weber JG. Clinical significance of pulmonary aspiration during the perioperative period. Anesthesiology [Internet] 1993;78(1):56–62. Available from: http://www.ncbi.nlm.nih.gov/pubmed/17122571\nhttp://www.ncbi.nlm.nih.gov/pubmed/8424572.
16. Mahajan V, Hashmi J, Singh R, Samra T, Aneja S. Comparative evaluation of gastric pH and volume in morbidly obese and lean patients undergoing elective surgery and effect of aspiration prophylaxis. J Clin Anesth. 2015;27(5):396–400.
17. Apfelbaum JL, C a H, R a C, Blitt CD, Connis RT, Nickinovich DG, et al. Practice guidelines for management of the difficult airway. Anesthesiology. 2003;98(2):1269–77.
18. Frerk C, Mitchell VS, McNarry AF, Mendonca C, Bhagrath R, Patel A, et al. Difficult Airway Society 2015 guidelines for management of unanticipated difficult intubation in adults. Br J Anaesth. 2015;115:827–48.
19. Chung F, Yegneswaran B, Liao P, Chung SA, Vairavanathan S, Islam S, et al. STOP Questionnaire. Anesthesiology. 2008;108(5):812–21.

20. Toshniwal G, McKelvey GM, Wang H, Chung SA, Yuan H, Chung F, et al. STOP-Bang and prediction of difficult airway in obese patients. J Clin Anesth [Internet]. Elsevier; 2014 Aug [cited 2016 Jun 20];26(5):360–7. Available from: http://linkinghub.elsevier.com/retrieve/pii/S0952818014000968.
21. Langeron O, Masso E, Huraux C, Guggiari M, Bianchi A, Coriat P, et al. Prediction of difficult mask ventilation. Anesthesiology. 2000;92(5):1229–36.
22. Kheterpal S, Han R, Tremper KK, Shanks A, Tait AR, O'Reilly M, et al. Incidence and predictors of difficult and impossible mask ventilation. Anesthesiology. 2006;105(5):885–91.
23. Juvin P, Lavaut E, Dupont H, Lefevre P, Demetriou M, Dumoulin J-L, et al. Difficult tracheal intubation is more common in obese than in lean patients. Anesth Analg. 2003;97(2):595–600.
24. Ezri T, Medalion B, Weisenberg M, Szmuk P, Warters RD, Charuzi I. Increased body mass index per se is not a predictor of difficult laryngoscopy. Can J Anaesth. 2003;50(2):179–83.
25. Brodsky JB, Lemmens HJM, Brock-Utne JG, Vierra M, Saidman LJ. Morbid obesity and tracheal intubation. Anesth Analg [Internet]. 2002;94(3):732–6. Available from: http://content.wkhealth.com/linkback/openurl?sid=WKPTLP:landingpage&an=00000539-200203000-00047
26. Kheterpal S, Martin L, Shanks AM, Tremper KK. Prediction and outcomes of impossible mask ventilation: a review of 50,000 anesthetics. Anesthesiology. 2009;110(4):891–7.
27. Samsoon GL, Young JR. Difficult tracheal intubation: a retrospective study. Anaesthesia [Internet]. 1987 May [cited 2016 Sep 30];42(5):487–90. Available from: http://www.ncbi.nlm.nih.gov/pubmed/3592174.
28. Gonzalez H, Minville V, Delanoue K, Mazerolles M, Concina D, Fourcade O. The importance of increased neck circumference to intubation difficulties in obese patients. Anesth Analg. 2008;106(4):1132–6.
29. Nicholson A, Cook TM, Smith AF, Lewis SR, Reed SS. Supraglottic airway devices versus tracheal intubation for airway management during general anaesthesia in obese patients. Cochrane Database Syst Rev [Internet]. 2013 [cited 2016 Aug 28];(9):CD010105. Available from: http://www.ncbi.nlm.nih.gov/pubmed/24014230.
30. Saito T, Chew STH, Liu WL, Thinn KK, Asai T, Ti LK. A proposal for a new scoring system to predict difficult ventilation through a supraglottic airway. Absalom AR, editor. Br J Anaesth [Internet]. Oxford University Press; 2016 Sep [cited 2016 Aug 28];117(Suppl 1):i83–6. Available from: http://bja.oxfordjournals.org/lookup/doi/10.1093/bja/aew191.
31. Greenland KB, Edwards MJ, Hutton NJ, Challis VJ, Irwin MG, Sleigh JW. Changes in airway configuration with different head and neck positions using magnetic resonance imaging of normal airways: a new concept with possible clinical applications. Br J Anaesth [Internet]. 2010 Nov [cited 2016 Aug 27];105(5):683–90. Available from: http://www.ncbi.nlm.nih.gov/pubmed/20846964.
32. Levitan RM, Mechem CC, Ochroch EA, Shofer FS, Hollander JE. Head-elevated laryngoscopy position: improving laryngeal exposure during laryngoscopy by increasing head elevation. Ann Emerg Med. 2003;41(3):322–30.
33. Collins JS, Lemmens HJM, Brodsky JB, Brock-Utne JG, Levitan RM. Laryngoscopy and morbid obesity: a comparison of the "sniff" and "ramped" positions. Obes Surg. 2004;14(9):1171–5.
34. Dixon BJ, Dixon JB, Carden JR, Burn AJ, Schachter LM, Playfair JM, et al. Preoxygenation is more effective in the 25 degrees head-up position than in the supine position in severely obese patients: a randomized controlled study. Anesthesiology. 2005;102(6):1110–5; discussion 5A
35. Cattano D, Melnikov V, Khalil Y, Sridhar S, Hagberg CA. An evaluation of the rapid airway management positioner in obese patients undergoing gastric bypass or laparoscopic gastric banding surgery. Obes Surg [Internet]. Springer-Verlag; 2010 Oct 24 [cited 2016 Aug 27];20(10):1436–41. Available from: http://link.springer.com/10.1007/s11695-009-9885-8.
36. Rao SL, Kunselman AR, Schuler HG, DesHarnais S. Laryngoscopy and tracheal intubation in the head-elevated position in obese patients: a randomized, controlled, equivalence trial. Anesth Analg [Internet]. 2008 Dec [cited 2016 Aug 27];107(6):1912–8. Available from: http://www.ncbi.nlm.nih.gov/pubmed/19020138.
37. Gander S, Frascarolo P, Suter M, Spahn DR, Magnusson L. Positive end-expiratory pressure during induction of general anesthesia increases duration of nonhypoxic apnea in morbidly obese patients. Anesth Analg. 2005;100(2):580–4.
38. Langeron O, Birenbaum A, Le Saché F, Raux M. Airway management in obese patient. Minerva Anestesiol [Internet]. 2014;80(3):382–92. Available from: http://www.ncbi.nlm.nih.gov/pubmed/24122033
39. Vennila R, Hall A, Ali M, Bhuiyan N, Pirotta D, Raw DA. Remifentanil as single agent to facilitate awake fibreoptic intubation in the absence of premedication. Anaesthesia. 2011;66(5):368–72.
40. Wieczorek PM, Schricker T, Vinet B, Backman SB. Airway topicalisation in morbidly obese patients using atomised lidocaine: 2% compared with 4%. Anaesthesia. 2007;62(10):984–8.
41. Marrel J, Blanc C, Frascarolo P, Magnusson L. Videolaryngoscopy improves intubation condition in morbidly obese patients. Eur J Anaesthesiol [Internet]. 2007;24(12):1045–9. Available from: http://www.ncbi.nlm.nih.gov/pubmed/17608975
42. Motamed C, Brain A, Honneur GD. Intubating laryngeal mask airway in morbidly obese and lean patients: a comparative study. J Am Dent Soc Anesthesiol. 2005;102(6):1106–9.
43. Hernandez MR, Klock PA, Ovassapian A. Evolution of the extraglottic airway. Anesth Analg [Internet]. 2012 Feb [cited 2016 Aug 29];114(2):349–68. Available from: http://content.wkhealth.com/

linkback/openurl?sid=WKPTLP:landingpage&an=00000539-201202000-00016.
44. Lamb A, Zhang J, Hung O, Flemming B, Mullen T, Bissell MB, et al. Accuracy of identifying the cricothyroid membrane by anesthesia trainees and staff in a Canadian institution. Can J Anaesth. 2015;62(5):495–503.
45. You-Ten KE, Desai D, Postonogova T, Siddiqui N. Accuracy of conventional digital palpation and ultrasound of the cricothyroid membrane in obese women in labour. Anaesthesia. 2015;70(11):1230–4.
46. Langeron O, Birenbaum A, Le Saché F, Raux M. Airway management in obese patient. Minerva Anestesiol. 2014;80(3):382–92.
47. DAS extubation guidelines|Difficult Airway Society [Internet]. Available from: https://www.das.uk.com/guidelines/das-extubation-guidelines1.
48. Murphy GS, Brull SJ. Residual neuromuscular block: lessons unlearned. Part I: definitions, incidence, and adverse physiologic effects of residual neuromuscular block. Anesth Analg [Internet]. 2010 Jul [cited 2016 Sep 3];111(1):120–8. Available from: http://www.ncbi.nlm.nih.gov/pubmed/20442260.
49. Leoni A, Arlati S, Ghisi D, Verwej M, Lugani D, Ghisi P, et al. Difficult mask ventilation in obese patients: analysis of predictive factors. Minerva Anestesiol. 2014;80(2):149–57.
50. Cattano D, Katsiampoura A, Corso RM, Killoran PV, Cai C, Hagberg CA. Predictive factors for difficult mask ventilation in the obese surgical population. F1000Research. 2014;3:239.

Positioning the Bariatric Surgical Patient

13

Jay B. Brodsky

Introduction

The perioperative management of an obese patient differs in many aspects from that of a normal-weight patient undergoing a similar operation. This is especially true when positioning an obese patient for surgery [1]. Placing an obese patient in a non-physiologic position can further impair their already reduced cardiopulmonary function, often resulting in serious consequences. Proper positioning can also help to optimize airway management by increasing oxygen reserves, by facilitating bag-mask ventilation, and by improving conditions for tracheal intubation. Standard operating room tables are not safe for extremely obese patients, especially when moving the table or changing patient position during surgery. Obese patients also are more likely to suffer perioperative neurologic and muscle injuries, so special attention must be directed to insure that all pressure points are adequately padded and the patient's head, neck, and extremities are well supported. This chapter reviews important considerations for positioning obese patients during laparoscopic bariatric surgery.

J. B. Brodsky (✉)
Department of Anesthesia, Perioperative and Pain Medicine, Stanford University School of Medicine, Stanford, CA, USA
e-mail: Jbrodsky@stanford.edu

Position and Cardiopulmonary Function

Laparoscopic bariatric operations always require that the patient undergo a general anesthetic. Normally, induction of anesthesia is performed on a recumbent, often sedated, spontaneously breathing patient. This routine management approach must be avoided in obese patients.

When a patient of any size lies flat, their now dependent abdominal contents restrict diaphragmatic movement. This results in a reduction of functional residual capacity (FRC) and an increase in atelectasis [2]. These changes are markedly exaggerated in a supine obese patient. Expiratory reserve volume (ERV), a component of FRC, progressively decreases with increasing weight and body mass index (BMI) [3]. A supine, spontaneously breathing obese patient experiences proportionally greater decreases in FRC, pulmonary compliance, and larger ventilation/perfusion mismatch than a supine normal-weight patient [4]. These changes can result in reduced oxygen reserves and hypoxemia [5]. In addition, simply lying down increases venous blood return to the heart, cardiac output (CO), pulmonary blood flow, and arterial blood pressure. All these changes are magnified in the obese patient [6]. A supine obese patient will experience significant increases in metabolic oxygen demand and carbon dioxide production, combined with increases in CO and arterial and pulmonary artery pressure [7–8]. In a sedated obese patient with preexisting limited

J. Ettinger et al. (eds.), *Gastric Bypass*, https://doi.org/10.1007/978-3-030-28803-7_13

physiologic reserves, simply assuming the supine position can lead to acute fatal cardiorespiratory failure ("obesity supine death syndrome") [9–10].

Position and Safe Apnea Period (SAP)

A spontaneously breathing obese patient should never lie flat but should always be in a head-elevated position. A head-elevated position will "unload" the weight of the intra-abdominal contents from the diaphragm, in turn increasing pulmonary compliance and FRC and improving oxygenation [11].

Prior to induction of general anesthesia, obese patients in a head-elevated position should be pre-oxygenated with 100% oxygen until their oxyhemoglobin saturation (S_pO_2) is 100% and their end-tidal O_2 is >90%. Even after pre-oxygenation, the obese patient can still experience very rapid S_pO_2 desaturation due to their increased metabolic demands coupled with their limited oxygen reserves.

Since hypoxemia during induction of general anesthesia must be avoided, the duration of the obese patient's "safe apnea period" (SAP) must be increased as much as possible. The SAP is the length of time between onset of apnea following administration of a neuromuscular blocking agent until S_pO_2 falls to 90% or 92%. If there is difficulty with bag-mask ventilation or with tracheal intubation, prolonging the SAP will delay the onset of hypoxemia allowing more time to safely secure the airway.

Strategies to increase SAP start with appropriate patient positioning prior to induction of anesthesia. As previously noted, the usual supine position must always be avoided.

In one study morbidly obese patients were pre-oxygenated in either the supine or sitting position. Following paralysis both groups were placed supine for tracheal intubation [12]. After successful intubation the still apneic, non-ventilated patients remained supine until their S_pO_2 decreased to 90%. SAP was significantly longer (214 +/– 28 seconds) in patients initially pre-oxygenated while sitting compared to those who were supine during pre-oxygenation (162 +/– 38 seconds). To increase SAP, pre-oxygenation should always be performed in a head-elevated position, and the obese patient should remain in that position for tracheal intubation [13].

Which head-elevated position maximizes SAP? In another study super-obese patients (average BMI >56 kg/m^2) were pre-oxygenated in three different positions. Group 1 patients were flat with the OR table tilted 30° in reverse Trendelenburg, Group 2 patients were in the conventional supine position with the OR table flat, and Group 3 patients were in a 30° "back-up" Fowler position [14]. SAP was 178 +/– 55 seconds (Group 1), 123 +/– 24 seconds (Group 2), and 153 +/– 63 seconds (Group 3). SAP was longest, and S_pO_2 dropped the least and recovered to 97% fastest in patients on an OR table in 30° reverse Trendelenburg (Fig. 13.1).

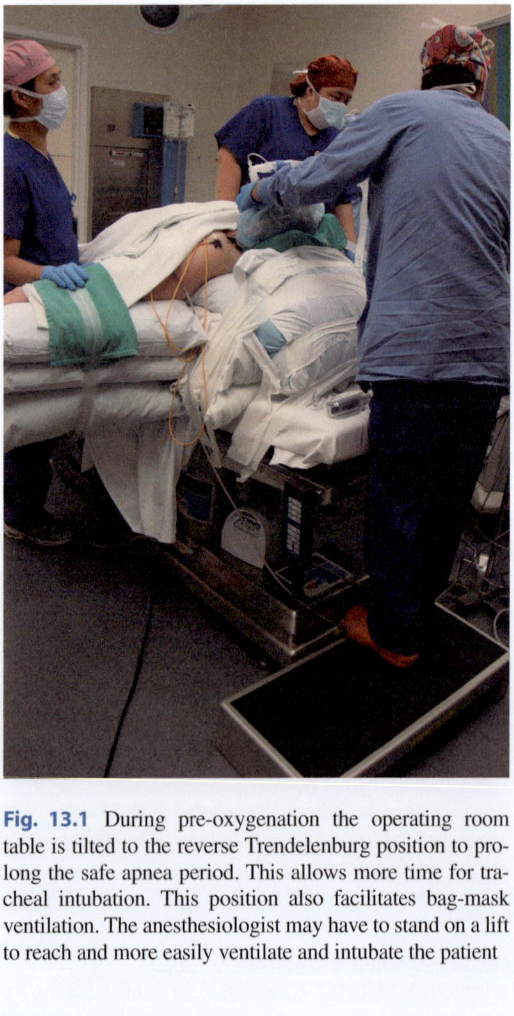

Fig. 13.1 During pre-oxygenation the operating room table is tilted to the reverse Trendelenburg position to prolong the safe apnea period. This allows more time for tracheal intubation. This position also facilitates bag-mask ventilation. The anesthesiologist may have to stand on a lift to reach and more easily ventilate and intubate the patient

Unless there is an increased risk for aspiration of gastric contents, bag-mask ventilation with 100% oxygen should be continued prior to laryngoscopy once the obese patient is rendered apneic. In addition to lengthening SAP, tilting the operating room table in reverse Trendelenburg will also facilitate bag-mask ventilation [15]. Although a patient in the reverse Trendelenburg position could potentially experience hypotension from venous pooling, in the absence of significant hypovolemia, no adverse cardiovascular changes have been reported with induction of anesthesia in that position.

Applying positive pressure mask ventilation can increase SAP by as much as 50% in morbidly obese patients [16]. Morbidly obese patients ventilated for 5 minutes before laryngoscopy with a ProSeal™ laryngeal mask airway (LMA) were compared to supine patients ventilated by facemask. After paralysis, SAP (defined as S_pO_2 = 92%) was 205 seconds (range 96–320) with bag-mask ventilation compared to 337 seconds (range 176–456) with the LMA [17].

Position and Direct Laryngoscopy

The tracheas of most obese patients can be successfully intubated using direct laryngoscopy [18–19]. The laryngoscopist's view of the vocal cords can be significantly improved when the obese patient's head, shoulders, and upper body are elevated (or "ramped") so that an imaginary horizontal line can be drawn from their sternum to their ear ("head-elevated laryngoscopy position", HELP) [20]. Improving laryngeal exposure reduces the time needed for successful tracheal intubation, potentially reducing the risk of hypoxemia in obese patients with short SAPs [21]. HELP also increases pulmonary compliance, thus further facilitating bag-mask ventilation. HELP has now become the standard position for direct laryngoscopy of obese patients [22].

HELP can be achieved with towels, blankets, and/or pillows placed under the patient's head, back, and shoulders (Fig. 13.2). Specially designed elevation pillows and other adjuncts are also commercially available [23–24]. Inflatable

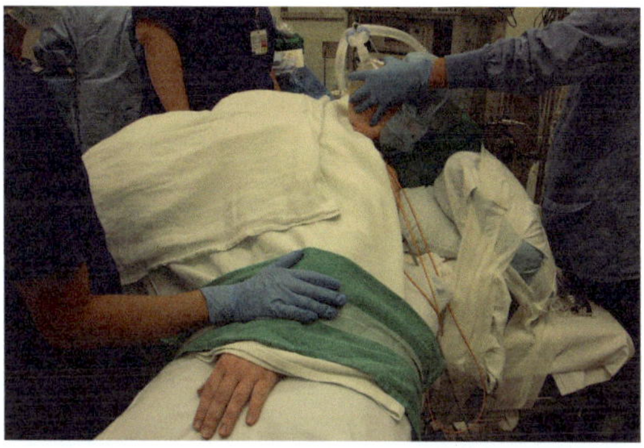

Fig. 13.2 Prior to the induction of anesthesia, the obese patient is placed in the "head-elevated laryngoscopy position" to facilitate the laryngoscopist's view of the vocal cords during direct laryngoscopy. Although special elevation devices are commercially available to ramp the head and upper body, pillows and towels can be used (as illustrated). All pressure points are padded, and the extremities are supported by pillows to prevent injury

devices allow initial HELP for intubation, can then be deflated during surgery, and re-inflated at the completion of the procedure prior to tracheal extubation [25–26]. HELP can also be achieved by flexing a flat OR table at the trunk-thigh hinge and raising only the back portion of the table, eliminating the expense of purchasing special positioning devices [27].

Position During Laparoscopic Bariatric Surgery

Once anesthetized, the patient's position may need to be changed to supine, lithotomy, Trendelenburg, or reverse Trendelenburg for surgical exposure. Spontaneously breathing morbidly obese patients do not tolerate any of these positions so assisted mechanical ventilation must always be provided. Supraglottic airways have been used during gynecologic laparoscopic procedures [28]. However, there is a high incidence of hypoxemia and gastric aspiration in obese patients ventilated with supraglottic airways [29], so an endotracheal tube is recommended [30].

Obese patients tolerate a head-down position even less than they do the supine position (Fig. 13.3). In Trendelenburg there is an autotransfusion of blood from the lower extremities

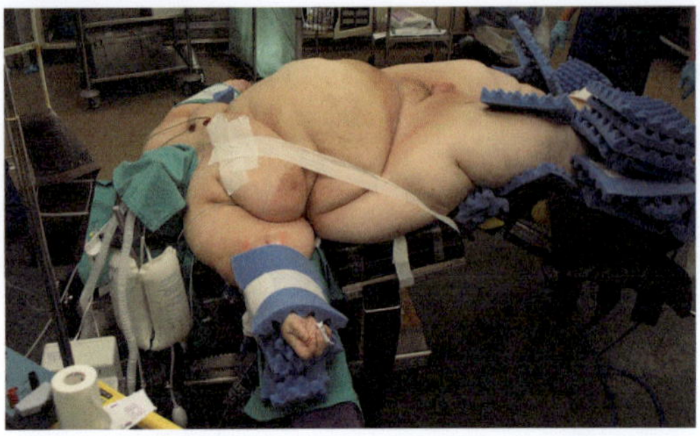

Fig. 13.3 With the operating room table tilted to the Trendelenburg position, there is a further decrease in lung volume leading to increased atelectasis and hypoxemia. Abdominal insufflation for laparoscopy combined with this position can cause displacement of the endotracheal tube into the right main bronchus

to the central and pulmonary circulation. The additional weight of the abdominal contents pressing on the diaphragm decreases total compliance and FRC even further, which in turn leads to increased atelectasis and hypoxemia. The combination of general anesthesia, laparoscopy with carbon dioxide pneumoperitoneum, and a 25°–30° Trendelenburg position increases central venous pressure, pulmonary capillary wedge pressure, and pulmonary arterial pressures and decreases cardiac output [31].

Abdominal insufflation for laparoscopy combined with changes in OR table position can also cause displacement of the endotracheal tube [32]. Advancement into the right bronchus can occur with the Trendelenburg position, and this causes a further reduction in pulmonary compliance and oxygenation.

The reverse Trendelenburg position generally improves ventilation and oxygenation during bariatric surgery [33]. This effect is less pronounced in older, obese male patients, presumably because central fat impedes diaphragmatic unloading. Addition of positive end-expiratory pressure (PEEP) can also improve oxygenation. Both PEEP and reverse Trendelenburg can reduce CO, but the hemodynamic effects are usually not clinically important [34].

Patient positioning can affect the surgical workspace. During laparoscopy the volume of intra-abdominal carbon dioxide was measured in morbidly obese patients. Five patient positions were studied. In Group 1 the OR table was horizontal with the patient supine; in Group 2 the OR table was in 20° reverse Trendelenburg with the patient's legs flat; in Group 3 the OR table was in 20° reverse Trendelenburg with the patient's legs flexed 45° upward at the hips (beach chair position); in Group 4 the OR table was flat with the patient's legs flexed 45° upward at the hips; and in Group 5 the OR table was in 20° Trendelenburg with the patient's legs flat. By increasing the workspace (i.e., greater volume), the Trendelenburg position was felt to be superior for lower abdominal exposure during laparoscopy, and the reverse Trendelenburg position with flexion of the legs at the hips was better for upper abdominal surgery [35].

If hemodynamically stable at the completion of surgery, the trachea should be extubated with the patient in a 30°–45° head-elevated position. The obese patient should then be transferred from the operating room either sitting or with the bed tilted in reverse Trendelenburg.

During the first postoperative 48 hours, especially after open abdominal surgery, the obese patient should never be supine but should recover in a semi-recumbent position to maximize arterial oxygenation [36].

Position and Injury

Obese patients are more likely to suffer physical injuries during surgery than normal-weight patients. Conventional OR equipment is not designed to accommodate the heavier patients now undergoing bariatric operations. OR tables become unstable and can tip over, especially when unlocked, and patients have been seriously injured after falling from tables during surgery [37].

Muscle breakdown (rhabdomyolysis, (RML)) occurs after long duration procedures when an obese patient is placed on a firm OR table [38]. Padding of all dependent pressure points is essential during operations of any length to reduce the chance of injury [39–40]. Although the majority of RML cases are subclinical and asymptomatic, fulminant RML with renal failure, compartment syndrome, neurologic injury, or even cardiac arrest and death have been reported. Maintaining adequate renal perfusion with intravenous fluids and diuretics, limiting the duration of surgery, and changing patient position both intra- and postoperatively may reduce the incidence of RML. A complete discussion of RML is found in another chapter in this book.

As with muscle injury, the incidence of skin pressure sores and neural compression injuries during surgery is higher in obese patients than in normal-weight patients [41]. For the diabetic obese patient, these risks are even greater. Prior to the induction of anesthesia, all potential pressure sites must be adequately padded and the padding maintained throughout the entire procedure.

Increased intra-abdominal pressure during laparoscopic surgery with the patient in reverse Trendelenburg can reduce femoral blood flow and increase venous stasis, in turn increasing the already high risk of pulmonary embolism [42]. The leg supports used during lithotomy can cause increases in intra-compartment pressure in the calf or knee compromising circulation. Because of the heavier weight of their lower extremities, obese patients in the lithotomy position are at increased risk for compartment syndrome [43]. The longer the patient is in lithotomy, the greater the chances of developing a lower extremity neuropathy or compartment syndrome.

Proper support to the arms and legs is essential to avoid stretch injury to nerves and joints. Bilateral brachial plexopathy has been reported during laparoscopic bariatric surgery, especially when the patient is placed in the reverse Trendelenburg position without proper arm supports [44].

Conclusion

Careful attention to patient position is extremely important during bariatric surgery. Spontaneously breathing obese patients should never be allowed to lie flat, whether prior to anesthetic induction, during surgery while anesthetized, or in the immediate postoperative period. Placing the OR table in reverse Trendelenburg increases the duration of SAP and facilitates bag-mask assisted ventilation. Ramping the upper body and head (HELP) improves the laryngoscopist's view, which in turn improves conditions for successful tracheal intubation. During laparoscopic surgery with a pneumoperitoneum, patient position can significantly affect cardiac and pulmonary function. Dependent pressure points must always be fully padded, and proper support of arms and legs must be maintained to avoid RML, pressure sores, and neurologic injuries.

References

1. Brodsky JB. Positioning the morbidly obese patient for anesthesia. Obes Surg. 2002;12:751–8.
2. Ike GM, Chan TC, Neuman T, et al. Spirometry in normal subjects in sitting, prone, and supine positions. Respir Care. 2000;45:407–10.
3. Biring MS, Lewis MI, Liu JI, et al. Pulmonary physiologic changes of morbid obesity. Am J Med Soc. 1999;318:293–7.
4. Pelosi P, Croci M, Ravagnan I, et al. Respiratory system mechanics in sedated, paralyzed, morbidly obese patients. J Appl Physiol. 1997;82:811–8.
5. Ferretti A, Giampiccolo P, Cavalli A, et al. Expiratory flow limitation and orthopnea in massively obese subjects. Chest. 2001;119:1401–8.
6. Alexander JK. Obesity and cardiac performance. Am J Cardiol. 1964;14:860–5.
7. Paul DR, Hoyt JL, Boutrous AR. Cardiovascular and respiratory changes in response to change in posture in the very obese. Anesthesiology. 1976;45:73–7.
8. Yap JC, Watson RA, Gilbey S, et al. Effects of posture on respiratory mechanics in obesity. J Appl Physiol. 1995;79:1199–205.
9. Tsueda K, Debrand M, Zeok SS, et al. Obesity supine death syndrome: reports of two morbidly obese patients. Anesth Analg. 1979;58:345–7.
10. Lemyze M, Guerry MJ, Mallat J, et al. Obesity supine death syndrome revisited. Eur Respir J. 2012;40:568–9.
11. Perilli V, Sollazzi L, Bozza P, et al. The effects of the reverse Trendelenburg position on respiratory mechanics and blood gases in morbidly obese patients during bariatric surgery. Anesth Analg. 2000;91:1520–5.
12. Altermatt FR, Munoz HR, Delfino AE, et al. Pre-oxygenation in the obese patient: effects of position on tolerance to apnoea. Br J Anaesth. 2005;95:706–9.
13. Dixon BJ, Dixon JB, Carden JR, et al. Preoxygenation is more effective in the 25° head-up position than in the supine position in severely obese patients. Anesthesiology. 2005;102:1110–5.
14. Boyce JR, Ness T, Castroman P, et al. A preliminary study of the optimal anesthesia positioning for the morbidly obese patient. Obes Surg. 2003;13:4–9.

15. De Jong A, Futier E, Millott A, et al. How to preoxygenate in operative room: healthy subjects and situations “at risk”. Ann Fr Anesth Reanim. 2014;33:457–61.
16. Gander S, Frascarolo P, Suter M, et al. Positive end-expiratory pressure during induction of general anesthesia increases duration of nonhypoxic apnea in morbidly obese patients. Anesth Analg. 2005;100:580–4.
17. Sinha A, Jayaraman L, Punhani D. ProSeal™ LMA increases safe apnea period in morbidly obese patients undergoing surgery under general anesthesia. Obes Surg. 2013;23:580–4.
18. Keller C, Brimacombe J, Kleinsasser A, et al. The Laryngeal Mask Airway ProSeal ™ as a temporary ventilatory device in grossly and morbidly obese patients before laryngoscope-guided tracheal intubation. Anesth Analg. 2002;94:737–40.
19. Brodsky JB, Lemmens HJ, Brock-Utne JG, et al. Morbid obesity and tracheal intubation. Anesth Analg. 2002;94:732–6.
20. Collins JS, Lemmens HJ, Brodsky JB, et al. Laryngoscopy and morbid obesity: a comparison of the “sniff” and “ramped” positions. Obes Surg. 2004;14:1171–5.
21. Brodsky JB, Lemmens HJ, Brock-Utne JG, et al. Anesthetic considerations for bariatric surgery: proper positioning is important for laryngoscopy. Anesth Analg. 2003;96:1841–2.
22. Schumann R. Anaesthesia for bariatric surgery. Best Pract Res Clin Anaesthesiol. 2011;25:83–93.
23. Rich JM. Use of an elevation pillow to produce the head-elevated laryngoscopy position for airway management in morbidly obese and large-framed patients. Anesth Analg. 2004;98:264–5.
24. Wong AB, Moore MSR. Positioning of obese patients in out-of-operating room locations. Anesth Analg. 2007;104:1306.
25. Nissen MD, Gayes JM. An inflatable, multichambered upper body support for the placement of the obese patient in the head-elevated laryngoscopy position. Anesth Analg. 2007;104:1305–6.
26. Cattano D, Melnikov V, Khalil Y, et al. An evaluation of the rapid airway management positioner in obese patients undergoing gastric bypass or laparoscopic gastric banding surgery. Obes Surg. 2010;20:1436–41.
27. Rao SL, Kunselman AR, Schuler HG, et al. Laryngoscopy and tracheal intubation in the head-elevated position in obese patients: a randomized, controlled, equivalence trial. Anesth Analg. 2008;107:1912–8.
28. Cooper RM. The LMA, laparoscopic surgery and the obese patient – can vs should. Can J Anaesth. 2003;50:5–10.
29. Cook TM, Woodall N, Frerk C. Fourth National Audit Project. Major complications of airway management in the UK: results of the Fourth National Audit Project of the Royal College of Anaesthetists and the Difficult Airway Society. Part 1: anaesthesia. Br J Anaesth. 2011;106:617–31.
30. Nightingale CE, Cousins J, Fox WT, et al. Comment on Fourth National Audit Project from the Society of Bariatric Anaesthetists. Br J Anaesth. 2011;107:272–3.
31. Hirvonen EA, Nuutinen LS, Kauko M. Hemodynamic changes due to Trendelenburg positioning and pneumoperitoneum during laparoscopic hysterectomy. Acta Anaesthesiol Scand. 1995;39:949–55.
32. Ezri T, Hazin V, Warters D, et al. The endotracheal tube moves more often in obese patients undergoing laparoscopy compared with open abdominal surgery. Anesth Analg. 2003;96:278–82.
33. Perilli V, Sollazzi L, Modesti C, et al. Determinants of improvement in oxygenation consequent to reverse Trendelenburg position in anesthetized morbidly obese patients. Obes Surg. 2004;14:866–7.
34. Perilli V, Sollazzi L, Modesti C, et al. Comparison of positive end-expiratory pressure with reverse Trendelenburg position in morbidly obese patients undergoing bariatric surgery: effects on hemodynamics and pulmonary gas exchange. Obes Surg. 2003;13:605–9.
35. Mulier JP, Dillemans B, Van Cauwenberge S. Impact of the patient’s body position on the intraabdominal workspace during laparoscopic surgery. Surg Endosc. 2010;24:1398–402.
36. Vaughan RW, Wise L. Postoperative arterial blood gas measurement in obese patients: effect of position on gas exchange. Ann Surg. 1975;182:705–9.
37. Booth RT, McAllister RK, Bittenbinder TM. Table tipping and a near-miss fall after unlocking a surgical table holding a morbidly obese patient. Proc (Baylor Univ Med Cent). 2016;29:145–6.
38. Ettinger JE, dos Santos PV Jr, Azari E, et al. Prevention of rhabdomyolysis in bariatric surgery. Obes Surg. 2005;15:874–9.
39. Bostanjian D, Anthone GJ, Hamoui N, et al. Rhabdomyolysis of gluteal muscles leading to renal failure: a potentially fatal complication of surgery in the morbidly obese. Obes Surg. 2003;13:302–5.
40. Pereira B, Heath D. Gluteal compartment syndrome following bariatric surgery: a rare but important complication. Ann Med Surg (Lond). 2015;4:64–6.
41. Gorecki PJ, Cottam D, Ger R, et al. Lower extremity compartment syndrome following a laparoscopic Roux-en-Y gastric bypass. Obes Surg. 2002;12:289–91.
42. Nguyen NT, et al. Duplex ultrasound assessment of femoral venous flow during laparoscopic and open gastric bypass. Surg Endosc. 2003;17:285–90.
43. Mizuni J, Takahashi T. Male sex, height, weight, and body mass index can increase external pressure to calf region using knee-crutch-type leg holder system in lithotomy position. Ther Clin Risk Manag. 2016;12:305–12.
44. Brunette KE, Hutchinson DO, Ismail H. Bilateral brachial plexopathy following laparoscopic bariatric surgery. Anaesth Intensive Care. 2005;33:812–5.

Developing the Laparoscopic Gastric Bypass

14

Cássio Renato Montenegro de Lima

Bariatric surgery remains the only effective and enduring treatment for morbid obesity. Since 1997, the number of bariatric surgical procedures in the United States has grown sevenfold as evidence has proven their safety and efficacy. Roux-en-Y gastric bypass (RYGB), which accounts for 88% of bariatric procedures in the United States, is considered a restrictive and malabsorptive procedure [1].

Gastric bypass has become the gold standard procedure in bariatric surgery. Mason and Ito [2] in 1967 developed the principles of gastric bypass surgery, as a variation of the Bilroth II reconstruction used after antrectomy in the treatment of peptic ulcer disease. They noticed that women were often underweight after this procedure.

Number of factors had led to the rising of bariatric surgery procedures, including technologic advances, like the introduction of laparoscopic approaches, that have improved safety, as well as shorter hospital stays [3]. In addition to technologic advances, increased awareness of the procedure among patients and physicians, media attention, celebrity patients' stories [4], and greater access through increased coverage by health insurance companies and third-party payers [5] have influenced the continued rise in bariatric surgical procedures since the first operations were introduced in the 1950s.

C. R. M. de Lima (✉)
Secretary of Health of Santa Catarina State, Florianópolis, Brazil

Bariatric surgery results in significant perioperative complications. A laparoscopic approach has significant potential to reduce perioperative complications and recovery time.

Since the introduction of laparoscopic cholecystectomy in the late 1980s, much has been learned about the profoundly positive impact of laparoscopic surgery on reducing perioperative complications. Patients undergoing bariatric surgery generally have more comorbidities and require more extensive incisions to complete the surgical procedure, compared with patients undergoing cholecystectomy. Because they are more vulnerable to cardiopulmonary and wound-related complications, laparoscopic access for bariatric surgery has a greater impact on reducing the perioperative complications related to the conventional access incision [6].

The popularity of the laparoscopic methodology for the performance of abdominal operations was extended to gastric bypass [7] and is now utilized in approximately 90% of gastric bypass procedures. The anatomic aspects of the gastric bypass itself are essentially the same as for open gastric bypass. Numerous high-quality studies have demonstrated the efficacy and safety of the procedure [8].

The advantages of the laparoscopic method are numerous and include reduced postoperative pain, decreased impairment due to pulmonary complications, faster recovery, diminished parameters of systemic injury, and a dramatic reduction in the frequency of wound infection and delayed ventral hernias [9].

J. Ettinger et al. (eds.), *Gastric Bypass*, https://doi.org/10.1007/978-3-030-28803-7_14

Laparoscopic gastric bypass is a technically feasible procedure, which can be accomplished with acceptable morbidity, reasonable operating times, and excellent clinical results. It deserves a place in the operative repertoire of modern bariatric surgeons [10].

The surgical community has also altered their perception of bariatric surgery. Advanced laparoscopy is now a growing field among surgical residents who are graduating [11]. For its minimally invasive approach, many patients and referring physicians incorrectly assume that bariatric surgery is linked to a minimal risk and is an easy solution to obesity, but bariatric surgery still has complications. It is important to seek additional training in bariatric laparoscopic surgery, like workshops and fellowships [12].

The gastric bypass operation for the treatment of morbid obesity was initially consisted of a loop gastrojejunostomy and a stapled pouch of approximately 10% of gastric volume. During the past years, numerous investigators have introduced modifications, including a Roux-en-Y gastrojejunostomy to prevent bile reflux, a reinforced staple line or an isolated gastric pouch to prevent disruption, a smaller pouch (15–30 mL), various lengths of Roux limb segments, and various types of banded pouch outlets [6].

The first laparoscopic approach to Roux-en-Y gastric bypass (LRYGB) was described by Wittgrove et al. [13]. They created a 15- to 30-mL gastric pouch isolated from the distal stomach, a 21-mm stapled, circular anastomosis, a 75-cm retrocolic, retrogastric Roux limb, and a stapled side-to-side jejunojenostomy. They developed a six-trocar technique.

The results were excellent, with a 500-patient study showing a 73% rate of excess body weight loss at 54 months. The overall complication rate was less than 10%, with a leakage rate about 2.2%, and comparable to the open procedure at that time [7].

Some bariatric surgeons require their patients to lose additional weight through diet and exercise between the time of initial bariatric surgery consultation and the date of operation. The laparoscopic approach is technically more difficult in superobese patients, especially those with extensive abdominal fat. This additional required preoperative weight loss is not correlated with comorbidity resolution or complication rates but is associated with shorter operative times and greater weight loss at 1 year after the surgery; therefore, it should be encouraged in all patients [14, 15].

Edholm et al. demonstrated that preoperative 4-week low-calorie diet reduces liver volume and intrahepatic fat and facilitates laparoscopic gastric bypass in morbidly obese, because it helps in the visualization of the area around the gastro-oesophageal junction, where the most complicated parts of the procedure is done [16].

The laparoscopic approach is technically challenging but with experience can be mastered. As with most complex laparoscopic procedures, the learning curve is steep, with long operating times [6], requiring stapling, handling of the small bowel, and construction of anastomoses. Wittgrove et al. [13] have found that with experience, operating times can be reduced to close to those for open RYGB.

Not only the surgeon but the whole team needs to be familiar with the special setting [17]. Stepaniak et al. [18] found that working with fixed teams, the duration of the laparoscopic bariatric surgery can be reduced, improving teamwork and safety climate.

Gastric bypass has evolved over the 30 years following its initial description to include multiple modifications.

In modern version, patient is placed supine in a gentle reverse Trendelenburg position.

To access the abdominal cavity, most bariatric surgeons use the established safe technique of placement of a bladeless optical view trocar with direct visualization by a laparoscope at Palmer's point, in favor of the periumbilical access location. Pneumoperitoneum (15–18 mmHg) can also be created using the Veress needle technique. Abiding by minimally invasive surgical principles, the four remaining trocars are placed in an arc pattern. Minor variations in trocar size and location are determined by surgical technique, patient body habitus, and stapling device to be used [19].

The size of the gastric pouch has gradually been reduced to the present 20–30-mL capacity. The gastric pouch is most commonly constructed by dividing the stomach to avoid potential creation of gastrogastric fistula. The development of devices that staple and divide the stomach simultaneously facilitated this advancement [8].

A small gastric pouch is believed to facilitate long-term weight loss and reduce the frequency of anastomotic ulcers in the acid-vulnerable jejunal mucosa [17].

Biliopancreatic limb of jejunum is confectioned typically 30–60 cm in length in most LRYGB procedures. This limb extends from the ligament of Treitz to the jejunojenostomy, which is the point at which the nutrient stream, the bile, and pancreatic secretions come together [8].

The Roux-en-Y limb may be transmitted to the small gastric pouch either anterior or posterior to the colon and stomach. Various lengths of small intestine have been used for construction of the Roux-en-Y limb.

Alimentary limb extends from the gastrojejunostomy to the jejunojenostomy. This limb transmits the ingested nutrients in the absence of bile and pancreatic juice. The length of this limb is typically 75–150 cm, although longer lengths may be used. A Roux or alimentary limb >150 cm is referred to as a long limb or distal gastric bypass, in an effort to achieve maximum outcomes of excess body weight loss.

Common channel is the remainder of the small bowel from the jejunojenostomy distally to the ileocecal valve. The length of this segment of bowel is typically not measured and is highly variable depending on the total length of the small bowel. The common channel usually constitutes the majority of the small bowel [8, 19].

There are varying techniques been performed to the construction of the anastomosis, including circular and linear stapler, or a totally hand-sewn gastrojejunal anastomosis. Roux limb can be transmitted by an antecolic or retrocolic orientation, and usually a stapled jejunojenostomy with hand-sewn common enterotomy closure is done. Other techniques used to perform jejunojenostomy are the double staple, which uses a stapled closure of the common enterotomy, and triple staple, involving both proximal and distal firing of linear stapling device with stapled closure of the common enterotomy [19].

Retrocolic orientation, which is the transmission of the Roux-en-Y limb to the small gastric pouch posterior to the colon, can be used and may reduce tension on the gastrojejunostomy anastomosis but has been associated with a significant increase in the internal hernia rate [20].

In antecolic technique, it is important to divide the omentum using an energy device, which reduces tension on gastrojejunal anastomosis [19].

Several methods to decrease leakage have been described, including staple line oversewing, fibrin glue and sealant application, and staple line reinforcements [21–23], but there is no prospective randomized evidence to suggest any method is effective [19].

Most bariatric surgeons use a form of intraoperative leak testing that allows for immediate repair [19]. There are two more commonly used techniques: blue dye instillation or air insufflation via endoscope or orogastric tube. In case of leak, the repair should be done and the leak test repeated. Routine drain placement at the gastrojejunal anastomosis is debated with proponents noting ability to diagnose and control leak [24] and opponents noting no benefit and potential increase in leak rate [19, 25].

Madan et al. [26] performed an online survey of American Society for Bariatric Surgery practicing surgeons and found that the percentage of those using the circular stapler, linear stapler, and hand sewing was 43%, 41%, and 21% for the gastrojejunal technique. Most surgeons (93%) routinely test the gastrojejunal intraoperatively, and 95% do not place a band around the pouch.

Studies have shown that hand-sewn gastrojejunostomy increased technical demand and operative time [17]. Linear stapler technique can reduce the frequency of strictures and surgical wound infections. A meta-analysis of comparative studies concluded that linear stapler technique may be safer than circular in gastrojejunal anastomosis for LRYGB [27].

Closure of the mesenteric defect is routine for most surgeons performing gastric bypass today. The three common sites of internal herniation are the mesojejunal site, trans-mesocolic associated with retrocolic Roux limb passage, and in the potential space between the Roux limb and the transverse mesocolon, also known as Petersen's hernia [19]. As the formation of adhesions is reduced compared to open surgery, the small bowel is more prone to slide into the opening [17]. Nonclosure and loss of mesenteric fat owing to postoperative weight loss can lead to mesojejunal herniation, the most common type [28].

Internal hernias are a significant cause of late complications (0.4–14.4%) [29]. They often present with vague symptoms, and computed tomography scanning has low sensitivity for diagnosis [30]. This finding can lead to delayed diagnosis, bowel strangulation, anastomotic dehiscence, gastric remnant dilation, and death [31].

The incidence of port site herniation is less than 2%. Closure should be attempted, usually with 0-absorbable suture passing device under laparoscopic visualization at the umbilicus and at any enlarged or dilated sites, although there is currently no evidence to support routine fascial closure in obese patients [19, 32].

Performing laparoscopic gastric bypass in public university hospitals has been difficult due to the high cost of the surgical staplers. This fact induced to look for different technical options, with low cost, maintaining the efficacy. LRYGB is viable with low cost; however, it is complex and requires ability mainly in laparoscopic hand-sewn sutures [33].

The weight loss results with LRYGB are very good to excellent, with patients now out to "long-term" follow-up. Resolution of the comorbidities is documented. The operation has an adequate track record to show effectiveness, and training programs should be established to maximize safety [7].

There are multiple complications associated with the LRYGB, including bleeding, infection, marginal ulceration, anastomotic leak, anastomotic stenosis or stricture, hypopharyngeal or esophageal injury, omental torsion or necrosis, pulmonary embolus, death, development of symptomatic cholelithiasis, inadequate weight loss, nutritional deficiencies, and symptomatic dumping syndrome [19].

Mortality was found to be lower for laparoscopic procedures than for open surgery, 0.16% and 0.41%, respectively [34].

In a study by Puzziferri et al. [9], the weight loss was similar between laparoscopic and open gastric bypass patients at 3-year (77% for laparoscopic versus 67% for open) and 4-year (76% for laparoscopic versus 71% for open) follow-up. Since the anatomic and physiologic principles of the gastric bypass operation were identical between the two techniques, it is not surprising that long-term weight loss was similar.

The major drawback of laparoscopic gastric bypass over the open approach is the steep "learning curve." LRYGB is currently one of the most challenging advanced laparoscopic operations. Because of its technical complexity, the learning curve for laparoscopic gastric bypass is longer than most other advanced laparoscopic operations. Many factors contribute to the extent of the learning curve for laparoscopic gastric bypass, including experience of the surgeon with other advanced laparoscopic operations, with open bariatric operations, and with laparoscopic suturing skill and intracorporeal knot tying techniques [9].

LRYGB can be done safely in patients over 60 years of age in an experienced bariatric program, even in patients with relatively high risk based on their comorbid conditions preoperatively. Resolution of associated comorbidities far exceeds that found with any other treatment modality [35].

Single incision laparoscopic surgery (SILS) is a minimally invasive technique which makes use of a single incision in performing RYGB. In this technique, a multichannel trocar is placed in the umbilical region, to reduce the number of trocars and improve cosmetics [36].

The first SILS was reported in 2009 by Huang et al. [37]. Compared with conventional LRYGB, SILS resulted in acceptable complications, the same recovery, comparative weight loss, and better patient satisfaction related to scarring [36].

The technique described by Fernández [38] for TUGB (transumbilical gastric bypass), with a single trocar, hand-sewn gastrojejunal anastomosis performed in two layers, and a stapled jejunojejunostomy, is a feasible procedure for surgeons who have previous experience with the transumbilical approach.

Studies have shown that single incision is safe and reproducible technique used as an access to complex surgeries like gastric bypass in carefully selected patients. However, the application of single incision laparoscopic surgery in bariatric patients has been limited to less complex procedures. Some potential benefits include less postoperative pain, improved cosmetics, and patient satisfaction. Randomized trials involving larger patient series with a longer follow-up and larger cohort studies and/or systematic reviews will be necessary to assess the extent of the benefits and limitations of single incision laparoscopic surgery (SILS) in bariatric surgery [39, 40].

Quality of life, as measured by the validated SF36 survey, improves greatly after LRYGB surgery. Preoperatively, morbidly obese patients score significantly lower than US population norms in the categories of general health, vitality, physical functioning, bodily pain, and emotional and social functioning. Three months following RYNGB, these same patients scored no differently than US norms in these categories [41].

LRYGB offers the afflicted patient a new option to achieve highly beneficial therapy, with optimally reduced morbidity and disability. Its potential for increased acceptance will allow improved management for an expanded set of suffering patients. Minimally invasive bariatric procedures should be performed only by bariatric surgeons who are experienced in laparoscopic techniques.

LRYGB produces excellent weight loss results, gratifying reduction of comorbidities, superior cosmetic effect, diminished recovery time, and rapid return to full activities. It can be accomplished within reasonable operating times. The long-term results, with respect to sustained weight loss, persistent benefits in relief of comorbidities, and incidence of incisional hernias, will continue to be observed. Surgeons who consider LRYGB to be the gold standard of obesity surgery should consider adding the laparoscopic access technique to their surgical armamentarium [10].

Many of the reported studies regarding morbidity and mortality had been completed prior to the many improvements in current surgical technique [41]. In addition, surgeon and hospital experience can mitigate the risks associated with weight loss surgery. The best demonstrated and most protective effect against complications is an experienced surgeon and hospital [42, 43]. Clearly, there is benefit in having this complex and demanding surgery performed by experienced and committed surgeons operating in a dedicated health-care facility.

None of the previously mentioned perioperative risk factors can be modified, with the exception of the volume status of the surgeon and hospital. For gastric bypass surgery, it has been demonstrated that a high-volume surgeon and high-volume hospital lead to decreased morbidity and mortality [42, 43].

In the United States, this volume outcome effect has been recognized by the Centers for Medicare and Medicaid Services, which now require Medicare patients to undergo surgery only at a Bariatric Surgery Center of Excellence [44]. Numerous criteria enable a center to become a Bariatric Surgery Center of Excellence, but the primary criteria are a surgeon volume of more than 50 cases and hospital volume exceeding 125 cases annually. Although a referral to a Bariatric Surgery Center of Excellence may lead to decreased morbidity and mortality, this referral pattern must be balanced with appropriate and sufficient access to care for a vulnerable population without other therapeutic options.

Conclusion

Patient safety and quality improvement have been part of bariatric surgery, including laparoscopic procedure, since its inception, and there have been significant improvements in outcomes of bariatric surgery over the past two decades [45].

The use of robotics is currently being implemented to perform RYGB. Transitioning from a laparoscopic to a robotic practice can be done safely; however, the initial operative times were longer, and the hospital cost was higher for robotic gastric bypass [46, 47].

References

1. Santry HP, Gillen DL, Lauderdale DS. Trends in bariatric surgical procedures. JAMA. 2005;294(15):1909–17.
2. Mason E, Ito C. Gastric bypass in obesity. Surg Clin North Am. 1967;47(6):1345–51.
3. Puzziferri N, Blankenship J, Wolfe BM. Surgical treatment of obesity. Endocrine. 2006;29:11–9.
4. Trus TL, Pope GD, Finlayson SRG. National trends in utilization and outcomes of bariatric surgery. Surg Endosc. 2005;19:616–20.
5. Tsai AG, Asch DA, Wadden TA. Insurance coverage for obesity treatment. J Am Diet Assoc. 2006;106:1651–5.
6. Schauer PR, Ikramuddin S, Gourash W, Ramanathan R, Luketich J. Outcomes after laparoscopic Roux-en-Y gastric bypass for morbid obesity. Ann Surg. 2000;232(4):515–29.
7. Wittgrove AC, Clark GW. Laparoscopic gastric bypass, Roux-en-Y – 500 patients: technique and results, with 3-60 month follow-up. Obes Surg. 2000;10:233–9.
8. Elder KA, Wolfe BM. Bariatric surgery: a review of procedures and outcomes. J Gastroenterol. 2007;132(6):2253–71.
9. Puzziferri N, Austrheim-Smith IT, Wolfe BM, Wilson SE, Nguyen NT. Three-year follow-up of a prospective randomized trial comparing laparoscopic versus open gastric bypass. Ann Surg. 2006;243:181–8.
10. Wittgrove AC, Clark GW, Schubert KR. Laparoscopic gastric bypass, Roux en-Y: technique and results in 75 patients with 3–30 months follow-up. Obes Surg. 1996;6:500–4.
11. Iordens GI, Klaassen RA, van Lieshout EM, Cleffken BI, van der Harst E. How to train surgical residents to perform laparoscopic Roux-en-Y gastric bypass safely. World J Surg. 2012;36(9):2003–10.
12. Cottam DR, Mattar S, Lord J, Schauer PR. Training and credentialing for the performance of laparoscopic bariatric surgery. Laparoscopy and SLS Report. 2003;2(1):15–21.
13. Wittgrove AC, Clark GW, Tremblay LJ. Laparoscopic gastric bypass, Roux-en-Y: preliminary report of five cases. Obes Surg. 1994;4:353–7.
14. Alvarado R, Alami RS, Hsu G, et al. The impact of preoperative weight loss in patients undergoing laparoscopic Roux-en-Y gastric bypass. Obes Surg. 2005;15:1282–6.
15. Harnisch MC, Portenier DD, Pryor AD, et al. Preoperative weight gain does not predict failure of weight loss or co-morbidity resolution of laparoscopic Roux-en-Y gastric bypass for morbid obesity. Surg Obes Relat Dis. 2008;4:445–50.
16. Edholm D, Kullberg J, Haenni A, Karlsson FA, Ahlström A, Hedberg J, Ahlström H, Sundbom M. Preoperative 4-week low-calorie diet reduces liver volume and intrahepatic fat, and facilitates laparoscopic gastric bypass in morbidly obese. Obes Surg. 2011;21:345–50.
17. Sundbom M. Laparoscopic revolution in bariatric surgery. World J Gastroenterol. 2014;20(41):15135–43.
18. Stepaniak PS, Heij C, Buise MP, Mannaerts GH, Smulders JF, Nienhuijs SW. Bariatric surgery with operating room teams that stayed fixed during the day: a multicenter study analyzing the effects on patient outcomes, teamwork and safety climate, and procedure duration. Anesth Analg. 2012;115:1384–92.
19. Berbiglia L, Zografakis JG, Dan AG. Laparoscopic Roux-en-Y gastric bypass: surgical technique and perioperative care. Surg Clin North Am. 2016;96(4):773–94.
20. Rondelli F, Bugiantella W, Desio M, et al. Antecolic or retrocolic alimentary limb in laparoscopic roux-en-Y gastric bypass? A meta-analysis. Obes Surg. 2016;26(1):182–95.
21. Silecchia G, Boru CE, Mouiel J, et al. Clinical evaluation of fibrin glue in the prevention of anastomosis leak and internal hernia after laparoscopic gastric bypass: preliminary results of a prospective randomized trial. Obes Surg. 2006;16:125–31.
22. Miller KA, Pump A. Use of bioabsorbable staple reinforcement material in gastric bypass: a prospective randomized clinical trial. Surg Obes Relat Dis. 2007;3(4):417–21.
23. Shikora SA. The use of staple-line reinforcement during laparoscopic gastric bypass. Obes Surg. 2004;14(10):1313–20.
24. Chousleb E, Szomstein S, Podkameni D, et al. Routine abdominal drains after laparoscopic Roux-en-Y gastric bypass: a retrospective review of 593 patients. Obes Surg. 2004;14(9):1203–7.
25. Kavuturu S, Rogers AM, Haluck RS. Routine drain placement in Roux-en-Y gastric bypass: an expanded retrospective comparative study of 755 patients and review of the literature. Obes Surg. 2012;22(1):177–81.
26. Madan AK, Harper JL, Tichansky DS. Techniques of laparoscopic gastric bypass: on-line survey of American Society for Bariatric Surgery practicing surgeons. Surg Obes Relat Dis. 2008;4:166–73.
27. Giordano S, Salminen P, Biancari F, Victorzon M. Linear stapler technique may be safer than circular in gastrojejunal anastomosis for laparoscopic Roux-en-Y gastric bypass: a meta-analysis of comparative studies. Obes Surg. 2011;21:1958–64.
28. Garrard CL, Clements RH, Nanney L, et al. Adhesion formation is reduced after laparoscopic surgery. Surg Endosc. 1999;13(1):10–3.
29. Delko T, Kraljevic M, Kostler T, Rothwell R, Droeser R, Potthast S, Oertli D, Zingg U. Primary non-closure of the mesenteric defects in laparoscopic Roux-en-Y gastric bypass: reoperations and intraoperative findings in 146 patients. Surg Endosc. 2016;30(6):2367–73.
30. Kawkabani MA, Denys A, Paroz A, Romy S, Suter M, Desmartines N, Meuli R, Schmidt S. The four

different types of internal hernia occurring after laparoscopic Roux-en-Y gastric bypass performed for morbid obesity: are there any multidetector computed tomography (MDCT) features permitting their distinction? Obes Surg. 2011;21:506–16.
31. Iliga KD, Ho T, Boone KB. Internal hernias after laparoscopic Roux-en-Y gastric bypass: incidence, treatment and prevention. Obes Surg. 2003;13(3):350–4.
32. Phillips E, Santos D, Towfigh S. Working port site hernias: to close or not to close? Does it matter in the obese? Bariatric Times. 2011;8(6):24–30.
33. Campos JM, Godoy EP, Siqueira LT, Evangelista LFL, Vasconcelos CS, Ferraz AAB, FERRAZ EM. Laparoscopic gastric bypass with low use of stapler sutures. Arq Bras Cir Dig. 2008;21(2):73–6.
34. Buchwald H, Estok R, Fahrbach K, Banel D, Sledge I. Trends in mortality in bariatric surgery: a systematic review and meta-analysis. Surgery. 2007;142:621–32.
35. Wittgrove AC, Martinez T. Laparoscopic gastric bypass in patients 60 years and older: early postoperative morbidity and resolution of comorbidities. Obes Surg. 2009;19(11):1472–6.
36. Ahluwalia JS, Chang PC, Yeh LR, Lin HY, Chi SC, Huang CK. Single incision transumbilical laparoscopic Roux-en-Y gastric bypass-our technique. Obes Surg. 2014;24(9):1585.
37. Huang CK, Houng JY, Chiang CJ, Chen YS, Lee PH. Single incision transumbilical laparoscopic Roux-en-Y gastric bypass: a first case report. Obes Surg. 2009;19(12):1711–5.
38. Fernández JI, Ovalle C, Farias C, de la Maza J, Cabrera C. Transumbilical laparoscopic roux-en-Y gastric bypass with hand-sewn gastrojejunal anastomosis. Obes Surg. 2013;23(1):140–4.
39. Rogula T, Daigle C, Dua M, Shimizu H, Davis J, Lavryk O, Aminian A, Schauer P. Laparoscopic bariatric surgery can be performed through a single incision: a comparative study. Obes Surg. 2014;24(7):1102–8.
40. Zepeda Mejia IA, Rogula T. Laparoscopic single-incision gastric bypass: initial experience, technique and short-term outcomes. Ann Surg Innov Res. 2015;9:7.
41. Nguyen NT, Goldman C, Rosenquist CJ, Arango A, Cole CJ, Lee SJ, Wolfe BM. Laparoscopic versus open gastric bypass: a randomized study of outcomes, quality of life, and costs. Ann Surg. 2001;234(3):279–89.
42. Wolfe BM, Morton JM. Weighing in on bariatric surgery: procedure use, readmission rates, and mortality. JAMA. 2005;294:1960–3.
43. Livingston EH, Ko CY. Assessing the relative contribution of individual risk factors on surgical outcome for gastric bypass surgery: a baseline probability analysis. J Surg Res. 2002;105:48–52.
44. Nguyen NT, Morton JM, Wolfe BM, et al. The SAGES bariatric surgery outcome initiative. Surg Endosc. 2005;19:1429–38.
45. Azagury DE, Morton JM. Bariatric surgery: overview of procedures and outcomes. Endocrinol Metab Clin N Am. 2016;45(3):647–56.
46. Lyn-Sue JR, Winder JS, Kotch S, Colello J, Docimo S. Laparoscopic gastric bypass to robotic gastric bypass: time and cost commitment involved in training and transitioning an academic surgical practice. J Robot Surg. 2016;10(2):111–5.
47. Park CW, Lam EC, Walsh TM, Karimoto M, Ma AT, Koo M, Hammill C, Murayama K, Lorenzo CS, Bueno R. Robotic-assisted roux-en-Y gastric bypass performed in a community hospital setting: the future of bariatric surgery? Surg Endosc. 2011;25(10):3312–21.

Systemic Inflammation in the Morbidly Obese Patient

15

Antonio Jamel Coelho

Systemic Inflammation in the Morbidly Obese Patient

The obesity, induced by uncontrolled and excessive food intake, is associated with a chronic systemic inflammatory state of adipose tissue [1], characterized by elevated serum levels of acute phase inflammatory markers, including interleukin 6 (IL-6), tumor necrosis factor-α (TNF-α), interleukin 1 (IL-1), C-reactive protein (CRP), complement, and leptin, and low level of serum markers that attenuate the inflammation such as adiponectin and interleukin 10 (IL-10).Obese patients present alterations in quantity and function of leukocytes on peripheral blood including increased number of macrophages and increased production of oxygen free radicals. This systemic inflammatory condition, associated with obesity which has an extreme clinical significance, is caused by specific abnormalities on molecular, immunological, cellular, and anatomical characteristics which may determine metabolic changes such as hyperglycemia, hyperinsulinemia, insulin resistance, and dyslipidemia. These alterations can cause the metabolic syndrome, which is the root of the many serious complications of obesity, and can lead to respiratory disorders such as airflow obstruction, dyspnea, and hypoxemia and other disorders such as cardiovascular, neurological, pulmonary, musculoskeletal, joint pain, diabetic retinopathy, and low self-esteem [2–6]. Although it is known that excessive fat accumulation is the cause of several diseases, not all obese individuals have important metabolic changes [7].

The term "metabolic syndrome" has been proposed to indicate a group of interrelated factors, such as abdominal obesity, insulin resistance (IR), hypertension, and dyslipidemia. Individuals who exhibit these conditions have increased risk to develop type 2 diabetes mellitus (T2DM) and cardiovascular disease. The metabolic syndrome has been defined as presenting three or more of the following: fasting plasma glucose of 5.6–6.9 mmol/L; waist circumference >102 cm (in men) or >88 cm (in women); fasting triglycerides ≥1.7 mmol/L; high-density lipoprotein cholesterol <1.0 mmol/L (in men) or <1.3 mmol/L (in women); and blood pressure ≥130/85 mmHg or current treatment for hypertension [8, 9]. Studies about the relationship between insulin resistance and diabetes showed that there is an association between inflammation and other diseases associated with diabetes, such as atherosclerosis, hypertension, hepatic steatosis, sleep apnea and allergic diseases, stroke, some types of cancer, and changes in skeletal muscle [10–12]. Barbarroja et al. [13] found that the development of insulin resistance associated with obesity depends on the inflammatory cascade activation. Interleukin 6 (IL-6), IL-1β, ERK (extracellular signal-regulated kinase ½), and nuclear

A. J. Coelho (✉)
Department of Emergency, Hospital Barra D'Or, Rio de Janeiro, Brazil

J. Ettinger et al. (eds.), *Gastric Bypass*, https://doi.org/10.1007/978-3-030-28803-7_15

factor-kappa β (NF-kβ) appear to be important mediators of inflammatory effects by promoting insulin resistance.

Inflammation Related to Adipose Tissue

Although the peripheral blood findings show the initial clinical condition, the inflammatory obesity disease begins in adipose tissue, before it can be seen in another organ and before the systemic metabolic disease. Adipose tissue, either in the lean individual or in the obese individual, is a complex organ, with endocrine and immunological activity, being composed by the extracellular matrix, adipocytes, fibroblasts, endothelial cells, preadipocytes, and cells of the immune system [14]. The number of leukocytes is increased in obesity at the expense of macrophages, T cells, and natural killer cells, among which are the adipose tissue macrophage (ATM), the main mediators of inflammation. In addition to their increased numbers, these macrophages express increased levels of inflammatory cytokines (TNF-α, IL-6, inducible nitric oxide synthase – iNOS) and chemokine receptors. Adipose tissue macrophages interact with other lymphocytes, adipocytes, and endothelial cells inducing the release of inflammatory cytokines, adipokines, reactive oxygen species, and chemokines all of which can contribute to inflammation and systemic metabolic disease. Adipose tissue macrophages have an important role in insulin resistance, caused by the cytokines that they release. Insulin resistance may lead to hyperglycemia and hyperlipidemia that may interfere with metabolic reactions and cause type 2 diabetes mellitus (T2DM), a disease closely associated with obesity. In turn, obesity has been shown to have great influence in the development of insulin resistance and the progress for T2DM. Type 2 diabetes mellitus is different from type 1 diabetes which is an autoimmune disease that mainly affects children and occurs due to the pancreatic β cells' inability to produce insulin. Adipose tissue macrophages are also involved in other metabolic diseases such as atherosclerosis, hepatic steatosis, sleep apnea, and asthma. Although adipose tissue macrophage plays an important role, it is not the only cause of inflammatory response and metabolic disease; other immune cells also play a role in the pathogenesis of these metabolic alterations.

Cytokines and Adipocytokines

Cytokines and adipocytokines are the main factor of the obesity-related inflammatory process. They were initially described due to their effects on inflammation and the regulation of body weight, but since then, it was shown that most cytokines and adipocytokines also control the glucose homeostasis. While some inflammatory cytokines control body weight, most of the adipocytokines have immunoregulatory properties. Phylogenetically and functionally, cytokines and adipocytokines are closely related. Consequently, physiologic systems that regulate inflammation, body weight, and metabolism were shown to have evolved though similar paths.

Previously, researchers believed that fat tissue was a static deposit of energy. However, now these structures are known as an endocrine organ that plays an important role in systemic and local homeostasis. Adipocytes secrete substances, such as cytokines and chemokines, called adipocytokines that have paracrine, autocrine, and endocrine (systemic) functions, including inflammatory mediators [17, 18]. The adipocyte is an important source of endogenous tumor necrosis factor-α (TNF-α). The secretion of TNF-α is stimulated by obesity [19, 20]. Fat cells also secrete other adipocytokines, such as interleukin-6 (IL-6), interleukin-1β (IL-1β), leptin, adiponectin, resistin, retinol-binding protein 4, visfatin, plasminogen activator-1 (PAI-1), monocyte chemoattractant protein-1, angiotensin, and fibrinogen [21, 22].

Obesity triggers an increase in the concentration of cytokines associated with the pathogenesis of the metabolic syndrome [12, 23]. Leptin, secreted by adipocytes, acts on the central nervous system and endocrine function, maintaining metabolic homeostasis by regulating appetite, physical activity, and stimulating insulin sensitivity [1, 24, 25].

The growth of adipocytes and accumulation of triglycerides causes an increase on the leptin production. The leptin concentration is an indicator of adipose tissue mass; thus if leptin levels in obese patients remain high for a long period, it will provoke leptin resistance [26], limiting satiety signals. The leptin action on the central nervous system can lead to normoglycemia independent of the action of pancreatic insulin [27]. Another adipocytokines, known as adiponectin, has its serum level lowered in obesity [28] and type 2 diabetes [29]. Adiponectin stimulates insulin sensitivity and has anti-inflammatory effects [30, 31]. Low serum levels of this cytokine are usually associated with the metabolic syndrome [32]. Both leptin and adiponectin protect peripheral tissues against lipotoxic injuries, because they stimulate fatty acids oxidation and increase insulin sensibility [24]. On the other hand, resistin, produced by macrophages, increases insulin resistance [33, 34]. Angiotensinogen production is increased in obesity because it is regulated by nutritional factors, decreasing during fasting and increasing during food intake [35, 36]. Adipose tissue also produces mediators of angiogenesis such as vascular endothelium growth factor (VEGF), matrix metalloproteinase-2 (MMP-2), matrix metalloproteinase-9 (MMP-9), and hepatocyte growth factor (HGF) [37]

Macrophages

Obesity is characterized by the progressive infiltration of immune cells in adipose tissue. It is thought that most cytokines released by the fat tissue are derived from adipose tissue macrophages. The recruitment and activation of these cells are necessary for the development of complications associated with obesity [38, 39]. Studies in obese mice have shown a marked infiltration of macrophages in white adipose tissue [40, 41]. It has been demonstrated that macrophages' accumulation is directly related to the size of the fat cells and body mass index [14, 41], as well as the size of adipocytes located in the omentum and in the subcutaneous. This process has a negative correlation to metabolic health [42, 43].

The progression of obesity increases the number of macrophages in adipose tissue that may correspond up to 50% of the tissue cells [44]. On the other hand, the reduction of the adipose tissue results in a significant decrease in the number and the distribution of macrophages, leading to a decreased expression of inflammatory markers [45]. Macrophage infiltration increases the process of low-grade inflammation of the white adipose tissue (WAT) [46]. It is important to note that the macrophage, mostly located in the dead adipocytes, become the predominant producer of adipocytokines in white adipose tissue [47] and its infiltration in adipose tissue is stimulated by changes in the signal sent by the altered adipocyte, resulting from its necrosis or death. In general, M1 macrophages have pro-inflammatory activity, while M2 macrophages have anti-inflammatory activity and perform remodeling and tissue repair. In regard to the microenvironment of adipose stromal cells: the M2 macrophages that reside in the fat tissue have a scattered distribution, maintaining its anti-inflammatory activity and preserving the insulin sensitivity in the liver and adipose tissue; M1 macrophages infiltrates the fat tissue, forming "crown-like structures" around the dying adipocytes, leading to inhibition of insulin sensitivity, which can cause systemic insulin resistance [47–50].

Features of the Adipose Tissue Damaged by Inflammation

Importance of Central Obesity

Vague was the first to draw attention to the importance of adipose tissue distribution. It was found that lower body obesity or subcutaneous is characterized by a "pear-shaped" body, and it is more common in women, whereas the central or abdominal obesity has an "apple-shaped" body and is more common in men. Thus, two designations were proposed: "gynecoid obesity" to express the accumulation of adipose tissue in the hip and thighs, loosely associated with metabolic complications, and "android obesity" to express the adipose tissue usually accumulated in the upper body area, closely associated with the metabolic syndrome and cardiovascular disease [51–53]. The distribution of adipose tissue is an indicator of metabolic and cardiovascular risk more important than the obesity in general. Additionally, the inability of subcutaneous fat deposit to grow when there is a positive energy balance can lead to cardiovascular complications [54]. The amount of intra-abdominal fat is closely related to metabolic syndrome [55] and with low levels of adiponectin, an insulin sensitizer adipocytokines [56]. The visceral white adipose tissue (WAT) is associated with hepatic steatosis and hepatic IR, and it is a risk factor for impaired glucose tolerance, independent of BMI and extension of subcutaneous depot [57, 58], although some reports say that SAT can generate a systemic flow of FFA greater than visceral or retroperitoneal fat, also capable of stimulating the development of IR [59]. Visceral fat storage capacity is relatively low compared to subcutaneous. Without available storage, lipids resulting from insufficient adipogenesis in the prediabetic obese individuals are delivered to the liver, heart, skeletal muscle, kidneys, and pancreas, causing accumulation of ectopic fat in these organs and cellular hypoxia [60–62], which can cause harmful metabolic changes. Obese and lean individuals are born with a limited number of adipocytes. In obese individuals, the WAT growth is thought to be achieved through hypertrophy and not hyperplasia [63]. The adipocytes are individually wrapped by extracellular matrix (ECM) support, with specific collagens. The remodeling of the extracellular matrix and specially the degradation/redeposition cycles of collagen are essential to the expansion of adipocytes and adipose tissue [64]. However, in obese adipose tissue, excessive and unregulated deposition of collagen and other components of ECM (fibrosis) eventually restricts the expansion of adipocytes, thereby causing changes in these cells, and activation of inflammatory/stress kinase, resulting in adipose tissue disorganization and systemic metabolic dysfunction [65, 66]. Collagen VI actively participates in the pathophysiology of adipose tissue fibrosis and metabolic dysfunction associated with obesity, and in obese patients with insulin resistance, collagen VI deposition is increased in WAT. Collagen VI deposition and adipose tissue fibrosis in the WAT coincide with the presence of activated adipose tissue macrophages (ATMs) that promote ECM remodeling and wound healing [43].

Adipose Tissue Distribution

Obesity is characterized by excess body fat, and it is classified by the body mass index (BMI), a relation between the body weight and the square of the height (kg/m^2). According to BMI, general population is classified into five categories: underweight (BMI <18.5 kg/m^2); normal weight (BMI 18.5–24.9 kg/m^2); class I obesity, overweight (BMI 25.0–29.9 kg/m^2); class II obesity, obesity (BMI 30.0–39.9 kg/m^2); and class III obesity, extreme obesity (BMI >40 kg/m^2) [29, 67].

The use of BMI as a unit of measure takes into account that adipose tissue has the same distribution throughout the body, as it does not consider different sites of body fat accumulation among individuals. Therefore, BMI does not represent dysfunctional adipose tissue and is not considered an accurate measure of metabolic disease. There are many individuals that present hyperglycemia, hyperinsulinemia, IR, hyperlipidemia, and hypertension despite having a lean body and a normal BMI. People with this phenotype are called "metabolically obese normal weight" [68, 69]. On the other hand, many people classified as obese, because of their high BMI, do not present the components of MS and have lower cardiovascular risk when compared to the general population; these individuals are called "metabolically healthy obese." [71], and these "paradoxical obesity" groups represent a topic of divergence amid the scientific community [71].

Subcutaneous adipose tissue (SAT) distribution, common in women, is related to metabolic protection, unlike central or intra-abdominal obesity, typical of men, that often causes MS [72, 73]. Considering the importance of fat distribution in metabolic disease, waist circumference

(WC) is considered a more reliable indicator of cardiometabolic risk than BMI. Waist circumference ≥88 cm, in women, and WC ≥102 cm, in men, is considered an independent risk factor for the development of cardiovascular diseases and atherogenic dyslipidemia and determinates the degree of IR.

There is no explanation to how the adipose tissue distribution occurs in the body regions. Several factors seem to interfere with the adipose tissue deposition, such as age, physical activity, nutritional status, growth hormone, glucocorticoids, sex steroids, sex, ethnicity, and genetic susceptibility.

Metabolically Obese Normal Weight and Metabolically Healthy Obese

Considering the body fat composition and its distribution, four obesity phenotypes were described: normal weight obese (NWO), metabolically obese normal weight (MONW), metabolically healthy obese (MHO), and metabolically unhealthy obese (MUO).

Obese individuals called "metabolically healthy obese" (MHO) [77–79] do not present the metabolic disorders typical of obesity; thus they present a normal risk for CVD, atherosclerosis, hypertension, type 2 diabetes, dyslipidemia, and hyperuricemia [75, 76].

Initially, it was claimed that these patients had lower to no risk of developing CVD when compared to metabolically healthy normal weight (MHNW) patients. However, this is being questioned because there is some doubt about MHO phenotype prognosis. Studies have shown that metabolically healthy obese have an equal or lower risk of developing CVD [80–82], while other studies demonstrated that these individuals have a higher risk of developing CVD [83, 84]. Ultrasonography studies have shown thickening of the common carotid artery intima-media layers and decreased flow-mediated dilatation of the brachial artery in these patients, suggesting deterioration of endothelial function and onset of atherosclerosis [85]. Moreover, HMO and *metabolically unhealthy normal weight* (MUNW) individuals show a greater inflammatory level when compared to metabolically healthy normal weight (MHNW) individuals, although this response is not as severe as in metabolically unhealthy obese (MUHO) individuals [86].

The "normal but metabolically obese" phenotype (MONW) was first described by Ruderman et al. in 1981 and revised in 1998 [68, 87]. Although they present normal body weight and BMI, these individuals present obesity-related characteristics, such as hyperinsulinemia, hyperglycemia, premature insulin resistance, impaired glucose tolerance, hypercholesterolemia, and hypertriglyceridemia, and they will probably develop T2DM and CVD [88].

References

1. Shoelson SE, Lee J, Goldfine AB. Inflammation and insulin resistance. J Clin Invest. 2006;116(7):1793–801.
2. Nigro E, Scudiero O, Monaco ML, Palmieri A, Mazzarella G, Costagliola C, Bianco A, Daniele A. New insight into adiponectin role in obesity and obesity-related diseases. Biomed Res Int. 2014;2014:658913 . [PMID: 25110685]. https://doi.org/10.1155/2014/658913.
3. Grundy SM, Bryan Brewer H Jr, Cleeman JI, Smith SC Jr, Lenfant C. Definition of metabolic syndrome: report of the National Heart, Lung, and Blood. Institute/American Heart Association Conference on scientific issues related to definition. Circulation. 2004;109:433–8. https://doi.org/10.1161/01.CIR.0000111245.75752.C6.
4. Bays HE, González-Campoy JM, Bray GA, Kitabchi AE, Bergman DA, Schorr AB, Rodbard HW, Henry RR. Pathogenic potential of adipose tissue and metabolic consequences of adipocyte hypertrophy and increased visceral adiposity. Expert Rev Cardiovasc Ther. 2008;6:343–68 . [PMID: 18327995]. https://doi.org/10.1586/14779072.6.3.343.
5. Kushner RF, Roth JL. Assessment of the obese patient. Endocrinol Metab Clin North Am. 2003;32:915–33. [PMID:14711068]
6. Shore SA. Environmental perturbations: obesity. Compr Physiol. 2011;1(1):263–82. https://doi.org/10.1002/cphy.c100017.
7. Vrbíková J, Cibula D, Dvoráková K, Stanická S, Sindelka G, Hill M, Fanta M, Vondra K, Skrha J. Insulin sensitivity in women with polycystic ovary syndrome. J Clin Endocrinol Metab. 2004;89:2942–5.
8. Grundy SM, Cleeman JI, Daniels SR, Donato KA, Eckel RH, Franklin BA, Gordon DJ, Krauss RM, Savage PJ, Smith SC Jr, Spertus JA, Costa F. American Heart Association, diagnosis and management of the

metabolic syndrome: an American Heart Association/National Heart, Lung, and Blood Institute Scientific Statement. Circulation. 2005;112:2735–52, Erratum in: Circulation 112, e297–8

9. Janiszewski, P.M., Ross, R. Effects of weight loss among metabolically healthy obese men and women. Diabetes Care. 2010;33:1957–9. Kahn SE, Zinman B, Haffner SM, O'Neill MC, Kravitz BG, Yu D, Freed MI, Herman WH, Holman RR, Jones NP, Lachin JM, Viberti GC. 2006.
10. Van Gaal LF, Mertens IL, De Block CE. Mechanisms linking obesity with cardiovascular disease. Nature. 2006;444:875–80.
11. Guh DP, Zhang W, Bansback N, Amarsi Z, Birmingham CL, Anis AH. The incidence of co-morbidities related to obesity and overweight: a systematic review and meta-analysis. BMC Public Health. 2009;9:88.
12. Xu H, Barnes GT, Yang Q, Tan G, Yang D, Chou CJ, Sole J, Nichols A, Ross JS, Tartaglia LA, Chen H. Chronic inflammation in fat plays a crucial role in the development of obesity-related insulin resistance. J Clin Invest. 2003;112(12):1821–30. [PubMed: 14679177]
13. Barbarroja N, López-Pedrera R, Mayas MD, García-fuentes E, Garrido-Sánchez L, Macías-González M, El Bekay R, Vidal-Puig A, Tinahones FJ. The obese healthy paradox: is inflammation the answer? Biochem J. 2010;430:141–9. https://doi.org/10.1042/BJ20100285.
14. Curat CA, Miranville A, Sengenès C, et al. From blood monocytes to adipose tissue-resident macrophages. Induction of diapedesis by human mature adipocytes. Diabetes. 2004;53(5):1285–92.
15. Wellen KE, Hotamisligil GS. Inflammation, stress, and diabetes. J Clin Invest. 2005;115:1111–9. [PubMed: 15864338]
16. Odegaard JI, Chawla A. Connecting type 1 and type 2 diabetes through innate immunity. Cold Spring Harb Perspect Med. 2012;2:a007724. [PubMed: 22393536]
17. Mraz M, Haluzik M. The role of adipose tissue immune cells in obesity and low-grade inflammation. J Endocrinol. 2014;222(3):R113–27.
18. Rosen ED, Spiegelman BM. What we talk about when we talk about fat. Cell. 2014;156(1–2):20–44.
19. Hotamisligil GS, Arner P, Caro JF, Atkinson RL, Spiegelman BM. Increased adipose tissue expression of tumor necrosis factor-α in human obesity and insulin resistance. J Clin Invest. 1995;95(5):2409–15.
20. Hotamisligil GS, Shargill NS, Spiegelman BM. Adipose expression of tumor necrosis factor-α: direct role in obesity-linked insulin resistance. Science. 1993;259(5091):87–91.
21. Rosen ED, Spiegelman BM. Adipocytes as regulators of energy balance and glucose homeostasis. Nature. 2006;444(7121):847–53.
22. Chakraborti CK. Role of adiponectin and some other factors linking type 2 diabetes mellitus and obesity. World J Diabetes. 2015;6(15):1296–308.
23. Lumeng CN, Saltiel AR. Inflammatory links between obesity and metabolic disease. J Clin Invest. 2011;121(6):2111–7.
24. Flachs P, Rossmeisl M, Bryhn M, Kopecky J. Cellular and molecular effects of n-3 polyunsaturated fatty acids on adipose tissue biology and metabolism. Clin Sci. 2009;116(1):1–16.
25. Havel PJ. Update on adipocyte hormones: regulation of energy balance and carbohydrate/lipid metabolism. Diabetes. 2004;53(Suppl 1):S143–51.
26. Scarpace PJ, Zhang Y. Leptin resistance: a predisposing factor for diet-induced obesity. Am J Physiol Regul Integr Comp Physiol. 2009;296:R493–500. [PubMed: 19091915]
27. Ueno N, Inui A, Kalra PS, Kalra SP. Leptin transgene expression in the hypothalamus enforces euglycemia in diabetic, insulin-deficient nonobese Akita mice and leptin-deficient obese ob/ob mice. Peptides. 2006;27(9):2332–42.
28. Arita Y, et al. Paradoxical decrease of an adipose-specific protein, adiponectin, in obesity. Biochem Biophys Res Commun. 1999;257:79–83. [PubMed: 10092513]
29. Hajer GR, van Haeften TW, Visseren FLJ. Adipose tissue dysfunction in obesity, diabetes, and vascular diseases. Eur Heart J. 2008;29(24):2959–71 . [PMID: 18775919]. https://doi.org/10.1093/eurheartj/ehn387.
30. Yamauchi T, et al. The fat-derived hormone adiponectin reverses insulin resistance associated with both lipoatrophy and obesity. Nat Med. 2001;7:941–6. [PubMed: 11479627]
31. Ouchi N, Walsh K. Adiponectin as an anti-inflammatory factor. Clin Chim Acta. 2007;380:24–30.
32. Vasseur F, Meyre D, Froguel P. Adiponectin, type 2 diabetes and the metabolic syndrome: lessons from human genetic studies. Expert Rev Mol Med. 2006;8:1–12. [PubMed: 17112391]
33. Steppan CM, Bailey ST, Bhat S, Brown EJ, Banerjee RR, Wright CM, et al. The hormone resistin links obesity to diabetes. Nature. 2001;409(6818):307–12.
34. Patel L, et al. Resistin is expressed in human macrophages and directly regulated by PPAR gamma activators. Biochem Biophys Res Commun. 2003;300:472–6. [PubMed: 12504108]
35. Einstein FH, Atzmon G, Yang XM, Ma XH, Rincon M, Rudin E, et al. Differential responses of visceral and subcutaneous fat depots to nutrients. Diabetes. 2005;54(3):672–8.
36. Kalupahana NS, et al. Overproduction of angiotensinogen from adipose tissue induces adipose inflammation, glucose intolerance, and insulin resistance. Obesity (Silver Spring). 2012;20:48–56. [PubMed: 21979391]
37. Fain JN. Release of inflammatory mediators by human adipose tissue is enhanced in obesity and primarily by the nonfat cells: a review. Mediators Inflamm. 2010;2010:513948. [PubMed: 20508843]
38. Kamei N, Tobe K, Suzuki R, et al. Overexpression of monocyte chemoattractant protein-1 in adipose

tissues causes macrophage recruitment and insulin resistance. J Biol Chem. 2006;281(36):26602–14.
39. Kanda H, Tateya S, Tamori Y, et al. MCP-1 contributes to macrophage infiltration into adipose tissue, insulin resistance, and hepatic steatosis in obesity. J Clin Invest. 2006;116(6):1494–505.
40. Soukas A, Cohen P, Socci ND, Friedman JM. Leptin-specific patterns of gene expression in white adipose tissue. Genes Dev. 2000;14(8):963–80.
41. Weisberg SP, McCann D, Desai M, Rosenbaum M, Leibel RL, Ferrante AW Jr. Obesity is associated with macrophage accumulation in adipose tissue. J Clin Invest. 2003;112:1796–808. [PubMed: 14679176]
42. Klöting N, Fasshauer M, Dietrich A, Kovacs P, Schön MR, Kern M, Stumvoll M, Blüher M. Insulin-sensitive obesity. Am J Physiol Endocrinol Metab. 2010;299:E506–15.
43. Spencer M, Yao-Borengasser A, Unal R, Rasouli N, Gurley CM, Zhu B, Peterson CA, Kern PA. Adipose tissue macrophages in insulin-resistant subjects are associated with collagen VI and fibrosis and demonstrate alternative activation. Am J Physiol Endocrinol Metab. 2010;299:E1016–27.
44. Weisberg SP, et al. CCR2 modulates inflammatory and metabolic effects of high-fat feeding. J Clin Invest. 2006;116:115–24. [PubMed: 16341265]
45. Cancello R, Henegar C, Viguerie N, et al. Reduction of macrophage infiltration and chemoattractant gene expression. Changes in white adipose tissue of morbidly obese subjects after surgery-induced weight loss. Diabetes. 2005;54(8):2277–86.
46. Ferrante AW Jr. Obesity-induced inflammation: a metabolic dialogue in the language of inflammation. J Intern Med. 2007;262(4):408–14.
47. Cinti S, Mitchell G, Barbatelli G, et al. Adipocyte death defines macrophage localization and function in adipose tissue of obese mice and humans. J Lipid Res. 2005;46(11):2347–55.
48. Lumeng CN, Bodzin JL, Saltiel AR. Obesity induces a phenotypic switch in adipose tissue macrophage polarization. J Clin Invest. 2007;117:175–84. [PubMed: 17200717]
49. Lumeng CN, DelProposto JB, Westcott DJ, Saltiel AR. Phenotypic switching of adipose tissue macrophages with obesity is generated by spatiotemporal differences in macrophage subtypes. Diabetes. 2008;57:3239–46. [PubMed: 18829989]
50. Odegaard JI, et al. Alternative M2 activation of Kupffer cells by PPARdelta ameliorates obesity induced insulin resistance. Cell Metab. 2008;7:496–507. [PubMed: 18522831]
51. Vague J. La differenciation sexuelle: facteur determinant des formes: de l'obesite. Presse Med. 1947;55:339–40.
52. Vague J. The degree of masculine differentiation of obesities: a factor determining predisposition to diabetes, atherosclerosis, gout, and uric calculous disease. Am J Clin Nutr. 1956;4:20–34. [PMID: 13282851]
53. Donahue RP, Abbott RD, Bloom E, Reed DM, Yano K. Central obesity and coronary heart disease in men. Lancet. 1987;1:821–4.
54. Gealekman O, Guseva N, Hartigan C, Apotheker S, Gorgoglione M, Gurav K, Tran KV, Straubhaar J, Nicoloro S, Czech MP, Thompson M, Perugini RA, Corvera S. Depot-specific differences and insufficient subcutaneous adipose tissue angiogenesis in human obesity. Circulation. 2011;123:186–94 . [PMID: 21200001]. https://doi.org/10.1161/CIRCULATIONAHA.110.970145.
55. Després J-P, Nadeau A, Tremblay A, Ferland M, Moorjani S, Lupien PJ, Thériault G, Pinault S, Bouchard C. Role of deep abdominal fat in the association between regional adipose tissue distribution and glucose tolerance in obese women. Diabetes. 1989;38:304–9.
56. Côté M, Mauriège P, Bergeron J, Alméras N, Tremblay A, Lemieux I, Després JP. Adiponectinemia in visceral obesity: impact on glucose tolerance and plasma lipoprotein and lipid levels in men. J Clin Endocrinol Metab. 2005;90:1434–9.
57. Bergman RN, Kim SP, Catalano KJ, Hsu IR, Chiu JD, Kabir M, Hucking K, Ader M. Why visceral fat is bad: mechanisms of the metabolic syndrome. Obesity (Silver Spring). 2006;14(Suppl 1):16S–9S.
58. Pouliot M-C, Després J-P, Nadeau A, Moorjani S, Prud'Homme D, Lupien PJ, Tremblay A, Bouchard C. Visceral obesity in men. Associations with glucose tolerance, plasma insulin and lipoprotein levels. Diabetes. 1992;41:826–34.
59. Patel P, Abate N. Body fat distribution and insulin resistance. Nutrients. 2013;5:2019–27 . [PMID: 23739143]. https://doi.org/10.3390/nu5062019.
60. Trayhurn P, Wang B, Wood IS. Hypoxia and the endocrine and signalling role of white adipose tissue. Arch Physiol Biochem. 2008;114(4):267–76.
61. Trayhurn P. Hypoxia and adipose tissue function and dysfunction in obesity. Physiol Rev. 2013;93(1):1–21.
62. Castro AVB, Kolka CM, Kim SP, et al. Obesity, insulin resistance and comorbidities? Mechanisms of association. Arq Bras Endocrinol Metabol. 2014;58(6):600–9.
63. Spalding KL, Arner E, Westermark PO, Bernard S, Buchholz BA, Bergmann O, Blomqvist L, Hoffstedt J, Näslund E, Britton T, Concha H, Hassan M, Rydén M, Frisén J, Arner P. Dynamics of fat cell turnover in humans. Nature. 2008;453:783–7.
64. Chun TH, Hotary KB, Sabeh F, Saltiel AR, Allen ED, Weiss SJ. A pericellular collagenase directs the 3-dimensional development of white adipose tissue. Cell. 2006;125:577–91.
65. Halberg N, Khan T, Trujillo ME, Wernstedt-Asterholm I, Attie AD, Sherwani S, Wang ZV, Landskroner-Eiger S, Dineen S, Magalang UJ, Brekken RA, Scherer PE. Hypoxia-inducible factor 1alpha induces fibrosis and insulin resistance in white adipose tissue. Mol Cell Biol. 2009;29:4467–83.

66. Khan T, Muise ES, Iyengar P, Wang ZV, Chandalia M, Abate N, Zhang BB, Bonaldo P, Chua S, Scherer PE. Metabolic dysregulation and adipose tissue fibrosis: role of collagen VI. Mol Cell Biol. 2009;29:1575–91.
67. Physical status: the use and interpretation of anthropometry. Report of a WHO Expert Committee. World Health Organ Tech Rep Ser 854, 1995. p. 1–452. [PMID: 8594834].
68. Ruderman NB, Schneider SH, Berchtold P. The "metabolically-obese," normal weight individual. Am J Clin Nutr. 1981;34(8):1617–21. [PMID: 7270486]
69. Ruderman N, Chisholm D, Pi-Sunyer X, et al. The metabolically obese, normal weight individual revisited. Diabetes. 1998;47(5):699–713.
70. Samocha-Bonet D, Dixit VD, Kahn CR, et al. Metabolically healthy and unhealthy obese–the 2013 Stock Conference report. Obes Rev. 2014;15(9):697–708.
71. Poirier P. Adiposity and cardiovascular disease: are we using the right definition of obesity? Eur Heart J. 2007;28:2047–8. [PMID: 17673449]
72. Snijder MB, Visser M, Dekker JM, et al. Low subcutaneous thigh fat is a risk factor for unfavourable glucose and lipid levels, independently of high abdominal fat. The Health ABC Study. Diabetologia. 2005;48(2):301–8.
73. Wajchenberg BL. Subcutaneous and visceral adipose tissue: their relation to the metabolic syndrome. Endocr Rev. 2000;21(6):697–738.
74. Tchernof A, Despre's J-P. Pathophysiology of human visceral obesity: an update. Physiol Rev. 2013;93(1):359–404.
75. Bonora E, Willeit J, Kiechl S, Oberhollenzer F, Egger G, Bonadonna R, Muggeo M. U-shaped and J-shaped relationships between serum insulin and coronary heart disease in the general population. The Bruneck study. Diabetes Care. 1991;21:221–30.
76. Wildman RP, Muntner P, Reynolds K, McGinn AP, Rajpathak S, Wylie-Rosett J, Sowers MR. The obese without cardiometabolic risk factor clustering and the normal weight with cardiometabolic risk factor clustering: prevalence and correlates of 2 phenotypes among the US population (NHANES 1999–2004). Arch Intern Med. 2008;168:1617–24.
77. Velho S, Paccaud F, Waeber G, Vollenweider P, Marques-Vidal P. Metabolically healthy obesity: different prevalences using different criteria. Eur J Clin Nutr. 2010;64(10):1043–51.
78. Blüher M. The distinction of metabolically 'healthy' from 'unhealthy' obese individuals. Curr Opin Lipidol. 2010;21(1):38–43.
79. Karelis AD. Obesity: to be obese—does it matter if you are metabolically healthy? Nat Rev Endocrinol. 2011;7(12):699–700.
80. Katzmarzyk PT, Janssen I, Ross R, Church TS, Blair SN. The importance of waist circumference in the definition of metabolic syndrome: prospective analyses of mortality in men. Diabetes Care. 2006;29(2):404–9.
81. Ogorodnikova M, Kim A, McGinn P, Muntner P, Khan U, Wildman RP. Incident cardiovascular disease events in metabolically benign obese individuals. Obesity. 2012;20(3):651–9.
82. Meigs JB, Wilson PWF, Fox CS, et al. Body mass index, metabolic syndrome, and risk of type 2 diabetes or cardiovascular disease. J Clin Endocrinol Metabol. 2006;91(8):2906–12.
83. Ärnlöv J, Ingelsson E, Sundström J, Lind L. Impact of body mass index and the metabolic syndrome on the risk of cardiovascular disease and death in middle-aged men. Circulation. 2010;121(2):230–6.
84. Flint AJ, Hu FB, Glynn RJ, et al. Excess weight and the risk of incident coronary heart disease amongmen andwomen. Obesity. 2010;18(2):377–83.
85. Oflaz H, Ozbey N, Mantar F, Genchellac H, Mercanoglu F, Sencer E, Molvalilar S, Orhan Y. Determination of endothelial function and early atherosclerotic changes in healthy obese women. Diabetes Nutr Metab. 2003;16:176–81.
86. Sameer Shaharyar, Lara L. Roberson, Omar Jamal, et al. Obesity and metabolic phenotypes (metabolically healthy and unhealthy variants) are significantly associated with prevalence of elevated C-reactive protein and hepatic steatosis in a large healthy Brazilian population. J Obes. 2015;2015:178526, 6 pages. https://doi.org/10.1155/2015/178526.
87. Ruderman N, Chisholm D, Pi-Sunyer X, Schneider S. The metabolically obese, normal-weight individual revisited. Diabetes. 1998;47:699–713. [PMID: 9588440]
88. Dvorak RV, DeNino WF, Ades PA, Poehlman ET. Phenotypic characteristics associated with insulin resistance in metabolically obese but normal-weight young women. Diabetes. 1999;48(11):2210–4.

16

Banded Gastric Bypass by Fobi Ring: Technique and Results

Mohit Bhandari, Hemant Kumar Nautiyal, Winni Mathur, and Susmit Kosta

Why banded gastric bypass? Banded gastric bypass was devised by Prof Fobi. Gastric bypass had incident of weight recidivism in many studies conducted in the past. At most studies it was documented that gastric bypass had a 50% excess weight loss at 5 years with some studies showing less than 30% weight loss as 5 years [1, 2].

Studies conducted by Fobi and Marc Bessler showed sustained weight loss with banded gastric bypass as compared to non-banded patients [3].

The banding of pouch was essential as the natural history of gastric pouch was dilatation, widening of anastomoses and patient eating into the Roux limb [4–6]. This resulted in weight regain and recurrence of comorbidities. Prof Fobi used a silicon ring to reinforce the gastric pouch [7]. The concept was that by reinforcing the pouch with a ring, the reservoir capacity of the pouch will be preserved, and dilatation of pouch can be stalled.

We have been performing banded procedures since 2011 at our centre.

Technique

The gastric pouch has to be a lesser curvature-based pouch made over a 36 fr bougie. The length of the pouch is 8 cm and breadth is 2.5 cm. The volume of the pouch is 30–50 ml. Just below the second gastric vein, the pars flaccida is opened with harmonic shear. Once the lesser sac is opened, a blue or purple load of size 6 cm is fired (Fig. 16.1). A gastric tube of size 36 fr is placed, and vertical blue load is fired over the tube. The pad of fat over the stomach close to the left crus is dissected, and the two firings complete the gastric pouch.

A perigastric space is created 2.5 cm below the gastroesophageal junction, and the ring (GABp ring) of size 7 is placed loose around the pouch. The ring is placed in position with a stay suture at the staple line (Fig. 16.2).

An 80 cm biliopancreatic limb from the ligament of Treitz was measured and transected. A Roux limb, 120 cm, was measured, and a side-to-side 3–4-cm-wide entero-enterostomy anastomosis was formed.

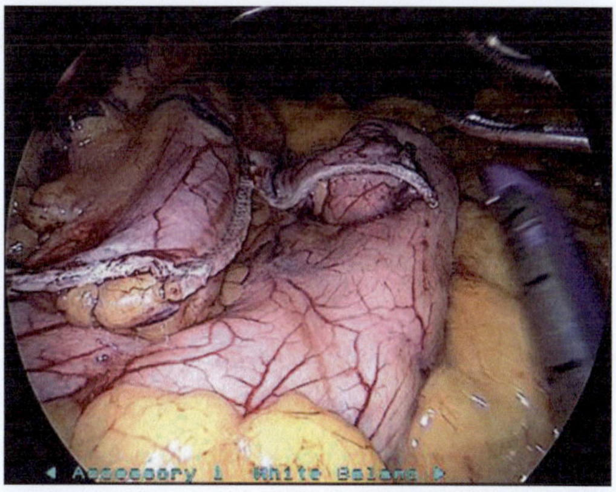

Fig. 16.1 Creating small pouch

M. Bhandari (✉) · H. Kumar Nautiyal · W. Mathur
S. Kosta
Department of Surgery, Mohak Bariatrics and Robotics Surgical Center, Indore, India

J. Ettinger et al. (eds.), *Gastric Bypass*, https://doi.org/10.1007/978-3-030-28803-7_16

Gastro-jejunal anastomoses of size 2.5 cm are made with the Roux limb with a blue load, and the defects are closed with absorbable suture (Figs. 16.3 and 16.4). Both Peterson's

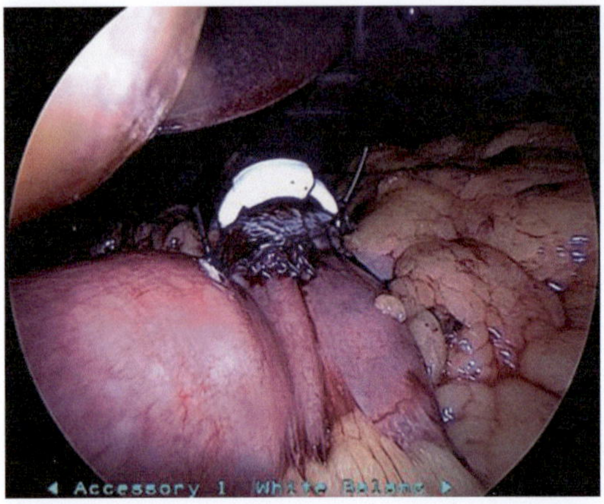

Fig. 16.2 Banding pouch with Fobi ring

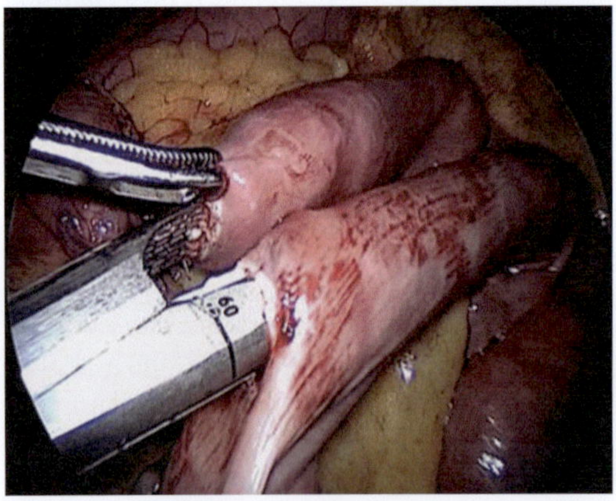

Fig. 16.3 Stapled Jejunojejunostomy

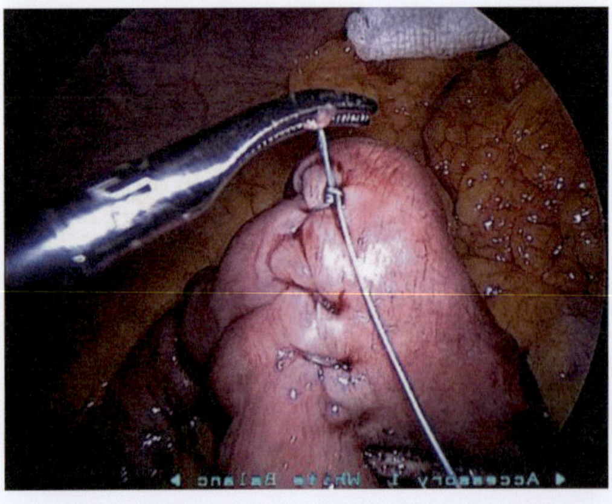

Fig. 16.4 Suture closure of enterotomy

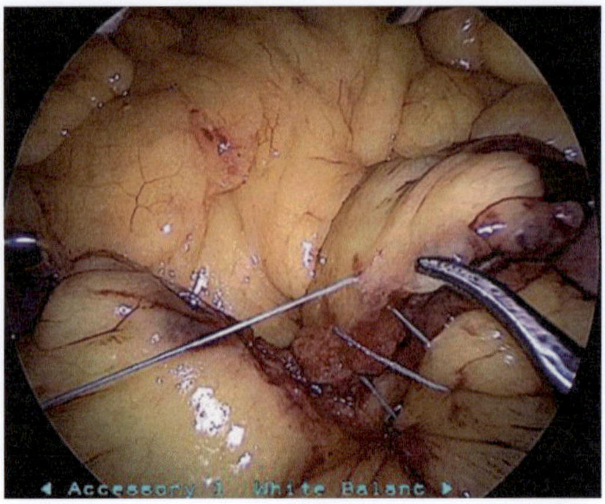

Fig. 16.5 Mesenteric defect closure

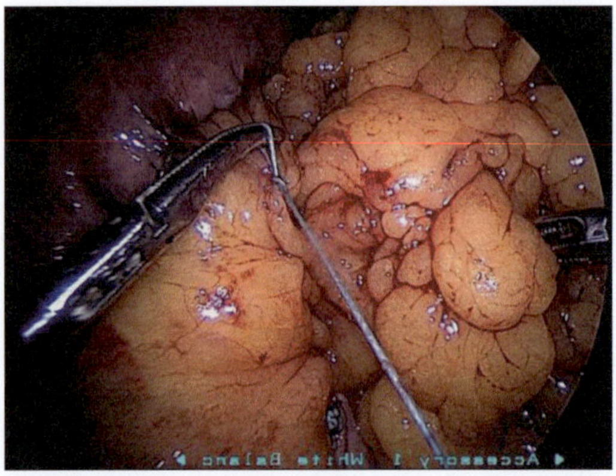

Fig. 16.6 Petersen's defect closure

and mesenteric defects are closed with non-absorbable sutures (Figs. 16.5 and 16.6).

Our Centres' Experience with Banded Gastric Bypass

Results/Complications

On 5-year follow-up of our patients, our banded RYGB patients have 71.5% EBWL and 30.5% TWL, though %EBWL and %TWL at 3 years was slightly more (Fig. 16.7). These results are significantly more than our results of non-banded RYGB which is 60.6% EBWL and 24% TWL at 5-year follow-up.

Similar results were shown by Luc Lemmen with 74% EWL in banded RYGB and 65.2% in

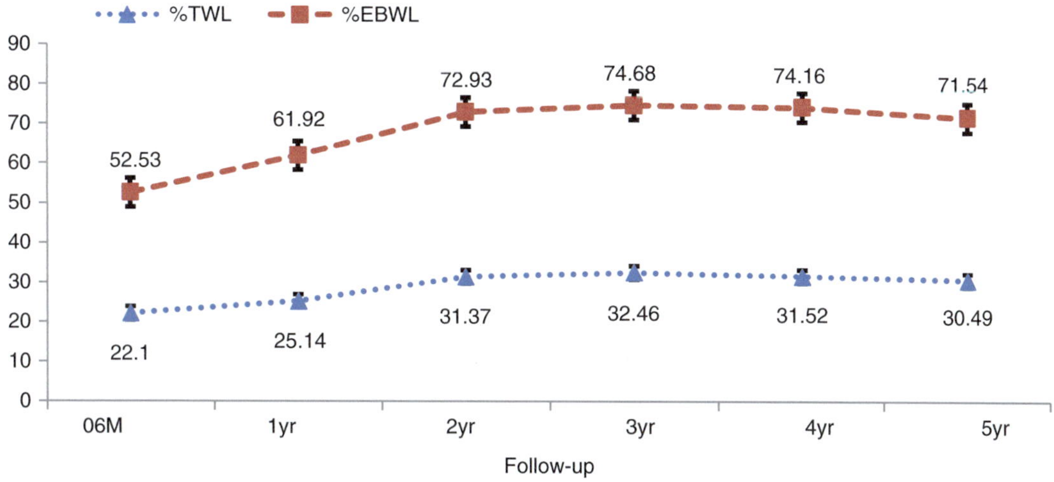

Fig. 16.7 %TWL and %EBWL post surgery with five years follow-up

non-banded at 5 years with significant weight regain in non-banded RYGB patients [8].

In long-term follow-up of 10 years, banded RYGB fared significantly better than non-banded RYGB, 82% and 63%, respectively, in study by William Awad [9]. Meta-analysis by Buchwald has also shown 72.5% EBWL at 5 years [10].

At 5-year follow-up, we achieved 80% resolution of T2DM, 56% hypertension, 40% sleep apnoea, and 56% resolution of dyslipidemia similar to our non-banded RYGB patients. Ten-year follow-up studies by William Awad have also shown 75% T2DM, 75% apnoea, and 66% dyslipidemia resolution which is significantly more than their non-banded RYGB patients [9]. Buchwald's meta-analysis has also shown resolution rates for T2DM from 75.0% to 92.0%, with an overall rate of 84.2%, dyslipidemia resolution rates ranged from 33.6% to 76.7%, with an overall rate 39.8%. Respective overall resolution rates for obstructive sleep apnoea and hypertension were 91.4% and 58.0% [10].

In our experience RYGB patients whether banded or non-banded perform significantly better than mini-gastric bypass or other more radical bypass procedure like SADI regarding long-term malnutrition. We had 19% anaemia, 10% hypoalbuminaemia, 30% vitamin B12, and 45.6% calcium deficiency at 5-year follow-up, which were corrected by dietary supplementation.

We have gradually simplified and perfected our technique which has led to very low complication rate. So far we have already done 2771 non-banded RYGB and 585 banded RYGB till October 2018. In perioperative period only one patient had to be reoperated for acute intestinal obstruction. Three patients had intra-abdominal bleeding which was managed conservatively by blood transfusion in two patients and one patient required re-laparoscopy. There was no case of documented marginal ulcer though many patients had complaint of pain abdomen in their follow-up period. As in most of these patients, they had already taken proton-pump inhibitors, which could have led to healing of early marginal ulcer. Among long-term complications, one patient had ring erosion which got extruded intraluminally spontaneously. In two patients we had to remove the gastric ring due to persistent dysphagia, though there was no mechanical obstruction due to ring. Two patients underwent revision surgery for regain of weight. In one patient we did lengthening of biliopancreatic limb, and in second case stomal narrowing was done with argon plasma coagulation and reinforcement suture for gastrojejunal stomal dilatation. There was no mortality. Various studies have shown wide range of early (up to 26%) and late complications up to 79% [11]. With complication rate of

1.19% and similar revision rate in our study, banded RYGB is an excellent procedure with sustained weight loss results.

References

1. Christou NV, Look D, Maclean LD. Weight gain after short- and long-limb gastric bypass in patients followed for longer than 10 years. Ann Surg. 2006;244(5):734–40.
2. Magro DO, Geloneze B, Delfini R, Pareja BC, Callejas F, Pareja JC. Long-term weight regain after gastric bypass: a 5-year prospective study. Obes Surg. 2008;18(6):648–51.
3. Bessler M, Daud A, Kim T, DiGiorgi M. Prospective randomized trial of banded versus non-banded gastric bypass for the super obese: early results. Surg Obes Relat Dis. 2007;3:480–4.
4. Capella JF, Capella RF. An assessment of vertical banded gastroplasty-Roux-en-Y gastric bypass for the treatment of morbid obesity. Am J Surg. 2002;183:117–23.
5. Halverson JD, Koehler RE. Assessment of patients with failed gastric operations for morbid obesity. Am J Surg. 1983;145:357–3.
6. Heneghan HM, Yimcharoen P, Brethauer SA, Kroh M, Chand B. Influence of pouch and stoma size on weight loss after gastric bypass. Surg Obes Relat Dis. 2012;8:408–15.
7. Fobi M. Why the operation I prefer is Silastic ring vertical gastric bypass. Obes Surg. 1991;1:423–6.
8. Lemmens L. Banded gastric bypass: better long-term results? A Cohort study with minimum 5-year follow-up. Obes Surg. 2017;27(4):864–72. https://doi.org/10.1007/s11695-016-2397-4.
9. Awad W, Garay A, Martinez C. Ten year's experience of banded gastric bypass: does it make a difference? Obes Surg. 2012;22(2):271–8. https://doi.org/10.1007/s11695-011-0555-2.
10. Buchwald H, Buchwald JN, McGlennon TW. Systematic review and meta-analysis of medium-term outcomes after banded Roux-en-Y gastric bypass. Obes Surg. 2014;24(9):1536–51. https://doi.org/10.1007/s11695-014-1311-1.
11. Bessler M, Daud A, Kim T, DiGiorgi M. Prospective randomized trial of banded vs nonbanded gastric bypass for the super obese: early results. Surg Obes Relat Dis. 2007;3:480–5.

17 Mini-Gastric Bypass and One-Anastomosis Gastric Bypass: Rationale

Mervyn Deitel, Cesare Peraglie, and David Hargroder

Introduction

The mini-gastric bypass (MGB) was devised by Robert Rutledge in the USA in 1997. As a trauma surgeon, he was faced with an abdominal gunshot wound where a duodenal exclusion with a Billroth II anastomosis was an appropriate reconstruction. This was the inspiration that led Rutledge to perform the MGB on consenting bariatric patients, constructing a *long* lesser curvature channel which prevents reflux [1, 2]. There was some initial skepticism of this new operation.

The authors of this chapter have been advocates of the MGB since 2002. The MGB has since increased throughout the world [3–14]. With the decrease in gastric banding, the MGB in 2016 is the third most common bariatric operation internationally [15] and the most common gastric bypass in India, Egypt, and Israel.

M. Deitel (✉)
Mini-Gastric Bypass–One Anastomosis Gastric Bypass Club, Toronto, ON, Canada
e-mail: book@obesitysurgery.com

C. Peraglie
Department of Surgery, Heart of Florida Regional Medical Center, Davenport, FL, USA

D. Hargroder
Department of Surgery, Mercy Hospitals, Joplin, MO, USA

Method of MGB

The laparoscopic MGB (Fig. 17.1) has two components: (1) a lesser-curvature *long* gastric pouch, serving as a slightly restrictive conduit, and (2) a 180–200 cm jejunal bypass with a wide antecolic gastrojejunal (GJ) anastomosis, which leads to carbohydrate and especially fat malabsorption.

Creation of the Pouch

After making a window into lesser sac, the lesser curvature of the stomach is stapler-divided at a right-angle distal to the incisura angularis (i.e., 2–3 cm distal to the crow's foot). A 28–40 Fr bougie is passed by the anesthesiologist, and the stomach is then stapler-divided proximally, parallel to lesser curvature. At the gastroesophageal (GE) junction, the surgeon divides this gastric conduit a few mm *lateral* to the angle of His; the cardia and left crus are explicitly avoided and *not* dissected, to prevent the leaks associated with the laparoscopic sleeve gastrectomy (LSG) operation [16, 17].

Thus, a low-pressure gastric conduit is constructed, unlike the high-pressure conduit of the LSG [18]. Attention is given to avoid any twist at the GJ anastomosis.

J. Ettinger et al. (eds.), *Gastric Bypass*, https://doi.org/10.1007/978-3-030-28803-7_17

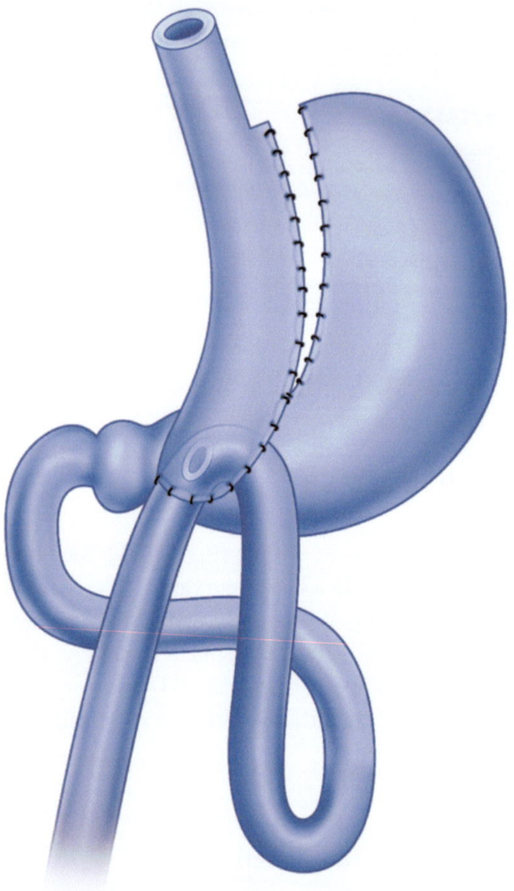

Fig. 17.1 MGB created by horizontal division *distal to* crow's foot, and then vertical division upwards (~18 cm length), extending to the left of the angle of His. A 4-cm wide antecolic gastrojejunostomy is performed 200 cm (varied with the BMI) distal to Treitz' ligament, providing malabsorption

Creation of the Malabsorptive Jejunal Bypass

Attention is turned to the left gutter. The greater omentum is retracted medially to identify the ligament of Treitz. The jejunum is run to 180 cm (Peraglie) or 200 cm (Hargroder) distal to Treitz' ligament. Peraglie traces the jejunum with 2.5 cm grasps hand over hand to 180 cm. Hargroder uses the width of his paddle retractor (3.5″, 8.75 cm) to measure the 200 cm.

In super-obese patients, up to 250 cm of proximal jejunum may be bypassed. However, with lesser BMI with comorbidities such as diabetes, a shorter jejunal limb (150 cm) may be bypassed [19–22].

At the selected site, the tip or adjacent posterior wall of the gastric pouch is anastomosed antecolic to the jejunum (can be fully stapled, hand-sewn or hybrid, and can be end to side or side to side), constructing a wide (3–4 cm) anastomosis under easy view. The GJ anastomosis should be at least 300 cm proximal to the ileocecal valve, to avoid protein malnutrition.

If a hiatal hernia (HH) is present, it is not repaired at the time of the MGB operation. If needed, HH repair can be performed 12–18 months later. However, experience has shown that the MGB is very effective in resolving GE reflux disease (GERD). This is due to traction that the GJ provides on the gastric pouch, reducing the cardia into the abdomen, plus the decreasing postoperative obesity.

However, if a large HH is present with adherence to the gastric fundus, it is dissected and repaired at the time of MGB; otherwise, a large bulbous fundus could be left. In this instance, a few plicating sutures are placed to approximate the crura posteriorly (or occasionally anteriorly).

Thus, a nonobstructed sleeve conduit is created, allowing slight restriction but adequate oral intake, accompanied by fat/carbohydrate malabsorption. Because the patient avoids carbohydrate which could produce rapid dumping, the intake has mainly fat malabsorption. The pouch in the MGB develops minimal dilatation, because there is no outlet narrowing by a stoma or pylorus [18]. There is slight increase in the number of stools per day (generally from 1 to 2), of no significance. Prasad and Bhandari perform the MGB using robotics, which is advantageous [23, 24].

Modifying the MGB

After the standard MGB, if ever necessary for inadequate or excess weight loss, the MGB can be modified by moving the GJ anastomosis distally or proximally, as a brief simple procedure [25]. The MGB can also be easily reversed in rare cases of intractable hypoalbuminemia or significant exccss weight loss; reversal entails stapler division along the GJ anastomosis (carefully inspecting the jejunal side), linear anastomosis of the gastric pouch to the matched bypassed stomach, and closing the defect at the bottom of the gastric pouch with running suture [22].

The One-Anastomosis Gastric Bypass (OAGB)

In 2002, after reading Rutledge's initial paper showing the simplicity and safety of the MGB [1], Profs. Miguel A. Carbajo and Manuel Garciacaballero in Spain (who had performed the RYGB for >10 years) began their variant of the MGB – the OAGB (BAGUA or *bypass gastrico de una anastomosis*) (Fig. 17.2) – which has a similar malabsorptive component [26, 27]. Because of suspicion by others of potential reflux and cancer, they designed a MGB variant with side-to-side anastomosis of the biliopancreatic limb to the gastric pouch (rising on the remnant stomach), to facilitate emptying of biliopancreatic juice toward the efferent limb and thus prevent reflux. The common limb (distal to the bypass) must always be ≥300 cm, to prevent malabsorption. In >3000 patients, Dr. Carbajo has not needed to revise any OAGB for reflux.

Thousands of OAGBs have been performed in Spain, Mexico, some Latin American countries, and Europe, and it currently represents 20% of the single-anastomosis gastric bypasses. The MGB itself, with the *long* gastric conduit, has a GE bile reflux problem in 0.7% of patients [14] (which may be treated conservatively or by a Braun jejuno-jejunostomy or RYGB). There has been no reported study comparing the OAGB to the MGB (which has the long conduit) with respect to GE reflux. The OAGB does take slightly longer to perform and is slightly more difficult to reverse than the MGB.

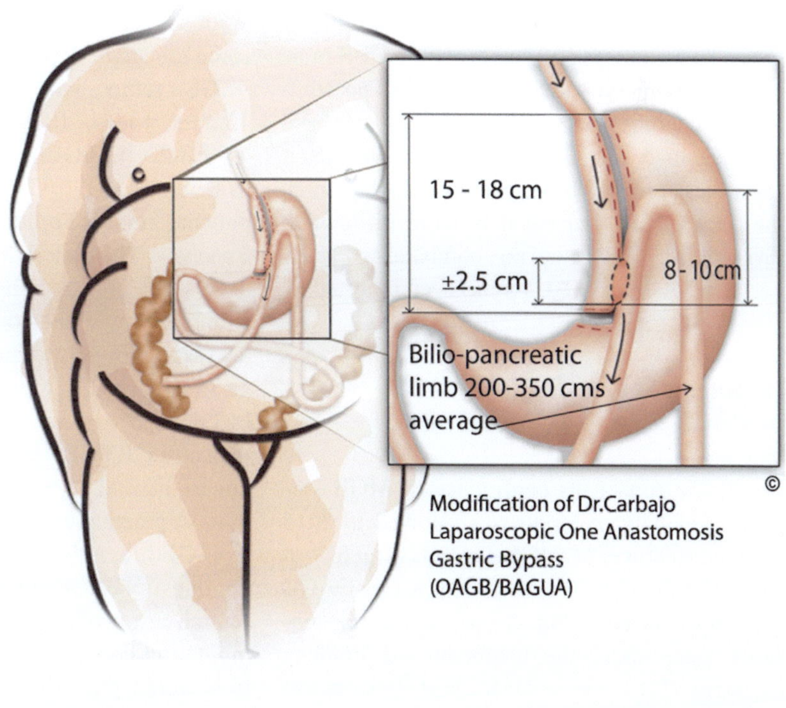

Fig. 17.2 OAGB with gastric pouch (~15 cm) and an antecolic 2.5 cm latero-lateral anastomosis between pouch and afferent jejunal loop which is suspended about 8–10 cm above the anastomosis through an initial continuous suture which secures the loop to the gastric pouch's staple line and with final fixation of the loop's apex to the bypassed stomach. Biliopancreatic limb averages 200–350 cm. (Diagram provided with the permission of Dr. Miguel A Carbajo; Modification of Dr. Carbajo Laparoscopic One Anastomosis Gastric Bypass (OAGB/ BAGUA))

Revision to MGB for Lap-Band or LSG Failure

The MGB is being commonly used as a salvage procedure for weight regain after the lap-band or LSG [4, 28]. If there is long-term follow-up after LSG, sleeve dilatation and weight regain are often found, particularly after 4 years [29]. Also, GE reflux may become troublesome in >30% of LSG patients [30].

In revision of LSG to MGB, it is very important *not* to construct a short gastric pouch (like the small pouch of the RYGB). A short, high gastric pouch with bile near the esophagus could lead to bile reflux esophagitis, as occurred occasionally after the old Mason horizontal loop gastric bypass [31]. Rather, for the MGB, a *long* gastric pouch must be constructed *below* crow's foot.

Advantages of MGB over the Single-Anastomosis Duodeno-Ileal Bypass with Sleeve Gastrectomy (SADI-S)

At the 2015 MGB Conclave [24], a number of surgeons had previous experience with the SADI-S (a one-anastomosis modification of the duodenal switch) [32]. They found SADI-S to be a longer operation: (1) SADI-S had the possibility of leak at the top of the SG; (2) it did not have the advantage of simple midline exposure; (3) it was necessary to mobilize proximal duodenum in the right gutter; and (4) it is more difficult to revise [33]. However, no comparative study between MGB and SADI-S has been reported.

Rationale for Performing MGB or OAGB

In 2014, a consensus conference of MGB surgeons was held in Montreal, followed in 2015 by a conference of MGB-OAGB surgeons at IFSO Vienna [34, 35] where the MGB-OAGB Club was formed (Fig. 17.3). These consensuses were under the leadership of Pradeep Chowbey (President of OSSI, past President of IFSO), Jean-Marc Chevallier (President of SOFCO), Robert Rutledge, K.S. Kular, and M. Deitel. A SurveyMonkey® questionnaire was filled out by 49 very experienced MGB-OAGB surgeons before the 2015 meeting. These surgeons reported past experience with the other operations – RYGB, banding, and LSG. The survey identified 22,988 MGBs-OAGBs, with average preoperative BMI 46.1 (range 35–63). Mean operating time was 60.7 minutes (range 35–127). Average hospital stay was 3.0 ± 1.6 days (range 1–5) and decreased with experience. Leak was reported in 8 patients (0.03%) (usually at the GJ), which is less than the troublesome proximal leaks following LSG [16]. Patients were usually ambulatory a few hours after surgery. Postoperative bleeding was reported in 9 patients (0.035%) and appears to be avoided by holding the stapler compressed for >30 seconds before firing. With hypertension, it may be advisable to reinforce the staple-line.

Fig. 17.3 Logo of the MGB-OAGB Club (www.mgb-oagb-club.com) which currently has >300 members

GE reflux was found preoperatively in 15.3 ± 14.2% (SD) and postoperatively in 4.6 ± 8.2%, i.e., GERD improved after the MGB, as demonstrated by Tolone [18]. About 1.5% of patients noticed bilious vomiting once every 3 months. The underlying cause may be an ulcer or a short pouch. It had been very rare for a Braun jejuno-jejunostomy or RYGB to become necessary for bile reflux (0.7%) with the long gastric pouch [14]. Marginal ulcers were reported in 1.4 ± 1.8% (range 0–5), which is slightly less than after RYGB [36, 37]. Bowel obstruction due to internal hernia has been exceedingly rare in most practices.

If GE bile reflux does occur, patients should be questioned about smoking and NSAIDs (which are prohibited), alcohol, eating late at night, and consuming a lot of fried foods [22]. It is noted that alcohol after MGB (as after RYGB) is absorbed rapidly. If persisting dyspepsia occurs, *H. pylori* or pouch kinking should be ruled out.

H. pylori (HP) stool antigen or breath test is checked preoperatively and treated if positive. HP is eradicated with helikit control before surgery. However, Rutledge has stated that reinfection with HP may negate the value of preoperative eradication therapy.

The MGB Conclave in India in July 2015 had 275 attendees [24]. It was reported that after MGB, EWL at 1 year was 76%, 2 years 85%, 3 years 78%, 4 years 75%, 5 years 70%, later 70%. The 30-day mortality has been low – 0.2%. Many of the MGB patients were high-risk [12, 24].

In the USA, the second author of this paper (CP) has had no operative deaths (i.e., within 30 days) out of 1800 MGBs over 13 years; the third author (DEH) has had no operative deaths in 1450 patients over 13 years of MGB. Both surgeons were trained by Dr. Rutledge. There have been deaths of patients for other reasons in later years. Peraglie found no deaths in his super-obese patients [21] and in those age >60 [38].

Intake Requirements

If there is indigestion, a proton pump inhibitor (PPI) may be prescribed. A PPI is important in treating marginal ulcer, as is eradication of *H. pylori* if present.

After MGB and OAGB, supplements consist of multivitamins, calcium (preferably dairy or calcium citrate), yogurt, vitamin D_3 1000 IU twice daily, and an intestinally absorbed iron supplement (Proferrin® – heme intestinal peptides). The duodenum where most iron absorption normally occurs is bypassed in the MGB-OAGB (as in the RYGB). Thus, in 5% of menstruating women, iron deficiency develops and requires increased oral iron or rarely IM or IV iron [39]. If B_{12} levels fall, replacement by sublingual crystalline B_{12} or injection becomes necessary.

Fruits and salads are well tolerated. Foods containing protein are important, e.g., meats, seafood, nuts, and dairy. Patients prevent "dumping" (weakness, sweating, diarrhea) by avoiding high-glycemic sugary foods. No intractable hypoglycemia has been reported. Fried, greasy, and fatty foods cause cramps and diarrhea (steatorrhea) and are thus avoided.

Vegetarians must take protein – legumes (lentils, beans, chick peas, peanuts, quinoa), yogurt, milk, soy (tofu) or whey protein, bran, brown rice, etc. Vegetables have incomplete protein, but multiple vegetables provide total amino acid requirements. In vegetarians and the elderly, it is usually wise not to bypass >200 cm of jejunum to avoid hypoalbuminemia [20].

Fear of Development of Cancer Unwarranted

After RYGB, lap-band or LSG, carcinoma of the gastric pouch and lower esophagus was reported in 46 patients [40–42]. After LSG, Barrett's esophagus may occur [43]. After MGB or OAGB, no carcinoma in the gastric pouch or esophagus has been reported. However, in the Far East where the incidence of gastric carcinoma remains high, one gastric carcinoma in Taiwan 9 years after MGB has been reported in the bypassed stomach, but not in the pouch [44]. Although some workers have compared the MGB to the Billroth II operation performed for peptic ulcer and cancer for 100 years, studies for development of gastric carcinoma after the Billroth II have found a decreased incidence [45–47], even though *H. pylori* was unknown and thus untreated. Furthermore, after performing >1000 vagotomy and pyloroplasties (V&P) by the first author (MD) in the 1960s–1970s for then-prevalent duodenal ulcer (with postoperative bile in the distal stomach), no gastric carcinoma has developed.

There was also fear of development of gastric cancer due to the effects of bile and other irritants in studies on the rat's stomach. However, Frantz [48] and Proctor [49] showed that bile led to hyperplasia and neoplasia in the proximal two-thirds of the unique rodent's stomach (which is *squamous-cell),* but not in the distal *glandular* third (which corresponds to the human stomach).

Advantages over Other Bariatric Operations

After LSG [29] and RYGB, variable weight regain has been found in the long-term [50, 51]. Comparative studies have documented more durable weight loss after the MGB [3, 13, 20, 52–55]. Also, better quality of life has been found after MGB [56, 57]. Regarding diabetes type 2, Lee reported greater elevation of GLP-1 after MGB than after RYGB [56].

Diabetes, hypertension, and lipid abnormalities have shown superior remission after MGB [58, 59]. Diabetes resolved in 75–95% [20, 60–62]. Kular found in diabetic patients with BMI <35 that HbA1c at 7 years was 5.7 ± 1.8% [63]; earlier intervention resulted in higher remission rates. In the Indian population, comorbidities of the metabolic syndrome often start at BMI 25. About 800 Canadians of Indian descent with metabolic syndrome (especially type 2 diabetes) have undergone MGB in India, with excellent resolution [34].

After the Spanish OAGB (BAGUA), the same resolution of type 2 diabetes and other comorbidities has been found [64, 65], including in the massively obese adolescent [66].

Conclusions

The MGB-OAGB has been found to be rapid, technically simpler and safer than other mainstream procedures. Very rare leaks or bleeding have occurred, and a single nonobstructing antecolic GJ anastomosis enables easy reversal or revision. The jejunal bypass length is modifiable with the BMI, and the MGB and OAGB have shown durable weight loss and comorbidity resolution. There should be surveillance for possible hypoalbuminemia and iron deficiency anemia. However, the foregoing advantages provide the rationale for these bariatric operations.

Acknowledgments The authors thank Prof. Miguel Carbajo (Member of International Committee for the European Accreditation Council for Bariatric Surgery of IFSO); Robert Rutledge, MD, FACS; and Kuldeepak S. Kular, President of the MGB-OAGB Club, for review and suggestions with this chapter.

Conflict of Interest The authors have no conflicts of interest to disclose.

References

1. Rutledge R. The mini-gastric bypass: experience with the first 1,274 cases. Obes Surg. 2001;11:276–80.
2. Rutledge R, Walsh W. Continued excellent results with the mini-gastric bypass: six-year study in 2,410 patients. Obes Surg. 2005;15:1304–8.
3. Lee WJ, Yu PJ, Wang W, Chen TC, Wei PL, Huang MT. Laparoscopic Roux-en-Y versus mini-gastric bypass for the treatment of morbid obesity: a prospective randomized controlled clinical trial. Ann Surg. 2005;42:20–8.
4. Rutledge R. Revision of failed gastric banding to mini-gastric bypass. Obes Surg. 2006;16:521–3.
5. Noun R, Riachi E, Zeidan S, Abboud B, Chalhoub V, Yazigi A. Mini-gastric bypass by mini-laparotomy: a cost-effective alternative in the laparoscopic era. Obes Surg. 2007;17:1482–6.
6. Chakhtoura G, Zinzindohou F, Ghanem Y, Ruseykin I, Dutranoy JC, Chevallier JM. Primary results of laparoscopic mini-gastric bypass in a French obesity-surgery specialized university hospital. Obes Surg. 2008;18:1130–3.
7. Chevallier J-M, Chakhtoura G, Zinzindohoue F. Laparoscopic mini-gastric bypass. In: Deitel M, Gagner M, Dixon JB, Himpens J, Madan A, editors. Handbook of obesity surgery. Toronto: FD-Communications; 2010. p. 78–84.
8. Piazza L, Ferrara F, Leanza S, Coco D, Sarvà S, Bellia A, et al. Laparoscopic mini-gastric bypass: short-term single-institute experience. Updates Surg. 2011;63:239–42.
9. Noun R, Skaff J, Riachi E, Daher R, Antoun NA, Nasr M. One thousand consecutive mini-gastric bypass: short and long-term outcome. Obes Surg. 2012;22:697–703.
10. Peterko AC, Mazul-Sunko B, Mirosevic G, Bekavac-Beslin M. Combined sleeve gastrectomy and mini-gastric bypass in a new bariatric procedure of mini-gastric bypass and proximal sleeve gastrectomy. Acta Clin Croat. 2013;52:316–20.
11. Musella M, Sousa A, Greco F, De Luca M, Manno E, Di Stefano C, et al. The laparoscopic mini-gastric bypass: the Italian experience: outcomes from 974 consecutive cases in a multi-center review. Surg Endosc. 2014;28:156–63.
12. Kular KS, Manchanda N, Rutledge R. A 6-year experience with 1,054 mini-gastric bypasses – first study from Indian subcontinent. Obes Surg. 2014;24:1430–5.

13. Musella M, Milone M, Gaudioso D, Bianco P, Palumbo R, Bellini M, et al. A decade of bariatric surgery. What have we learned? Outcome in 520 patients from a single institution. Int J Surg. 2014;12(Suppl 1):S183–8.
14. Chevallier JM, Arman GA, Guenzi M, Rau C, Bruzzi M, Beaupel N, et al. One thousand single anastomosis (omega loop) gastric bypasses to treat morbid obesity in a 7-year period: outcomes show few complications and good efficacy. Obes Surg. 2015;25:951–8.
15. Deitel M. Letter to the editor: bariatric surgery worldwide 2013 reveals a rise in mini gastric bypass. Obes Surg. 2015;25:2165.
16. Moszkowicz D, Arienzo R, Khettab I, Rahmi G, Zinzindohoue F, Berger A, et al. Sleeve gastrectomy severe complications: is it always a reasonable surgical option? Obes Surg. 2013;3:676–86.
17. Sakran N, Assalia A, Keidar A, Goitein D. Gastrobronchial fistula as a complication of bariatric surgery: a series of 6 cases. Obes Facts. 2012;5:538–45.
18. Tolone S, Cristiano S, Savarino E, Lucido FS, Fico DI, Docimo L. Effects of omega-loop bypass on esophagogastric junction function. Surg Obes Relat Dis. 2016;12:62–9.
19. Lee WJ, Wang W, Lee YC, Huang MT, Ser KH, Chen J. Laparoscopic mini-gastric bypass: experience with tailored bypass limb according to body weight. Obes Surg. 2008;18:294–9.
20. Jammu GS, Sharma R. A 7-year clinical audit of 1107 cases comparing sleeve gastrectomy, Roux-en-Y gastric bypass and mini-gastric bypass, to determine an effective and safe bariatric and metabolic procedure. Obes Surg. 2016;26:928–32.
21. Peraglie C. Laparoscopic minigastric bypass (LMGB) in the super-super obese: outcomes in 16 patients. Obes Surg. 2008;18:1126–9.
22. Rutledge R, Kular KS, Deitel M. Laparoscopic mini-gastric (one-anastomosis) bypass surgery. In: Agrawal S, editor. Obesity, bariatric and metabolic surgery: a practical guide. Cham: Springer; 2016. p. 415–25.
23. Prasad A. Robotic one anastomosis (omega loop/mini) gastric bypass for morbid obesity. J Robotic Surg. 2014;8:371–4.
24. Deitel M, Prasad A, Kular KS, Rutledge R. Report on the mini-gastric bypass conclave, India. Bariatric News. 2015;(26):33.
25. Lee WJ, Lee YC, Ser KH, Chen SC, Su YH. Revisional surgery for laparoscopic minigastric bypass. Surg Obes Relat Dis. 2011;7:486–91.
26. Garcia-Caballero M, Carbajo M. One anastomosis gastric bypass: a simple, safe and efficient procedure for treating morbid obesity. Nutr Hosp. 2004;19:372–5.
27. Carbajo M, Garcia-Caballero M, Toledano M, Osorio D, Garacia-Lanza C, Carmona JA. One-anastomosis gastric bypass by laparoscopy: results of the first 209 patients. Obes Surg. 2005;5:398–404.
28. Weiner RA, Theodoridou S, Weiner S. Failure of laparoscopic sleeve gastrectomy – further procedure? Obes Facts. 2011;(Suppl 1):42–6.
29. Golomb I, Ben David M, Glass A, Kolitz T, Keidar A. Long-term metabolic effects of laparoscopic sleeve gastrectomy. JAMA Surg. 2015;150:1051–7.
30. Thereaux J, Barsamian C, Bretault M, Dusaussoy H, Lamarque D, Bouillot J-L, et al. pH monitoring of gastro-oesophageal reflux before and after laparoscopic sleeve gastrectomy. Br J Surg. 2016;103:399–406.
31. Mason EE, Ito C. Gastric bypass. Ann Surg. 1969;170:329–39.
32. Sánchez-Pernaute A, Rubio MA, Pérez Aguirre E, Barabash A, Cabrerizo L, Torres A. Single-anastomosis duodenoileal bypass with sleeve gastrectomy: metabolic improvement and weight loss in first 100 patients. Surg Obes Relat Dis. 2013;9:731–5.
33. Summerhays C, Cottam D, Cottam A. Internal hernia after revisional laparoscopic loop duodenal switch surgery. Surg Obes Relat Dis. 2016;12:e13–5.
34. Deitel M, Kular KS. Mini-gastric (one-anastomosis) bypass course. Bariatric News. 2014;(22):8.
35. Deitel M, Kular KS, Musella M, Carbajo M, Luque-de-Leon E. A new organization – The MGB/OAGB Club. Bariatric News. 2016;(26):9.
36. El-Hayek K, Timratana P, Shimizu H, Chand B. Marginal ulcer after Roux-en-Y gastric bypass: what have we really learned? Surg Endosc. 2012;26:2789–96.
37. Gumbs AA, Duffy AJ, Bell RL. Incidence and management of marginal ulceration after laparoscopic Roux-en-Y gastric bypass. Surg Obes Relat Dis. 2006;2:460–3.
38. Peraglie C. Laparoscopic mini-gastric bypass in patients age 60 and older. Surg Endosc. 2016;30:38–43.
39. Chen MC, Lee YC, Lee WJ, Liu HL, Ser KH. Diet behavior and low hemoglobin level after laparoscopic mini-gastric bypass surgery. Hepatogastroenterology. 2012;59:2530–2.
40. Scozzari G, Trapani R, Toppino M, Morino M. Esophagogastric cancer after bariatric surgery: systematic review of the literature. Surg Obes Relat Dis. 2013;9:133–42.
41. Scheepers AF, Schoon EJ, Nienhuijs SW. Esophageal cancer after sleeve gastrectomy. Surg Obes Relat Dis. 2011;7(4):e11–2.
42. Angrisani L, Santonicola A, Iovino P. Gastric cancer: a de novo diagnosis after laparoscopic sleeve gastrectomy. Surg Obes Relat Dis. 2014;10:186–7.
43. Braghetto I, Csendes A. Prevalence of Barrett's esophagus in bariatric patients undergoing sleeve gastrectomy. Obes Surg. 2016;26:710–4.
44. Wu CC, Lee WJ, Ser KH, Chen JC, Tsou JJ, Chen SC, et al. Gastric cancer after mini-gastric bypass surgery: a case report. Asian J Endosc Surg. 2013;6:303–6.
45. Schafer LW, Larson DE, Melton LJ III. The risk of gastric carcinoma after surgical treatment for benign ulcer disease: a population-based study in Olmsted County, Minnesota. N Engl J Med. 1983;309:1210–3.
46. Luukkonen P, Kalima T, Kivilaako E. Decreased risk of gastric stump carcinoma after partial gastrectomy. Hepatogastroenterol. 1990;37:392–4.

47. Bassily R, Smallwood RA, Crotty R. Risk of gastric cancer is not increased after partial gastrectomy. J Gastroenterol Hepatol. 2000;15:762–5.
48. Frantz JD, Bretton G, Cartwright ME, Crissman JW, Macklin AW, Maronpot RR. Proliferative lesions of the non-glandular and glandular stomach of rats. In: Guides for Toxicologic Pathology STP/ARP/AFIP. Washington, DC: Society of Toxicologic Pathologists; 1991. p. 1–20. https://www.toxpath.org/docs/SSNDC/StomachProliferativeRat.pdf.
49. Proctor DM, Gatto NM, Hong SJ, Allamneni KP. Mode-of-action framework for evaluating the relevance of rodent forestomach tumors in cancer risk assessment. Toxicol Sci. 2007;98:313–26.
50. Christou NV, Look D, MacLean LD. Weight gain after short- and long-limb gastric bypass in patients followed for longer than 10 years. Ann Surg. 2006;244:734–40.
51. Hsieh T, Zurita L, Grover H, Bennett A, Farrokhyar F, Gmora S, et al. 10-year outcomes of the vertical transected gastric bypass for obesity: a systematic review. Obes Surg. 2014;24:456–61.
52. Padwal R, Klarenbach S, Wiebe N, Birch D, Karmali S, Manns B, Sharma AM, Tonelli M. Bariatric surgery: a systematic review and network meta-analysis of randomized trials. Obes Rev. 2011;12:602–21.
53. Lee WJ, Ser KH, Lee YC, Tsou JJ, Chen SC, Chen JC. Laparoscopic Roux-en-Y vs. mini-gastric bypass for the treatment of morbid obesity: a 10-year experience. Obes Surg. 2012;22:1827–34.
54. Disse E, Pasquer A, Espalieu P, Poncet G, Gouillat C, Robert M. Greater weight loss with the omega loop bypass compared to Roux-en-Y gastric bypass: a comparative study. Obes Surg. 2014;24:841–6.
55. Kular KS, Manchanda N, Rutledge R. Analysis of the five-year outcomes of sleeve gastrectomy and mini gastric bypass: a report from the Indian sub-continent. Obes Surg. 2014;24:1724–8.
56. Lee WJ, Chong K, Lin YH, Wei JH, Chen SC. Laparoscopic sleeve gastrectomy versus single anastomosis (mini-) gastric bypass for the treatment of type 2 diabetes mellitus: 5-year results of a randomized trial and study of incretin effect. Obes Surg. 2014;24:1552–62.
57. Bruzzi M, Rau C, Voron T, Guenzi M, Berger A, Chevallier JM. Single anastomosis or mini-gastric bypass: long-term results and quality of life after a 5-year follow-up. Surg Obes Relat Dis. 2015;11:321–6.
58. Georgiadou D, Sergentanis TN, Nixon A, Diamantis T, Tsigris C, Psaltopoulou T. Efficacy and safety of laparoscopic mini-gastric bypass. A systematic review. Surg Obes Relat Dis. 2014;10:984–91.
59. Milone M, Lupoli R, Maletta P, Di Minno A, Bianco P, Ambrisoni P, et al. Lipid profile changes in patients undergoing bariatric surgery: a comparative study between sleeve gastrectomy and mini-gastric bypass. Int J Surg. 2015;14:28–32.
60. Milone M, Di Minno MN, Leongito M, Maietta P, Bianco P, Taffuri C, Gaudioso D, Lupoli R, et al. Bariatric surgery and diabetes remission: sleeve gastrectomy or mini-gastric bypass? World J Gastroenterol. 2013;19:6590–7.
61. Musella M, Apers J, Rheinwalt K, Ribeiro R, Manno E, Greco F, et al. Efficacy of bariatric surgery in type 2 diabetes mellitus remission: the role of mini gastric bypass/one anastomosis gastric bypass and sleeve gastrectomy at 1 year of follow-up. A European survey. Obes Surg. 2016;26:933–40.
62. Quan Y, Huang A, Ye M, Xu M, Zhuang B, Zhang P, et al. Efficacy of laparoscopic mini gastric bypass for obesity and type 2 diabetes mellitus: a systematic review and meta-analysis. Gastroenterol Res Pract. 2015;2015:13. https://doi.org/10.1155/2015/152852.
63. Kular SK, Manchanda N, Cheema GK. Seven years of mini-gastric bypass in type II diabetes patients with a body mass index <35 kg/m^2. Obes Surg. 2016;26:1457–62.
64. Garcia-Caballero M, Valle M, Martinez-Moreno JM, Miralles F, Toval JA, Mata JM, et al. Resolution of diabetes mellitus and metabolic syndrome in normal weight 24-29 BMI patients with one anastomosis gastric bypass. Nutr Hosp. 2012;27:623–31.
65. Carbajo MA, Jimenez JM, Castro MJ, Ortiz-Solorzano J, Arango A. Outcomes and weight loss, fasting blood glucose and glycosylated hemoglobin in a sample of 415 obese patients, included in the database of the European Accreditation Council for Excellence Centers for bariatric surgery with laparoscopic one anastomosis gastric bypass. Nutr Hosp. 2014;30:1032–8.
66. Carbajo MA, Vazquez-Pelcastre R, Aparicio-Ponce R, Luque de Lyon E, Jimenez JM, Ortiz-Solarzano J, et al. 12-year old adolescent with super morbid obesity, treated with laparoscopic one anastomosis gastric bypass (LOAGB/BAGUA): a case report after 5-year follow-up. Nutr Hosp. 2015;31:2327–32.

Simplified Gastric Bypass: The Brazilian Technique

18

Almino Cardoso Ramos
and Eduardo Lemos de Souza Bastos

Introduction

Despite the exponential growth of laparoscopic sleeve gastrectomy (LSG) indications in recent years, which now accounts for about 50% to 60% of all bariatric procedures [1, 2], Roux-en-Y gastric bypass (RYGB) is still considered the "gold standard" operation for morbid obesity based on its better long-term weight loss and control of comorbidities. Since the original description more than 50 years ago [3], gastric bypass (GB) underwent several technical changing and improvements over time, resulting in the current concept of small vertical gastric pouch, narrow gastrojejunostomy, and Roux-en-Y reconstruction with longer limbs. After so many technical proposals, the expected result is the absence of a universally accepted step-by-step systematization [4]. Gastric pouch size, restriction ring placement, gastrojejunostomy stapled or hand-sewn and calibrated or non-calibrated, intestinal time before or after the gastric pouch construction, transmesocolic or antecolic pathway, lengths of the alimentary and biliopancreatic limbs, closure of the mesenteric spaces, staple-line reinforcement, and drainage of the peritoneal cavity are just some topics still under debate. However, some principles such as the use of the laparoscopic approach, the creation of a small vertical pouch, Roux-en-Y reconstruction, and longer limbs appear to be widely accepted and commonly practiced by most surgeons nowadays.

Since the end of the year 2001, the excellence team in Bariatric and Metabolic Surgery at Gastro Obeso Center (Sao Paulo, Brazil) started to perform the laparoscopic RYGB with a more simplified systematization, whose safety and feasibility were presented in 2004 with more than 500 patients operated [5], and a large series involving 12,000 patients was subsequently published [6]. This standardization became known as "simplified gastric bypass" or "simplified Brazilian gastric bypass technique" and has since been adopted as technique of choice by several other bariatric surgeons [7–10].

The main purpose of simplified gastric bypass is to make the procedure technically easier and more reproducible, shortening the learning curve and contributing to the expansion of the laparo-

A. C. Ramos
International Federation for the Surgery of Obesity and Metabolic Disorders (IFSO), Naples, Italy

Gastro-Obeso-Center – Advanced Institute for Metabolic Optimization, São Paulo, Brazil

Brazilian Society of Bariatric and Metabolic Surgery (SBCBM), São Paulo, Brazil

E. L. de S. Bastos (✉)
International Federation for the Surgery of Obesity and Metabolic Disorders (IFSO), Naples, Italy

Gastro-Obeso-Center – Advanced Institute for Metabolic Optimization, São Paulo, Brazil

Division of Gastrointestinal Surgery, Marilia School of Medicine, São Paulo, Brazil

Brazilian Society of Bariatric and Metabolic Surgery (SBCBM), São Paulo, Brazil

J. Ettinger et al. (eds.), *Gastric Bypass*, https://doi.org/10.1007/978-3-030-28803-7_18

scopic RYGB. To date, the excellence team in Bariatric and Metabolic Surgery at Gastro Obeso Center has already submitted more than 20,000 morbidly obese patients to simplified gastric bypass, being arguably one of the most expressive experiences in the laparoscopic RYGB technique worldwide. More recently, simplified gastric bypass has also been performed through robotic platforms [11], but the step-by-step technique is quite similar to the traditional laparoscopic approach.

Laparoscopic Simplified Gastric Bypass: Step-by-Step Technique

Position the Patient and the Surgical Team

The operation is performed with the patient in horizontal dorsal decubitus with open legs and pronounced reverse Trendelenburg position (35–45 degrees). Fixation on the operating table is accomplished by placing a leather belt below the waist line. In addition, the lower limbs are also attached to the surgical table using bandages at the level of the thighs and knees. The surgeon remains between the legs of the patient (Fig. 18.1), with the first assistant, who manipulates the camera and the auxiliary tweezers, and the instrumentator on his right side. Typically, bladder catheterization is not performed. Antibiotic prophylaxis is routinely used. The prevention of thromboembolism is made using graduated compression stockings, pneumatic boots of intermittent compression, and administration of low molecular weight heparin, which is maintained for 10 days after discharge. A 32-gauge Fouchet-type gastric probe is placed in the stomach by the anesthesiologist before the onset of pneumoperitoneum.

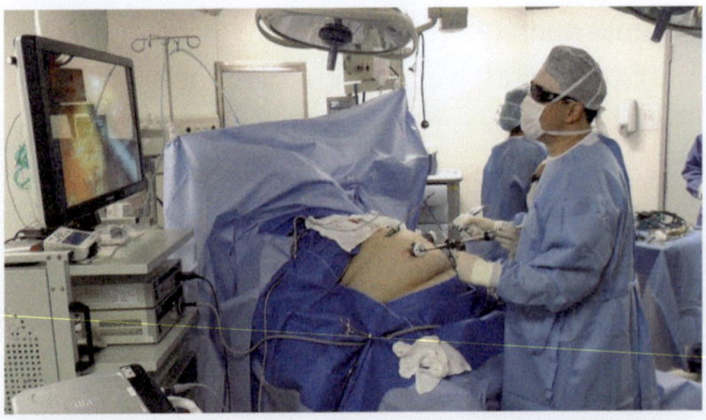

Fig. 18.1 Patient's position: pronounced reverse Trendelenburg position with the surgeon in between patient's legs

Pneumoperitoneum and Placement of the Trocars

The pneumoperitoneum is routinely performed with direct puncture with a Veress needle in the left upper quadrant, near the costal margin at the level of the midclavicular line (Palmer's point). The initial pressure is set at 16 mmHg and maintained till the expected pressure (from 15 to 16 mmHg) is reached. The laparoscopic approach of the abdominal cavity is initiated through trocar number 1, permanent 10 mm, placed at mesogastrium, 12–15 cm below the xiphoid process and 3 cm to the left of the midline, and used for the insertion of a 30-degree optic/camera. The trocar number 2 (5 mm, permanent) is placed near the xiphoid process for the liver retractor, which is usually a stick/probe attached to the surgical field with the aid of Backhaus forceps and surgical dressing. The trocar number 3, 12-mm disposable, used by the surgeon's left hand, is placed on the right side of the patient in an intermediate position between the two anterior and 3–5 cm laterally to the midline. The trocar number 4, also 5-mm permanent, is placed along the left costal margin in the anterior axillary line and used by the first assistant. Lastly, the trocar number 5, 12-mm disposable, is placed adjacent to the left costal margin in the hemiclavicular line to surgeon's right hand manipulation. The pneumoperitoneum is usually maintained by trocar number 5 (Fig. 18.2).

Gastric Pouch Construction

The preparation to create the gastric pouch is initiated with the dissection of the esophagogastric angle (His) and the opening of the left gastro-

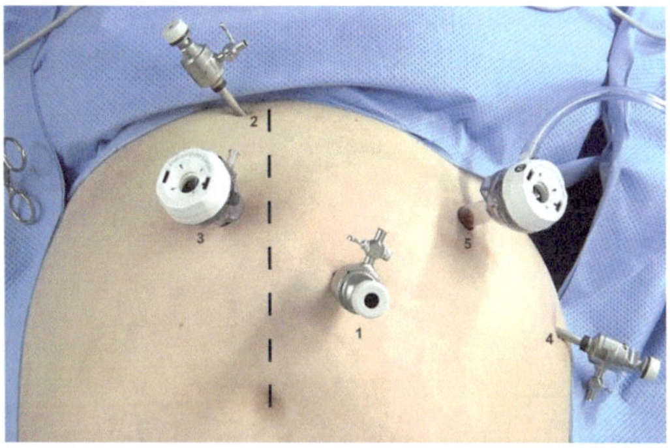

Fig. 18.2 Trocars set placement position

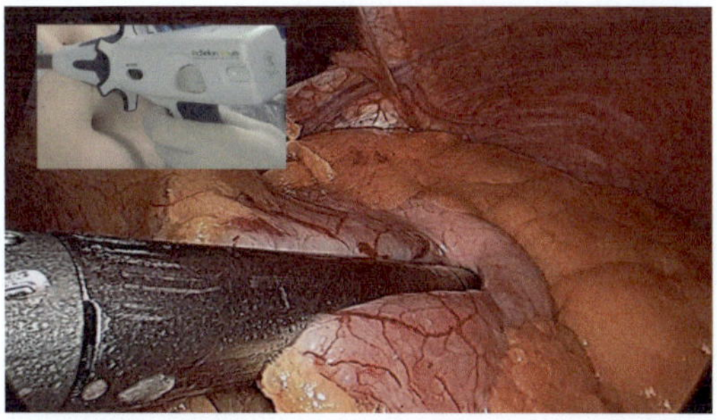

Fig. 18.3 Pouch construction: first stapling, horizontal, starting in the second vessel in the lesser gastric curvature

phrenic ligament with ultrasound scissors, so as to expose the lateral aspect of the left diaphragmatic pillar. Then, the exeresis of the fat pad of the esophagogastric junction (Belsey's fat) is done. The lesser curvature is opened between the second and third gastric vessel, also with Ultracision®, getting access to the posterior gastric wall. The first firing of the linear cutting stapler is performed through trocar number 3 in the horizontal direction loaded with a 45 mm blue cartridge (Fig. 18.3). Then, the retrogastric space is dissected until complete visualization of the left diaphragmatic crus, and a vertical staple-line is performed through trocar number 5 in cranial direction, also with blue cartridges of 45 mm, finishing the gastric pouch, always keeping safe distance from the esophagus of at least 0.5 cm from gastric tissue to esophagogastric angle (Fig. 18.4). The staple-lines of both bypassed stomach (Fig. 18.5), and gastric pouch are submitted to continuous and transfixing suture reinforcement of absorbable sutures (3-0 Caprofyl®).

Gastrojejunostomy

Aiming the ascent of the jejunal loop to the supramesocolic area, the greater omentum is mobilized to the upper abdomen and completely divided caudo-cranially using ultrasound scissors. This maneuver allows easy access to duodenojejunal angle to define the length of biliopancreatic limb, usually 100 cm for BMI up to 50 kg/m^2 or 200 cm for super-obese patients. Keeping the proximal part of the jejunum always to the right side of the surgeon, the jejunal loop is moved to the upper abdomen without division, similarly to the isoperistaltic Billroth II reconstruction. In this way, the surgeon can set the length of preference for biliopancreatic limb and the gastrojejunostomy (GJ) accomplishment. After doing two small holes with ultrasound scissors – one on the jejunal loop and the other on the posterior surface of the gastric pouch – the GJ is performed using a 45 mm linear cutting stapler loaded with white cartridge, introduced by trocar number 3. A calibrated GJ is carried out using only the final portion of the stapler (15 mm) (Fig. 18.6). The aperture was sutured with running absorbable seromuscular suture (Caprofyl® 3-0), having a 32-Fr Fouchet probe type for calibration. Interrupted seromuscular sutures with nonabsorbable thread (Ethibond® 2-0) are routinely applied at the GJ angles in order to decrease the tension in the anastomosis and to collaborate with maintaining the original diameter in the long term (Fig. 18.7).

Petersen Space Closure

With cranial traction of the mesocolon – close to the medial part of the transverse colon toward to the liver –, the Petersen space is closed with continuous double layer of nonabsorbable suture (Ethibond® 2-0), starting close to transverse colon border toward the lower angle of the space and returning to the starting point with the same unabsorbable thread, similar to a gastrointestinal anastomosis in two layers (Fig. 18.8). This technique aims to avoid small

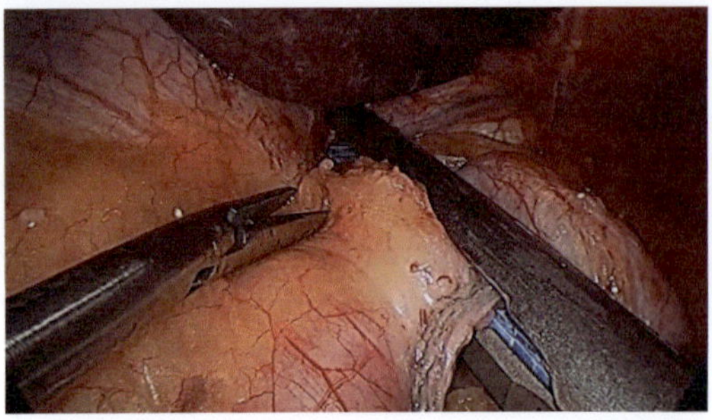

Fig. 18.4 Pouch construction: last vertical stapling, with perfect visualization of the tip of the blue cartridge, keeping a safe distance from the esophagus

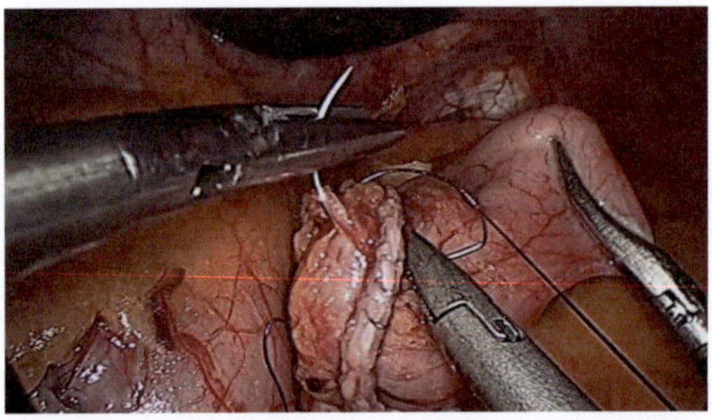

Fig. 18.5 Running absorbable transfixant reinforcement suture at the bypassed stomach

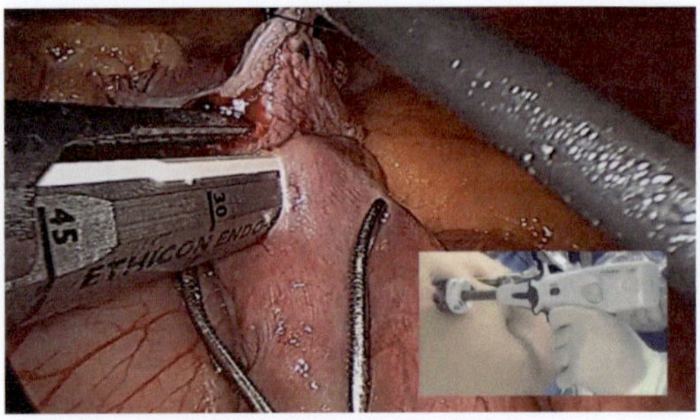

Fig. 18.6 Stapler positioned for GJ calibrated to 15 mm with white cartridge

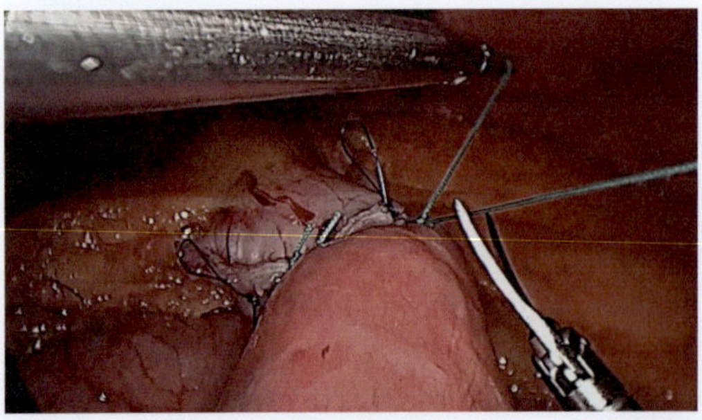

Fig. 18.7 GJ angle reinforcement

holes between the suture loops, especially after large visceral fat losses. It is worth noting that a good exposure of the surgical field greatly facilitates the technical execution of the complete closure of the Petersen space, with low risk of complications.

Entero-entero Anastomosis (EEA)

From the GJ, in distal jejunum direction and according to the surgeon's preference, a segment of 1 m of jejunum was measured to be anastomosed to the biliopancreatic limb on the afferent portion of the GJ, thereby determining the length of the alimentary limb (Roux limb) (Fig. 18.9).

The EEA is performed in the anisoperistaltic way, with 45 mm white cartridge stapler. After reviewing the possibility of internal bleeding on the stapler line, the aperture made for stapler jaws placement is closed with running seromuscular absorbable suture (3-0 Caprofyl®). The new-created mesenteric defect between the mesentery of the biliopancreatic limb and common channel is also routinely closed with continuous nonabsorbable suture (2-0 Ethibond®).

After finishing the EEA, about 250 ml of saline solution stained with 10 ml of methylene blue are introduced through Fouchet probe to verify the integrity of both anastomoses previously performed (GJ and EEA) and still connected through double omega reconstruction. Then, the portion corresponding to biliopancreatic limb is sectioned close to the GJ to convert the initial format of double omega to Roux-en-Y technique (Fig. 18.10).

When it is rarely necessary, a tubular silicone drain is exteriorized through the trocar number 4. The trocars, then, are removed under direct visualization and in case of bleeding the corresponding incision was closed with Vicryl® 0. All skin incisions are closed with absorbable intradermal interrupted sutures (Monocryl® 3-0).

In summary, after 18 years of experience and over 20,000 patients operated only at Gastro Obeso Center, the simplified gastric bypass remains a feasible and safe technique with a low

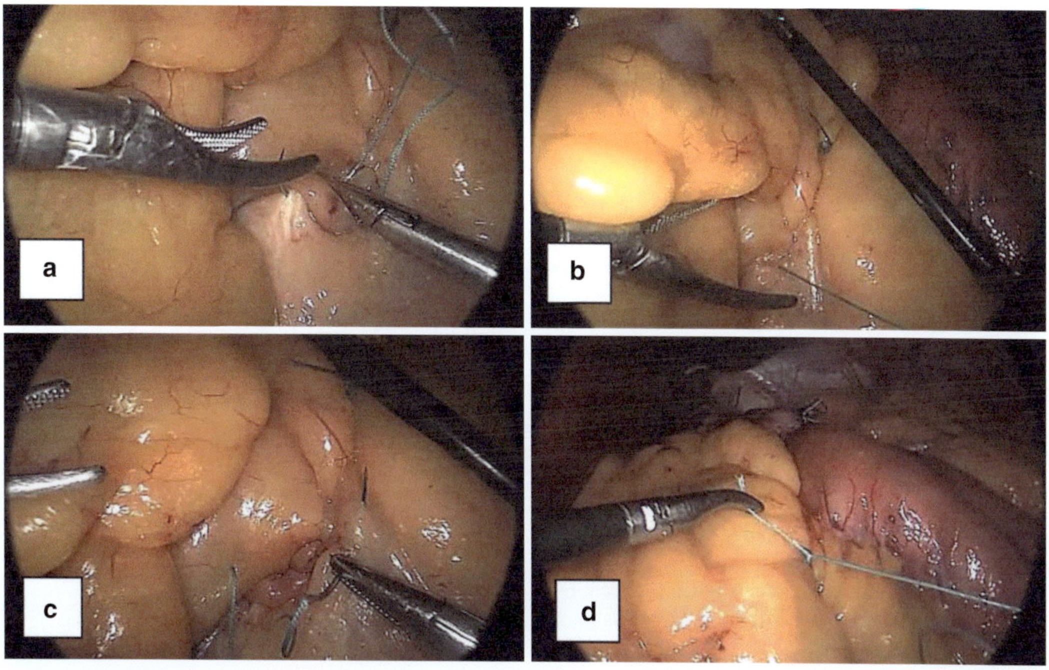

Fig. 18.8 Technical sequence of the continuous double layer Petersen space closure. (**a**) Starting the running suture close to transverse colon edge; (**b**) first layer finished; (**c**) backing to the starting point with the second layer of continuous nonabsorbable suture; (**d**) finishing the Petersen space closure

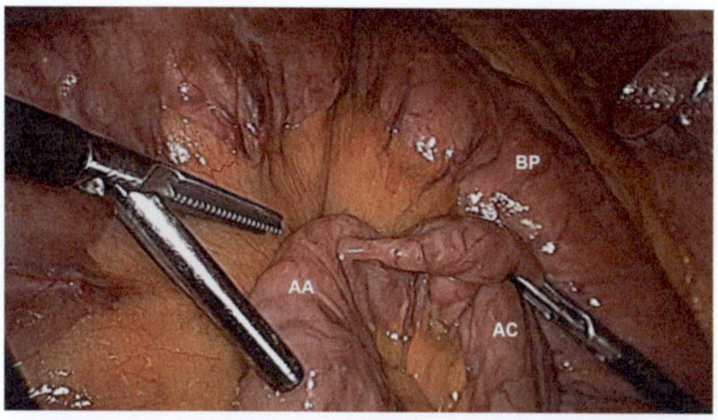

Fig. 18.9 Lengthening the alimentary limb for an omega side-to-side anastomosis with the biliopancreatic limb

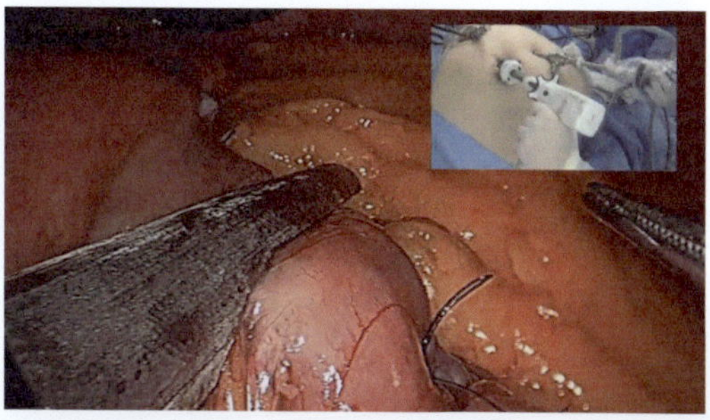

Fig. 18.10 Final section of the biliopancreatic limb close to GJ, converting the initial double omega reconstruction to a final Roux-en-Y fashion

rate of complications. In addition, the high reproducibility provided by this simplified step-by-step technique is especially interesting for training and teaching in bariatric surgery, shortening the learning curve.

References

1. English WJ, DeMaria EJ, Brethauer SA, Mattar SG, Rosenthal RJ, Morton JM. American Society for Metabolic and Bariatric Surgery estimation of metabolic and bariatric procedures performed in the United States in 2016. Surg Obes Relat Dis. 2018;14(3):259–63.
2. Angrisani L, Santonicola A, Iovino P, Vitiello A, Higa K, Himpens J, et al. IFSO worldwide survey 2016: primary, endoluminal, and revisional procedures. Obes Surg. 2018;28(12):3783–94.
3. Mason EE, Ito C. Gastric bypass in obesity. Surg Clin North Am. 1967;47:1345–51.
4. Madan AK, Harper JL, Tichansky DS. Techniques of laparoscopic gastric bypass: on-line survey of American Society for Bariatric Surgery practicing surgeons. Surg Obes Relat Dis. 2008;4(2):166–72.
5. Cardoso RA, Galvão NM, Carlo A. Simplified gastric bypass – 522 initial cases. Rev Mexicana Cir Endosc. 2004;5(Suppl 1):36.
6. Ramos AC, Silva AC, Ramos MG, Canseco EG, Galvão-Neto Mdos P, Menezes Mde A, et al. Simplified gastric bypass: 13 years of experience and 12,000 patients operated. Arq Bras Cir Dig. 2014;27(Suppl 1):2–8.
7. Prieto-Aldape MR, Martinez-Meldrano A, Vargas-Maldonado E, Aceves Velázquez E, Aceves Ávalos M. Bypass Gástrico Simplificado – 150 casos. Cir Gen. 2010;32(2):76–82.
8. Hernández-Miguelana L, Maldonado-Vázquez A, Cortés-Romano P, Rios-Cruz D, Marín-Domínguez R, Castillo-González A. Bypass Gástrico laparoscópico Simplificado. Experiência inicial. Cir Cir. 2014;82(3):262–7.
9. Palermo M, Serra E. Simplified laparoscopic gastric bypass with gastrojejunal linear mechanical anastomosis: technical aspects. Arq Bras Cir Dig. 2016;29(Suppl 1):91–4.
10. Quevedo MDP, Palermo M, Serra E, Ackermann MA. Metabolic surgery: gastric bypass for the treatment of type 2 diabetes mellitus. Transl Gastroenterol Hepatol. 2017;2:58.
11. Ramos AC, Domene CE, Volpe P, Pajecki D, D'Almeida LA, Ramos MG, et al. Early outcomes of the first Brazilian experience in totally robotic bariatric surgery. Arq Bras Cir Dig. 2013;26(Suppl 1):2–7.

Roux-en-Y Gastric Bypass in the Elderly Patient

19

Denis Pajecki, Andre Morrell, and Marco Aurelio Santo

Introduction

The problem of obesity as a disease in the elderly began to draw the attention of the medical community for about two decades [1]. Since then, we have noted the continued increase in life expectancy of the population and, in parallel, the significant increase in the prevalence of obesity in all age groups and in particular the elderly. In the United States, the rate of obesity in men and women aged 60 or more jumped from 12.3% and 16.5%, respectively, between 1976 and 1980 to 36.6% and 42.3% between 2009 and 2010 [2]. In Brazil, the population over 60 has doubled in the last 20 years. The prevalence of overweight and obesity in this age group has also increased, reaching 57.8% and 19.8% of subjects, respectively [3].

Excess body fat in the elderly is associated with increased incidence of metabolic (type II diabetes, dyslipidemia) and cardiovascular diseases (hypertension, coronary insufficiency), orthopedic (osteoarthritis), and even increased risk of dementia [4]. Moreover, it can lead to worsening of functionality, understood as the individual's ability to perform daily activities independently [5]. Functionality can be measured through simple questionnaires that assess an individual's ability to exercise these activities. The reduction in functionality relates to worsening of quality of life, frailty, and increased risk of mortality [6]. Frailty is a concept that describes the reduction of physiological and functional reserve of the individual, and in the elderly it is characterized by weakness, exhaustion, and slow activity. In this context, obesity in the elderly population has a significant impact on public health, with increased spending related to treatment and care for these patients in the final stage of their lives [7]. Therefore, there is a growing concern with the treatment of obesity in older adults in recent years.

The goals of obesity treatment may vary according to age groups: while in the youth population, prevention of systemic complications, risk reduction, and treatment of comorbidities such as diabetes, hypertension, and dyslipidemia are the main goals; in the elderly priority is to improve the quality of life and increase survival with less disability. In this context, reducing the amount of medication to control chronic diseases, the improvement of mechanical aspects related to mobility and functionality are outcomes related to those purposes [8]. Sarcopenia is the process of replacement of lean body mass by body fat that affects the elderly, especially from 65, to a greater or lesser degree. It is characterized by increased visceral fat and loss of peripheral muscles, which leads to reduced strength and performance (ability to walk in a certain rhythm) which, therefore,

D. Pajecki (✉) · A. Morrell · M. A. Santo
Bariatric and Metabolic Surgery Unit – Gastroenterology Department – Surgical Division, Hospital das Clínicas – University of São Paulo, São Paulo, Brazil
e-mail: pajecki@netpoint.com.br

J. Ettinger et al. (eds.), *Gastric Bypass*, https://doi.org/10.1007/978-3-030-28803-7_19

affect the functionality. For a long time, it was considered that the treatment of obesity in the elderly could be harmful, because it could lead to excessive muscle loss in individuals who already have some degree of sarcopenia, functional deterioration, and even increased risk of falls and fractures [9–11]. It's been established then that the candidates for treatment should be individuals who had poorly controlled medical comorbidity and functional impairment, with the objectives of the loss of visceral fat with the preservation of skeletal muscle mass. Diet, physical activity, and lifestyle modification are the pillars of the clinical treatment of obesity in these individuals [12]. Several studies have shown that this association promotes satisfactory weight loss with preservation of lean body mass and functionality in elderly subjects with mild obesity (Grade I). Furthermore, it's been already shown that this type of intervention increases survival [13]. The use of specific medication for obesity in the elderly should be done with extreme caution, because of side effects and the risk of drug interactions, considering the frequent use of polypharmacy in this population [14].

Bariatric surgery in the elderly has always been a paradigm. Although indications for adult patients is well established and has its well-defined rules, the same is not true for elderly patients. The first directive establishing the bariatric surgery indication criteria, published by the National Institute of Health (NIH) of the United States in 1991 and used as a reference for this practice since, has not set strict age limits for the elderly [15]. It was recommended, however, that patients older than 65 years should be assessed individually and carefully in order to establish the benefit/risk of surgical treatment. A review by the American Society of Bariatric Surgery in 2004 made the statement based on age more liberal. In Brazil, the resolution of the Federal Council of Medicine of 2005 specified that the elderly could only be operated by special precautions and reviews of "cost-benefit ratio" [16]. In an article reviewing the criteria of the NIH, Yermilov et al., in 2009, proposed that for patients over 65 years, the indications for surgery should be more rigid, only for patients with a BMI above 40 kg/m^2 and with more severe degrees of diabetes, hypertension, sleep apnea, or chronic joint pain [17]. However, little importance was given to the worsening of quality of life as an indication factor. More recently, IFSO (International Federation of Obesity Surgery) published guidelines highlighting the importance of assessing risks and benefits of surgical treatment in these patients and that the ultimate goal would be to improve the quality of life, not really expecting significant increase in survival [18]. In the other hand, Perry et al. [19], in 2008, had already demonstrated the increased survival of morbidly obese patients operated with more than 65 years when compared to nonoperated ones. Nevertheless, currently, the surgical treatment of obesity in patients over 65 years remains controversial, with a lack of specific criteria or outcomes that characterize the potential benefits.

The increased surgical risk in patients over 65 years is certainly a limiting factor for the broader indication of bariatric surgery in this population [6]. The use of specific risk scores, such as the Obesity Surgery Mortality Risk Score (OS-MRS), may be useful in selecting patients and has been used by some authors [20]. The choice of conventional or laparoscopic approach and the surgical technique is also related to it. The advantages of laparoscopy in this particular situation are evident. Among the most used surgical techniques, sleeve gastrectomy (SG) and Roux-en-Y gastric bypass (RYGBP) are the most frequent. In Brazil, RYGBP is still the surgical technique most commonly used for the treatment of morbid obesity and has been, currently, the most used in the elderly population.

Regarding the benefits, most studies evaluate the usual outcomes of bariatric surgery as weight loss and control of metabolic and cardiovascular comorbidities. In general, older people lose less weight than younger adults do but have similar levels of comorbidity resolution [21, 22]. Particular endpoints in the elderly, such as improved functionality, reduced frailty, and improved quality of life, have not been studied [7, 8]. The presence of sarcopenia can be one of the factors that compromise the effectiveness of weight loss in this population. On the other hand, the great weight loss in these individuals may increase the risk of falls and fractures leading paradoxically to a worsening of functioning and quality of life. Therefore, the goal of weight loss in the elderly undergoing surgical treatment should be different.

Evaluation of the elderly for bariatric surgery should be done from the geriatrics perspectives, which includes several of the issues mentioned here and serves to a better understanding of the overall health of the individual [23]. In our unit, we have applied the comprehensive geriatric assessment (AGA), an instrument used for the evaluation of elderly, which aims to identify diseases, functional and cognitive limitations, as well as physical and psychosocial weaknesses to generate approach strategies and more effective treatments, considering functional loss and mortality. A study of patients over 60 years in preparation for bariatric surgery has shown that there was significant reduction in functionality in those with a BMI above 47 kg/m^2 [24].

We also believe that the preoperatively assessment of bone mass and body composition in these individuals is essential. This can be done by bioimpedance absorptiometry or dual energy X-ray absorptiometry (DEXA) [25]. Postoperatively, special attention should be given to nutritional supplementation to ensure adequate intake of protein and adequate physical activity for their age, preventing excessive loss of muscle mass. Follow-up with functional tests and body composition should be routinely performed.

The benefits of bariatric surgery in the elderly, with regard to the control of comorbidities, improved quality of life, and increased life expectancy, have already been shown in midterm follow-up. Longer follow-up with the implementation of comprehensive geriatric assessment is needed for more comprehensive and systematic assessment of the benefits of this treatment in the overall health of the elderly.

Results from the Surgical Treatment

Surgical morbidity in patients over 60 years undergoing laparoscopic or conventional gastric bypass is no different from that observed in younger subjects. Dunkle-Blatter et al. [26] reported the same rates of major complications and mortality in 30 and 90 days. Similar results were reported by Hazzan et al. [27] and St Peter et al. [21]. In Medicare patients, who usually wait longer for surgery and have more comorbidities, Hollowell et al. [28] have also reported the same results.

When we analyze patients over 65 years operated by open surgery, the scenario is a bit different. A survey in US database (National Hospital Discharge Survey and National Inpatient Survey), analyzing more than 25,000 bariatric surgeries, revealed mortality of 3.2% in the elderly subjected to open RYGBP (against 0.2 to 0.7% in the younger population) and adverse outcomes in 32.3% (against 21.6% in the younger) [29]. Nelson et al. [30] reported a 4% mortality and risk of surgical complications up to 20% of patients. More recently, O'Keefe et al. [22] analyzed 157 patients over 65 years undergoing laparoscopic RYGB in specialized centers of high surgical volume in the United States ("Centers of Excellence") and reported major complications in 7% and minor complications in 33.1%. In comparison to the younger population subjected to the same surgical technique in the same centers, the elderly had similar complication rate but higher mortality (1.3% versus zero to 0.4%). Nevertheless, the study considered the procedure safe and effective for patients over 65 years and suggests that age should not be a barrier for patients with severe obesity. Dorman et al. [31] concluded that the age over 65 alone was not a predictor of surgical complications nor corresponds to longer hospital stays compared to the adult-young people. In a recent systematic review, Chow et al. [32] showed that bariatric surgery performed laparoscopically in patients over 65 years is safe, with an average mortality of 0.14%.

Regarding the control of comorbidities, Nelson et al. [30] reported resolution of 100% of cases of type 2 diabetes and GERD in patients undergoing gastric bypass, in addition to improvement reported in frames of AOS, arthropathy, and hypertension, 77%, 91%, and 67%, respectively. Besides, a decrease in the number of medications used to treat comorbidities was observed in 50% of patients. Quebbemann et al.

[33] also reported significant improvement in quality of life and reduced medication use in elderly patients undergoing LRYGB.

In a study conducted in our unit [34], a retrospective evaluation of patients over 60 years undergoing open RYGB, the average follow-up time was 5.9 years (71 months). Thirty patients were between 60 and 65 years and had 16 over 65 years at the time of operation. The average excess weight loss was 71.8%, similar to the result observed in younger individuals with no difference between patients with more or less 65 years. The resolution rate of comorbidities such as type II diabetes and hypertension was similar to those seen in younger populations. However, patients with more than 65 years had a higher rate of complications (26.6% × 37.5%), including wound infection and incision hernias. On the other hand, the incidence of nutritional deficiencies in the medium and long term was very low, because of the high adherence rate of this group of patients to postoperative follow-up and regular use of vitamin and micronutrients supplements.

The results of surgical treatment with published RYGB by different authors are listed in Tables 19.1,19.2, and 19.3.

Few studies compared the different surgical techniques in this population. Most of them are retrospective or prospective nonrandomized or have analyzed only one technique [37]. Recently, Moon et al. [43] concluded that, in elderly, weight loss with RYGB was higher but Sleeve's surgical morbidity was lower and there was no difference in the resolution of comorbidities between the two techniques. Garofalo et al. [44] performed the sleeve gastrectomy in 27 individuals, mean age 67.2 years and mean BMI of 44.1; the loss of excess weight was 53.8 + − 19% in 12 months and 52.9 + − 21% in 36 months, and there was no mortality in the series. He also noted that BMI >45 and the presence of type II diabetes were relevant factors for inadequate weight loss and weight regain in a short time. Pequignot et al. [45] also demonstrated that the Sleeve is a safe technique for patients over 60 years, with complication rates up to 30 days similar to younger adults (17.9% and 17.6%).

Table 19.1 RYGB outcomes in the elderly

Author	Mean age	Preoperative BMI	Intervention	Mean follow-up	Excess weight loss %	Mortality
Nelson 2006 [30]	68 + −1	50 + −3 (PRE)	OGBP	9 months	45% + −7	4% (90 DAYS)
Blatter 2007 [26]	62	49.3 + −7,5	OGBP	13.8 months	54.9% + −16.6	1.64% (30/90 DAYS)
Thereaux 2015 [35]	62.6 + −2.3	45.6 + − 6.4	LGBP	36 months	63% + −18.7	2.1% (30 DAYS)
Pajecki 2015 [34]	64	49,63	OGBP	5,9 years	72%	4,3% (90 DAYS)
Montastier 2016 [36]	61.9	43.9 + −5.3	LGBP	24 months	31.8% + −7.2	–
Huang 2015 [37]	58.88 + −2.6	40.5 + −7.3	LGBP	80.3 months	–	2.3%
Chow 2015 [32]	67.6	46.2	LGBP	26.6 months	66.2%	0,14% (30 DAYS)
Sosa 2004 [38]	64.4	48.5	OGBP	12 months	65%	4,3%
Wittgrove 2009 [39]	63.4	45.2	LGBP	12 months	–	0%
Willkomm 2010 [40]	68	45	LGBP	24 months	83.4%	0%
Giordano 2015 [41]	59.43 + −3.81	46.21 + − 7.47	LGBP	–	64.48% + −18.44	0% (30 DAYS)
Robert 2014 [42]	61.7	41.3 + −1	LGBP	12 months	73.7% + −4.5	4%

Table 19.2 Postoperative complications following 30/90 days

Author	Bleeding	Fistula/Leak	Obstruction	Acute pulmonary embolism	Deep venous thrombosis	Incisional hernia
Blatter 2007 [26]	3.28%/1.64%	0%/3.8%	1.64%/0%	0%	0%	0/3.28%
Pajecki 2015 [34]	4,3%	4,3%	4,3%	2,2%	2,2%	10,8%
Huang 2015 [37]	–	6.8%	4.6%	–	–	–
Chow 2015 [32]	1.94%	–	1.53%	2.96%	–	–
Sosa 2004 [38]						
Wittgrove 2009 [39]	2,5%	0%		0%		0,85%
Willkomm 2010 [40]	1%	–	–	3%	–	–
Giordano 2015 [41]	3,7%	0,7%	–	1,4%	–	–
Robert 2014 [42]	4%	0%	4%	0%	–	–

Table 19.3 Resolution of comorbidities

Author	Diabetes	Hypertension	OSA	Joint pain	GERD
Nelson 2006 [30]	100% (remission)	67% (remission/ improve)	77% (remission/ improve)	91% (improve)	100% (remission)
Blatter 2007 [26]	53.5% remission/97.7% improve	30% remission/76% improve			–
Thereaux 2015 [35]	53.3% remission/80% improve	18.8% remission/75% improve	60.6% remission /87.9% improve	42.1% remission /73.1% improve	–
Pajecki 2015 [34]	77% remission/23% improve	30% remission/26% improve	–	–	–
Montastier 2016 [36]	59% remission	27% remission	80% remission	–	–
Huang 2015 [37]	69.2% remission	56% remission	–	–	–
Sosa 2004 [38]	75% remission	91% remission / improve	67% remission	–	–
Wittgrove 2009 [39]	75% remission	88% remission	94% remission	–	–
Willkomm 2010 [40]	63% remission	23% remission	–	–	–
Giordano 2015 [41]	25% remission	5% remission	–	–	–
Robert 2014 [42]	37% remission/58% improve	45% remission/50% improve	–	–	–

Conclusions

Roux-en-Y gastric bypass can be safely performed in the elderly, but laparoscopic RYGB is particularly safer than open RYGB in patients over 65 years. Evaluation of body composition, bone health, and functionality should be performed before and after surgical treatment in these patients. More data about long-term outcomes of bariatric surgery in this population is necessary before we have more clear guidelines indicating which patients should or should not go to surgical treatment.

References

1. Rossner S. Obesity in the elderly – a future matter of concern? Obes Rev. 2001;2:183–8.
2. Flegal KM, Carroll MD, Kit BK, Ogden CL. Prevalence of obesity and trends in distribution of BMI among US adults, 1999–2010. JAMA. 2012;307(5):491–7.
3. Brasil. Instituto Brasileiro de Geografia e estatística. Pesquisa de Orçamentos Familiares: 2008–2009. Antropometria e Estado Nutricional de Crianças, Adolescentes e Adultos no Brasil. Bibli. Do Minist. Do Planejamento e Gestão. 2010. p. 130.
4. Fontaine KR, Redden DT, Wang C, et al. Years of life lost due to obesity. JAMA. 2003;289(2):187–93.
5. Lang IA, Llewellyn DJ, Alexander K, et al. Obesity, physical function and mortality in older adults. JAGS. 2008;56:1474–8.
6. Scandrett KG, Zuckerbraun BS, Peitzman AB, et al. Operative risk stratification in the older adult. Sug Clin N Am. 2015;95:149–72.
7. Snih SA, Ottenbacher KJ, Markides KS, et al. The effect of obesity on disability vs mortality in older americans. Arch Intern Med. 2007;167:774–80.
8. Vliegen M, et al. Prevalence, pathophysiology, health consequences and treatment options of obesity in the elderly: a guideline. Obes Facts. 2012;5:460–83.
9. Mitchell RJ, Lord SR, Harvey LA, et al. Associations between obesity and overweight and fall risk, health status and quality of life in older people. Aust N Z J Public Health. 2014;38(1):13–8. https://doi.org/10.1111/1753-6405.12152.
10. Grabowski DC, Ellis JE. High body mass index does not predict mortality in older people: analysis of the Longitudinal Study of Aging. J Am Geriatr Soc. 2001;49(7):968–79.
11. Losonczy KG, Harris TB, Cornoni-Huntley J, et al. Does weight loss from middle age to old age explain the inverse weight mortality relation in old age? Am J Epidemiol. 1995;141(4):312–21.
12. Kennedy RL, Chokkalingham K, Srinivasan R. Obesity in the elderly: who should web e treating, and why, and how? Currnt Op Clin Nut Met Care. 2004;7:3–9.
13. Shea MK, et al. ADAPT study. J Gerontol A Biol Sci Med Sci. 2010;65(5):519–25.
14. Horie NC, Cercato C, Mancini MC, et al. Long term pharmacoterapy for obesity in the elderly patients. Drugs Aging. 2010;27:497–506.
15. NIH conference. Gastrointestinal surgery for severe obesity. Consensus Development Conference Panel. Ann Intern Med. 1991;115(12):956–61.
16. Brasil. Conselho Federal de Medicina RESOLUÇÃO CFM N° 1.766/05.
17. Yermilov I, McGory ML, Shekelle PW, et al. Appropriateness criteria for bariatric surgery: beyond the NIH guidelines. Obesity (Silver Spring). 2009;17(8):1521–7.
18. De Luca M, et al. Indications for surgery for obesity and weight-related diseases: position statements from the International Federation for the Surgery of Obesity and Metabolic Disorders (IFSO). Obes Surg. 2016;26:1659–96.
19. Perry CD, Hutter MM, Smith DB, et al. Survival and changes in comorbidities after bariatric surgery. Ann Surg. 2008;247(1):21–7.
20. Brolin RE, Cody RP, Marcella SW. Differences inn open versus laparoscopic gastric bypass mortality risk using the Obesity Surgery Mortality Risk Score (OS-MRS). SORD. 2015;11:1201–6.
21. St Peter SD, Craft RO, Tiede JL. Impact of advanced age, on weight loss and health benefits after laparoscopic gastric bypass. Arch Surg. 2005;140(2):165–8.
22. O'Keefe KL, Kemmeter PR, Kemmeter KD. Bariatric surgery outcomes in patients aged 65 years and older at an American Society for Metabolic and Bariatric Surgery Center of Excellence. Obes Surg. 2010;20(9):1199–205. https://doi.org/10.1007/s11695-010-0201-4.
23. Batsis JA, Dolkart KM. Evaluation of older adults with obesity for bariatric surgery: geriatrician's perspective. J Clin Geront Geriatr. 2015;6:45–53.
24. Pajecki D, Santo MA, Kanagi AL, et al. Functional assessment of older obese patients candidates for bariatric surgery. Arq Gastroenterol. 2014;51(1):25–8.
25. Otto M, et al. Handgrip strength as a predictor for post bariatric body composition. Obes Surg. 2014;24:2082–8.
26. Dunkle-Blatter SE, St Jean MR, Whitehead C, et al. Outcomes among elderly bariatric patients at a high-volume center. Surg Obes Relat Dis. 2007;3(2):163–9.
27. Hazzan D, Chin EH, Steinhagen E, et al. Laparoscopic bariatric surgery can be safe for treatment of morbid obesity in patients older than 60 years. Surg Obes Relat Dis. 2006;2(6):613–6.
28. Hallowell PT, Stellato TA, Schuster M, et al. Avoidance of complications in older patients and Medicare recipients undergoing gastric bypass. Arch Surg. 2007;142:506–10.
29. Livingston EH, Langert J. The impact of age and Medicare status on bariatric surgical outcomes. Arch Surg. 2006;141(11):1115–20.
30. Nelson LG, Lopez PP, Haines K, et al. Outcomes of bariatric surgery in patients > or =65 years. Surg Obes Relat Dis. 2006;2(3):384–8.
31. Dorman RB, Abraham AA, Al-Rafaie WB, et al. Bariatric surgery outcomes in the elderly: an ACS NSQIP study. J Gastrointest Surg. 2012;16:35–44.
32. Chow A, Switzer NJ, Gill RS, et al. Roux-en-Y gastric bypass in the elderly: a systematic review. Obes Surg. 2016;26:626–30.

33. Quebbemann BB, Engstrom DR, Siegfried T, et al. Bariatric surgery in patients older than 65 years is safe and effective. Surg Obes Relat Dis. 2005;1:389–93.
34. Pajecki D, Santo MA, Joaquim HD, et al. Bariatric surgery in the elderly: results of a mean follow-up of five years. Arq Bras Cir Dig. 2015;28(Suppl 1):15–8.
35. Thereaux J, Poitou C, Barsamian C, et al. Midterm outcomes of gastric bypass for elderly patients: a comparative study. Surg Obes Relat Dis. 2015;11:836–41.
36. Montastier E, Becouam G, Bérard E, et al. Gastric bypass in older patients: complications, weight loss and resolution of comorbidities at 2 years in a matched controlled study. Obes Surg. 2016;26:1806–13.
37. Huang CK, Garg A, Kuau HC, et al. Bariatric surgery in old age: a comparative study of laparoscopic Roux-en-Y gastric bypass and sleeve gastrectomy in an Asia center of excellence. J Biomed Res. 2015;29(2):118–24.
38. Sosa JL, Pombo H, Pallavicini H, et al. Laparoscopic gastric bypass beyond age 60. Obes Surg. 2004;14:1398–401.
39. Wittgrove AC, Martinez T, et al. Laparoscopic gastric bypass in patients 60 years and older: early postoperative morbidity and resolution of comorbidities. Obes Surg. 2009;19:1472–6.
40. Willkomm CM, Fischer TL, Barnes GS, et al. Surgical weight loss > 65 years old: is it worth the risk? Surg Obes Relat Dis. 2010;6:491–7.
41. Giordano S, Victorzon M, et al. Bariatric surgery in the elderly: a systematic review. Clin Interv Aging. 2015;10:1627–35.
42. Robert M, Pasquer A, Espalieu P, et al. Gastric bypass for obesity in the elderly: is it as appropriate as for young and middle-aged populations? Obes Surg. 2014;24:1662–9.
43. Moon RC, Kreimer F, Teixeira AF, et al. Morbidity rates and weight loss after Roux-en-Y gastric bypass, sleeve gastrectomy, and adjustable gastric banding in patients older than 60 years old: which procedure to choose? Obes Surg. 2016;26(4):730–6. https://doi.org/10.1007/s11695-015-1824-2.
44. Garofalo F, Denis R, Pescarus R, et al. Long-term outcome after laparoscopic sleeve gastrectomy in patients over 65 years old: a retrospective analysis. Surg Obes Relat Dis. 2017;13(1):1–6.
45. Peguinot A, Prevot F, Dharih A, et al. Is Sleeve Gastrectomy still contraindicated for patients aged >60 years? A case-matched study with 24 months of follow-up. Surg Obes Relat Dis. 2015;11(5):1008–13.

20 Gastric Bypass Reoperation for Weight Regain

Gustavo Peixoto Soares Miguel, Paulo Henrique Oliveira de Souza, Isaac Walker de Abreu, Luize Giuri Palaoro, and Thales Ribeiro dos Santos Vecci

Introduction

The World Health Organization estimates that about 13% of the world's adult population were obese in 2014 and 39% were overweight. It has been consolidated in the literature that bariatric surgery is the most efficient treatment to provide a sustained weight lost [1–3]. This factor associated with the increase of safety of procedure has contributed to an increase in the number of surgeries during the last decade. However, during 2013, only 0.01% of world's population underwent bariatric surgery, showing a significant difference between the number of procedures and the actual obese population [4].

The most commonly used technique in 2013 was the Roux-en-Y gastric bypass (RYGB); however, there is a trend in reducing its proportion worldwide, while sleeve gastrectomy is rising [4]. Due to its wide use and rates of weight regain or insufficient weight loss, RYGB patients with failure of treatment can become even more common, and bariatric surgeons should know how to correctly evaluate and conduct these patients.

G. P. S. Miguel (✉) · P. H. O. de Souza
I. W. de Abreu · L. G. Palaoro · T. R. dos Santos Vecci
Department of Surgical Clinics, Hospital Universitário Cassiano Antônio de Moraes – HUCAM/UFES, Vitória, ES, Brazil

Gastric Bypass Results

Laparoscopic RYGB (LRYGB) was first described by Wittgrove and Clark in 1994 [5], and of all bariatric surgeries in the world, 95.7% were performed laparoscopically [4]. Schroeder et al. (2011) observed a faster postoperative recuperation, a shorter hospital stay, and a lower incidence of surgical site complications, such as hernias and dehiscences in the laparoscopic approach [6]. Other advantages include a decreased impairment due to pulmonary complications, diminished parameters of systemic injury, and a dramatic reduction in the frequency of wound infection [7]. Thus, patients who were submitted to a laparoscopic surgery showed a better recuperation and an early return to the daily activities.

Gastric bypass can promote weight loss of 39% of preoperative weight, in the long term [8], and around 65% of excess of weight loss (%EWL), type 2 diabetes mellitus (T2DM) control and remission, and hyperlipidemia and hypertension remission [9]. This high efficacy to control T2DM (about 80% for RYGB) occurs by different mechanisms besides the known restrictive and malabsorptive components that include regulation of gut hormones with incretin effect [10, 11]. The remission of hypertension might be related to EWL itself, leading to an improvement in the cardiac autonomic control directed to the heart, which might be related to an increase in the

J. Ettinger et al. (eds.), *Gastric Bypass*, https://doi.org/10.1007/978-3-030-28803-7_20

parasympathetic modulation to the heart after bariatric surgery [12]. Therefore, associated with the benefit of EWL, RYGB can provide resolution of obesity-related comorbidities.

However, several studies show rates of up to 54% of failure to lose weight or weight recidivism. RYGB patients can have 23% of weight regain from nadir weight [8].

Some technical aspects of the RYGB operation are being modified intending to prevent relapse of obesity and comorbidities. These changes can modify the restrictive (size of the gastric pouch) or disabsorptive component (length of intestinal limbs). Too much care is taken in gastric pouch construction, since technical error during this step can promote postoperative pouch dilation. A large pouch allows a return to the erroneous alimentary habits like overfeeding and smaller weight loss [13–15]. To provide a higher food restriction, a silicone ring around the new gastric pouch can be added [5, 6]. Gastrojejunostomy is also a concern, because it can limit gastric emptying and prevent overfeeding. Different techniques of this anastomosis can be used, and studies did not show any differences between anastomoses with circular stapler or linear stapler or hand sewn in relation to early complications and weight loss [16, 17]. Furthermore, the length of intestinal limbs can be altered to increase or reduce the degree of disabsorption and provide a better control of gut hormones involved in T2DM pathogenesis [18, 19]. There is a trend to a higher weight loss when a long limb RYGB was done in patients with a BMI greater than 50 kg/m^2, who present a higher rate of failure with the conventional surgery. However, these were based on heterogenous studies with conflicting data [18, 20].

Definition of Failure

There is no uniform or internationally recognized definition for what constitutes failure of bariatric surgery. A systematic review demonstrated the inconsistency in reporting and defining the reasons for failure of a primary bariatric procedure and that the majority of studies concerning revisional operations do not report their selection criteria [21]. However, the most commonly used criterion is an excess weight loss lower than 50%. Actually, this percentage may consider the technique used on bariatric procedure and should vary according to the expected EWL. Besides that, some authors described a failure of the procedure based on weight regain or in an inadequate excess weight loss. It is important to consider the resolution and recurrence of obesity comorbidities before indicating a surgical revision. The recurrence of comorbidities can indicate a failure of surgery, and, even in patients who present an adequate EWL, the lack of comorbidity improvement shows a possible necessity of reoperation.

Causes and Diagnosis of Failure

There are preoperative factors that can predict weight regain, such as very high BMI, age over than 50 years old, and the use of diabetes medications [22–24]. These findings might be related to metabolic changes associated with the aging process and the insulinemic and glycemic control in T2DM [23].

RYGB failure can be caused basically by mechanisms related to patient or surgery (Table 20.1).

Postoperative compliance is of paramount influence in the success in postoperative period. Postoperative compliance is linked to patients' motivation and results in regular medical, dietary, and surgical recommendations. A meta-analysis of studies that compared %EWL between follow-up compliant patients and less or noncompliant patients showed that there was an increase in the %EWL in those patients who were compliant

Table 20.1 Causes of weight regain and insufficient weight loss after RGBP

Patient related	Surgery related
Inappropriate diet Lack of nutritional counseling Mental health disorders Binge eating disorders No physical activity Hormonal/metabolic	Pouch dilation Band/ring removal Gastrojejunostomy dilation Gastrogastric fistula

with follow-up at 12-month postsurgery [25]. A study with adolescents also showed that the number of consultations per year was the only variable significantly associated with weight loss [26]. Factors that can predict patient compliance to clinical appointments and recommendations can be identified. Larjani et al. (2016) recently studied patient attendance rate of follow-up to clinical appointments after bariatric surgery and tried to identify predictive factors of adherence. Patients more than 25 years old, patients with obstructive sleep apnea, patients who live nearby bariatric clinic, and employed patients are more likely to attend follow-up consultations; however, only occupation status had statistical significance in a multivariate analysis [27].

When related to patient, the most significant factors include an improper feeding, sedentary lifestyle, and pathological eating behaviors. Furthermore, some studies show that alcohol abuse, depression, and other psychiatric disorders are related to weight regain [22, 28]. In this way, weight regain, in some cases, is related to potentially modifiable factors that should be aggressively assessed by a multidisciplinary team before a revisional surgery is thought. Nutritional habits and behavioral aspects should be taken into account.

Besides evaluating patient-related causes of weight regain or insufficient weight loss, one should rule out dilation of gastric pouch and/or gastrojejunostomy enlargement. Gastric pouch and gastrojejunal anastomosis dilation are considered the two major anatomic determinants of weight loss failure or weight regain after RYGB. Two methods are essential in this work out: esophagogastroduodenoscopy (EGD) and upper gastrointestinal (UGI) series. Both are realized in order to assess the size of gastric pouch and of stoma, gastrojejunostomy patency, presence of fistula, location of band/ring, and also presence of gastrogastric fistula. EGD allows direct visualization of gastric mucosa, and UGI can estimate gastric pouch emptying. Despite usefulness of those methods, they have inherent limitations, and there is no consensus on how gastric pouch volume must be measured [29]. Contrasted CT scan

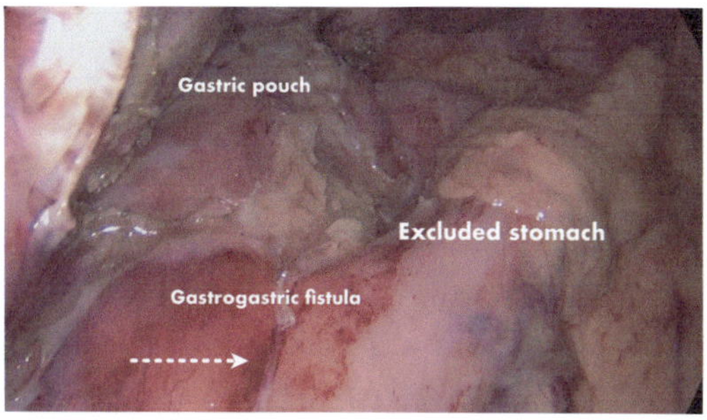

Fig. 20.1 Laparoscopic view of gastrogastric fistula (arrow)

exams can be used as a valuable tool to better understand pouch anatomy, and three-dimensional images can be obtained, revealing also staple lines and position of band, if it was placed in primary surgery [30].

Gastrogastric fistula is a rare complication that allows food to pass through the excluded stomach and proximal intestine and then permits ingestion of a bigger amount of food and diminishes hormonal effects of RYGB [31] (Fig. 20.1). There is a relatively frequent association of gastrogastric fistulas with marginal ulcers, and in those cases, the fistula tends to be more distal in the gastric pouch. Marginal ulcers can either be a result of gastrogastric fistulas or a cause itself. Patients can present only with weight regain and may have nonspecific symptoms [32].

Medical Management

The first step is to refer the patient to multidisciplinary team and reinforce importance of dietary and behavioral recommendations. Allied to nutritional and psychological counseling, endocrinology team also plays a crucial rule, since there are medical options to restore patient's weight and spare a surgical treatment, which has a higher morbimortality rates than compared to primary surgery.

The association of anti-obesity drugs is a common practice in the offices of endocrinologists, although there are few data on the long-term results of this kind of approach. Some studies have described the use of medications, but most of them are uncontrolled and retrospective, with a small number of patients and short follow-up [33].

Orlistat, a lipase inhibitor that prevents absorption of about one-third of ingested fat, was used after failed AGB, with good results [34]. In gastric bypass patients, this drug should be used carefully because it can worsen post-RYGB diarrhea. Topiramate is an antiepileptic drug which is associated with weight loss and has good effect in patients with binge eating disorder. Small studies have shown that post-bariatric patients can benefit from topiramate in a short-term period, in RYGB and AGB patients [35, 36]. Other drugs, such as fluoxetine and sertraline, can be used in binge eating patients.

The use of appetite suppressors, like phentermine, alone or in association with topiramate, in addition to diet and exercise, demonstrated weight loss in post-RYGB and LAGB patients who experienced weight recidivism and weight loss plateau [37].

Pajecki et al. (2013) published a small retrospective study using liraglutide, a synthetic analogue of the hormone GLP-1, as an option to treat weight regain after different bariatric surgery techniques. All 15 included patients had improvement of satiety and displayed weight loss, ranging from 2 to 18 kg. The use of these medications may be limited by their side effects, nausea, vomiting and hyperamylasemia, and their cost [38].

Surgical Treatment

When a period of 3 to 6 months with multidisciplinary approach fails, revision of surgery can be considered. Surgical options of RYGB revision are strictly related to the identified cause of failure of the initial treatment (Fig. 20.2). The options basically involve modifying a portion of the bypass anatomy or adding a component to the existing bypass anatomy. The surgical strategy

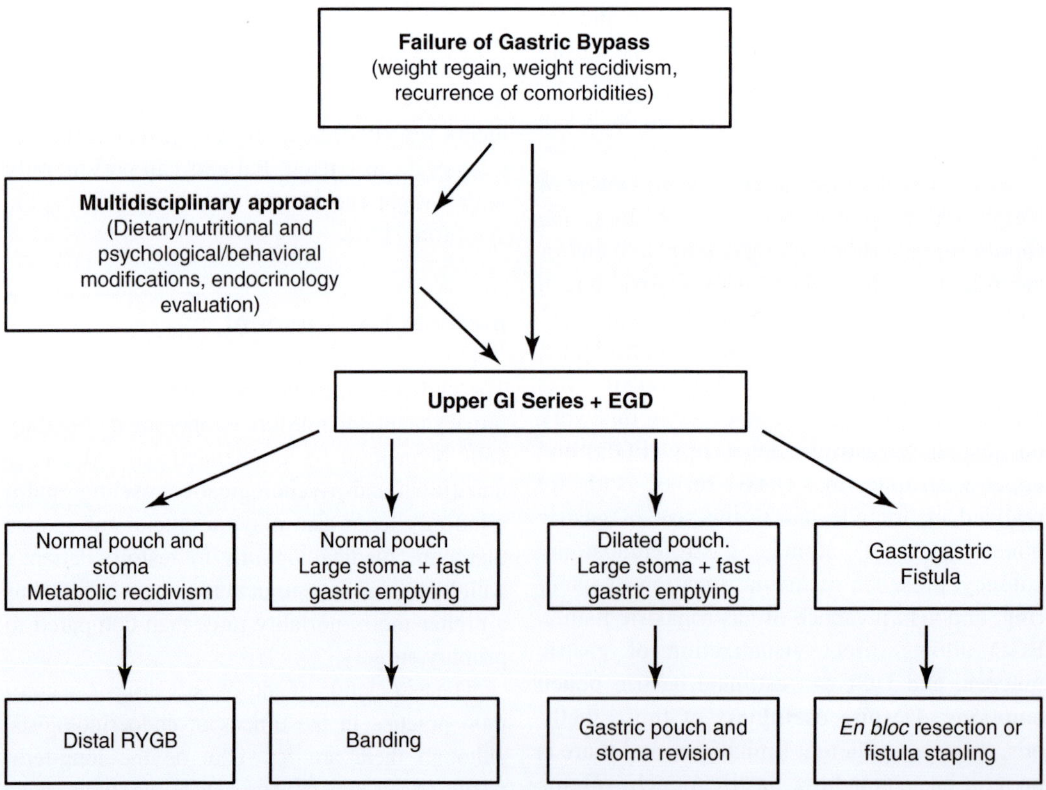

Fig. 20.2 Algorithm of surgical management of failed Roux-en-Y gastric bypass

requires a thorough review of the primary procedure and identification of a safe and feasible operative approach for revision, which can be technically challenging.

As it happens with the failure definition, there is no consensus in reporting post-revisional procedures results. Many authors take into account only the weight and BMI immediately before the second procedure, while others consider the initial clinical data.

Banding

Banded RYGB was much popular in the 1990s and early 2000s, and band/ring complications have decreased its use. Also due to superiority of other techniques, adjustable gastric band represents only 10% of all bariatric procedures [4]. However, as a revisional procedure after failed non-banded RYGB, in order to increase the restrictive component, with an advocated relatively low risk of surgical complications, one can indicate banding in cases of pouch dilation.

In the larger series of patients who underwent gastric banding as salvage procedure for patients with weight loss failure after Roux-en-Y gastric bypass, 44 patients were followed up for 12 months and presented a 17.6% EWL after LAGB, with a low rate of comorbidity amelioration [39]. In another series with similar number of patients, but a longer follow-up, there was a mean EWL of 31% and a decrease in BMI of 8.2 kg/m^2 [40]. Both studies reported a 30% of overall adverse event rate and a 15% to 21% of reoperations. Bessler et al. (2010) had better results in terms of EWL, but only eight patients were studied and presented a 44% EWL in 2-year follow-up after the revision and 62% when combined with the original surgery [41]. Some authors even report loose placing of a nonadjustable band placing, in order to reduce pouch's compliance, with good 1-year results [42].

Unfortunately, overall results are not consistent, and reported complication/reoperation rates are not so low as one could expect. So, banding a failed RYGB procedure may not be a good alternative as a sole procedure, and all cases should be carefully analyzed. For example, cases in which stoma is enlarged, with a rapid gastric pouch emptying and a preserved pouch volume, can fit to banding procedures.

Gastric Pouch and Anastomosis Revision

Also in order to increase restrictive component of primary surgery, gastric pouch and/or anastomosis revision are an option, usually due to pouch dilation and gastrojejunostomy enlargement. This dilated gastric pouch can be resized by a partial resection, and the enlarged gastrojejunostomy can be resected and redone. But gastric pouch dissection and anastomosis region may be challenging due to adhesions in the upper abdomen, previous band placement, interposed afferent intestinal limb, and retrocolic alimentary limb.

Al-Bader et al. (2015) reported a series of 32 laparoscopic pouch revisions, performed for dilated gastric pouch after RYGB, with a mean follow-up of 14 months. A new 20–25-cc gastric pouch was created by stapling the dilated Roux loop and across the gastrojejunostomy and gastric pouch up to the gastroesophageal junction. A median %EWL of 29.1% was observed, and the total weight loss and BMI reduction after the laparoscopic pouch revision were 13.9 kg and 5.5 kg/m^2, respectively. The overall complication and reoperation rates were 15.6% and 3.1%, respectively [43]. Another study reported 20 patients who underwent laparoscopic pouch revision in a similar fashion followed by 21 months. The authors reported a BMI of 29.6 kg/m^2 and %EWL of 68.6%, with almost complete resolution of comorbidities [29]. Parikh et al. (2011) also had good results with the so-called gastrojejunal sleeve reduction performed in 14 patients, who had, at 12 months postoperatively, mean BMI decrease of 2.7 kg/m^2, representing additional EWL of 12.8%, and overall EWL of 62.0%; however, only 22% patients experienced resolution of comorbidities [44]. All those studies used different sizes of bougies to calibrate the revisited pouch, a fact that can lead to different outcomes. Another point is that none had long-term results and remains the necessity of revaluate gastric pouch volume postoperatively, since it may become newly dilated, with consequent weight regain.

Another surgical strategy is to resize the gastric pouch by en bloc resection and recreate the gastrojejunostomy. An evaluation of 25 laparoscopic revisions showed that the peak of EWL postrevision (64.1%) was noted 1 year after surgery and it was comparable to that at the patients' nadir weight after primary RYGB [45]. Also in order to reduce the volume of gastric pouch and gastrojejunostomy, one can perform a plication of these structures, with no resection. In a small series of four patients, this procedure could reach a BMI loss and median %EWL of 4.9 kg/m^2 and 46.2%, respectively, with no complications or mortality [46].

There is a special concern about RYGB with ring that was considered the gold standard procedure for some years, especially in Brazil. The procedure consists of the insertion of a Silastic ring around the gastric pouch, usually made bigger than in the version without the ring [46]. Despite the encouraging results regarding weight loss and control of comorbidities [47], the intense restriction to solid food intake and the occurrence of complications with the ring (slip and extrusion) [48] lead to reduction in the number of cases using this variant technique around the country and also around the world.

A numerous proportion of surgeries for revisional RYGB performed nowadays in Brazil are of primary procedures with Silastic ring as consequent of a perigastric ring removal over a dilated pouch or of a ring extrusion into the pouch (some cases with gastrogastric fistula formation). In case of slipping or late intolerance, the ring removal can be performed by laparoscopy. In the extrusion, the removal is done through endoscopic methods. In both cases, the patient must receive more intense attention from the multidisciplinary team due to the potential of weight regain, since ring removal is associated with weight recidivism. In cases of progressive dilation, resection of both excess gastric pouch and the anastomosis is indicated.

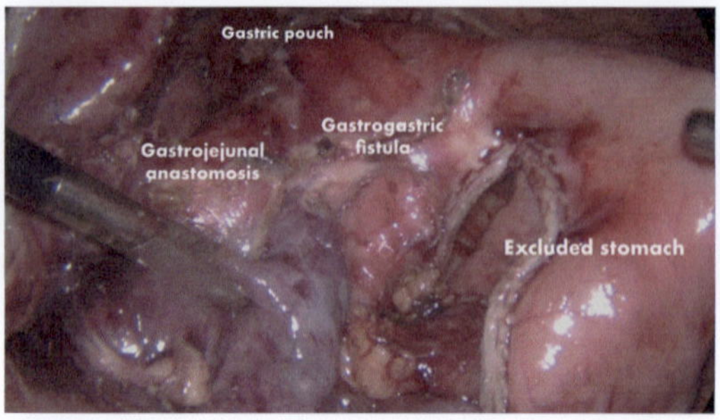

Fig. 20.3 Revisional surgery for gastric bypass with weight regain due to dilated pouch and gastrogastric fistula. En bloc resection of the alimentary limb, gastrogastric fistula, gastric pouch, and excluded stomach

Gastrogastric Fistula Treatment

Especially in banded RYGB, gastrogastric fistula can occur and be the cause of failure. When there is a gastrogastric fistula in association with failed RYGB, en bloc resection of the fistula with the excess gastric pouch, the anastomosis, and part of the excluded stomach, is performed (Fig. 20.3). This procedure is more efficient than the simple closure of the gastrogastric fistula, forming a new gastric bypass with a smaller pouch and a manual or stapled anastomosis calibrated by a 32 Fr boogie. In cases of very small gastric pouch or proximal gastrogastric fistulas, stapling or resection of fistula tract can be performed.

Conversion to Distal Gastric Bypass

Besides, to increase restrictive component of RYGB, the disabsorptive component can also be augmented. This alternative is applicable to patients whose cause of weight regain is not related to alimentary issues or in those with recidivism of metabolic diseases, such as T2DM and dyslipidemia.

There are numerous ways in which alimentary, biliopancreatic, and common limbs can be measured at the moment of primary RYGB. Distal RYGB is even performed in some cases as an initial operation in some cases of superobese patients [49]. The measurement distribution of intestinal loops is objective of many investigations regarding which one promotes a better outcome, and it seems that there is no significant impact of alimentary limb length on weight loss for patients with BMI <50 kg/m^2, but it may make a small difference for the superobese (BMI >50 kg/m^2). Furthermore, the degree of malabsorption after gastric bypass is especially influenced by the length of the common channel [18]. Even more controversial is the adequate length of limbs in a revisional set. Sugerman et al. (1996) reported the first description of distal RYGB as a revisional procedure in a 27 patient series, in which jejunojejunostomy was taken down at the alimentary side and re-anastomosed to the ileum at a point 150 cm proximal to the ileocecal valve, in 22 patients, and 50 cm proximal to ileocecal valve in 5 patients. The final result is an alimentary limb with its original size of 100–150 cm, the common channel at 150 or 50 cm, and a very long unmeasured BP limb. After 5 years of revision, BMI fell 13 kg/m^2 and the EWL was 69%. All the patients with a 50 cm common limb developed severe protein-calorie malnutrition that was refractory to high-protein liquid supplements as well as non-enteric-coated pancreatic enzymes and required reversal, and two died from hepatic failure. Three patients with a 150 cm common channel still required revision to a longer common tract because of malnutrition [50].

A variation was proposed by Brolin et al. (2007), in which the biliopancreatic limb was taken down at the jejunojejunostomy and re-anastomosed to a point 75–100 cm proximal to the ileocecal valve. The common channel was then measured at 75–100 cm, the biliopancreatic limb at its original, with a very long unmeasured Roux limb. The authors reported a 1-year %EWL higher than 50% in 47.9% of patients but 7.4% rate of protein-caloric malnutrition with 6% requirement of reversal [51].

The revision procedure proposed by Fobi et al. (2001) resulted in an average weight loss of 20 kg or an average decrease in BMI of 7 kg/m^2, but protein malnutrition occurred in 23.1%. The authors extended the length of the biliopancreatic limb by an additional 50% of the total common limb length, which was not measured, in 65 patients who underwent RYGB [52].

As observed in the aforementioned studies, a special care should be taken of nutritional deficiencies. Furthermore, a long-term follow-up study of distal RYGB as a revisional procedure after failed restrictive surgeries presented an 8.3% of hipoproteinemia and around 13% of malabsorption symptoms after 3 years. All patients were managed successfully with conservative measures, and none of the patients in this series needed lengthening of the common channel [53].

Conversion to BPD-DS

All aforementioned surgical options involved increasing either restrictive or malabsorptive components only. An alternative to get best long-term weight loss and control of comorbidities is conversion BPD-DS. This procedure is complex and technically challenging, because it requires taking down of the gastrojejunostomy and reestablishment of the gastrogastric continuity, followed by a sleeve gastrectomy. As originally, the procedure can be done in a single- or two-step manner. Laparoscopy is feasible and showed good results after 11 months, as shown by Parikh et al. (2007), who demonstrated dramatic weight after revision, with EWL of 62.7%, overall mean weight loss of 35.5 kg, and mean BMI decrease of 10.5 kg/m^2. The comorbidities resolved completely in all patients, and no mortality or reoperations for leakage or malnutrition were reported [54]. However, it has not gained wide acceptance due to the complexity of the procedure and the concern for long-term severe malnutrition.

Endoscopic Revision

Since surgical options are limited, with no well-established long-term results and, in some cases, technically difficult, endoscopic options for failed RYGB are rising, as endoscopic technologies are developed. The application of these ongoing procedures can also be adequate to high-risk patients, super-super obese patients, and patients who not fit for primary surgery. All the endoscopic techniques act over the restrictive component of the RYGB, in pouch reduction or narrowing gastrojejunostomy.

Endoscopic gastric plication (EGP) was first described in 2013, and it was conceived to simulate a sleeve gastrectomy using StomaphyX® device. However, it was applied for RYGB revision in 27 patients with lack of sustained weight loss after 1 year. Furthermore, most part of the plicated gastric fold became undone [55].

Other applicable techniques are transoral outlet reduction (TORe) and restorative obesity surgery endoscopy (ROSE) in which gastrojejunostomy anastomotic aperture is reduced. In TORe, a special endoscopic suture device is used, and thus the output of the distal stomach pouch is reduced. A single center experience of 150 cases had a EWL of 19.2% at 3-year follow-up and found no benefit to performing gastric pouch reduction concurrently with TORe [56]. Furthermore, RESTORe trial, a prospective, multicenter, randomized, blinded, sham-controlled trial, evaluated the effectiveness of TORe and showed that proportion of patients of TORe group and control group who achieved more than 20% of EWL (30% vs 14.8%, respectively) and the mean %EWL (15.9 vs 7.7, respectively) was greater in the procedure group, however, with no statistical significance. Both groups lost weight within the first 6 weeks after the procedure; however, control patients showed a trend toward weight regain after that; in contrast, the mean weight of the TORe group remained relatively stable [57].

In ROSE, tissue plications are created by opposing tissue and then deploying and anchoring full-thickness stitches. A multicentric series of 116 patients reported reduction in 50% of stoma diameter and loss of 32% of regained weight after RYGB [58].

Enlargement of gastric outlet can also be treated by other techniques, like endoscopic sclerotherapy, with a reported 6-month 4.5 kg weight loss [59], but the sclerosing substance is no longer commercially available. Argon plasma coagulation (APC) of margins of gastrojejunostomy results in scarring and consequently narrowing and decreased tissue compliance. Baretta et al. (2015) performed three sessions of APC and obtained a loss of 15 kg and reduction of 66% in the anastomotic diameter [60].

The available data show a short-term relative efficacy with acceptable risk of endoscopic procedures but with necessity of longer-term follow-up evaluation to determine if the effect will be sustained. Other limiting aspects of those procedures are the cost and need for special training and equipment for its execution. Nevertheless, endoscopic techniques can represent a promising tool, besides multidisciplinary approach with dietary and behavioral changes, to achieve a less invasive option to post-RYGB weight regain [61].

Robotic Revisional Bariatric Surgery

Bariatric revisional surgery is more difficult technically than primary operations. The presence of adhesions and cicatricial and inflammatory changes makes reoperations a challenge, with a greater possibility of complications such as bleeding and fistulas. In the revision procedures, there is a greater possibility of conversion from minimally invasive surgery to laparotomy, mainly due to the difficulty in performing some movements due to rigid instruments and two-dimensional vision [62]. Therefore, technologies such as robotic surgery, which allow three-dimensional vision, greater freedom and precision of movement, and greater ergonomics to the surgeon, have the potential to reduce complications and improve the outcome of reoperations.

Most of the studies in robotic revisional bariatric surgery have as primary outcome the cost, learning curve, time of hospitalization, and complications. The results of a systematic review showed that bariatric surgery, when performed with the use of robotics, had similar or lower complication rates compared with traditional laparoscopy [63] In addition, the learning curve appears to be shorter when robotic gastric bypass is compared with the traditional laparoscopic approach. Bariatric surgeons are doing more revisions to bypass and bypass revisions too, every year. Revising previous bariatric operations is difficult and time-consuming, but robotic revision surgery can be done safely and with good long-term weight loss results [64].

In a recent 27,997-patient meta-analysis study [65], there were no significant differences between robotic and laparoscopic bariatric surgery, regarding overall postoperative complications, the length of hospital stay, reoperation, conversion, and mortality. However, the incidence of anastomotic leak was lower in robotic procedures. Therefore, as we know that anastomotic leaks are more common in revisional procedures, the robotic platform might offer a cost saving alternative.

The common point of all studies evaluating the use of robot-assisted operations for revision bariatric surgery is the need for further studies [65]. Despite the potential advantages, there is a complete lack of prospective and comparative studies.

References

1. Jauno SS, Southall PJ. Bariatric surgery. Int J Surg. 2010;8:86–9.
2. Sjöstrom L, Narbro K, Sjöstrom CD, Karason K, Larsson B, Wedel H, et al. Effects of bariatric surgery on mortality in Swedish obese subjects. N Engl J Med. 2007;357:741–52.
3. Maggard MA, Shugaman LR, Suttorp M, Maglione M, Sugerman HJ, Livingston EH, et al. Meta-analysis: surgical treatment of obesity. Ann Intern Med. 2005;142:547–59.
4. Angrisani L, Santonicola A, Iovino P, Formisano G, Buchwald H, Scopinaro N. Bariatric surgery worldwide 2013. Obes Surg. 2015;25(10):1822–32.
5. Buchwald H, Buchwald JN. Evolution of operative procedures for the management of morbid obesity 1950–2000. Obes Surg. 2002;12:705–17.
6. Schroeder R, Garrison JM, Johnson MS. Treatment of adult obesity with bariatric surgery. Am Fam Physician. 2011;84(7):805–14.
7. Elder KA, Wolfe BM. Bariatric surgery: a review of procedures and outcomes. Gastroenterology. 2007;132(6):2253–71.
8. Cooper TC, Simmons EB, Webb K, Burns JL, Kushner RF. Trends in weight regain following Roux-en-Y Gastric Bypass (RYGB) bariatric surgery. Obes Surg. 2015;25(8):1474–81.
9. Puzziferri N, Roshek TB, Mayo HG, Gallagher R, Belle SH, Livingston EH. Long-term follow-up after bariatric surgery: a systematic review. JAMA. 2014;312(9):934–42.
10. Mingrone G, Panuzi S, De Gaetano A, Guidone C, Iaconelli A, Leccesi L, Nanni G, et al. Bariatric surgery versus conventional medical therapy for type 2 diabetes. N Engl J Med. 2012;366(17):1577–85.
11. Schauer PR, Kashyap SR, Wolski K, Brethauer SA, Kirwan JP, Pothier CE, et al. Bariatric surgery versus intensive medical therapy in obese patients with diabetes. N Engl J Med. 2012;366(17):1567–76.
12. Maser RW, Lenhard MJ, Peters MB, Irgau I, Wynn GM. Effects of surgically induce weight loss by Roux-en-Y gastric bypass on cardiovascular autonomic nerve function. Surg Obes Relat Dis. 2013;9:221–8.
13. Topart P, Becouarn G, Ritz P. Pouch size after gastric bypass does not correlate with weight loss outcome. Obes Surg. 2011;21(9):1350–4.
14. Edholm D, Ottosson J, Sundbom M. Importance of pouch size in laparoscopic Roux-en-Y gastric bypass: a cohort study of 14,168 patients. Surg Endosc Other Interv Tech. 2016;30(5):2011–5.
15. Roberts K, Duffy A, Kaufman J, Burrell M, Dziura J, Bell R. Size matters: gastric pouch size correlates with weight loss after laparoscopic Roux-en-Y gastric bypass. Surg Endosc. 2007;21(8):1397–402.
16. Bendewald FP, Choi JN, Blythe LS, Selzer DJ, Ditslear JH, Mattar SG. Comparison of hand-sewn, linear-stapled, and circular-stapled gastrojejunostomy in laparoscopic Roux-en-Y gastric bypass. Obes Surg. 2011;21(11):1671–5.
17. Langer FB, Prager G, Poglitsch M, Kefurt R, Shakeri-Leidenmühler S, Ludvik B, et al. Weight loss and weight regain – 5-year follow-up for circular- vs. linear-stapled gastrojejunostomy in laparoscopic roux-en-Y gastric bypass. Obes Surg. 2013;23(6):776–81.
18. Stefanidis D, Kuwada TS, Gersin KS. The importance of the length of the limbs for gastric bypass patients-an evidence-based review. Obes Surg. 2011;21(1):119–24.
19. Valezi AC, Marson AC, Merguizo RA, Costa FL. Roux-en-Y gastric bypass: limb length and weight loss. Arq Bras Cir Dig. 2014;27(1):56–8.
20. Orci L, Chilcott M, Huber O. Short versus long roux-limb length in roux-en-Y gastric bypass surgery for the treatment of morbid and super obesity: a systematic review of the literature. Obes Surg. 2011;21(6):797–804.
21. Mann JP, Jakes AD, Hayden JD, Barth JH. Systematic review of definitions of failure in revisional bariatric surgery. Obes Surg. 2015;25(3):571–4.
22. Yanos BR, Saules KK, Schuh LM, Sogg S. Predictors of lowest weight and long-term weight regain among Roux-en-Y gastric bypass patients. Obes Sug. 2015;25:1364–70.
23. Cazzo E, da Silva FP, Pareja JC, Chaim EA. Predictors for weight loss failure following Roux-en-Y gastric bypass. Arq Gastroenterol. 2014;51(4):328–30.
24. Still CD, Wood GC, Chu X, et al. Clinical factors associated with weight loss outcomes after Roux-en-Y gastric bypass surgery. Obesity (Silver Spring). 2014;22:888–94.

25. Kim HJ, Madan A, Fenton-Lee D. Does patient compliance with follow-up influence weight loss after gastric bypass surgery? A systematic review and meta-analysis. Obes Surg. 2014;24(4):647–51.
26. Khen-Dunlop N, Dabbas M, De Filippo G, Jais JP, Hervieux E, Télion C, et al. Primordial influence of post-operative compliance on weight loss after adolescent laparoscopic adjustable gastric banding. Obes Surg. 2016;26(1):98–104.
27. Larjani S, Spivak I, Hao Guo M, Aliarzadeh B, Wang W, Robinson S, et al. Preoperative predictors of adherence to multidisciplinary follow-up care postbariatric surgery. Surg Obes Relat Dis. 2016;12(2):350–6.
28. Amundsen T, Strommen M, Martins C. Suboptimal weight loss and weight regain after gastric bypass surgery—postoperative status of energy intake, eating behavior, physical activity, and psychometrics. Obes Surg. 2017;27(5):1316–23.
29. Iannelli A, Schneck AS, Hébuterne X, Gugenheim J. Gastric pouch resizing for roux-en-Y gastric bypass failure in patients with a dilated pouch. Surg Obes Relat Dis. 2013;9(2):260–7.
30. Blanchet M, Mesmann C, Yanes M, Lepage S, Marion D, Gelas P, et al. 3D gastric computed tomography as a new imaging in patients with failure or complication after bariatric surgery. Obes Surg. 2010;20:1727–33.
31. O'Brien CS, Wang G, McGinty J, Agénor KK, Dutia R, Colarusso A, et al. Effects of gastrogastric fistula repair on weight loss and gut hormone levels. Obes Surg. 2013;23:1294–301.
32. Corcelles R, Jamal MH, Daigle CR, Rogula T, Brethauer SA. Surgical management of gastrogastric fistula. Surg Obes Relat Dis. 2015;11(6):1227–32.
33. Heber D, Greemway FL, Kaplan LM, Livingston E, Salvador J, Still C, Endocrine Society. Endocrine and nutritional management of the post-bariatric surgery patient: an Endocrine Society Clinical Practice Guideline. J Clin Endocrinol Metab. 2010;95(11):4823–43.
34. Zoss I, Piec G, Horber FF. Impact of orlistat therapy on weight reduction in morbidly obese patients after implantation of the Swedish adjustable gastric band. Obes Surg. 2002;12(1):113–7.
35. Guerdjikova AI, Kotwal R, McElroy SL. Response of recurrent binge eating and weight gain to topiramate in patients with binge eating disorder after bariatric surgery. Obes Surg. 2005;15(2):273–7.
36. Zilberstein B, Pajecki D, De Brito ACG, Gallafrio ST, Eshkenazy R, Andrade CG. Topiramate after adjustable gastric banding in patients with binge eating and difficulty losing weight. Obes Surg. 2004;14(6):802–5.
37. Schwartz J, Suzo A, Wehr AM, Foreman KS, Mikami DJ, Needleman BJ, et al. Pharmacotherapy in conjunction with a diet and exercise program for the treatment of weight recidivism or weight loss plateau post-bariatric surgery: a retrospective review. Obes Surg. 2016;26(2):452–8.
38. Pajecki D, Halpern A, Cercato C, Mancini M, de Cleva R, Santo MA. Short-term use of liraglutide in the management of patients with weight regain after bariatric surgery. Rev Col Bras Cir. 2013;40(3):191–5.
39. Uittenbogaart M, Leclercq WK, Luijten AA, van Dielen FM. Laparoscopic adjustable gastric banding after failed Roux-En-Y gastric bypass. Obes Surg. [Internet]. 2016;27:381. Available from: https://doi.org/10.1007/s11695-016-2283-0.
40. Irani K, Youn HA, Ren-Fielding CJ, Fielding GA, Kurian M. Midterm results for gastric banding as salvage procedure for patients with weight loss failure after Roux-en-Y gastric bypass. Surg Obes Relat Dis. 2011;7(2):219–24.
41. Bessler M, Daud A, DiGiorgi MF, Inabnet WB, Schrope B, Olivero-Rivera L, et al. Adjustable gastric banding as revisional bariatric procedure after failed gastric bypass-intermediate results. Surg Obes Relat Dis. 2010;6(1):31–5.
42. Dapri G, Cadière GB, Himpens J. Laparoscopic placement of non-adjustable silicone ring for weight regain after roux-en-Y gastric bypass. Obes Surg. 2009;19(5):650–4.
43. Al-Bader I, Khoursheed M, Al Sharaf K, Mouzannar DA, Ashraf A, Fingerhut A. Revisional laparoscopic gastric pouch resizing for inadequate weight loss after Roux-en-Y gastric bypass. Obes Surg. 2015;25:1103–8.
44. Parikh M, Heacock L, Gagner M. Laparoscopic "gastrojejunal sleeve reduction" as a revision procedure for weight loss failure after Roux-En-Y gastric bypass. Obes Surg. 2011;21(5):650–4.
45. León F, Maiz C, Daroch D, Quezada N, Gabrielli M, Muñoz C, et al. Laparoscopic hand-sewn revisional gastrojejunal plication for weight loss failure after Roux-en-Y gastric bypass. Obes Surg. 2015;25(4):744–9.
46. Miguel GPS, Azevedo JLMC, De Souza PHO, De Siqueira Neto J, Mustafa F, Zambrana ÉS, et al. Erosive esophagitis after bariatric surgery: banded vertical gastrectomy versus banded Roux-en-Y gastric bypass. Obes Surg. 2011;21(2):167–72.
47. Costa RC, Yamaguchi N, Santo MA, Riccioppo D, Pinto-Junior PE. Outcomes on quality of life, weight loss and comorbidities after Roux-en-Y gastric bypass. Arq Gastroenterol. 2014;51(3):165–70.
48. Elias AA, Garrido-Junior AB, Berti LV, Oliveira MR, Bertin NTS, Malheiros CA, et al. Derivações gástricas em y- de- roux com anel de silicone para o tratamento da obesidade: estudo das complicações relacionadas com o anel. Arq Bras Cir Dig. 2011;24(4):290–5.
49. Tran DD, Nwokeabia ID, Purnell S, Zafar SN, Ortega G, Hughes K, et al. Revision of Roux-En-Y gastric bypass for weight regain: a systematic review of techniques and outcomes. Obes Surg. 2016;26(7):1627–34.
50. Sugerman HJ, Kellum JM, DeMaria EJ. Conversion of proximal to distal gastric bypass for failed gastric bypass for superobesity. J Gastrointest Surg. 1996;1(6):517–24; 526
51. Brolin RE, Cody RP. Adding malabsorption for weight loss failure after gastric bypass. Surg Endosc Other Interv Tech. 2007;21(11):1924–6.

52. Fobi MAL, Lee H, Igwe D, Felahy B, James E, Stanczyk M, et al. Revision of failed gastric bypass to distal Roux-en-Y gastric bypass: a review of 65 cases. Obes Surg. 2001;11(2):190–5.
53. Srikanth MS, Oh KH, Fox SR. Revision to malabsorptive Roux-En-Y gastric bypass (MRNYGBP) provides long-term (10 years) durable weight loss in patients with failed anatomically intact gastric restrictive operations: long-term effectiveness of a malabsorptive roux-En-Y gastric bypass. Obes Surg. 2011;21(7):825–31.
54. Parikh M, Pomp A, Gagner M. Laparoscopic conversion of failed gastric bypass to duodenal switch: technical considerations and preliminary outcomes. Surg Obes Relat Dis. 2007;3(6):611–8.
55. Ong'uti SK, Ortega G, Onwugbufor MT, Ivey GD, Fullum TM, Tran DD. Effective eight loss management with endoscopic gastric plication using StomaphyX device: is it achievable? Surg Obes Relat Dis. 2013;9:113–7.
56. Kumar N, Thompson CC. Transoral outlet reduction for weight regain after gastric bypass. Gastrointest Endosc. 2016;83(4):776–9.
57. Thompson CC, Chand B, Chen YK, Demarco DC, Miller L, Schweitzer M, et al. Endoscopic suturing for transoral outlet reduction increases weight loss after Roux-en-Y gastric bypass surgery. Gastroenterology. 2013;145(1):129–37.
58. Horgan S, Jacobsen G, Weiss D, Oldham JS Jr, Denk OM, Borao F, et al. Incisionless revision of post-Roux-en-Y bypass stomal and pouch dilation: multicenter registry results. Surg Obes Relat Dis. 2010;6:290–5.
59. Dayyeh BKA, Jirapinyo P, Weitzner Z, Barker C, Flicker MS, Lautz DB, et al. Endoscopic sclerotherapy for the treatment of weight regain after Roux-en-Y gastric bypass: outcomes , complications, and predictors of response in 575 procedures. Gastrointest Endosc. 2012;76(2):275–82.
60. Baretta GAP, Alhinho HCAW, Matias JEF, Marchesini JB, Lima JHF, Empinotti C, et al. Argon plasma coagulation of gastrojejunal anastomosis for weight regain after gastric bypass. Obes Surg. 2015;25:72–9.
61. Kumar N. Weight loss endoscopy: development, applications, and current status. World J Gastroenterol. 2016;22(31):7069–79.
62. Bindal V, Gonzalez-Heredia R, Elli EF. Outcomes of robot-assisted Rou-em-Y gastric bypass as a reoperative bariatric procedure. Obes Surg. 2015;25:1810–5.
63. Fourman MM, Saber AA. Robotic bariatric surgery: a systematic review. Surg Obes Relat Dis. 2012;8(4):483–8.
64. Snyder B, Wilson T, Woodruff V, Wilson E. Robotically assisted revision of bariatric surgeries is safe and effective to achieve further weight loss. World J Surg. 2013;37:2569–73.
65. Li K, Zou J, Tang J, Di J, Han X, Zhang P. Robotic versus laparoscopic bariatric surgery: a systematic review and meta-analysis. Obes Surg. 2016;26:3031–44.

21 Conversion from Sleeve to Bypass

Alcides José Branco Filho and André Thá Nassif

Introduction

With the progressive increase in the number of bariatric surgeries performed around the world, there is an increasing demand of patients who require revision surgery, either due to failure of results or complications [1]. Studies indicate that the revisional surgeries already represent between 5% and 10% of the total of the bariatric procedures currently performed [2].

Depending on the technique used primarily, the need for a revision procedure varies and may be very high as in the adjustable gastric band that reaches up to 26%. When we compare the two most performed surgeries today, the rate of reoperation after the sleeve gastrectomy (SG) is almost twice as high as after the Roux-en-Y gastric bypass (RYGB) (9.8% vs 4.9%, respectively) [1]. In an absolute number, revisional surgeries after RYGB and adjustable gastric banding are still the most performed ones [2, 3], but with the recent increase in SG's popularity, there is a tendency of this to become the primary surgery with the higher need for revision in the medium to long term [4].

The possible post-SG revision surgeries are the re-sleeve, the complement for doudenal switch (DS), and the conversion to RYGB [5]. The re-sleeve is indicated in cases of resultant failure in which there is a very important dilation of the remaining stomach. Deguines et al. attempted to estimate 225 cc as the exact number from which the chance of therapeutic failure increases [6]. Some services choose this reoperation option because it is technically less challenging [4, 7].

For the complementation to DS, it is necessary to perform a bowel bypass by connecting the distal ileum directly to the duodenum and leaving a common loop of 1 to 1.5 m. Despite providing one of the largest weight losses, this technique is becoming less common due to its high risk of malnutrition, chronic diarrhea, and hypovitaminosis [8]. A less aggressive surgery that is gaining ground in Europe as an alternative to DS in completing the SG is the single-anastomosis duodenoileal bypass (SADI) with a 250-cm common channel [9].

The other option, which is the focus of this chapter, is the conversion from SG to RYGB. It consists in approaching the stomach again for the creation of a small pouch and deviates the intestinal transit with a Roux-en-Y. It has become increasingly common because of its feasibility and good results [10].

Indications and Results

The most common indications of converting SG to RYGB are intractable gastroesophageal reflux disease (GERD), inadequate weight loss or regain, failure to treat metabolic diseases, and

A. J. B. Filho (✉) · A. T. Nassif
Department of Bariatric Surgery, Curitiba, Brazil

J. Ettinger et al. (eds.), *Gastric Bypass*, https://doi.org/10.1007/978-3-030-28803-7_21

Table 21.1 Indication of revisional surgery on articles that analyzed exclusively cases of conversions from sleeve to bypass

Author, year	Total N	GERD	Inadequate weight loss	Persistence of metabolic disease	Complications (fistula, stenosis)
Iannelli et al., 2016 [12]	40	11	29	0	0
Langer et al., 2010 [13]	8	3	5	0	0
Gautier et al., 2013 [14]	18	6	9	3	0
Abdemur et al., 2016 [11]	30	9	7	0	14

cases of complication following SG, as shown in Table 21.1 [5, 11].

Untreatable GERD

The sleeve gastrectomy (SG) is formed of a high-pressure gastric tube that is related both to the persistence of preoperative GERD symptoms and the risk of presenting new symptoms of GERD in the postoperative period in those who were asymptomatic [15]. In most cases, these symptoms can be managed clinically with proton pump inhibitors, but in the face of clinical intractability, it is necessary to indicate a revision surgery [16]. Conversion to RYGB makes the gastric reservoir smaller, with rapid emptying and low pressure, thus being very effective in the treatment of GERD. Studies are unanimous in demonstrating a 100% improvement in GERD symptoms after conversion and most often treat this as the main indication of this revisional surgery [12–14].

Failure to Lose Weight

The expected mean postoperative weight loss of the SG is between 50% and 70% of the excess weight or 30% to 40% of the total weight. The rate of regaining more than 10 kgs from the minimum weight is up to 20% [17].

A failure in weight loss is defined when the current BMI is greater than or equal to 35 while maintaining grade II obesity or when weight loss is less than 50% of the excess lost [18] and is directly related to a qualitatively bad alimentary habit [19].

Several studies documented effective weight loss after SG conversion to RYGB, maintaining an average loss of excess weight between 60% and 64% postoperatively [7, 12, 14]. But Nevo et al., when asked if it is worth converting SG to RYGB to this purpose, respond that although it significantly reduces the weight, this procedure kept 34% of the patients in the criterion of failure and emphasizes that it adds morbidities to patients in general [18].

It can be concluded that the conversion from SG to RYGB actually lowers weight, but it is not a large and sustained weight loss, and it does not happen in all patients and generates some morbidities that these patients did not previously have, such as anemia and hypovitaminosis. You should be aware of these factors prior to your appointment for this purpose.

Persistence of Metabolic Diseases

The fact of adding an intestinal deviation and the incretin effect of the RYGB presumably causes important benefits in the patients who maintained metabolic diseases after the SG.

In cases of persistent diabetes, conversion to RYGB may be an option. Gautier et al. reported three patients who maintained type 2 diabetes mellitus after the SG and were free of medication after reversal to RYGB [14]. Other studies show improvements in comorbidities after conversion but no more objective data [12].

Studies that objectively document the results of this conversion in metabolic diseases are lacking.

Complications After Sleeve

Acute cases of fistula after SG are usually treated through drainage of the cavity, endoscopy with esophageal-gastric prosthesis, passage of naso-enteral tube after the defect, and even jejunostomy sometimes [20].

In cases in which this fistula chronifies, there is a tendency of conversion to RYGB with resection of the fistulous path and placement of the alimentary loop just in the local of the fistula or to facilitate the emptying and decrease the pressure of the gastric tube [21–23].

If gastric tube stenosis happens due to the proximity of the angular incision staple or twist of the SG, we initially opt for endoscopic treatments such as dilatation, prosthesis placement, or septotomy. Usually they have good results, but in cases of failure, the conversion of this SG into RYGB is also presented as the best option [24].

Surgical Technique

The conversion of SG to RYGB is, among the revisional surgeries, one of the most feasible, but it requires a lot of respect precisely because the previous approach can turn it very difficult. Basically its accomplishment is similar to the techniques of the primary bypass RYGB with some special attentions [14]. Depending on the baseline indication and prioritization of one or another technical aspect, such as in an SG reversal because of GERD with hiatal hernia, the diaphragmatic crura should be well dissected and closed for a better end result.

Initially cautious access should be made, since the postoperative adhesion of an open primary surgery can be challenging. The first puncture is usually located in a supra-umbilical umbilical region, and a total of five portals is required. The release of adhesion is the first intra-abdominal step, and among those that form between the liver and the gastric tube are those that require greater care in handling to avoid bleeding. During access to the retrocavity of the small curvature, it is important to determine distance for esophagogastric transition and always leave a small pouch. Remember to remove the gastric fundus it is too large to decrease ghrelin secretion. There is controversy regarding removing or not routinely the antrum to avoid chronic pain, retained antrum syndrome, and gastric ulcer, which ends up being defined depending on the trans-operative conditions and the size of the remaining antrum. The intestinal deviation should be at least 50 cm of alimentary loop to avoid biliary reflux, and commonly 100 cm of alimentary limb and 100 cm of bileopancreatic limb is used. The jejuno-jejunostomy can be performed manually or mechanically, but it is very important to always close the intermesenteric gap. An option for ascending the alimentary limb with less tension is the bipartition of the large omentum, and the jejuno-gastrostomy again can be performed manually or stapled. For verification of patency and leak intraoperatively, a methylene blue test is performed through a 36 French Fouchet tube. Another gap that must be closed routinely is the Petersen space. Finally, drainage is optional depending on intraoperative aspects and surgeon's experience [18].

An alternative technique is the conversion of the SG into a simplified bypass, also called functional single-anastomosis or omega-loop bypass or minigastric bypass by bringing a unique loop to the gastric pouch. It is a surgery that grows very much today but with controversies on the results [25, 26]

Complications

The rate of complications expected for revision surgery is higher than for primary surgery, and this should always be analyzed before it's indicated [27]

When compared to a primary RYGB in a revision surgery, there are a higher number of patients: estimated blood loss, operative time, ICU stay, hospitalization time, intraoperative (hepatic, splenic, and intestinal) injuries, rehospitalization, and early reoperation [27].

Complications in a casuistry of 31 cases of revision surgery (RYGB or SG conversion) showed intraoperative complications in 17.65%, postoperative complications in 26.47%, and major complications in 8.2% % of the cases, including 5.8% of fistulas. Conversion to open surgery was required in one patient (2.94%) [28]

When speaking specifically of SG-to-RYGB conversion, an analysis of 40 cases identified 7 complications (16.7%), of which 5 were grade II and 2 grade IIIa of the classification of Clavien-Dindo. In 7.5% of cases, it was necessary to convert to open surgery [12]. Langer et al. documented one case of gastro-enteroanastomosis fistula of the eight revisionals performed but successfully treated with an endoscopic prosthesis [13].

There is no documented mortality increase after revision procedures. Despite increasing the chance of complications, the articles show that sleeve to bypass conversion is a safe procedure.

Conclusion

The conversion from SG to RYGB is a feasible, safe, and increasingly performed revision surgery option. It has a well-established indication in cases of intractable GERD or complications after the SG. It can also be used in postoperative weight loss failure and probably improves metabolic diseases but not with great evidences of success yet. It should always be weighted that it also adds morbidities and a higher chance of complications.

References

1. Altieri MS, Yang J, Nie L, Blackstone R, Spaniolas K, Pryor A. Rate of revisions or conversion after bariatric surgery over 10 years in the state of New York. Surg Obes Relat Dis [Internet]. 2018;14(4):500–7. https://doi.org/10.1016/j.soard.2017.12.019.
2. Shimizu H, Annaberdyev S, Motamarry I, Kroh M, Schauer PR, Brethauer SA. Revisional bariatric surgery for unsuccessful weight loss and complications. Obes Surg. 2013;23(11):1766–73.
3. Khoursheed MA, Al-Bader IA, Al-Asfar FS, Mohammad AI, Shukkur M, Dashti HM. Revision of failed bariatric procedures to Roux-en-Y gastric bypass (RYGB). Obes Surg. 2011;21(8):1157–60.
4. El Chaar M, Stoltzfus J, Claros L, Miletics M. Indications for revisions following 630 consecutive laparoscopic sleeve gastrectomy cases: experience in a single accredited center. J Gastrointest Surg [Internet]. 2017;21(1):12–16. Available at: https://doi.org/10.1007/s11605-016-3215-y
5. Ferrer-Márquez M, Belda-Lozano R, Solvas-Salmerón J, Ferrer-Ayza M. Revisional surgery after laparoscopic sleeve gastrectomy. Surg Laparosc Endosc Percutan Tech. 2015;25(1):6–9.
6. Deguines JB, Verhaeghe P, Yzet T, Robert B, Cosse C, Regimbeau JM. Is the residual gastric volume after laparoscopic sleeve gastrectomy an objective criterion for adapting the treatment strategy after failure? Surg Obes Relat Dis [Internet]. 2013;9(5):660–6. https://doi.org/10.1016/j.soard.2012.11.010.
7. Cheung D, Switzer NJ, Gill RS, Shi X, Karmali S. Revisional bariatric surgery following failed primary laparoscopic sleeve gastrectomy: a systematic review. Obes Surg. 2014;24(10):1757–63.
8. Homan J, Betzel B, Aarts EO, Van Laarhoven KJHM, Janssen IMC, Berends FJ. Secondary surgery after sleeve gastrectomy: Roux-en-Y gastric bypass or biliopancreatic diversion with duodenal switch. Surg Obes Relat Dis [Internet]. 2015;11(4):771–777. Available at: https://doi.org/10.1016/j.soard.2014.09.029
9. Sánchez-Pernaute A, Rubio MÁ, Conde M, Arrue E, Pérez-Aguirre E, Torres A. Single-anastomosis duodenoileal bypass as a second step after sleeve gastrectomy. Surg Obes Relat Dis [Internet]. 2015;11(2):351–5. https://doi.org/10.1016/j.soard.2014.06.016.
10. Ben AI, Debs T, Martini F, Elias B, Kassir R, Gugenheim J. Laparoscopic conversion of a sleeve gastrectomy to the Roux-en-Y gastric bypass. Obes Surg. 2015;25(8):1556–7.
11. Abdemur A, Han SM, Lo Menzo E, Szomstein S, Rosenthal R. Reasons and outcomes of conversion of laparoscopic sleeve gastrectomy to Roux-en-Y gastric bypass for nonresponders. Surg Obes Relat Dis [Internet]. 2016;12(1):113–8. https://doi.org/10.1016/j.soard.2015.04.005.
12. Iannelli A, Debs T, Martini F, Benichou B, Ben Amor I, Gugenheim J. Laparoscopic conversion of sleeve gastrectomy to Roux-en-Y gastric bypass: indications and preliminary results. Surg Obes Relat Dis [Internet]. 2016;12(8):1533–8. https://doi.org/10.1016/j.soard.2016.04.008.
13. Langer FB, Bohdjalian A, Shakeri-Leidenmühler S, Schoppmann SF, Zacherl J, Prager G. Conversion from sleeve gastrectomy to roux-en-y gastric bypass-indications and outcome. Obes Surg. 2010;20(7):835–40.
14. Gautier T, Sarcher T, Contival N, Le Roux Y, Alves A. Indications and mid-term results of conversion from sleeve gastrectomy to roux-en-Y gastric bypass. Obes Surg. 2013;23(2):212–5.
15. Carter PR, Leblanc KA, Hausmann MG, Kleinpeter KP, Debarros SN, Jones SM. Association between gastroesophageal reflux disease and laparoscopic sleeve gastrectomy. Surg Obes Relat Dis [Internet]. 2011;7(5):569–72. https://doi.org/10.1016/j.soard.2011.01.040.
16. Soricelli E, Iossa A, Casella G, Abbatini F, Calì B, Basso N. Sleeve gastrectomy and crural repair in obese patients with gastroesophageal reflux disease and/or hiatal hernia. Surg Obes Relat Dis. 2013;9(3):356–62.
17. Bohdjalian A, Langer FB, Shakeri-Leiden Mühler S, Gfrerer L, Ludvik B, Zacherl J, et al. Sleeve gastrectomy as sole and definitive bariatric procedure: 5-year results for weight loss and ghrelin. Obes Surg. 2010;20(5):535–40.

18. Nevo N, Abu-Abeid S, Lahat G, Klausner J, Eldar SM. Converting a sleeve gastrectomy to a gastric bypass for weight loss failure—is it worth it? Obes Surg. 2018;28(2):364–8.
19. Cena H, De Giuseppe R, Biino G, Persico F, Ciliberto A, Giovanelli A, et al. Evaluation of eating habits and lifestyle in patients with obesity before and after bariatric surgery: a single Italian center experience. Springerplus. 2016;5(1):1–9.
20. Praveenraj P, Gomes R, Kumar S, Senthilnathan P, Parthasarathi R, Rajapandian S, et al. Management of gastric leaks after laparoscopic sleeve gastrectomy for morbid obesity: a tertiary care experience and design of a management algorithm. J Minim Access Surg [Internet]. 2016;12(4):342. Available at: http://www.journalofmas.com/text.asp?2016/12/4/342/181285
21. Baltasar A, Serra C, Bengochea M, Bou R, Andreo L. Use of Roux limb as remedial surgery for sleeve gastrectomy fistulas. Surg Obes Relat Dis [Internet]. 2008;4(6):759–63. https://doi.org/10.1016/j.soard.2008.07.012.
22. Márquez MF, Ayza MF, Lozano RB, Del Mar Rico Morales M, García Díez JM, Poujoulet RB. Gastric leak after laparoscopic sleeve gastrectomy. Obes Surg. 2010;20(9):1306–11.
23. Thompson CE, Ahmad H, Lo Menzo E, Szomstein S, Rosenthal RJ. Outcomes of laparoscopic proximal gastrectomy with esophagojejunal reconstruction for chronic staple line disruption after laparoscopic sleeve gastrectomy. Surg Obes Relat Dis [Internet]. 2014;10(3):455–9. https://doi.org/10.1016/j.soard.2013.10.008.
24. Deslauriers V, Beauchamp A. Endoscopic management of post-laparoscopic sleeve gastrectomy stenosis. Surg Endosc. 2012;1:822–5.
25. Greco F. Conversion of vertical sleeve gastrectomy to a functional single-anastomosis gastric bypass: technique and preliminary results using a non-adjustable ring instead of stapled division. Obes Surg [Internet]. 2017;27(4):896–901. https://doi.org/10.1007/s11695-016-2392-9.
26. Moszkowicz D, Rau C, Guenzi M, Zinzindohoué F, Berger A, Chevallier JM. Laparoscopic omega-loop gastric bypass for the conversion of failed sleeve gastrectomy: early experience. J Visc Surg [Internet]. 2013;150(6):373–8. https://doi.org/10.1016/j.jviscsurg.2013.08.010.
27. Zhang L, Tan WH, Chang R, Eagon JC. Perioperative risk and complications of revisional bariatric surgery compared to primary Roux-en-Y gastric bypass. Surg Endosc. 2015;29(6):1316–20.
28. Victorzon M. Revisional bariatric surgery by conversion to gastric bypass or sleeve-good short-term outcomes at higher risks. Obes Surg. 2012;22(1):29–33.

22 Gastrojejunostomy Testing

Amador García Ruiz de Gordejuela
and Jordi Pujol Gebelli

Gastrojejunostomy is one of the key points for the Roux-en-Y gastric bypass (RYGB). This anastomosis is responsible for some of the most frequent complications after this procedure and, for the most complex and risk one, leaks. It is important to perform an adequate technique, respecting some rules that were examined in the previous chapters, but now we are going to discuss how we check the anastomosis is fine and if we need to do it.

We can test the anastomosis both during surgery and in the postoperative time. We will examine different methods for testing, with their pros and cons, and try to elucidate which is the actual recommendation according to the evidence.

Intraoperative Gastrojejunostomy Testing

Gastrojejunostomy is one of the most complex and critical steps of the RYGB procedure. It is the only anastomosis constructed with intention to be as small as possible by a general surgeon. It is also a technically demanding gesture independently the way it is constructed. The most feared complication is the leak. Leaks are responsible for at least 1% to 5% [1] of complications after RYGB.

The clinical and technical expertise, a good and well-trained technique, and some tips and tricks are the keys for a successful anastomosis. But, even if we construct the perfect anastomosis with the ideal conditions and the right steps, it may fail and lead to a leak. Several technical gestures and adjuvants have been discussed for the prevention of leaks, and even in the best of the conditions, do not lead to a 0% of postoperative leaks.

Historically, the checking of the anastomosis was the quality control checkpoint after every procedure. There are three different ways to check this anastomosis:

- Air test through an orogastric tube
- Methylene blue through an orogastric tube
- Intraoperative upper gastrointestinal endoscopy

Methylene Blue and Air Leak Test

Methylene blue and air leak test are easy-to-perform ways of testing the anastomosis. After the anastomosis is completed, the anesthetist introduces an orogastric tube (or uses the one that calibrated the anastomosis and/or the pouch) and flushes air and/or methylene blue. The surgeon clamps the bowel proximal to the suture in order to create some tension inside the lumen. This way we may observe some blue liquid or

A. García Ruiz de Gordejuela (✉) · J. Pujol Gebelli
Bariatric Surgery Unit, General Surgery Department, Bellvitge University Hospital, Barcelona, Spain

J. Ettinger et al. (eds.), *Gastric Bypass*, https://doi.org/10.1007/978-3-030-28803-7_22

bubbles between the stitches and detect the leak or any potential defect at the anastomosis.

Some authors prefer to use only air [2] because of several reasons. The main reason we may argue is that air can easily pass and may be more sensitive in detecting a leak. It may also detect leak where the suture is not seen as the bubbles will appear at any place. It is also less harmful than methylene blue and cheaper. Despite these potential advantages, there are not comparative trials between air and methylene blue, and we do not exactly know the sensitivity and specificity of both tests.

It is not common that a leak may be seen during surgery. It usually occurs in difficult cases such as in revisional surgeries. Most common locations to appear used to be corner and stapler intersections. Once the leak is diagnosed, the surgeon may decide how to treat it like oversewing or constructing a new anastomosis.

Intraoperative Endoscopy

Endoscopy testing uses the air that is insufflated during the procedure to check the watertightness of the new suture. The endoscopy also has a very interesting add-on to the testing: it is a live image of the anastomosis from inside, so we can check for bleeding, mucosal perfusion, and the real wide of the anastomosis [3].

Intraoperative endoscopy is not only a tool for anastomosis testing. It is also a very useful tool for complicated cases as revisional surgery, intraoperative complications, or difficult scenarios. In those occasions endoscopy may add or confirm information to the surgical team in order to safely complete the procedures.

The endoscopy requires both adequate equipment in the theater and trained surgeons to perform it during the surgery. Both conditions are not available everywhere, so its implementation tends to be complicated. Despite these limitations upper and lower gastrointestinal endoscopy should be part of the education of every surgeon, and in several countries, they are mandatory for every future surgeon.

Pros and Cons of Intraoperative Testing

Both intraoperative endoscopy and methylene blue-air leak testing are useful for technical defects, but they are not usually useful for late-onset leaks. These leaks usually are related to ischemic or blood supply difficulties that methylene blue-air leak will not be able to check and that endoscopy may fail to clearly evaluate. These difficulties may be solved with new image technologies that may add image filters to facilitate interpretation about blood supply to the tissues. Despite these innovations, there is not clear correlation yet between adequate or no blood supply at the time of the surgery and the appearance or not of a leak in the near future.

Both procedures also may be harmful. During the insertion of the orogastric tube, tears can be done over the esophagus or the anastomosis itself due to malpractice. Also excessive pressure during the instillation of the methylene blue or the air may arrive to harm the suture. The endoscope itself also may cause lesions during its manipulation or related to the insufflation at any time of the testing.

Nowadays there are several authors that begin to discuss it as a mandatory step at every surgery. There are just a very few positive testings, and even if a test is negative, it does not prevent a leak. So these authors defend that those intraoperative testings should be abandoned as a routine practice and to keep them for difficult cases or complicated scenarios. It is also argued that positive intraoperative testings only diagnose technical failures, but will not prevent for other causes of leaks as ischemia. Even with a good endoscopy that may not show any sign of ischemia at the time of surgery, this finding is no guarantee for a good healing.

Postoperative Testing

At the beginning of the bariatric surgery, the complications of the patients themselves and the difficulties for the surgical procedures kept all the surgeons with more than 100% of attention at their patients. This way, several testings of the most complex anastomosis were developed. Nowadays we have moved to keep only the easiest testings or reserve all this armamentarium to selective indications.

There are different tests to be done:

- Methylene blue
- Radiological examinations
  - Contrast swallow studies
  - Double-contrast CT scan

Methylene blue at the postoperative time requires an intraabdominal drain after the surgery. If there is a leak, the drain would collect the methylene blue as soon as it goes out from the lumen. This is the easiest test we may perform but requires a drain in place and permeable. Since the introduction of the enhanced recovery programs, the use of drains has declined, and just a few surgeons use them routinely. The low morbidity rate justifies that most of the drains are useless. Moreover, it is mandatory that the drain keeps in place, close to the anastomosis, and they also move after surgery, not always remaining at the place we left them during the surgery.

Contrast swallow series were very common at the beginnings of the bariatric surgery and at the introduction of the laparoscopy. They give an anatomic view of what was constructed at the theater and were very useful for the diagnosis of stenosis or leak after the surgery. Despite their pros, the sensitivity and specificity were not very high, with a high rate or false-negative tests [4]. Oral soluble contrasts usually move too fast inside the lumen, so they may fail to properly diagnose a leak, especially if it is very small. Barium has a higher sensitivity but also higher complications, and it is quite worse tolerated. Despite this, these contrast studies still are better than just clinical signs to detect a leak [5].

Double-contrast CT scan studies have the higher sensitivity for the diagnosis of a leak [6, 7] but they are more expensive, they may be not be available for heavier patients (limitations of the table, the circumference of the detectors, or both), and they require higher doses of radiation for the diagnosis. Specificity is better than swallow studies, but not very high. CT scan with intravenous contrast may also give some information about the perfusion status of the pouch and the anastomosis. It also may show other indirect signs to detect the leak as pneumoperitoneum (bigger than expected for the postoperative day or at an unusual location) or fluid collections at some locations.

Endoscopy can be also used for the diagnosis of a leak after surgery. It may check complications from inside the anastomosis, and it can be also therapeutic. Finally, surgical revision is, in some cases, the only effective tool to clearly diagnose, and then to treat, the leak.

Nowadays, most of the authors recommend selective indications of these tests. The best tool for the postoperative diagnosis of a leak is clinical suspicious plus an adequate imaging. The first sign is usually just a non-justified tachycardia followed by other clinical and analytical signs and symptoms, like changes in blood tests. In those cases, a CT scan or an early endoscopic examination may clearly diagnose the leak. The most recent papers clearly demonstrate that routine examinations are not needed; they only make the process more expensive, may add morbidity, and do not prevent or advance the diagnosis of the leak [8–10].

References

1. Quezada N, Maiz C, Daroch D, Funke R, Sharp A, Boza C, et al. Effect of early use of covered self-expandable endoscopic stent on the treatment of postoperative stapler line leaks. Obes Surg. 2015;25:1816. https://doi.org/10.1007/s11695-015-1622-x.
2. Amarasinghe DC. Air test as an alternative to methylene blue test for leaks. Obes Surg. 2002;12:295–6. https://doi.org/10.1381/096089202762552557.
3. Al Hadad M, Dehni N, Elamin D, Ibrahim M, Ghabra S, Nimeri A. Intraoperative endoscopy decreases postoperative complications in laparoscopic Roux-en-Y gastric bypass. Obes Surg. 2015;25:1711–5. https://doi.org/10.1007/s11695-015-1604-z.
4. Schiesser M, Guber J, Wildi S, Guber I, Weber M, Muller MK. Utility of routine versus selective upper gastrointestinal series to detect anastomotic leaks after laparoscopic gastric bypass. Obes Surg. 2011;21:1238–42. https://doi.org/10.1007/s11695-010-0284-y.

5. Madan AK, Stoecklein HH, Ternovits CA, Tichansky DS, Phillips JC. Predictive value of upper gastrointestinal studies versus clinical signs for gastrointestinal leaks after laparoscopic gastric bypass. Surg Endosc. 2007;21:194–6. https://doi.org/10.1007/s00464-005-0700-x.
6. Yu J, Turner MA, Cho S-R, Fulcher AS, DeMaria EJ, Kellum JM, et al. Normal anatomy and complications after gastric bypass surgery: helical CT findings. Radiology. 2004;231:753–60. https://doi.org/10.1148/radiol.2313030546.
7. Lyass S, Khalili TM, Cunneen S, Fujita F, Otsuka K, Chopra R, et al. Radiological studies after laparoscopic Roux-en-Y gastric bypass: routine or selective? Am Surg. 2004;70:918–21.
8. White S, Han SH, Lewis C, Patel K, McEvoy B, Kadell B, et al. Selective approach to use of upper gastroesophageal imaging study after laparoscopic Roux-en-Y gastric bypass. Surg Obes Relat Dis. 2008;4:122–5. https://doi.org/10.1016/j.soard.2007.10.007.
9. Sethi M, Zagzag J, Patel K, Magrath M, Somoza E, Parikh MS, et al. Intraoperative leak testing has no correlation with leak after laparoscopic sleeve gastrectomy. Surg Endosc. 2015;30:883. https://doi.org/10.1007/s00464-015-4286-7.
10. Nelson L, Moon RC, Teixeira AF, Jawad MA. Methylene blue or upper GI, which is more effective for detecting leaks in gastric bypass patients? Surg Laparosc Endosc Percutan Tech. 2015;25:451–4. https://doi.org/10.1097/SLE.0000000000000191.

23 Closing the Mesenteric Defects

Mariano Palermo, Pablo A. Acquafresca, and Edgardo Serra

Among all the bariatric procedures, the Roux-en-Y gastric bypass (RYGB) is the most frequently performed, accounting for approximately 45% of all bariatric procedures [1]. Nowadays sleeve gastrectomy is increasing and probably has similar frequency than gastric bypass, but this last continues being the gold standard in bariatric surgery procedures. Together with the growing popularity of RYGB, there has been an increase in the incidence of internal herniation. This occurs when the small bowel herniates through the defects in the intermesenteric spaces created when the Roux limb is being mobilized to the newly created pouch.

The gaps that are created when performing a RYGB are the transverse mesocolic, the Petersen's space, and the jejunojejunostomy mesentery (Fig. 23.1). Whether to close or not these gaps, it's a matter of debate that we will discuss in this chapter.

It is not possible to talk about the topic of the closure of the mesenteric defect without talking about internal hernias. The most common causes of small bowel obstruction following laparoscopic RYGB are related to internal hernias [2–4] which are a feared and well-recognized complication, with a reported prevalence as high as 14% [5].

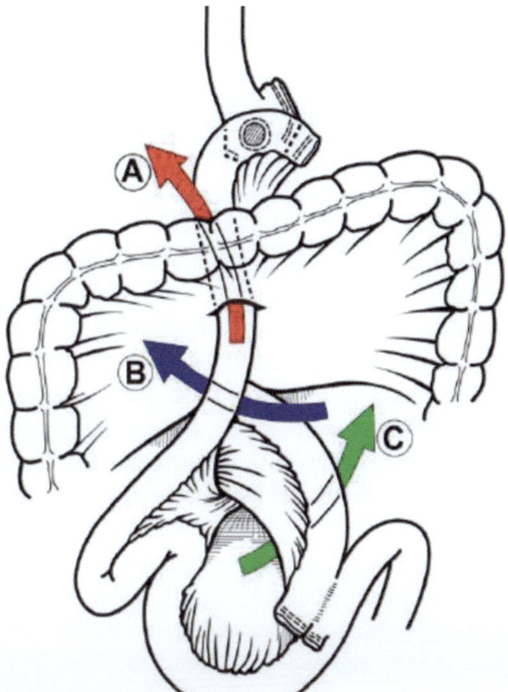

Fig. 23.1 Mesenteric defects: (**a**) transverse mesocolic, (**b**) Petersen's space, and (**c**) jejunojejunostomy mesentery

An internal hernia can be defined as a protrusion of the intestine through a defect within the abdominal cavity. Most internal hernias present later in the postoperative period rather than early.

When making the decision to close or not the mesenteric defect, it's also important to take into account the approach type, open or laparoscopic.

M. Palermo (✉) · P. A. Acquafresca · E. Serra
Division of Bariatric Surgery Centro CIEN – DIAGNOMED, Affiliated Institution to the University of Buenos Aires and DAICIM Foundation, Buenos Aires, Argentina

J. Ettinger et al. (eds.), *Gastric Bypass*, https://doi.org/10.1007/978-3-030-28803-7_23

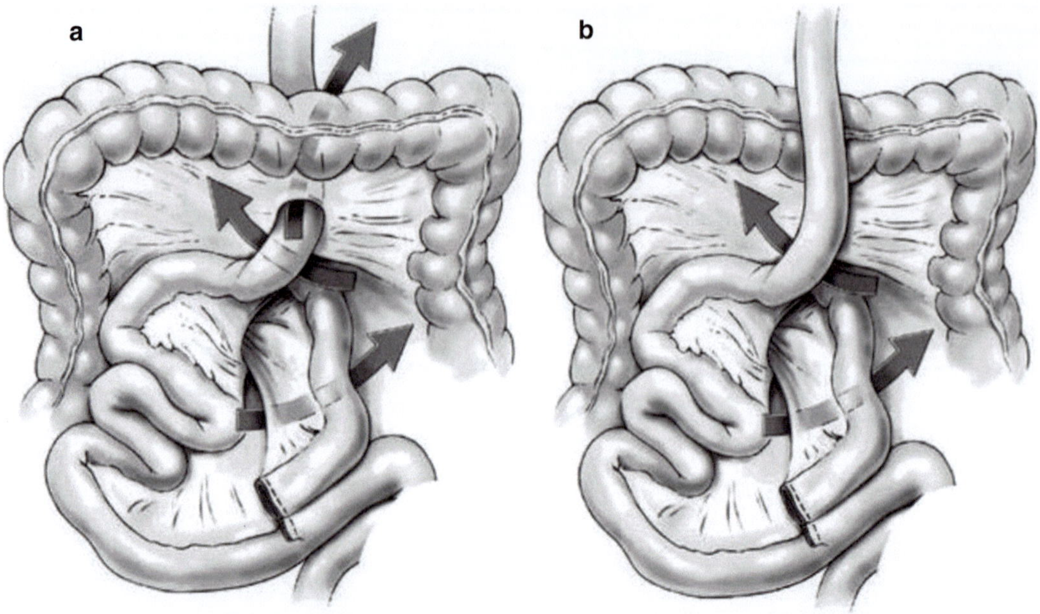

Fig. 23.2 (**a**) Retrocolic approach creating three defects. (**b**) Antecolic approach creating two defects

Compared with the open approach, the incidence of internal hernia is greater after laparoscopic RYGB, estimated between 3% and 4.5% [6]. Some hypotheses postulate that the laparoscopic approach reduces the bowel manipulation and peritoneal irritation, so it generates fewer postoperative adhesions and therefore less fixation of the small bowel to adjacent structures [3]. In addition, rapid weight loss after laparoscopic RYGB results in reduced intraperitoneal fat and larger mesenteric defects [7].

Bowel obstruction secondary to internal hernias usually presents in the later postoperative period, while early small bowel obstructions (in less than 1 month) usually result from technical problems with the Roux limb (e.g., complete blockage or partial narrowing of the gastrojejunostomy or jejunojejunostomy, acute angulation of the Roux limb, and narrowing of the Roux limb at the level of the transverse mesocolon).

RYGB can be accomplished using either an antecolic or retrocolic approach. Depending on the chosen approach, a number of potential mesenteric defects are created. The retrocolic approach creates three defects: one in the transverse mesocolon, one at the site of the jejunojejunostomy, and a Petersen defect (a space created between the Roux limb and the transverse mesocolon), while the antecolic approach creates only two mesenteric defects, one at the jejunojejunostomy and the Petersen defect (Fig. 23.2).

The most common location for internal hernias and its relation to Roux limb configuration have been a subject of debate. Understandably, mesocolic defect hernias are unique to a retrocolic approach and are not seen with an antecolic approach.

In some reports, mesocolic defects were the most common among all internal hernias [8]. Some authors reported that transverse mesocolic hernias were the most common, followed by jejunojejunostomy and Petersen's space hernias [6]. In an antecolic approach, however, both Petersen's and jejunojejunostomy mesenteric defect hernias are reported, with hernias at the jejunojejunostomy defect being more common in some other series [3]. Other investigators report a higher incidence of Petersen's and jejunojejunostomy hernias with a retrocolic approach [4]. A significant decrease in small bowel obstruction has been reported by some authors after switching from a retrocolic to an antecolic technique [3].

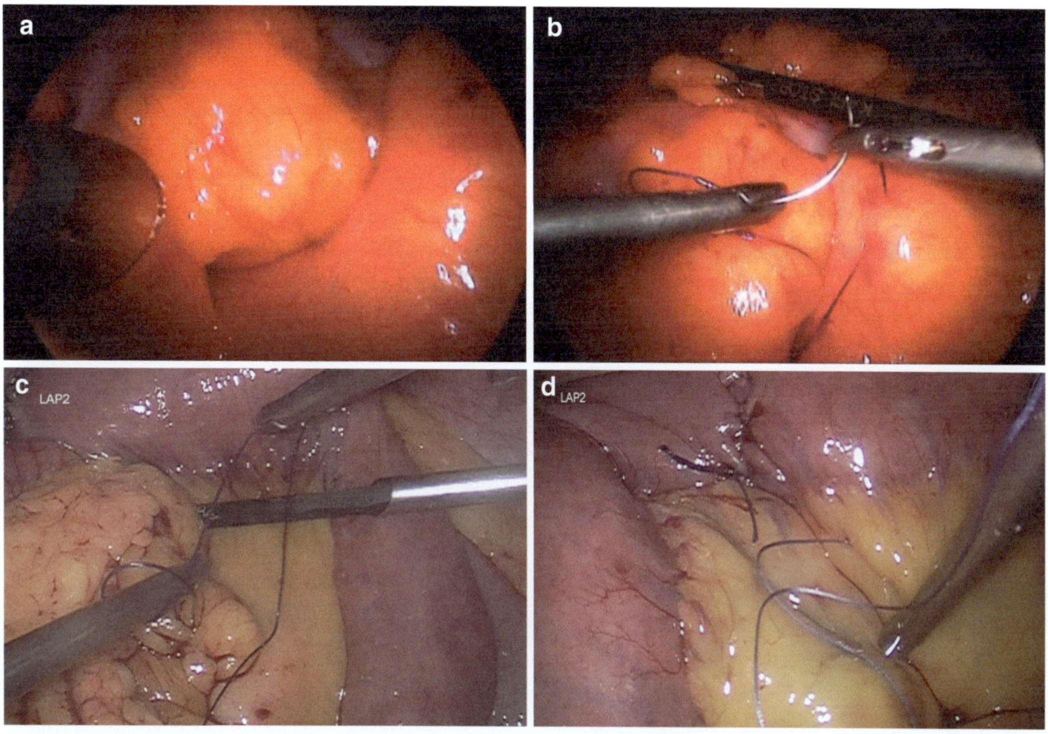

Fig. 23.3 Closure of mesenteric defects with an absorbable suture. Petersen and mesentery

Internal hernias can have devastating results when the diagnosis is delayed, and this can occur due to its presentation. Dull abdominal pain with or without intestinal obstruction is the most common presentation. Usually the presentation is delayed, occurring several months to years after the operation, but it can occur in the immediate postoperative period.

Due to the previously discussed (the severe adverse outcome and the easy way to prevent it), most authors concur that specific measures should be taken to avoid bowel obstruction after gastric bypass. The main measure that can be taken is the routine closure of the mesenteric defect at the jejunojejunostomy, transverse mesocolon mesenteric defect, and the Petersen defect (Fig. 23.3a, b). A drop on the internal hernia incidence from 3.5% to 1.7% has been reported after closing the mesenteric defects [9].

Whether to use absorbable or nonabsorbable, running or interrupted suture has been also a matter of debate, and it's not clear yet which technique contributes with less adverse outcomes. Some authors who have modified their technique from absorbable to nonabsorbable sutures and from an interrupted to a running technique have reported a reduction in the incidence of internal hernias [10].

Another technique that has been described to close the defects uses 4.8 mm staplers (Fig. 23.4). A pair of graspers can be used to expose the defects, and the staples can be partially extended presenting "hooks" that facilitate the catching and adaptation of the mesenteric serosa. To avoid vascular injury, it is important not to press the clip applicator too deeply. This technique has proved to be effective to prevent internal hernias (results showed that the internal hernia rate dropped from 5% to 0.6%) and doesn't add much surgical time (average time used for closing mesenteric defects of 1 min and 49 seconds) [11, 12].

Other authors, having in mind the fact that the internal hernia incidence is lower in the open approach due to adhesions generated by the peritoneal irritation, have described a more "physiological" way to close the defects. The mesenteric irritation technique is performed after closure of the jejunojejunal mesenteric defect with a running 2-0 silk suture. In this technique, an unfolded gauze X-ray detectable is introduced with a laparoscopic grasper through an already placed periumbilical port site. The gauze is then rubbed against the closed visceral peritoneal mesentery, over the silk suture closure, until petechiae are visualized on the surface of the mesentery confirming adequate irritation and removal of the visceral peritoneal surface of the mesentery (Fig. 23.5). With this technique the internal hernia incidence dropped from 5.3% to 1.4%; however this was not statistically significant [13].

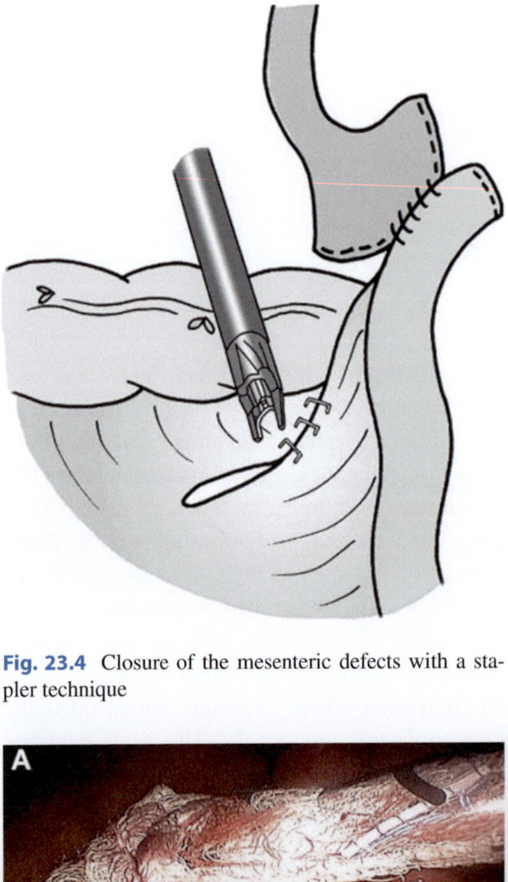

Fig. 23.4 Closure of the mesenteric defects with a stapler technique

On the other hand, it is important to mention that some authors have criticized the closure of mesenteric defects during the RYGB due to prolonging the procedure and thereby increasing the operative risks [14, 15]; and they emphasize that risks associated with closing the defect may be underreported. Furthermore, closure of the internal hernia may create kinking near the jejunojejunostomy which will lead to dilatation of the alimentary limb or the biliopancreatic limb with the subsequent increased risk of "blowout" of the bypassed stomach (gastric rupture) [13, 16]. In conclusion, having into account the risk versus the benefit of closing the mesenteric defects, one should close these defects as a routine. We strongly recommend closing routinely the defects using absorbable sutures.

References

1. Buchwald H, Oien DM. Metabolic/bariatric surgery worldwide 2011. Obes Surg. 2013;23:427–36.
2. Himpens J, Verbrugghe A, Cadière G-B, Everaerts W, Greve JW. Long-term results of laparoscopic Roux-en-Y gastric bypass: evaluation after 9 years. Obes Surg. 2012;22:1586–93.
3. Champion JK, Williams M. Small bowel obstruction and internal hernias after laparoscopic Roux-en-Y gastric bypass. Obes Surg. 2003;13(4):596–600.
4. Capella RF, Iannace VA, Capella JF. Bowel obstruction after open and laparoscopic gastric bypass surgery for morbid obesity. J Am Coll Surg. 2006;203(3):328–35.
5. Rodríguez A, Mosti M, Sierra M, Pérez-Johnson R, Flores S, Dominguez G, et al. Small bowel obstruction

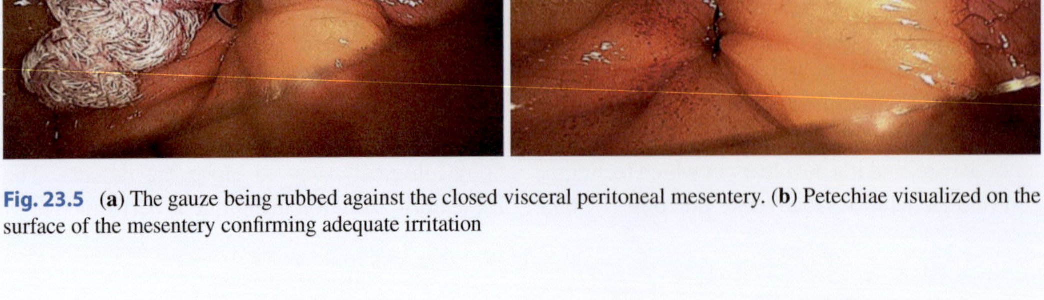

Fig. 23.5 (**a**) The gauze being rubbed against the closed visceral peritoneal mesentery. (**b**) Petechiae visualized on the surface of the mesentery confirming adequate irritation

after antecolic and antegastric laparoscopic Roux-en-Y gastric bypass: could the incidence be reduced? Obes Surg. 2010;20:1380–4.
6. Garza E Jr, Kuhn J, Arnold D, et al. Internal hernias after laparoscopic Roux-en-Y gastric bypass. Am J Surg. 2004;188(6):796–800.
7. Schneider C, Cobb W, Scott J, Carbonell A, Myers K, Bour E. Rapid excess weight loss following laparoscopic gastric bypass leads to increased risk of internal hernia. Surg Endosc. 2011;25:1594.
8. Rogula T, Yenumula PR, Schauer PR. A complication of Roux-en-Y gastric bypass: intestinal obstruction. Surg Endosc. 2007;21(11):1914–8. Epub 2007 Sep 22
9. Chowbey P, Baijal M, Kantharia NS, Khullar R, Sharma A, Soni V. Mesenteric defect closure decreases the incidence of internal hernias following laparoscopic Roux-En-Y gastric bypass: a retrospective Cohort study. Obes Surg. 2016;26:2029. https://doi.org/10.1007/s11695-016-2049-8.
10. Higa KD, Ho T, Boone KB. Internal hernias after laparoscopic Roux-en-Y gastric bypass: incidence, treatment and prevention. Obes Surg. 2003;13(3):350–4.
11. Aghajani E, Jacobsen HJ, Nergaard BJ, et al. Internal hernia after gastric bypass: a new and simplified technique for laparoscopic primary closure of the mesenteric defects. J Gastrointest Surg. 2012;16:641–5.
12. Aghajani E, Jacobsen HJ, Nergaard BJ, Hedenbro JL, Leifson BG, Gislason H. Internal hernia after gastric bypass: a new and simplified technique for laparoscopic primary closure of the mesenteric defects. J Gastrointest Surg. 2012;16:641–5.
13. Walker AS, Bingham JR, Causey MW, Sebesta JA. Mesenteric irritation as a means to prevent internal hernia formation after laparoscopic gastric bypass surgery. Am J Surg. 2014;207:739–42.
14. Cho M, Pinto D, Carrodeguas L, et al. Frequency and management of internal hernias after laparoscopic antecolic antegastric Roux-en-Y gastric bypass without division of the small bowel mesentery or closure of mesenteric defects: review of 1400 consecutive cases. Surg Obes Relat Dis. 2006;2:87–91.
15. Bauman RW, Pirrello JR. Internal hernia at Petersen's space after laparoscopic Roux-en-Y gastric bypass: 6.2% incidence without closure – a single surgeon series of 1047 cases. Surg Obes Relat Dis. 2009;5:565–70.
16. Sjöström CD. Surgery as an intervention for obesity. Results from the Swedish obese subjects study. Growth Hormon IGF Res. 2003;13(Suppl A):S22–6.

Preventing Complications

24

Felipe de la Cruz Vigo, José Luis de la Cruz Vigo, Elías Rodríguez Cuéllar, Pilar Gómez Rodríguez, and José María Canga Presa

Introduction

Bariatric surgery has always been considered difficult to do, because of the patients' physical characteristics, and with a high risk of complications that, due to the physiological characteristics of the morbid obese patient, often involve unusual severity. The incorporation of laparoscopy into this discipline has increased its difficulty and, thus, the possibility of complications, especially during the learning curve [1].

Gastric bypass is one of the most complex laparoscopic procedures, with a learning curve of 75 to 150 cases [2–4], though some surgeons think the figure is closer to 500 consecutive cases [5]. In a study conducted among expert laparoscopic surgeons, the major complication rate fell significantly from 13% in the first 75 cases to 3% in the next 75 procedures [4]. In our own experience, the incidence of major complications was 7.3% in the first 150 cases, falling to 2.8% in the next 250 [6]. In any case, laparoscopic gastric bypass today has become an elective approach with a lower mortality 0.22% than open gastric bypass 0.82% (p <0.001), as shown by Rausa et al. [7] in a meta-analysis and meta-regression on 69,494 patients.

Laparoscopic gastric bypass involves significant technical difficulties that can be the cause of different complications: the need to work in both supra- and inframesocolic compartments, the need to carry out digestive anastomoses, and the creation of mesenteric and, sometimes, mesocolic defects. Therefore, the standardization of the technique and its frequent repetition are the most important factors in reducing its risks [1, 5].

Many complications have their origin in inappropriate or incorrect intraoperative manoeuvres as well as in accidents, detected or not, during the intervention. In a study of 26,173 patients receiving laparoscopic gastric bypass surgery by the Swedish Obesity Surgery Registry (SOReg), adverse intraoperative events (AIEs) were, along with the conversion to open surgery, the most determining factors of postoperative complications [1]. The prospective multicentre study of six centres of excellence in bariatric surgery by the Longitudinal Assessment of Bariatric Surgery included 5882 patients, who received surgery between March 2005 and April 2009. The interventions were 1608 adjustable gastric bands (AGB), 3770 laparoscopic gastric bypasses (LGB), and 504 open gastric bypasses (GB). This is a prospective record of data with a protocol defined to indicate adverse intraoperative events. It is probably the first in this category to be published. Collected AIEs

F. de la Cruz Vigo (✉) · E. R. Cuéllar
P. G. Rodríguez
General, Digestive and Transplantation Surgery Department, 12 de Octubre University Hospital, Madrid, Spain

J. L. de la Cruz Vigo · J. M. C. Presa
Laparoscopic Surgery Department, San Francisco Hospital, León, Spain

J. Ettinger et al. (eds.), *Gastric Bypass*, https://doi.org/10.1007/978-3-030-28803-7_24

were wounds to organs (liver, spleen, blood vessels, intestine, and diaphragm), bleeding of over 2 U of transfusion, anastomosis revisions (gastrojejunostomy, jejunojejunostomy), equipment or instrument failure (staplers), and anaesthesia-related events (multiple intubation attempts, maintained hypoxia, maintained arrhythmia, hypoxia, hypotension, or prolonged hypercarbia). AIEs were detected in 3% of AGB, 5.5% of LGB and 7.3% of GB. The major post-operative complication rate was 8.8% in the AIE group and 3.9% if there was no AIE (p <0.001). The multivariable analysis revealed that patients with an AIE had 90% more risk of major complication than those without an AIE [8].

The purpose of this chapter is to describe the problems that can happen during the execution of a laparoscopic gastric bypass and to propose how they can be prevented and/or resolved.

Injuries Caused by Trocar Punctures

The three possible methods for the insertion of the first trocar in the execution of a gastric bypass – creation of pneumoperitoneum with a Veress needle, direct entry with an optical trocar, and open entry with the Hasson technique [9] – must be assessed by studying the injuries caused in this initial phase of the operation.

The injury can affect the great vessels, sometimes with retroperitoneal bleeding without clear exteriorization to the peritoneal cavity. It must be suspected in the face of severe intraoperative hemodynamic instability, especially if it is accompanied by the bulging of the retroperitoneum. It requires a laparotomy and retroperitoneal exploration. In the study of 11,744 LRYGBs by the SOReg and the National Patient Register of 2009–2010, five aortic injuries were recorded, representing a global risk of 0.043% and of 0.091% using an optical trocar, since the five injuries occurred with this kind of trocar [10].

Bowel injuries are not frequent due to their mobility and lubrication, unless there are intraperitoneal adhesions. Nevertheless, a distended stomach caused by insufflation during a difficult intubation can easily be perforated, which can be avoided if the anaesthetist has placed a gastric tube. These injuries are usually resolved with a suture.

Solid organ injuries are more frequent in the liver, more so if there is hepatomegaly; less so in the spleen, especially in patients with splenomegaly; and very rare in the pancreas. Spontaneous haemostasis in the liver is usual, but complex haemostatic manoeuvres may be required in the spleen or pancreas.

Other intra-abdominal structures that can be injured are the greater omentum or the mesentery, but this is usually easily resolved with any of the coagulation instruments or a suture. In 17,446 LRYGBs of the SOReg, from 2012 to 2014, 12 intra-abdominal injuries caused by a trocar (0.07%) were collected. Access was carried out using the Veress technique in 59% (10,338 cases), counting 8 injuries (0.077%), 5 bleedings (3 in the omentum or mesentery and 2 in the liver), and three intra-abdominal organ injuries (2 in the stomach and 1 in the small intestine). In 30% (5187), an optical trocar was used, with 4 events being detected (0.077%), 3 bleedings from the omentum or mesentery and 1 small bowel wound. In the remaining 11% (1921), the Hasson technique was used with no injury or bleeding observed. This study observed a change in preference from the optical trocar to the Veress technique [11].

Though the Veress needle can also injure any intra-abdominal structure, this is usually less serious. Kosuta et al. [12] mention a colon perforation upon inserting the needle into the upper left quadrant. When inserting the Veress needle, the insertion site is particularly important, our preference being the left hypochondrium under the rib cage border in Palmer's point or very close thereto. Using direct entry with a bladed non-optical trocar, Ertugrul et al. [13] report two mesenteric injuries in 39 patients. Using direct entry with a bladed optical trocar, Sabeti et al. [14] collected 4 vascular injuries (0.18%) in 2207 bariatric surgeries that occurred in entries separated from the midline. Using the same system, Bernante et al. [15] had no vascular or visceral injuries in 200 patients. Rosenthal et al. [16], using direct entry with a bladeless optical trocar, had no injuries in 849 LRYGBs.

This kind of complication usually occurs with the first blind puncture, which is why it is obligatory for Veress needles and trocars to be provided with safety mechanisms or be bladeless, threaded or radially expandable [17]; and it is recommended to make the first entry into the left hypochondrium. The use of optical trocars, designed to reduce risk, has provided controversial results [10], with the general precautions adopted in the insertion of any trocar having to be observed, as well as be separated from the umbilical region in the cranial direction and directed towards the left hypochondrium. Another option for entry is the open Hasson technique considered the safest, though there is also a reported case of aortic injury with this trocar [18].

The abdominal wall can also be the cause of post-operative bleeding, sometimes serious, due to any parietal vessel wound that has been occluded during the intervention by the trocar itself (Figs. 24.1 and 24.2). When it is removed, the holes must be carefully looked at inside, to carry out a haemostasis, if necessary. There is no consensus on whether to close such holes or on the option to plug them with prosthetic or haemostatic material [19].

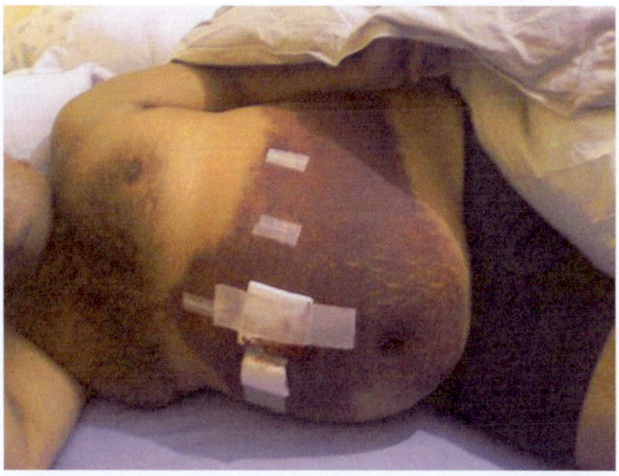

Fig. 24.1 Abdominal wall hematoma originated in the left subcostal trocar puncture

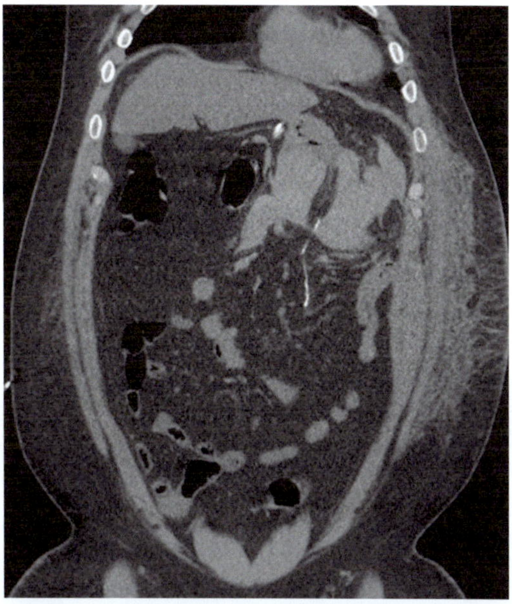

Fig. 24.2 CT scan showing blood infiltration of the abdominal wall by trocar puncture bleeding

Adverse Intraoperative Events

Visceral Injuries

Besides trocar puncture wounds, abdominal structures can be injured during the operation. Digestive injuries can occur at different levels. The hypopharynx and the oesophagus, cervical or cervicothoracic, have been described especially in relation to the oral insertion of the anvil, to carry out a circular-stapler gastrojejunal anastomosis [20]. The distal oesophagus can also be injured in the dissection of a hiatal hernia, especially paraoesophageal, or acting simultaneously with a Heller myotomy, due to coincident achalasia, or in cases of prior hiatal surgery. The stomach is less susceptible to injury since it has a more resistant wall.

An excessive dissection of the oesophagogastric junction or a too tight stapling to the angle of His can give rise to the subsequent appearance of a leak at this level; therefore it is recommended to move away the stapler 1 cm to the greater curvature. A rather inflexible orogas-

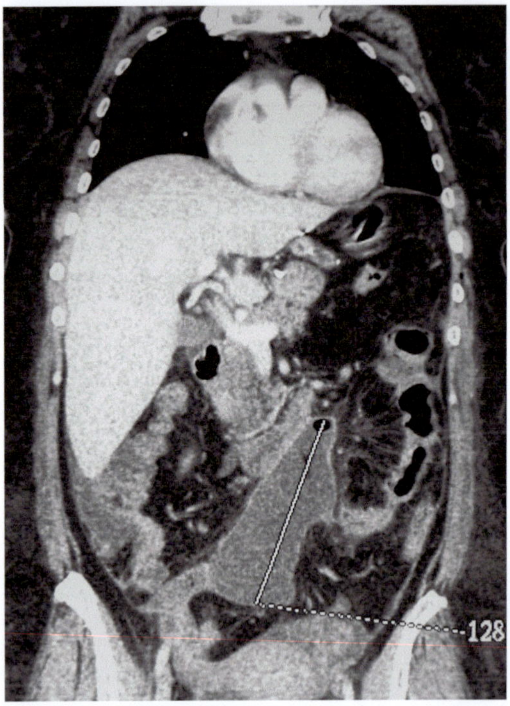

Fig. 24.3 Intermesenteric abscess secondary to bowel instrumental perforation

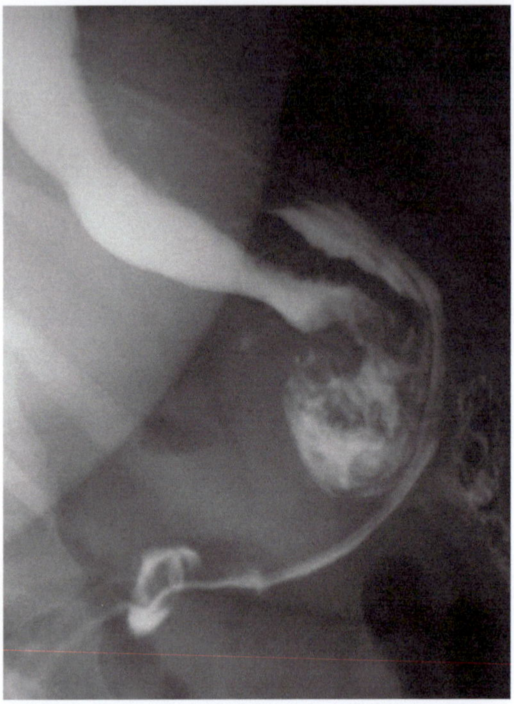

Fig. 24.4 Leak at the gastrojejunal anastomosis, diagnosed by gastrografin swallow and surgically treated 24 hours after surgery. Uneventful recovery

tric tube handled roughly can cause tearing in the gastric reservoir. If the bypass is carried out adding a band or ring, the passing of instruments through the posterior face of the gastric pouch, while placing it, risks perforating or eroding the posterior gastric surface.

The Roux-en-Y jejunojejunal anastomosis does not usually lead to big problems, but roughly grasping the adjacent intestine or using traumatic instruments sometimes causes perforation, which can be immediately detected and repaired or, if not, can appear during the post-operative period as a peritonitis (Fig. 24.3). This eventuality is also possible while measuring the loops, which are more fragile on their mesenteric edge.

Instrument Failure

Technology has made possible the implementation of minimally invasive surgery in obesity surgery but has also created a dependence on instruments that are increasingly complex and specific. The use of mechanical staplers has become universal in laparoscopic procedures and, in the case of laparoscopic gastric bypass, is widespread. Even though stapling instruments, both linear and circular, are very reliable, the frequency of their use and the severity of the consequences of a malfunction are necessary to be prepared for potential failures. The FDA has a voluntary notification system for medical instrument problems, the Manufacturer and User Facility Device Experience (MAUDE), but most incidents are not reported. Nonetheless, bariatric surgeons are those who report more cases of stapler failure.

The true incidence of this problem is not known, but 1.7% [21] rate of malfunction in the use of these devices has been published and up to 45% of cases are associated with morbi-mortality [22]. Sixty-six percent of surgeons mention having had some kind of problem with staplers, and in 25% of cases this led to a change in the initially scheduled surgical procedure. In many cases, it is necessary to change to open surgery to resolve it. There are many problems caused by staplers documented in literature, including stapler block before or after shooting (33%); cutting but partially stapling (16%); faulty staple line (12%); unstapled division (12%); inadequate closure (7%); detachment of the cartridge (7%) [23]; partial or absent cut; damage to nearby tissue during insertion, extraction, or handling of the stapler; perforation or trapping of the tissue in the stapler during fastening; etc.

Early identification of the problem and having the necessary resources and tools to solve it, usually in an intraoperative way, is very important. Failure can be due to a fault in the manufacture of the stapler or its inappropriate use. It is estimated that only 0.3% to 0.003% of cases are due to manufacturing faults; therefore, it is very important for the surgeon to receive appropriate training and to be perfectly familiar with the opening, closure, and shooting mechanisms of the stapler. The personnel responsible for handling and changing the cartridges must also have the necessary knowledge. These devices must always be handled carefully within the abdominal cavity, and their correct positioning must be verified on all their sides, as well as the inclusion of tissue that does not need to be stapled and the absence of foreign bodies (clips, tubes). Examples of incorrect use include not completely removing the blade before opening the stapler, shooting the device when there is something metallic (a haemostatic clip) between the mandibles or using a fired cartridge (the safety block can be broken by applying excessive force). The surgeon must know the resistance and normal touch of the tissue when closing and stapling, so that any abnormality, such as excessive difficulty in shooting, must raise suspicion.

The most frequent problem is that the stapler does not open, before or after shooting. In these cases, provided it is possible, new trocars must be placed, and a stapling done parallel to both sides, extracting the tissue trapped by the blocked machine. In stapling vascular structures or in anatomical places where there are limited segments for handling, such as the creation of the gastric reservoir in LRYGB, the solution is more complex. In vascular structures the vessel must be clamped and haemostatic clips and sutures be used as recourse. In the case of the gastric pouch, the edges must be sectioned, manual sutures be done, reinforcement be added, or, if possible, a new stapling be done. In these cases, a high risk of leak has been described.

With today's staplers, mechanized or not, the possibility of the actual device failing has radically decreased. This was not uncommon with the first prototypes, with Higa et al. [24] reporting this problem in 6 (1.5%) of his first 400 patients. In our first 400 cases, we saw stapler failure in 5 patients (1.2%), 2 in the gastrojejunostomy, 2 in the reservoir, and 1 in the jejunojejunostomy. Everyone was resolved with manual laparoscopic suture, with one case, in the gastrojejunostomy, developing a leak [6] (Fig. 24.4).

Bleeding

The incidence of intraoperative bleeding is hard to assess, since on many occasions they are not reflected in the intraoperative incidence record. Perhaps the most reliable study is the one by the Longitudinal Assessment of Bariatric Surgery database, collected prospectively and aimed specifically at detecting AIEs. Most intraoperative bleeding comes from organ injury, the next cause being instrument failure (0.9%), responsible not only for bleeding but also for the revision of anastomoses [8].

The incidence of bleeding after laparoscopic gastric bypass fluctuates between 0.6% and 4.4% [25–28]. There is a series of factors that can increase the risk of bleeding, such as cirrhosis of the liver, hepatosplenomegaly, undetected coagulation factor deficiencies, prior abdominal surgery [27], super obesity, certain drugs and anticoagulation [29].

Bleeding is a significant complication that not only increases morbidity (by 35%) or the hospital stay (in 87% of patients) [27] but can also cause mortality (7.1% in those who bled compared with 0.9% in those who did not) [30]. Patients can bleed out of the gastrointestinal tract, to the peritoneal cavity, extraluminal bleeding, or to the digestive tube lumen, intraluminal bleeding.

Extraluminal Bleeding

Solid Organs

In the Longitudinal Assessement of Bariatric Surgery (LABS) [8], the incidence of visceral injuries in the laparoscopic gastric bypass (LGB) group is 1.9% (intestine 1.2%, liver 0.4%, spleen 0.2%, vessels 0.1%). In the open gastric bypass (GB) group, the incidence of organ injury is 2% (intestine 1%, spleen 0.6%, liver 0.2%, vessels 0.2%).

Solid organs most often injured are the liver and the spleen. The liver can be lacerated by the hepatic retractor or other instrument, more easily if it suffers steatosis and/or hepatomegaly. The subsequent bleeding makes seeing difficult, but it is usually self-restricting or ceases with compression. The spleen can be decapsulated when retracting an adherent omentum or be perforated by an instrument or by the stapler while constructing the reservoir. The spleen injury can be more difficult to control and usually requires the use of hemostatic substances and more rarely a partial or total splenectomy.

Undoubtedly, the incidence of splenectomy in open gastric bypass is greater than when it is carried out using laparoscopy, reaching figures as high as 4.9% (34 splenectomies in 700 interventions) [31]. In Podnos et al. [32] meta-analysis, the incidence of iatrogenic injury of the spleen was 0.4% in open gastric bypass compared with 0% when the intervention was carried out using laparoscopy. It has been indicated that the pressure exerted by the pneumoperitoneum can have a certain haemostatic effect [33].

Visceral and solid organ injuries must be prevented by carefully handling the tissue, using the appropriate instruments, better reusable than disposable, that must be handled within view of both the surgeon and the assistant and revising the grasping zones. Any injury to the digestive tract that makes us wonder about its evolution must be repaired with a suture.

Staple Line Bleeding

One of the potential sites of intraperitoneal bleeding includes the various staple lines.

Nonetheless, the selection of the staple height in accordance with the tissue in which it is used is still very important, generally 2.5 mm for the small intestine and 3.5 mm for the stomach [20]. In the event of conversions from another technique, it is necessary to use higher staples, such as 3.8 mm or 4.2 mm. The staple lines must be revised after each shot and when completing the intervention, since rebleeding after an initial haemostasis is not uncommon, especially in the gastric remnant. To achieve the haemostasis, we use clips, since we do not advocate monopolar or bipolar coagulation due to their thermal effect that may encourage disruption of the stapling. In the case of the gastric remnant, it is occasionally necessary to use a running absorbable suture. In the gastric reservoir, we systematically use this kind of suture, not only with haemostatic character but also to prevent the appearance of leaks in the post-operative period. Sajid et al. [34] meta-analysis, on the reinforcement of the staple line, does not find that it is better at controlling bleeding, though it does reduce the number of haemostatic clips used and reduces the incidence of leaks and post-operative complications. In Heneghan et al. [27] study, 33% of early post-operative intra-abdominal bleedings were related to the staple line, 30% at the gastrojejunostomy, 40% at the gastric remnant, and 30% at the jejunojejunostomy.

Intraluminal Bleeding

The most frequent cause of intraluminal bleeding is the actual staple line of anastomoses, both gastrojejunal and jejunojejunal, which must always be inspected and haemostasized, if applicable. We use clips in both. There are surgeons who use intraoperative endoscopy both for the diagnosis and to achieve the haemostasis with epinephrine, sclerosing substances or endoscopic clips [35]. In the circular suture, direct inspection is not feasible, since a higher incidence of bleeding complications has been described with this kind of suture. Steffen et al. [36] reported 7 post-operative bleedings in 76 patients (9.2%), achieving the endoscopic haemostasis in them all. The 2 cm devascularization of the lesser curvature and of the posterior face of the reservoir is a manoeuvre we carry out systemically in our linear anastomosis, which has also been indicated as effective in preventing bleeding in circular stapling [36]. In a study that compared the rate of post-operative complications in gastric bypass with mechanical linear anastomosis, when the neurovascular bundle in the lesser gastric curvature was sectioned, there was post-operative bleeding in 12 out of 407 (2.7%), compared with 5 out of 366 (1.4%) when the perigastric dissection was carried out with the preservation thereof [37].

Most intraoperative bleeding will be definitively resolved during surgery, but some will cause complications in the immediate post-operative period.

The Gastric Pouch

Preservation of the Neurovascular Axis

The pouch formation is one of the most demanding parts in Roux-en-Y gastric bypass surgery. We, as well as other surgeons, try to preserve the integrity of the neurovascular axis, which includes the anterior and posterior branches of the vagus nerve of Latarjet, though this step entails greater technical difficulty, especially in men and patients with a high body mass index (BMI), in whom the perigastric dissection in the lesser curvature is difficult, and with a risk of bleeding or even perforation. However, other surgeons believe that the division of this neurovascular axis, in addition to facilitating the surgery, has no adverse consequences for the patient.

Perathoner et al. [38] study 47 patients with laparoscopic gastric bypass split into Group 1 ($n = 25$) with vagal nerve preservation and Group 2 ($n = 22$) with vagal nerve section. They evaluate clinical, functional (oesophageal transit, endoscopy, pH-metry and manometry) and laboratory (ghrelin and gastrin) parameters. No significant differences are found in weight loss, overall satisfaction, feeling of hunger or satiety, dumping and ghrelin or gastrin levels. He concludes that the section of the vagal trunks facilitates the formation of the gastric pouch without having adverse effects.

Frantzides et al. [39] study 108 patients split into two groups, with transection of the lesser omentum ($n = 48$) and with preservation of the lesser omentum ($n = 64$). Two years after the laparoscopic Roux-en-Y gastric bypass, they were given a questionnaire with 17 symptoms, 11 of which were more frequent in the transection group ($p < 0.05$). The interpretation is that the symptoms in this group, above all dumping, are due to a vagotomy when sectioning the fibres contained in the lesser omentum. The recommendation is to change to the preservation of the vagal axis, if a large incidence of dumping symptoms occurs in patients with transection of the lesser omentum.

Van Wezenbeek et al. [37], studying the theory that, in humans, the vagal block reduces ghrelin levels, thereby increasing satiety, reducing food ingestion and promoting greater weight loss, analyse 773 consecutive patients with laparoscopic gastric bypass in two groups, with transection of the neurovascular axis (NBT, $n = 407$) and with preservation of the neurovascular axis (NBP, $n = 366$). The operating time of the two groups was, respectively, 67.7 minutes and 60 minutes ($p = 0.001$). 81.2% of the patients had 1 year's follow-up, and 49 patients (6.3%) developed complications (NBT 8.8% vs NBP 3.6%, $p = 0.003$). The incidence of complications varied according to the group, NBT or NBP, and also according to the type of event: fistula (3.3% vs 1.4%, $p = 0.09$), bleeding (2.7% vs 1.4%, $p = 0.19$), or intra-abdominal abscess (4.4% vs 1.6%, $p = 0.026$). However, weight loss did not increase in the transection group.

The authors have systematically carried out the preservation of the neurovascular axis since the start of their experience with open gastric bypass in 1998 and then since starting laparoscopic gastric bypass in 1999.

Trapping of the Gastric Tube

Complications relating to the nasogastric or orogastric tube, calibration bougie or temperature sensors are rare, but in the case of bariatric surgery and specifically LRYGB, they are complications to be feared and occasionally hard to resolve. Between 1.2% and 5% of tube-related complications [40, 41] in patients receiving LRYGB interventions has been published.

The most important thing about these complications is that they can be prevented by limiting the use of tubes, in number and time, not simultaneously using more than one tube and, when using the orogastric calibration tube, making sure that the anaesthetist removes it or moves it, if a stapling or anastomosis is going to be carried out. Communication between the surgeon and the anaesthesiologist is, therefore, very important to limit the use of tubes in the stomach; their correct movement, provided it is necessary; and the performance of a leak test to confirm the watertightness of the sutures. Some authors recommend an intraoperative endoscopy to avoid the use of calibration bougies [42].

In LRYGB, tube-related complications occur when the gastric pouch is created or, more frequently, when the gastrojejunal anastomosis is carried out. In general, they are detected during the operation, and up to 22% [43] require conversion to open surgery. The tube can be stapled or sutured during the anastomosis or reinforcement stitches. The surgeon must discover this complication intraoperatively. He must be able to detect, through the touch of the stapler, any anomaly (use of excessive force, resistance to the stapling, difficulty in closing the device, bleeding or deformity in the staple line, etc.). If they are handsewn sutures, resistance to the passage of the needle may indicate, though not always, the suture of the tube.

If the tube is stapled, it is necessary to dissect and release it with the subsequent resection of the stapled area. If it is an anastomosis, it is advisable to redo it completely. A high fistula incidence when defects created to remove the tube are sutured has been published. The rate of postoperative fistulas (17.6%) and general complications (29%) are higher after these repairs [44]. If the gastric reservoir is too small, it may be necessary to carry out an oesophageal-jejunal anastomosis. Attempts to manually or mechanically resuture the anastomosis usually achieve worse results. Drains must be left, it being advisable to place a nasojejunal feeding tube through the gastrojejunal anastomosis or a gastrostomy feeding tube in the remaining stomach as well as prolong post-operative fasting.

Gastrojejunal Anastomosis

There is no consensus in the bariatric surgery field on the best way to carry out gastrojejunal (GJ) anastomosis in the laparoscopic gastric bypass. Generally, a narrow anastomosis is constructed, which can favour the appearance of stenosis. Calibration procedures, with or without bougies, are usually used to avoid this complication.

The handsewn anastomosis, proposed by Higa et al. [24], is the most technically difficult to master, and it has the longest learning curve. In this kind of anastomosis, non-absorbable sutures can lead to the appearance of an ulcer, in addition to the development of a bezoar. The two-layer suture has a greater risk of ischemia, in addition to the narrowing due to the invagination it produces. The running suture, by being tied with tension, if it is not done on a tube that calibrates the anastomosis, can reduce its perimeter [43]. Vasquez et al. [44] mention fewer complications from gastrojejunal anastomosis in their series of 315 gastric bypasses, if the reinforcement suture used on the circular 25 mm stapling is done with absorbable thread. Ruiz de Adana et al. [45], in his prospective cohort study of 242 LGB with manual anastomosis, obtains 9.5% stenosis in the gastrojejunal anastomosis with absorbable braided suture group and 0.7% in the group done with absorbable monofilament thread.

The technique of the circular-stapler anastomosis was originally proposed by Wittgrove et al. [46], using the orogastric technique. The size of the anvil conditions a certain anastomotic opening; therefore, the circular 21 mm stapler provides an internal opening diameter of 11.8 mm, while the 25 mm stapler gives an internal diameter of 15.3 mm [47]. Several studies have shown a high risk of stenosis when the 21 mm stapler was used [43, 48, 49]. In Suggs et al. [50] study of 438 patients, those LRYGB carried out with a 25 mm stapler had 2.9% stenosis, compared with 9.4% with a 21 mm stapler. Fischer et al. [51], in a prospective randomized blind study of 200 patients, comparing both diameters, find 17% stenosis with 21 mm and 7% with 25 mm. Baccaro et al. [52], in another study of 639 patients, find that the rate of stenosis is 7.12% with the 21 mm stapler, compared with 1.09% with the 25 mm stapler ($p < 0.0004$). The analysis of 5 studies and 1217 patients (393 with a circular 21 mm stapler and 824 with a 25 mm one) shows a significant increase in stenosis with the 21 mm stapler ($p = 0.0001$) [53]. However, Frutos et al. [54], in 676 LRYGB with the 21 mm stapler anastomosis, obtain 3.4% stenosis.

The linear-stapled anastomosis technique, popularized by Williams and Champion [55] and by Schauer et al. [56], requires the manual suturing of the enterotomy. In a meta-analysis of 7 comparative or randomized studies that brought together 808 patients, the rate of stenosis in the linear-stapled anastomosis fluctuated between 0% and 10%, with an average of 4.6% [57]. In a retrospective study on 1291 patients with linear-stapled anastomosis, stenosis was recorded in 7.3% [58]. The orientation of the handsewn closure of the enterotomy is very important; it can be done lengthwise, stomach with stomach and jejunum with jejunum, or crosswise, stomach with jejunum. In a study [59] on 197 patients, 97 with lengthwise closure and the rest with crosswise closure, the rate of stenosis of the anastomosis was 16%, compared with 0%, respectively (p <0.0001). Our own experience [60, 61], in 1271 banded gastric bypass with linear-stapled gastrojejunal anastomosis and crosswise closure technique of the enterotomy with monofilament absorbable suture, the stenosis rate was 2.3%.

Stenosis of the Gastrojejunal Anastomosis

The definition of stenosis of GJ anastomosis is variable, the most accepted being that the 9.8 mm endoscopy cannot be inserted through the stoma [62, 63].

The incidence of stenosis of the GJ anastomosis after laparoscopic gastric bypass fluctuates between 0% and 26.8% [49, 60, 63–65]. Among other considerations, the learning curve is also important; therefore, in our first 100 cases, with linear-stapled anastomosis and handsewn suture of the enterotomy opening, the incidence of stenosis was 9% [61], falling to 2.3% in the next 1271 cases [60].

Different technical factors can cause or facilitate the appearance of stenosis in gastrojejunal anastomosis, such as the type of suture, manual, absorbable or non-absorbable, one-layer or two-layer, mechanical circular or linear stapler, the tension in the anastomosis, its irrigation, the use of the antecolic or retrocolic route for the Roux-en-Y loop [66], a marginal ulcer [48, 67], a submucosal hematoma that evolves into ischemic cicatricial fibrosis [68], the scarring of an anastomotic fistula [69], endoscopic hemostatic scleroses and their possible retraction [43, 64], etc.

There are different studies that compare the three primary methods of performing gastrojejunostomy, the main purpose being the rate of stenosis:

- *Manual* vs *circular-stapled suture*. Abellan et al. [70] prospective randomized study of 238 patients comparing handsewn suture vs circular-stapled suture finds that there was no difference in the rate of stenosis.
- *Manual* vs *linear-stapled suture*. Awad et al. [63] compare the results of two surgeons trained in bariatric surgery with 366 patients (linear suture = 144 and manual suture = 222). The rate of stenosis that required dilatation was 7.7% in the manual suture vs 0% in the linear suture (p <0.001).
- *Linear-stapled* vs *circular-stapled suture*. Data from 8 studies and 1321 patients is analysed by Giordano et al. [71]. There is a significant difference in favour of linear anastomosis in terms of a lower rate of stenosis. In another study from a single centre, in 55 patients the rate of stenosis of gastrojejunal anastomosis was 14.7% with a circular 21 mm stapler versus 3.2% with a linear stapler ($p = 0.001$) [60].

- *Manual* vs *circular-stapled* vs *linear-stapled suture*. In Lee et al. study [72] of 426 patients (manual = 174, circular-stapled = 110 and linear-stapled = 142), there were no significant differences in the incidence of stenosis among the three techniques, though the linear suture was the one that required a lesser number of post-operative dilatations. In Jiang et al. [73] recent meta-analysis which includes 13,626 patients (manual = 3.309, circular-stapled = 6791 and linear-stapled = 3526), there were no differences as for the risk of stenosis (manual vs circular-stapled: OR, 1.80; 95% CI, 0.66–4.87; $p = 0.67$ and manual vs linear stapled: OR, 1.23; 95% CI, 0.62–2.44; $p = 0.56$).

In those studies, in which there were significant differences regarding the incidence of stenosis, this was not the case about weight loss in the short-medium term; that is, more stenosis does not lead to greater weight loss.

Anastomotic stenosis responds well to endoscopic dilatations, albeit with a certain risk of perforation [74]. With 6% stenosis, 61 out of 1012 patients reported by Ukleja et al. [75] received 128 dilatations which in all of them resolved the issue. Though three showed radiological perforation criteria, they were not confirmed in the laparoscopic exploration and were resolved with drainage, antibiotics and gut rest, with no further complications.

The Jejunal Loop

Error in the Measurement of the Loop

Though in proximal gastric bypass, which is the most often used, a certain margin of variability in the length of the alimentary loop is not particularly significant, which is why it is usually approximately calculated. However, in the distal gastric bypass, the common loop must be scrupulously measured, for which the most suitable thing is to use clamps marked at a known distance.

Roux-en-O Configuration

The anastomosis, in error, of the biliopancreatic loop to the gastric reservoir involves the formation of a "Roux-en-O", a closed circuit that, if it occurs unnoticed during the operation, causes gastric distension and bilious vomiting and can produce a dehiscence of the anastomosis. When it is diagnosed, the gastrojejunal anastomosis must be undone and redone correctly. Shermann et al. [76] advise using a short biliopancreatic loop, identifying the ligament of Treitz and creating the Roux-en-Y immediately after sectioning the jejunum. Our preference is to start with the jejunojejunal anastomosis of the Roux-en-Y, always keeping the end of the biliopancreatic loop held with a clamp from the time of the transection, during the measurement of the alimentary loop and until the anastomosis is completed.

Position of the Alimentary Loop

Internal hernia is the most frequent late complication, which can reach 16% [77]. Most of the authors start, in the late 1990s, by carrying out laparoscopic gastric bypass with the Roux-en-Y loop passed through the retrocolic route [3, 6, 25, 78–81]. With this technique, most internal hernias are caused in the mesocolic window through which the loop passes [6, 79, 80] (Figs. 24.5 and 24.6). In our own experience, in the first 276 retrocolic laparoscopic gastric bypass cases, we had an internal hernia incidence of 1.8% ($n = 5$), 4 of which occurred in the mesocolic breach. Changing the position of the Roux-en-Y loop from retrocolic to antecolic, the internal hernia incidence fell from 4% to 0.5% [74] and from 7% to 2% [73], respectively. Since then, most bariatric surgeons switched to this technique (Fig. 24.7). Steele et al. [82] report 2.6% of internal hernias in retrocolic and none in antecolic, closing all defects in both ways.

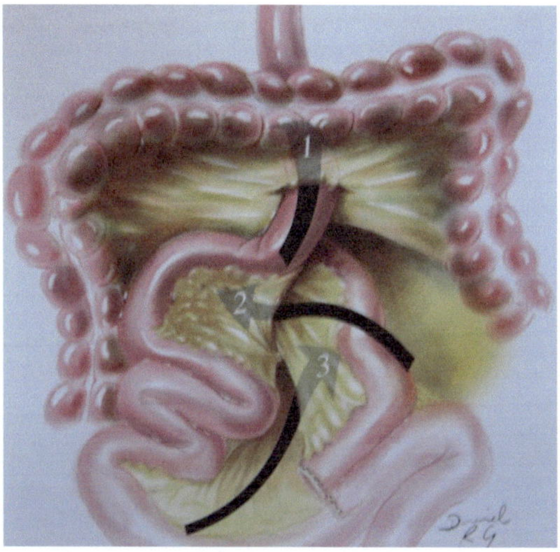

Fig. 24.5 Internal hernia sites. (1) Mesocolic defect. (2) Petersen's space. (3) Mesenteric defect

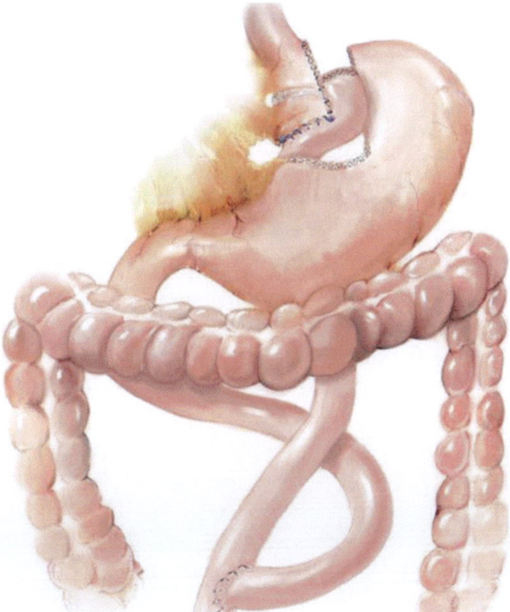

Fig. 24.6 Authors' first banded LRYGB technique. Retrocolic and retrogastric

Kinking of the Loop

This eventuality is more likely if the retrocolic-retrogastric route is used to lift the alimentary loop towards the reservoir, since it is hidden behind the stomach. One safety manoeuvre is to open a window onto the gastrocolic omentum to

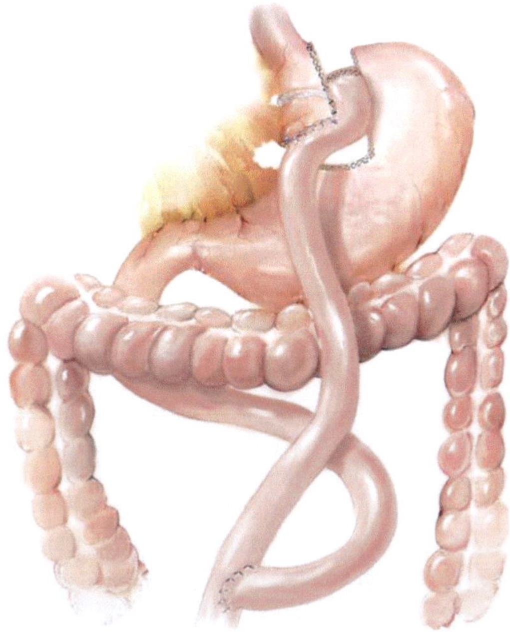

Fig. 24.7 Authors' current banded LRYGB technique. Antecolic and antegastric

display its position before carrying out the gastrojejunal anastomosis. In the antecolic-antegastric route, this kinking is very rare, since the loop is always visible. If the passage or vascularization of the loop is compromised, it will be necessary to redo the anastomosis with the loop in the correct position. If not, it is not strictly necessary.

Mesenteric defect closure manoeuvres, in addition to preventing the formation of internal hernias, can show the unnoticed incorrect position of the loop.

Orientation of the Antecolic Roux-en-Y Loop

In addition to the upward route and the suture of the mesenteric defects as the most determining factors in the reduction in the number of internal hernias, there are others that have not been sufficiently studied. Quebbemann et al. [83], in 2005, indicate that the orientation of the distal tip of the antecolic alimentary loop, in the gastrojejunal anastomosis, notably affects the internal hernia incidence in laparoscopic gastric bypass

(Fig. 24.8). They analyse two consecutive series of 200 patients each: A (distal tip of the loop towards the lesser curvature) and B (opposite orientation). An internal hernia occurred in 9% of Group A compared with 0.5% in Group B. Follow-up was 2.1 and 1.6 years, respectively. A more recent study [82] insists on the significance of the orientation of the Roux-en-Y loop, but with a different result, since in its 86 cases with the end cut of the Roux-en-Y towards the lesser curvature, only 1 internal hernia was detected.

Nandipati et al. [84] publish the comparative results from 444 antecolic laparoscopic gastric bypass patients, split into two groups: Group 1 with 291 patients with a clockwise rotation of the Roux-en-Y loop (Fig. 24.9) and Group 2 with 151 patients with an anti-clockwise rotation (Fig. 24.9). The global internal hernia incidence is 6.9% and 0.6%, respectively. Eighty-one percent of hernias occur in Petersen's space, and there continue to be differences for this location among Groups 1 and 2 (5.5% vs 0.6%, $p = 0.0089$). There is still a significant difference between Groups 1 and 2 when Petersen's space closed (Group 1, 4/54 (7%); Group 2, 0/63 (0%) ($p = 0.043$)) and a difference, albeit insignifi-

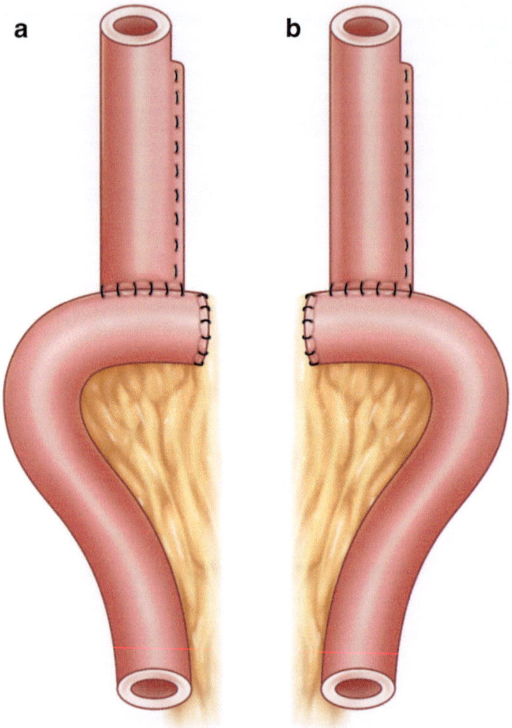

Fig. 24.8 (a) Tip of the alimentary limb oriented opposite to the lesser curvature. (b) Tip of the alimentary limb oriented to the lesser curvature

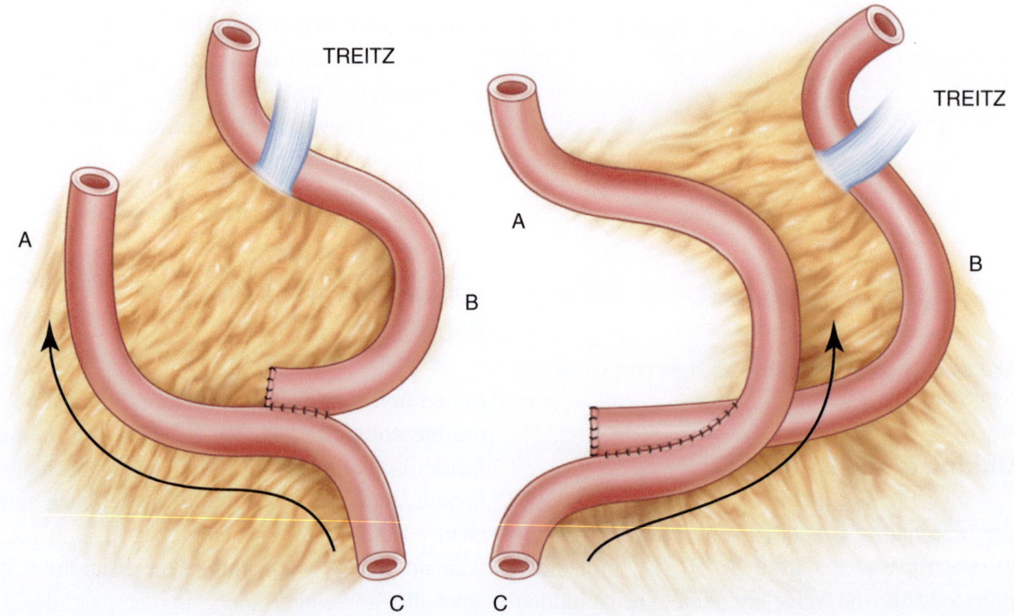

Fig. 24.9 Position of the alimentary limb at the jejunojejunostomy. (Left) Anti-clockwise. (Right) Clockwise. A: Alimentary limb. B: Biliopancreatic limb. C: Common limb

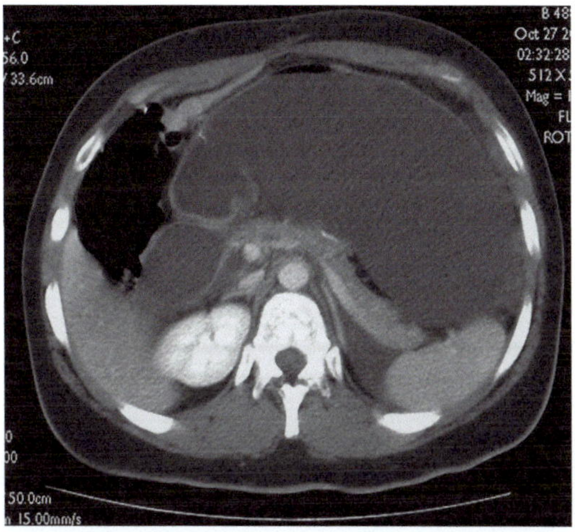

Fig. 24.10 CT scan showing gastric dilation by acute post-operative obstruction secondary to Petersen's internal hernia

cant, when this was not sutured: 12/237 (5.1%) vs 1/88 (1.1%) (p = 0.12). According to the authors, this is probably due to the scant number of patients in this subgroup. The conclusion is that the construction of the antecolic Roux-en-Y loop with an anti-clockwise rotation of the bowel, in such a way that both the jejunojejunal anastomosis and the ligament of Treitz are to the left of the axis of the mesentery, significantly reduces the internal hernia incidence, regarding the clockwise rotation of the intestine.

From the beginning of our experience, we have used the anti-clockwise orientation and the closure of the mesenteric defect with an internal hernia rate, in the antecolic laparoscopic gastric bypass of 1% (14/1479) and with a minimal follow-up of 30 months. In the first 777 patients, Petersen's space was not closed, and the internal hernia incidence was 1.8% (14/777) (Fig. 24.10), while in the remaining 702, in whom it was closed with a continuous non-reabsorbable suture, there was no internal hernia (0/702) (p = 0.0003) (Cruz Vigo JL&F, 2017, unpublished data).

Jejunojejunostomy

In the laparoscopic Roux-Y gastric bypass technique, whether it be retrocolic or antecolic, a jejunojejunostomy can be carried out prior to creating the gastric pouch, after having constructed it or after the gastrojejunal anastomosis has been performed. Most surgeons use for this anastomosis a 45 mm or 60 mm linear stapling device. The closure of the enterotomy can also be done with a linear stapler or with a handsewn running suture. When this closing suture is done with the linear stapler, the suture is orientated crosswise with regard to the jejunojejunal staple line, with different incidences with this technique having been described, both in open and laparoscopic Roux-Y-gastric bypass. Brolin et al. [85] describe obstruction in the jejunojejunostomy in 3 out of 393 cases (0.76%), caused by folding from the distal loop to the anastomosis on itself at the level of said cross stapling, and describe an "anti-obstructive" stitch to avoid it. Hwang et al. [78] publish stenosis or kinking of the anastomosis in 4 and 9 cases, respectively (0.76%, 13/1715), with closure of the enterotomy using a linear stapler and 2 or 3 "anti-obstruction" stitches. In 12 out of the 13 cases, the obstruction was diagnosed in the first 3 weeks, with reoperation being necessary in the great majority.

Problems with jejunojejunal anastomoses seem to be largely due to technical matters, and, in that respect, we think that the technique described by Lönroth et al. [86] increases the difficulties and risks of this anastomosis. Briefly, the technique consists in creating an antecolic-antegastric omega loop gastrojejunal anastomosis. The jejunojejunal anastomosis is performed afterwards in the supramesocolic compartment, sometimes involving considerable difficulties. Finally, the omega loop is transformed into a Roux-en-Y loop by transecting the biliopancreatic loop next to the gastrojejunal anastomosis. In the Lönroth series published on 150 patients, one early obstruction was detected in the jejunojejunal anastomosis, which required reoperation, and another patient died on the third day from acute gastric dilatation and perforation of the gastric remnant, due to biliopancreatic limb obstruction secondary to stenosis at the level of the jejunojeunal anastomosis.

Stenberg et al. study [87] is the largest randomized study published on the closure of mesenteric defects in laparoscopic Roux-en-Y gastric bypass with the Lönroth technique [86]. Twelve centres in Sweden participated, gathering 2507 patients split up into two groups, one with closure of mesenteric defects (mesentery and Petersen's space) and the other without closure, with a 2-year follow-up in 99.8% of patients. It was concluded that, after 3 years, the closure of mesenteric defects with a running, braided, non-absorbable suture significantly reduces the need for late reoperation (after 30 days) due to intestinal obstruction, whose most frequent cause (68%) is internal hernia, with a significantly different incidence between both procedures (2.1% with closure of defects vs 7.1% without closure of defects). However, the number of early major complications within 30 days of surgery, according to the Clavien-Dindo classification, was 4% when mesenteric defects were closed compared with 3%, when they were not (p = 0.027). The most frequent cause of intestinal obstruction in the early postoperative period was kinking and stenosis of the jejunojejunostomy with 16 cases, when the defect was closed, compared with 3 cases of which it was not. As a possible explanation, it is indicated that, though all the surgeons were experts in laparoscopic gastric bypass, it was not with respect to mesenteric defects closure and this could cause unfavourable consequences due to the learning curve.

In the authors' experience of over 2000 jejunojejunal anastomoses carried out in the inframesocolic compartment, with closure of the insertion hole with handsewn running monofilament absorbable suture orientated lengthwise, in the same direction as the staple line not crosswise thereto, there was no obstruction, kinking, stenosis or other complication, neither early (<30 days) nor late (>30 days), in this jejunojejunal anastomosis. In no case was anti-obstruction stitch used.

In summary, close attention to technical details and laparoscopic surgical manoeuvres, using delicate and precise surgical instruments, besides surgeon's experience and skillfulness, based on a tutorized learning, are the best preventive measures of LRYGB post-operative complications.

Disclosure The authors declare that they have no conflicts of interest concerning this chapter.

References

1. Stenberg E, Szabo E, Agren G, et al. Early complications after laparoscopic gastric bypass surgery: results from the Scandinavian Obesity Surgery Registry. Ann Surg. 2014;260(6):1040–7.
2. Shin RB. Evaluation of the learning curve for laparoscopic Roux-en-Y gastric bypass surgery. Surg Obes Relat Dis. 2005;1:91–4.
3. Schauer P, Ikramuddin S, Hamad G, et al. The learning curve for laparoscopic Roux-en-Y gastric bypass is 100 cases. Surg Endosc. 2003;17:212–5.
4. Oliak D, Ballantyne GH, Weber P, et al. Laparoscopic Roux-en-Y gastric bypass. defining the learning curve Surg Endosc. 2003;17:405–8.
5. El-Kadre L, Tinoco AC, Tinoco RC, et al. Overcoming the learning curve of laparoscopic Roux-en-Y gastric bypass: a 12-year experience. Surg Obes Relat Dis. 2013;9(6):867–72.
6. Cruz Vigo JL, Cruz Vigo F, Sanz de la Morena P, Canga Presa JM. By-pass gastrique "bandé" par laparoscopie. Technique et résultats des 400 premiers cas. Le Jour de Celio-chir. 2004;50:26–36.
7. Rausa E, Bonavina L, Asti E, et al. Rate of death and complications in laparoscopic and open Roux-en-Y gastric bypass. A meta-analysis and meta-regression analysis on 69,494 patients. Obes Surg. 2016;26(8):1956–63.
8. Greenstein AJ, Wahed AS, Adenji A. Prevalence of adverse intraoperative events during obesity surgery and their sequelae. J Am Coll Surg. 2012;215(2):271–7.
9. Kassir R, Blanc P, Lointier P, et al. Laparoscopic entry techniques in obese patient: Veress needle, direct trocar insertion or open entry technique? Obes Surg. 2014;24:2193–4.
10. Sundbom M, Hedberg J, Wanhainen A, et al. Aortic injuries during laparoscopic gastric bypass for morbid obesity in Sweden 2009–2010: a nationwide survey. Surg Obes Relat Dis. 2014;10(2):203–7.
11. Sundbom M, Ottosson J. Trocar injuries in 17.446 laparoscopic gastric bypass – a nationwide survey from the Scandinavian Obesity Surgery Registry. Obes Surg. 2016;26:2127–30.
12. Kosuta M, Palmisano S, Piccinni G, et al. Safety of Veress needle insertion in laparoscopic bariatric surgery. Surg Laparosc Endosc Percutan Tech. 2014;24(1):e1–4.
13. Ertugrul I, Kayaalp C, Yagci MA, et al. Comparison of direct trocar entry and Veress needle entry in laparoscopic bariatric surgery: randomized controlled trial. J Laparoendosc Adv Surg Tech A. 2015;25(11): 875–9.
14. Sabeti N, Tarnoff M, Kim J, et al. Primary midline peritoneal access with optical trocar is safe and

effective in morbidly obese patients. Surg Obes Relat Dis. 2009;5(5):610–4.
15. Bernante P, Foletto M, Toniato A. Creation of pneumoperitoneum using a bladed optical trocar in morbidly obese patients: technique and results. Obes Surg. 2008;18(8):1043–6.
16. Rosenthal RJ, Szomstein S, Kennedy CI, et al. Direct visual insertion of primary trocar and avoidance of fascial closure with laparoscopic Roux-en-Y gastric bypass. Surg Endosc. 2007;21(1):124–8.
17. Johnson WH, Fecher AM, McMahon RL, et al. VersaStep trocar hernia rate in unclosed fascial defects in bariatric patients. Surg Endosc. 2006;20(10):1584–6.
18. Pring CM. Aortic injury using the Hasson trocar: a case report and review of the literature. Ann R Coll Surg Engl. 2007;89(2):W3–5.
19. Moreno-Egea A. How to prevent trocar-site hernia? A totally atraumatic endoscopic mini-IPOM-plug technique (with extra-lightweight titanium-coated mesh and glue). Surg Laparosc Endosc Percutan Tech. 2015;25(3):106–8.
20. Nguyen NT, Wolfe BM. Hypopharyngeal perforation during laparoscopic Roux-en-Y gastric bypass. Obes Surg. 2000;10:64–7.
21. Chan D, Bishoff JT, Ratner L, et al. Endovascular gastrointestinal stapler device malfunction during laparoscopic nephrectomy: early recognition and management. J Urol. 2000;164:319–21.
22. Deng DY, Meng MV, Nguyen HT, et al. Laparoscopic linear cutting stapler failure. Urology. 2002;60(3):415–9; discussion 419–20
23. Kwazneski D, Six C, Stahlfeld K. The unacknowledged incidence of laparoscopic stapler malfunction. Surg Endosc. 2013;27:86.
24. Higa K, Boone K, Ho T. Laparoscopic Roux-en-Y gastric bypass for morbid obesity: technique and preliminary results of our first 400 patients. Arch Surg. 2000;135:1029–33.
25. Nguyen NT, Rivers R, Wolfe BM. Early gastrointestinal haemorrhage after laparoscopic gastric bypass. Obes Surg. 2003;13:62–5.
26. Higa KD, Boone KB, Ho T. Complications of the laparoscopic Roux-en-Y gastric bypass: 1,040 patients what have we learned? Obes Surg. 2000;10(6):509–13.
27. Heneghan HM, Meron-Eldar S, Yenumula P, et al. Incidence and management of bleeding complications after gastric bypass surgery in the morbidly obese. Surg Obes Relat Dis. 2012;8(6):729–35.
28. Mehran A, Szomstein S, Zundel N, et al. Management of acute bleeding after laparoscopic Roux-en-Y gastric bypass. Obes Surg. 2003;13:842–7.
29. Mourelo R, Kaidar-Person O, Fajnwaks P, et al. Haemorrhagic and thromboembolic complications after bariatric surgery in patients receiving chronic anticoagulation therapy. Obes Surg. 2008;18(2):167–70.
30. Dick A, Byrne TK, Baker M, et al. Gastrointestinal bleeding after gastric bypass surgery: nuisance or catastrophe? Surg Obes Relat Dis. 2010;6(6):643–7.
31. Murphy K, McCracken JD, Ozment KL. Gastric bypass for obesity. Am J Surg. 1980;140:747–50.
32. Podnos YD, Jimenez JC, Wilson SE, et al. Complications after laparoscopic gastric bypass. Arch Surg. 2003;138:957–61.
33. Papp A, Vereczkei LJ, et al. The effect of different levels of peritoneal CO_2 pressure on bleeding time of spleen capsule injury. Surg Endosc. 2003;17:1125–8.
34. Sajid MS, Khatri K, Singh K, et al. Use of staple-line reinforcement in laparoscopic gastric bypass surgery: a meta-analysis. Surg Endosc. 2011;25(9):2884–91.
35. Madan AK, Martinez JM, Lo Menzo E, et al. Omental reinforcement for intraoperative leak repairs during laparoscopic Roux-en-Y gastric bypass. Am Surg. 2009;75:839–42.
36. Steffen R. Early gastrointestinal haemorrhage after laparoscopic gastric bypass. Obes Surg. 2003;13:466–7.
37. Van Wezenbeek MR, Van Oudheusden TR, Smulders JF, et al. Transection versus preservation of the neurovascular bundle of the lesser omentum in primary Roux-en-Y gastric bypass surgery. Surg Obes Relat Dis. 2016;12:283–9.
38. Perathoner A, Weiss H, Santner W, et al. Vagal nerve dissection during pouch formation in laparoscopic Roux-Y-gastric bypass for technical simplification: does it matter? Obes Surg. 2009;19:412–7.
39. Frantzides CT, Carlson MA, Shostrom VK, et al. A survey of dumping symptomatology after gastric bypass with or without lesser omental transection. Obes Surg. 2011;21:186–93.
40. Sanchez BS, Safadi BY, Kieran JA, et al. Orogastric tube complications in laparoscopic Roux-en-Y gastric bypass. Obes Surg. 2006;16(4):443–7.
41. Abu-Gazala S, Donchin Y, Keidar A. Nasogastric tube, temperature probe, and bougie stapling during bariatric surgery: a multicenter survey. Surg Obes Relat Dis. 2012;8(5):595–600; discussion 600–1
42. Higa G, Szomstein S, Rosenthal R. Stapling of orogastric tube during gastrojejunal anastomosis: an unusual complication after conversion of sleeve gastrectomy to laparoscopic Roux-en-Y gastric bypass. Surg Obes Relat Dis. 2012;8(1):116–8.
43. Campillo-Soto A, Torralba-Martínez JA, Martín-Lorenzo JG, et al. Gastrojejunal anastomosis stricture after laparoscopic gastric bypass. Our experience with 62 patients. Rev Esp Enferm Dig. 2010;102:187–92.
44. Vasquez JC, Wayne Overby D, Farrell TM. Fewer gastrojejunostomy strictures and marginal ulcers with absorbable suture. Surg Endosc. 2009;23:2011–5.
45. Ruiz de Adana JC, Hernández Matías A, Hernández Bartolomé M, et al. Risk of gastrojejunal anastomotic stricture with multifilament an monofilament sutures after hand-sewn laparoscopic gastric bypass: a prospective cohort study. Obes Surg. 2009;19:1274–7.

46. Wittgrove AC, Clark GW. Combined laparoscopic/endoscopic anvil placement for the performance of the gastroenterostomy. Obes Surg. 2001;11(5):565–9.
47. Himpens JM. The gastrojejunostomy in laparoscopic Roux-en-Y gastric bypass. Semin Laparosc Surg. 2004;11(3):171–7.
48. Gonzalez R, Lin E, Venkatesh KR, et al. Gastrojejunostomy during laparoscopic gastric bypass: analysis of 3 techniques. Arch Surg. 2003;138:181–4.
49. Nguyen NT, Stevens CM, Wolfe BM. Incidence and outcome of anastomotic stricture after laparoscopic gastric bypass. J Gastrointest Surg. 2003;7(8):997–1003.
50. Suggs WJ, Kouli W, Lupovici M, et al. Complications at gastrojejunostomy after laparoscopic Roux-en-Y gastric bypass: comparison between 21- and 25-mm circular staplers. Surg Obes Relat Dis. 2007;3:508–14.
51. Fischer BL, Atkinson JD, Cottam D. Incidence of gastroenterostomy stenosis in laparoscopic Roux-en-Y gastric bypass using 21- or 25-mm circular stapler: a randomized prospective blinded study. Surg Obes Relat Dis. 2007;3:176–9.
52. Baccaro LM, Vunnamadala K, Sakharpe A, et al. Stricture rate after laparoscopic Roux-en-Y gastric bypass with a 21-mm circular stapler versus a 25-mm linear stapler. Bariatr Surg Pract Patient Care. 2015;10:33–7.
53. Markar SR, Penna M, Venkat-Ramen V, et al. Influence of circular stapler diameter on postoperative stenosis after laparoscopic gastrojejunal anastomosis in morbid obesity. Surg Obes Relat Dis. 2012;8:230–5.
54. Frutos MD, Luján J, García A, et al. Gastrojejunal anastomotic stenosis in laparoscopic gastric bypass with a circular stapler (21 mm): incidence, treatment and long term follow-up. Obes Surg. 2009;19:1631–5.
55. Williams MD, Champion JK. Linear technique of laparoscopic Roux-en-Y gastric bypass. Surg Technol Int. 2004;13:101–5.
56. Schauer PR, Ikramuddin S, Hamad G, et al. Laparoscopic gastric bypass surgery: current technique. J Laparoendosc Adv Surg Tech A. 2003;13:229–39.
57. Penna M, Markar SR, Venkat-raman V, et al. Linear-stapled versus circular-stapled laparoscopic gastrojejunal anastomosis in morbid obesity: meta-analysis. Surg Laparosc Endosc Percutan Tech. 2012;22:95–101.
58. Carrodeguas L, Szomstein S, Zundel N, et al. Gastrojejunal anastomotic strictures following laparoscopic Roux-en-Y gastric by- pass surgery: analysis of 1291 patients. Surg Obes Relat Dis. 2006;2:92–7.
59. Mueller CL, Jackson TD, Swanson T, et al. Linear-stapled Gastrojejunostomy with transverse hand-sewn enterotomy closure significantly reduces strictures for laparoscopic Roux-en-Y gastric bypass. Obes Surg. 2013;23:1302–8.
60. de-la-Cruz-Vigo F, de-la-Cruz-Vigo JL. Stenosis in gastric bypass for morbid obesity. Rev Esp Enferm Dig. 2010;102:151–8.
61. Cruz Vigo F, Cruz Vigo JL. La obesidad: problema del siglo XXI. En: Cruz Vigo F, Cruz Vigo JL, editores. Bypass gástrico por laparoscopia. Cáceres: Centro de Cirugía de Mínima Invasión; 2005. pp. 21–33.
62. Yimcharoen P, Heneghan H, Chand B, et al. Successful management of gastrojejunal strictures after gastric bypass: is timing important? Surg Obes Relat Dis. 2012;8:151–7.
63. Awad S, Aguilo R, Agrawal S, et al. Outcomes of linear-stapled versus hand-sewn gastrojejunal anastomosis in laparoscopic Roux en-Y gastric bypass. Surg Endosc. 2015;29:2278–83.
64. Espinel J, De-la-Cruz JL, Pinedo E, et al. Stenosis in laparoscopic gastric bypass: management by endoscopic dilation without fluoroscopic guidance. Rev Esp Enferm Dig. 2011;103:508–10.
65. Caro L, Sanchez C, Rodriguez P, Bosch J. Endoscopic balloon dilation of anastomotic strictures occurring after laparoscopic gastric bypass for morbid obesity. Dig Dis. 2008;26:314–7.
66. Ribeiro-Parenti L, Arapis K, Chosidow D, et al. Gastrojejunostomy stricture rate: comparison between antecolic and retrocolic laparoscopic Roux-en-Y gastric bypass. Surg Obes Relat Dis. 2015;11:1076–84.
67. Cruz Vigo JL, Cruz Vigo F, Sanz de la Morena P, et al. Consideraciones técnicas para minimizar las complicaciones. Cir Esp. 2004;75:292–8.
68. De Moura EG, Orso IR, Aurélio EF, et al. Factors associated with complications or failure of endoscopic balloon dilation of anastomotic stricture secondary to Roux-en-Y gastric bypass surgery. Surg Obes Relat Dis. 2016;12(3):582–6.
69. Campos JM, Ferreira Filho HA, Galvao Neto MP, et al. Estenosis de la anastomosis gastroyeyunal. En: Campos JM, Galvao Neto MP, Moura EGH, editores. Endoscopia en cirugía de la obesidad. Caracas: Amolca; 2009. pp. 215–227.
70. Abellán I, López V, Lujan J, et al. Stapling versus hand suture for gastroenteric anastomosis in Roux-en-Y gastric bypass: a randomized clinical trial. Obes Surg. 2015;25:1796–801.
71. Giordano S, Salminen P, Biancari F, et al. Linear stapler technique may be safer than circular in gastrojejunal anastomosis for laparoscopic Roux-en-Y gastric bypass: a meta-analysis of comparative studies. Obes Surg. 2011;21:1958–64.
72. Lee S, Davies AR, Bahal S, et al. Comparison of gastrojejunal anastomosis techniques in laparoscopic Roux-en-Y gastric bypass: gastrojejunal stricture rate and effect on subsequent weight loss. Obes Surg. 2014;24:1425–9.
73. Jiang HP, Lin LL, Jiang X, et al. Meta-analysis of hand-sewn versus mechanical gastrojejunal anastomosis during laparoscopic Roux-en-Y gastric bypass for morbid obesity. Int J Surg. 2016;32:150–7.
74. Espinel J, Pinedo E. Stenosis in gastric bypass: endoscopic management. World J Gastrointest Endosc. 2012;4:290–5.

75. Ukleja A, Afonso BB, Pimentel R, et al. Outcome of endoscopic balloon dilation of strictures after laparoscopic gastric bypass. Surg Endosc. 2008;22(8):1746–50.
76. Sherman V, Dan AG, Lord JM, et al. Complications of gastric bypass: avoiding the Roux-en-O configuration. Obes Surg. 2009;19(8):1190–4.
77. Higa K, Ho T, Tercero F, et al. Laparoscopic Roux-en-Y gastric bypass. 10 years' follow-up. Surg Obes Relat Dis. 2011;7:516–25.
78. Hwang RF, Swartz DE, Felix EL. Causes of small bowel obstruction after laparoscopic gastric bypass. Surg Endosc. 2004;18:1631–5.
79. Champion JK, Williams M. Small bowel obstruction and internal hernias after laparoscopic Roux-en-Y gastric bypass. Obs Surg. 2003;13:596–600.
80. Higa KD, Ho T, Boone KB. Internal hernias after laparoscopic Roux-en-Y gastric bypass: incidence, treatment and prevention. Obes Surg. 2003;13:350–4.
81. Wittgrove AC, Endres JE, Davis M, et al. Perioperative complications in a single surgeon's experience with 1000 consecutive laparoscopic Roux-en-Y gastric bypass operations for morbid obesity. Obes Surg 2002;12:457–8(abst L4).
82. Steele KE, Prokopowicz GP, Magnuson T, et al. Laparoscopic antecolic Roux-en-Y gastric bypass with closure of internal defects leads to fewer internal hernias than the retrocolic approach. Surg Endosc. 2008;22(9):2056–61.
83. Quebbemann BB, Dallal RM. The orientation of the antecolic Roux limb markedly affects the incidence of internal hernias after laparoscopic gastric bypass. Obes Surg. 2005;15:766–70.
84. Nandipati KC, Lin E, Husain F, et al. Counter clockwise rotation of Roux-en-Y limb significantly reduces internal herniation in laparoscopic Roux-en-Y gastric bypass (LRYGB). J Gastrointest Surg. 2012;16:675–81.
85. Brolin RE. The antiobstruction stitch in stapled Roux-en-Y enteroenterostomy. Am J Surg. 1995;169:355–7.
86. Olbers T, Lonroth H, Fagevik-Olsen M, et al. Laparoscopic gastric bypass: development of technique, respiratory function, and long-term outcome. Obes Surg. 2003;13:364–70.
87. Stenberg E, Szabo E, Ågren G, et al. Closure of mesenteric defects in laparoscopic gastric bypass: a multicentre, randomised, parallel, open-label trial. Lancet. 2016;387:1397–404.

Laparoscopic Gastric Bypass: Tricks and Tips

25

Fábio Almeida, Juliana Moura, and Antonio Alves Jr.

Purpose

The objective of this chapter is to demonstrate and review the main steps for the accomplishment of laparoscopic gastric bypass surgery to allow for standardization, reproducibility, and performance with fewer difficulties and complications.

Introduction

The laparoscopic gastric bypass is currently one of the most frequently used procedures in metabolic and bariatric surgery [5, 6, 8, 12–14, 16, 17]. The laparoscopic approach to this procedure was initially published by Allan Wittgrove, followed by Gagner, Schauer, and others [5, 6, 9]. It was quickly accepted by the bariatric community, recognized as being a safe and feasible technique, with high efficacy and low morbidity and mortality [17, 18, 22]. To assure the safety of the procedure, adequate training and the use of specific materials for better performance are imperative [7, 10].

This chapter presents the technical aspects of the operation and ways to facilitate its implementation. Several factors, such as appropriate surgical preparation, anesthesia, patient positioning, surgical team, appropriate materials, trocar positions, and standardization of the surgical steps, are critical to the safety of the procedure [1, 10].

The most common variables are addressed here: types of anastomoses [5, 9–11], better access to the upper mesocolic, anastomosis size [9], and the technical details of the anastomosis [2–5, 10]. The intent is make this procedure as safe as possible.

The robotic and single port approach can be used, but should be considered only if the benefits to the patient are clear enough to justify the higher costs and increased operative time.

Adequate Preoperative Preparation

In addition to adequate clinical, nutritional, and psychological preparation, the anesthetic protocol (see specific chapters) must be evaluated.

One of the most important factors is weight loss by the patient, which should occur during the period of preoperative preparation [19]. The loss of 5–10% of the initial body weight provides improved lung and cardiac reserve during surgery and postoperative recovery [17]. Furthermore, this approach optimizes the surgery, because it is specifically related to loss of intraabdominal fat mass and a consequent reduction in liver size and mesenteric fat. Thus, access to the retrogastric cavity is less demanding and there is a clear reduction of tension in the gastrojejunal anastomosis.

F. Almeida (✉) · J. Moura · A. Alves Jr.
SIGO – Serviço Integrado de Gastroenterologia e Obesidade and Unit of Bariatric Surgery of University Hospital of Universidade Federal de Sergipe, Aracaju, Sergipe, Brazil

J. Ettinger et al. (eds.), *Gastric Bypass*, https://doi.org/10.1007/978-3-030-28803-7_25

Surgical Room Checklist

Safe Surgery

Check the clinical protocol to be adopted, which must always be strictly followed, to ensure that it includes all items of the checklist for safe surgery: identification of allergy and bleeding history; control of the patient's body and room temperature; recognition by all staff of the type of surgery to be performed; adequate materials and the patient's examination results are available in the surgical suite; and prevention of infection and thromboembolic events. Hypothermia can be prevented by using a thermal blanket and heated infusion liquids. The verification of blood glucose before, during, and after surgery may be particularly important for obese patients with insulin resistance or those who are already suffering from diabetes. Antibiotic prophylaxis must include the use of antibiotics immediately before and during the course of surgery only. There is no consensus in the literature on when, where, and for how long thromboembolism prevention should be continued. Our group routinely administers enoxaparin at 40 mg per day, beginning the day before surgery and continuing for 10 days, associated with mechanical prevention measures such as the use of progressive compression leg stockings (not pneumatic) and early ambulation.

Equipment and Instruments

Special attention must be given to the choice of equipment and instruments for working with obese patients. A proper automatic and wider surgical table allows generous inclination and good fixation of the patient. Suitable laparoscopy devices include cameras, preferably high-definition, and a high-flow insufflator. Appropriate surgical instruments include graspers for the digestive tract, needle holders of appropriate size for each surgical step, and available intestinal clamps; staplers with the appropriate cartridge for each tissue being operated; access trocars; and above all, with well-trained staff.

Staff Position

The position of the table and the surgical staff should be as familiar as possible with laparoscopic procedures in the gastric esophageal transition. We choose to keep the patient in the supine position, slightly inclined; the surgeon and the assistant with the camera are on the right side of the patient, and the monitor, second auxiliary, and scrub nurse are on the left side. If there is only one monitor, place it on the left side of the patient, in a region close to the shoulder. If two monitors are available, the second will be positioned at the height of the right shoulder and within sight of the auxiliary and the scrub nurse. It is very important to position the patient between 15° and 30° of inclination before beginning the incisions and the pneumoperitoneum.

Intraoperative Technical Steps

Access and Trocars

Many surgeons opt, if available, for trocars with direct view of the abdominal cavity. The first access may be done blindly or guided by these instruments. Trocars with a disabled blade or without a blade are widely used, which has been linked to lower rates of bleeding complications. The preparation of the pneumoperitoneum can be made with a Veress needle. Some groups work with direct puncture using disposable trocars, and have not reported complications using this access. The other trocars should always be passed under direct vision. We use five incisions for gastric bypass, one being compatible with the type of stapler to be used. If a 5 mm optical is available, only one trocar greater than 5 mm is required, the one for stapler use, and should be compatible to that use (Fig. 25.1).

TIP 1 Do not perform the first incision with the patient in the horizontal supine position. If the patient is placed in the inclined position before this incision, the surgeon's working angle will be better. If this is the trocar with which staplers will be used, it should be compatible with the type of load to be used (typically 12 mm). Articulated staplers are preferable. The surgery can also be

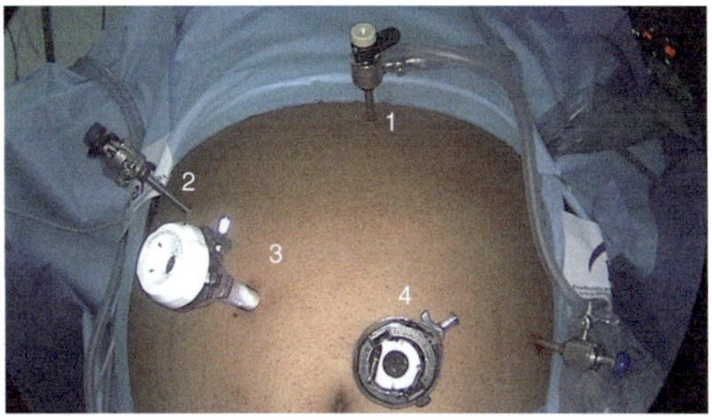

Fig. 25.1 Position of the access trocars. (*1*) Subxyphoid (5 mm) for liver elevator. (*2*) Right hypochondrium (5 mm) for surgeon's left hand. (*3*) Right midclavicular line (10 mm) for optical (if you have 5 mm optics, replace for compatible trocar). (*4*) Medial border of the left abdominal rectal muscle (12 mm) about 20 cm below the xiphoid process trocar for stapler. (*5*) Left midclavicular line trocar (5 mm) to auxiliary

performed with straight staplers, but the steps can become more complex.

TIP 2 Before the first incision, make sure that the anesthesiologist has already passed a nasogastric or orogastric tube for full stomach emptying, sometimes filled with air for a difficult intubation or one that is more time consuming.

With the trocar subxiphoid of 5 mm, it may be a good option to use a grasping clamp that is set on the right arm of the diaphragmatic crus. This maneuver usually does not need any other type of incidental exposure. Some choose to use static retractors; however, we must be absolutely certain that the patient remains in a completely anesthetized state, at risk of extensive liver damage.

TIP 3 In cases of fatty liver with a high level of steatosis, a 10 mm trocar may be used with a clamp of the same size or even two clamps of 5 mm each.

Making the Gastric Pouch

Ask your auxiliary to remove the perisplenic fat and omenta to complete exposure of the gastric esophageal transition safely. Make sure the stomach is completely empty and there is no more intragastric bougie.

Identify the left angle of the gastrophrenic ligament and section with an ultrasound or bipolar scalpel, or similar, to expose the left side of the diaphragmatic crus and perirenal fat. Clean the gastric esophageal transition fat carefully. At this time observe the esophageal hiatus. If there is sign of hernias that might insinuate the pouch into the mediastinum, especially after weight loss, it is appropriate to adjust the esophageal hiatus by performing hiatoplasty.

Ask your helper to position the clamp to expose the small gastric curvature below the hepatic branch of the vagus nerve.

TIP 4 The assistant supports the stomach with a clamp on its anterior wall near the lesser curvature, pushing it up and toward the left.

Identify a remote location 4–6 cm from the cardia and section at least one vessel of the lesser curvature, pulling it with the left-hand clamp in the transverse direction and up. With the right hand, the ultrasonic or advanced bipolar scalpel is used to dissect in the posterior direction to the stomach until the gastric retrocavity. Perform maneuvers gently at this time to avoid lacerations with bleeding (Fig. 25.2). Some surgeons use monopolar energy, but this type of energy can cause electric accidents.

After viewing the free retrogastric space, position the stapler in the transverse direction to the stomach with slight cephalic angulation (Fig. 25.3).

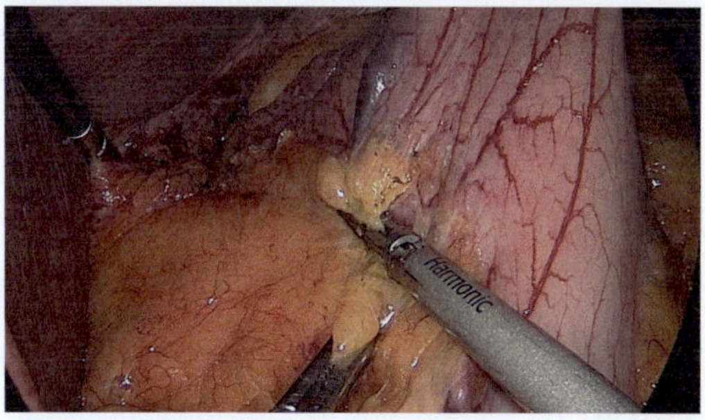

Fig. 25.2 First entry in the small gastric curvature. The auxiliary pulls the stomach laterally. The surgeon gently pulls the vessels of the small curvature with his left hand, and seals and cuts one or two vessels to access the retrogastric cavity

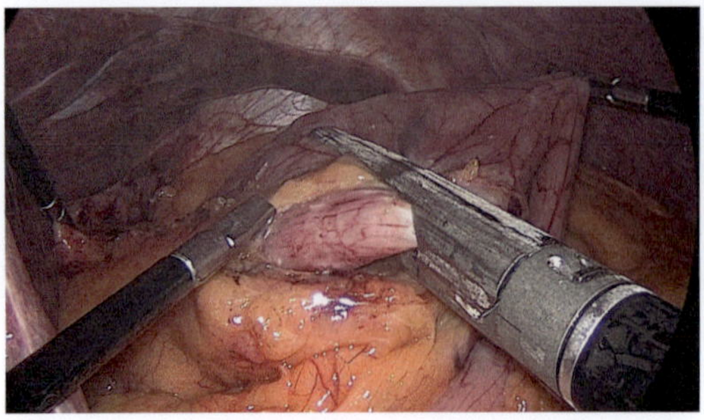

Fig. 25.3 Stapler positioned for first shot. Maintain an angle of approximately 60° in relationship to the dissected small curvature. Use appropriate cartridge. Generally, it is not necessary to articulate the stapler in this position. Observe that the Fouchet is not in the stomach

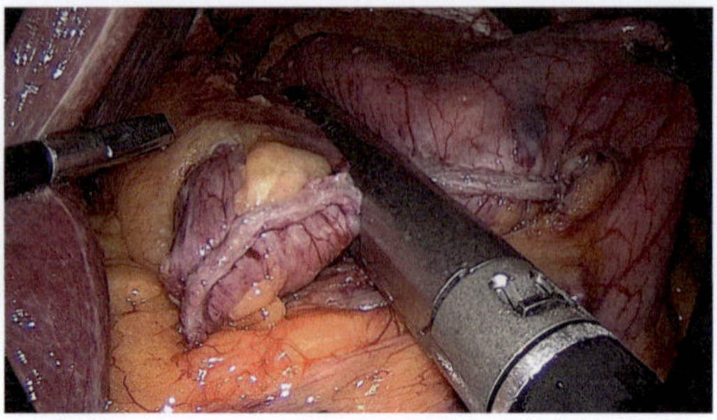

Fig. 25.4 Second stapler firing. If there is possibility of variable size load use, choose 60 mm. Keep the stapler straight, adjusted to the Fouchet 32F or similar. Avoid twisting at this time. Follow up to complete septation

TIP 5 Ensure, with the anesthetist, that there is no intragastric bougie at this time.

TRICK A small cephalic angulation by stapler articulation will create a point at the pouch that will facilitate the introduction and fitting of the Fouchet tube.

With the left hand, firmly pull the right angle of the gastric stapling edge, positioning the stapler, now with a new cartridge (45 or 60 mm), in the cardia region direction. Ask the anesthetist to pass a Fouchet (number 32 or 36). Position the bougie in the lesser curvature, trying to fit it into the tip of the first stapling. Avoid gripping the staple lines. After proper placement of the bougie, ask the anesthesiologist to keep it in place under tension. If possible, partially dissect the left side of the region of the right crus, visualized by the retrogastric face. Place the stapler against the Fouchet tube (thus the Fouchet is the approximate size of the new stomach). Fire the stapler and replace the cartridge (Fig. 25.4).

TIP 6 Request the anesthetist to gently mobilize the bougie to avoid clipping it and make sure it is free.

TRICK Be careful not to kink the pouch. So this does not happen, note the symmetry between the anterior and posterior wall of the pouch. A good reference is to observe the entry of vessels in the gastric wall and keep the tube pressed against the first row of staples.

To complete the gastric section and formation of the pouch, it is possible to dissect with the stapler from the region behind the pouch until there is exposure of the same region of the gastrophrenic ligament dissected at the start of surgery.

TRICK The tip of the stapler often serves as a 'finger' of the surgeon, with gentle maneuvers that allow good blunt dissection at that time.

Angle the stapler slightly to the left of the patient and fire. Make sure there was complete section of the stomach and creation of the small gastric pouch. Review hemostasis. Some groups neither do nor recommend suturing. Because a transfixing hemostatic suture may be made with the new staplers and suture line protection devices, most likely this maneuver will no longer be required.

Intestinal Time and Anastomosis

Reduce the patient's position to 10° cephalic slope. Locate the greater omentum in a less thick spot. Section it with an ultrasonic scalpel or similar device (bipolar with built-in scissors is a good choice) near the transverse colon. The help of the auxiliary clamp is very important at this time (Fig. 25.5).

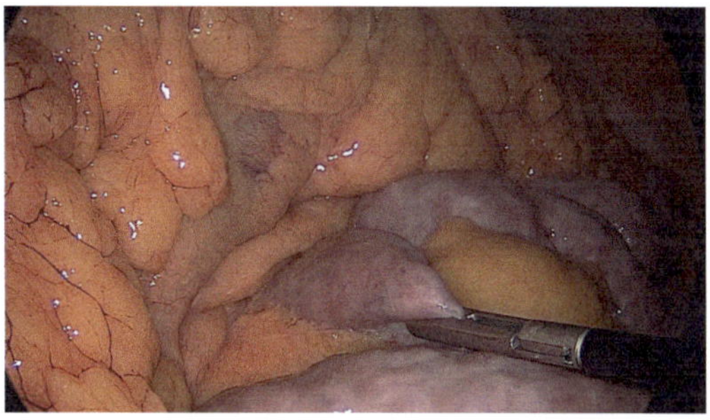

Fig. 25.5 Elevation of transverse mesocolon by the auxiliary, after septation of the greater omentum. Location of Treitz angle. Check fixed jejunum and middle colic artery

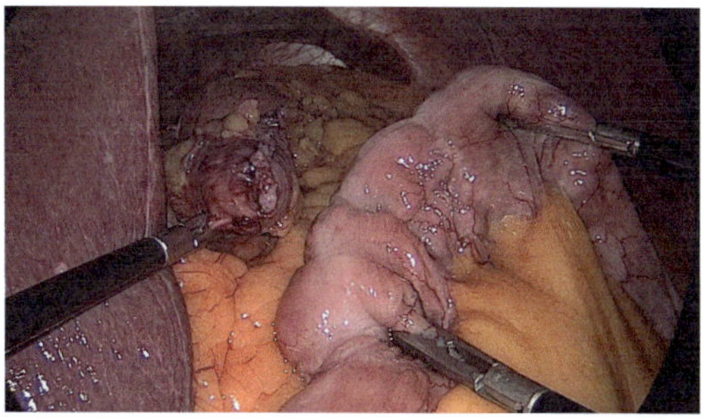

Fig. 25.6 After measuring 1 m biliopancreatic limb to be positioned at the patient's left, keeping an omega limb, analyze if the mesentery is sufficiently loose to perform anastomosis. If necessary, make small adjustments

TIP 7 In general, the spot of better access is more to the left of the patient.

Locate the transverse mesocolon. The same must be fixed with the clamp of the auxiliary to the left of the Treitz angle as near as possible to the transverse colon without grasping the colon and with traction in the superior way and cranially. Identify the Treitz angle to the root of the transverse mesocolon.

TIP 8 To confirm the first jejunal loop and the angle of Treitz, try to identify the ligament and the passage of the mesenteric vein.

From the Treitz angle, measure the jejunal loop to make a excluded limb (called the biliary-pancreatic limb). Measure 1 m using two clamps with marks of 5 or 10 cm, always being sure to leave the excluded limb to the *left* side of the patient. After measuring 1 m, locate a lower tension point and ask the assistant to hold this limb, elevating it to the top position of the abdomen.

TRICK The best way to hold this limb will always be using tweezers, firmly, with the jaws perpendicular to the small intestine.

Place the limb on OMEGA scan through the pre-colic so that it exposes the edge against the mesentery to the surgeon (Fig. 25.6).

Perform with ultrasonic scalpel, mono- or bipolar, a hole in the gastric pouch, on the right side, toward the Fouchet, outside the staple line. Never pierce the line of staples, especially if using monopolar energy. There is risk of power dissipation by parallel staplers, compromising the staple line. It is essential to maintain the bougie on this site.

TIP 9 At the time of completion of the hole in the gastric pouch, ask the anesthesiologist to maintain the Fouchet tube in place with some tension, so it can serve as a support against the pressure of the ultrasonic scalpel in making the hole.

Make a hole also in the jejunal loop supported by the auxiliary. Dilate slightly with a Maryland forceps. Place the stapler with blue load, introducing a 3.0 cm cartridge on the pouch. This maneuver is much easier if instead of pushing the stapler, we choose to pull the gastric pouch gently, rotating the stapler slightly toward its axis. For this technique, the stapler need not be articulated at this time. Use the stapler area that receives the staples for smooth introduction into the neo-gastric pouch, aided by a light draw Fouchet tube, which will serve as a guide for introduction of the stapler in the neo-stomach (Fig. 25.7).

TIP 10 For the introduction of the stapler in the gastric pouch, support the stapler in the Fouchet through the hole previously made and ask the anesthesiologist to retrocede the bougie slowly as the stapler is being introduced.

Double check that the edges of the anastomosis are aligned; avoid misaligned edges of the limb or the gastric pouch. If possible leave the initial staple line between the lines of anastomo-

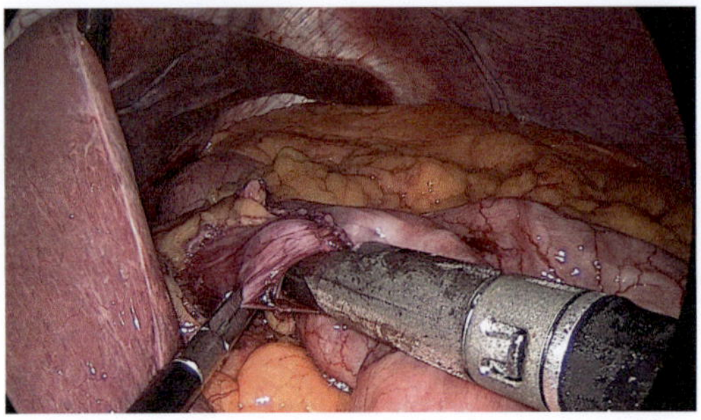

Fig. 25.7 Accomplishment of mechanical terminolateral anastomosis, linear, with 3 cm stapling. Use care to maintain alignment of the stapler jaws. If possible, leave staple line of gastric pouch positioned anteriorly

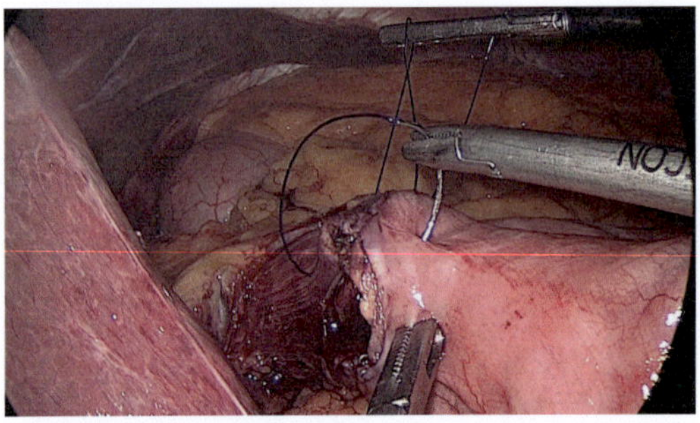

Fig. 25.8 Suture closure of stapling gap. We began on the *left* side angle of anastomosis with continuous transfixing suture, encompassing stomach and jejunum, until end of gap created to insert the stapler. On open gap, use seromuscular extramucosal suture

sis. Fire the stapler. Pass the Fouchet through the anastomosis, leaving it positioned in the alimentary limb to protect the anastomosis from being accidentally occluded in the suture closure of the stapling gap. Make an extramucosal continuously running suture until the gap is completely closed (Fig. 25.8).

TIP 11 Make a stitch with PDS 3-0 in the left angle of the anastomosis and ask the auxiliary to pull in the anterior left direction; this symmetrically exposes the area to be closed, preventing kinks.

Then expose the transverse mesocolon, with the auxiliary's help, and locate the mesentery of the alimentary limb for viewing the Petersen space. Close the space carefully, starting from the base of the transverse mesocolon, laterally to the middle colic artery (Figs. 25.9 and 25.10) [2–4].

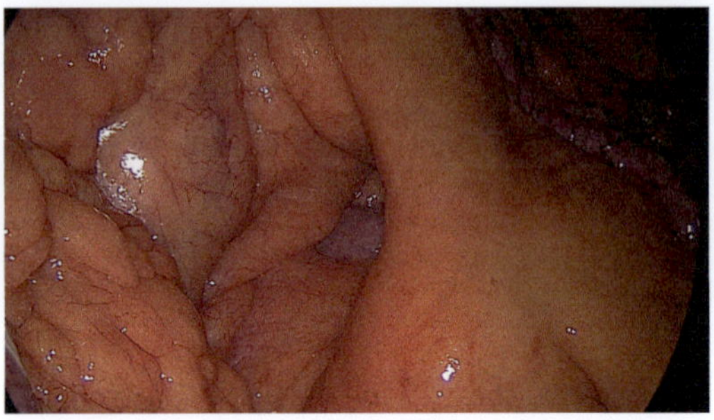

Fig. 25.9 Petersen space exposition. The auxiliary lifts the transverse mesocolon closest to the edge of the colon. Start a continued suture with preformed loop, suturing the transverse mesocolon to the mesentery food limb. Avoid close proximity to the vascular pedicle and avoid leaving small open spaces at this time. Finalize approach of the colon

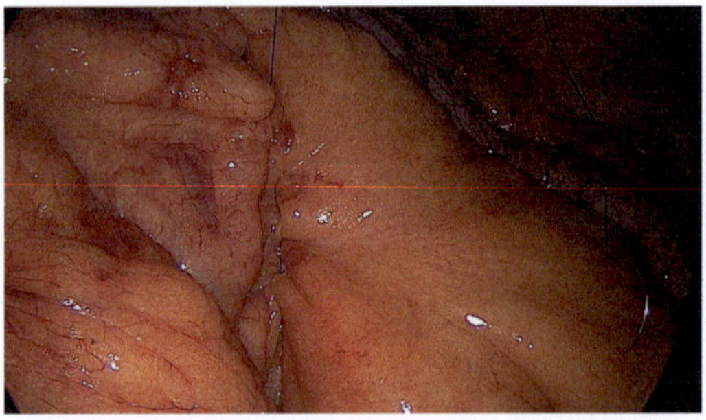

Fig. 25.10 Detail of Petersen space closure

TIP 12 Use a wire with a loop at the end, and pass all the sutures homogeneously without twists. Usually four to five continuous points are sufficient. Either nonabsorbent or slow absorption wire can be used.

Ask your helper to hold the bilio-pancreatic limb. Create a mesenteric gap in the pancreatic-bilio portion of the intestine 1–2 cm apart from the anastomosis that will serve to pass one of the stapler jaws. Use stapling for creation of an excluded loop with 45 mm load (usually white or beige load). At this time, turn the stapler, causing the load (thickest area) to be free, and the stapler receptacle is passed in the bowel in a minimum space, avoiding opening the bowel too much (Fig. 25.11).

In most cases the limb turns easily without the need to expand the mesentery section. Turn the excluded limb in the flow direction, and from that moment, it does not need to be maintained by the auxiliary.

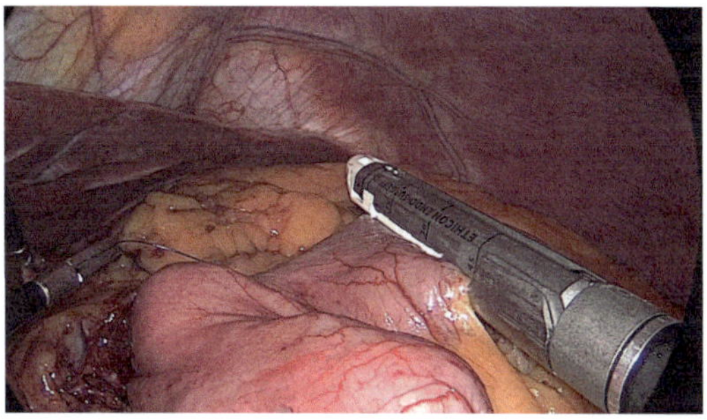

Fig. 25.11 Make small gap in the mesentery of the biliopancreatic loop, which simply allows passage of the stapler. At this time, we chose to use the load anteriorly and the staple receiving jaw posteriorly: this facilitates introduction and viewing of this operative time. Maintain distance of 2 cm from gastrojejunal anastomosis

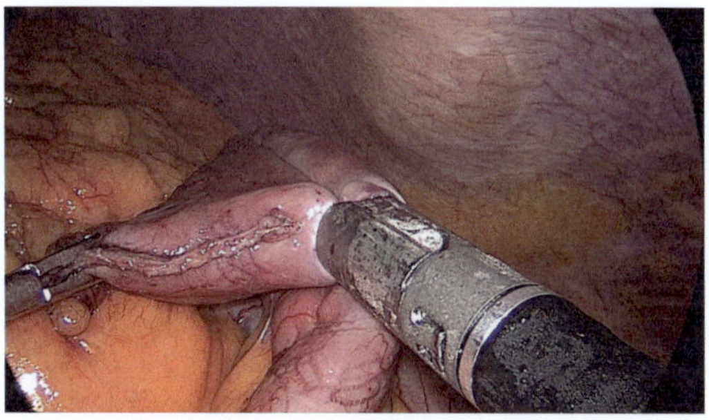

Fig. 25.12 After measuring the alimentary limb with 1.7 m positioned to *left* of patient, we prepared for mechanical anastomosis, antimesenteric, anisoperistaltic. Use stapler of 45 mm or 30 mm if available

Starting from the gastrojejunal anastomosis, measure between 1 and 2.5 m of the jejunum, taking care to place the alimentary limb on the right side of the patient. Fix the site measured with the aid of the clamp holding the alimentary limb [20, 21]. As already described, make a hole in each limb with an ultrasonic scalpel, dilate with Maryland forceps, and introduce a white load of 30 or 45 mm. The cartridge is positioned in the alimentary limb, and the part receiving the staples is excluded. Fire the stapler and review hemostasis (see Fig. 25.12).

Start closing the hole (caused by the passage of the stapler) from the left edge of the hole so that the auxiliary can pull on the thread during closure. Perform an extramucosal running suture with PDS 3-0 (Fig. 25.13).

Keep the auxiliary pulling the edge of the anastomosis to expose the mesenteric defect (Fig. 25.14). Close the defect with continuous suture Ethibond or PDS 2-0. Use care to prevent bleeding in the mesentery as well as twisting of the anastomosis (Fig. 25.15).

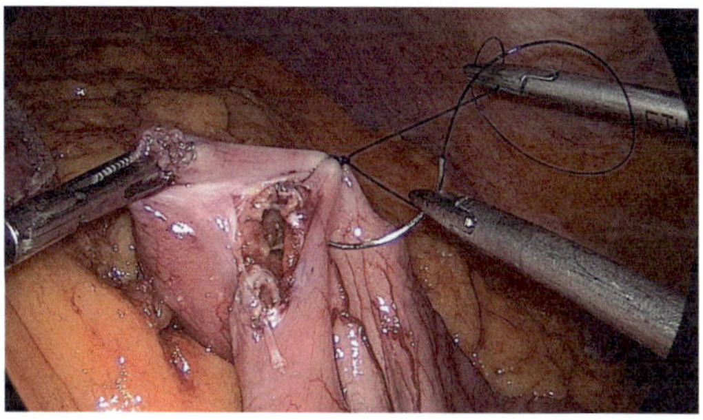

Fig. 25.13 Begin closing stapler gap. Note auxiliary pulling anterocranially to the *left*, exposing the gap. Continue extramucosal seromuscular suture, initiated in default, until complete occlusion of gap

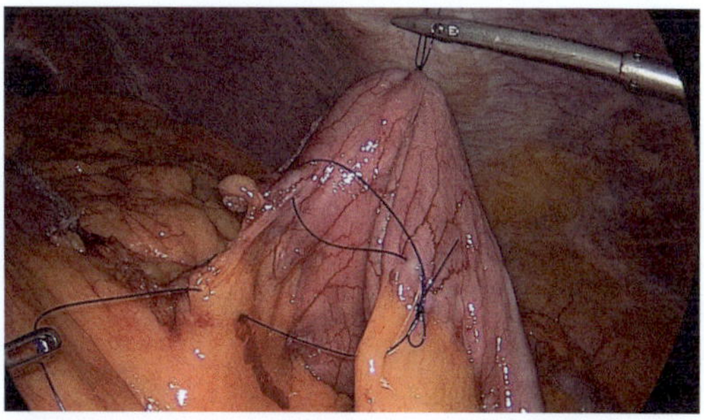

Fig. 25.14 After closing the enteroenterostomal gap, we request that the auxiliary pull on the last thread of the suture for exposure of the mesenteric gap that will be occluded with simple suture, started in serous layer, until complete closure

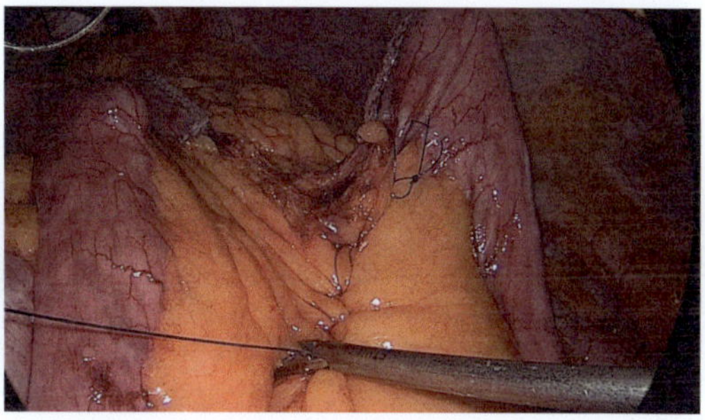

Fig. 25.15 Detail of final closure of mesenteric defect

In the option of manual anastomosis, these procedures may be performed in the same way, always starting from the most distal side in rela-

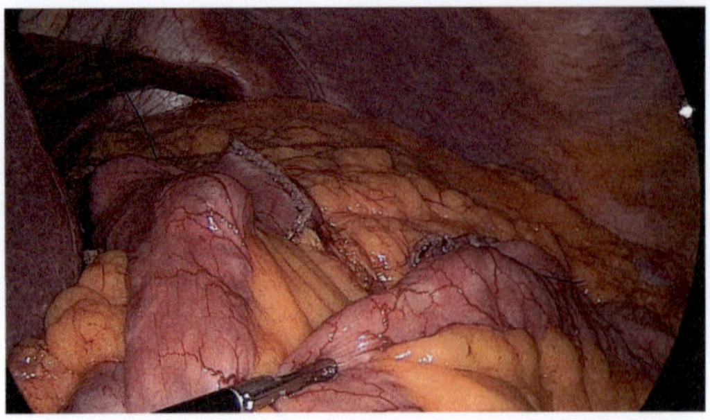

Fig. 25.16 Final aspect of procedure. The two anastomoses are seen with good aspect, accessible, and without twists or angulation

tionship to the surgeon: this is valid for the two anastomoses, gastrojejunal and jejuno-jejunal.

Suture Test and Conclusion of the Procedure

With the use of a clamp to occlude the alimentary limb, introduced by the auxiliary (lower left trocar), at a distance of 20–30 cm from the gastrojejunostomy, reposition the patient slightly.

Introduce saline solution until the pouch and the gastrojejunal anastomosis are submerged. Ask your anesthesiologist to inject air by Fouchet (50–60 ml) and verify that the gastrojejunostomy is airtight and there are no leaks (air leak).This test can be performed with methylene blue; however, there are reports of adverse drug reactions.

Aspirate the saline solution, and review hemostasis. Currently, it is considered unnecessary to use a drain in the cavity, except in special situations (Fig. 25.16; final appearance).

Remove the trocars with special attention to bleeding. Whenever possible, close the trocar insertion sites of 12 mm. When opting to use a 15 mm trocar, closure of the aponeurosis is required.

Postoperative

After extubation by the anesthesiologist, we suggest the patient should remain in the postanesthesia recovery room. Despite some different approaches in current services, we do not indicate intensive routine support therapy for laparoscopic gastric bypass (if there is no complication). Specific cases or possible complications intra- or postoperatively may require hospital care.

Early ambulation should be encouraged. A liquid diet may be introduced between 6 and 12 h after surgery, and the patient may be discharged at 48 h.

References

1. Czeczko LE, Cruz MA, Klostermann FC, Czeczko NG, Nassif PAN, Czeczko AEA. Correlação entre a endoscopia digestive alta pre e pos-operatoria em pacientes submetidos ao bypass gastrojejunal em y-Roux. ABCD Arq Bras Cir Dig. 2016;29(1):33–7.
2. Ahmed AR, Rickards G, Husain S, et al. Tendências na incidência de hérnia interna após laparoscópica Roux-en-Y bypass gástrico. Obes Surg. 2007;17(12):1563–6.
3. Capella RF, Iannace VA, Capella JF. Obstrução interstinal após a cirurgia de bypass gástrico aberta e laparoscópica para a obesidade mórbida. J Am Coll Surg. 2006;203(3):328–35.
4. Schneider C, Cobb W, Scott J, Carbonell A, Myers K, Bour E. Rápida perda de excesso de peso após bypass gástrico laparoscópico leva ao aumento do risco de hérnia interna. Surg Endosc. 2011;25(5):1594–8. https://doi.org/10.1007/s00464-010-1444-9. Epub 12 de novembro de 2010.
5. Wittgrove AC, Facs MD, Clark GW. Laparoscopic gastric bypass, Roux en-Y: 500 patients. Technique and results, with 3–60 month follow-up. Obes Surg. 2000;10:233–9.
6. Wittgrove AC, Clark GW. Laparoscopic gastric bypass, Roux-en-Y: preliminary report of five cases. Obes Surg. 1994;4:353–7.
7. Hamad MD, Giselle G. Operating room setup and instrumentation. In: Inabnet WB, Demaria EJ, Ikramuddin S, editors. Laparoscopic bariatric surgery. Philadephia: Lippincott Williams & Wilkins; 2005. p. 55–60.
8. Miller K. Adjustable gastric banding in the treatment of obesity. In: Weiner RA, editor. Collection on laparoscopic in bariatrics: Moby Dick; 2009. p. 8–19.
9. Wittgrove A. Laparoscopic gastric bypass: circular stapler technique. In: Pitombo C, Jones KB, Higa KD, Paeja JC (e), editors. Obesity surgery: principles and practice. Albany: McGraw-Hill; 2008. p. 189–93.
10. Higa KD, Higa JE. Laparoscopic gastric bypass: hand sewn. In: Pitombo C, Jone KB, Higa KD, Paeja JC, editors. Obesity surgery: principles and practice. Albany: McGraw-Hill; 2008. p. 189–93.
11. Fobi MA. Vertical banded gastroplasty vs. gastric bypass: ten years follow-up. Obes Surg. 1993;3:369.

12. Capella JF, Capella RF. The weight reduction operation of choice: vertical banded gastroplasty or gastric bypass. Am J Surg. 1996;171:74.
13. Capella RF, Capella JF, Mandac H. Vertical banded gastroplasty. Gastric bypass: preliminary report. Obes Surg. 1991;1:389–95.
14. Capella JF, Capella RF. An assessment of vertical banded gastroplasty Roux-en-Y gastric bypass for the treatment of morbid obesity. Am J Surg. 2002;183:117–23.
15. World Health Organization [homepage na internet]. Obesity and overweight. Fact sheet no. 311, Updated January 2015. Disponível em: http://www.who.int/mediacentre/factsheets/fs311/en/.
16. World Health Organization (WHO) World health statistics 2012. Geneva, 2012. [acessado em 2 de setembro de 2016]. Disponível em: http://apps.who.int/iris/bitstream/10665/44844/1/9789241564441_.
17. Consenso Bariátrico. Sociedade Brasileira de Cirurgia Bariátrica e Metabólica. 2008:8–14. [acessado em 04 de setembro de 2016]. Disponível em: http://www.sbcbm.org.br/membros_consenso_bariatrico.php.
18. Westling A, Gustavsson S. Laparoscopic vs. open Roux-en-Y gastric bypass: a prospective, randomized trial. Obes Surg. 2001;11(3):284–92.
19. Costa TMRL, Paganoto M, Radominski RB, Borba VZC. Impacto da deficiência nutricional na massa óssea após cirurgia bariátrica. Arq Bras Cir Dig. 2016;29(1):38–42.
20. Sampaio-Neto J, Branco-Filho AJ, Nassif LS, Nassif AT, Mais FDJ, Ximenez DR. Proposta de cirurgia revisional para o tratamento de hipoglicemia hiperinsulinêmica não insulinomaapós by-pass gástrico. ABCD Arq Bras Cir Dig. 2015;28(4):278–81.
21. Ramos RJ, Mottin CC, Alves LB, Benzano D, Padoin AV. Effect of size of intestinal diversion in obese patients with metabolic syndrome submitted to gastric bypass. ABCD Arq Bras Cir Dig. 2016;29(suppl 1):15–9.
22. Stoll A, Rosin L, Dias MF, Marquiotti B, Gugelmin G, Stoll GF. Early postoperative complications in Roux-en-Y gastric bypass. ABCD Arq Bras Cir Dig. 2016;29(suppl 1):72–4.

Psychiatric Assistance in Bariatric Surgery

26

Adriano Segal and Debora Kinoshita Kussunoki

Introduction

Pinpointing behavioral and psychological/psychiatric predictive factors in bariatric surgery (BS) has been a major concern throughout surgical teams around the world. Despite the extensive research history and considerable amount of data obtained on this particular area, its scientific literature still remains somehow contradictory.

In this chapter, we will provide a brief review of persisting dilemmas in modern BS practice, examining its main controversies and non-consensual points of view. We will also discuss the bias toward psychiatric disorders (PD).

It is very likely that some points discussed in this chapter for bariatric surgeries will prove to be very similar and valid in metabolic surgeries. However, the data on the interface of this form of treatment and the psychiatric area are very scarce.

A. Segal (✉) · D. K. Kussunoki
Obesity and Diabetes Center, German Hospital Oswaldo Cruz, São Paulo, Brazil

Obesity and Metabolic Syndrome Outpatient Clinic, Service of Endocrinology and Metabolism-HCFMUSP/SP, São Paulo, Brazil

Brazilian Society of Bariatric and Metabolic Surgery, São Paulo, Brazil

Brazilian Association for the Study of Obesity and Metabolic Syndrome, São Paulo, Brazil

Segal Clinic, São Paulo, Brazil

Obesity and Prejudice

To the present, obesity is not classified as a PD [1, 2]. However, it is frequently studied from a similar theoretical standpoint, since it shares several of PD's characteristics, such as chronicity, multifactorial etiologies, some common pathophysiological pathways, and a strong and widespread associated social stigma, in addition to being frequently a comorbid situation as will be cited ahead.

Therefore, obese patients with mental disorders are usually subject to twice the discrimination faced by regular psychiatric patients, a fact which often jeopardizes their global treatment.

The prejudice endured by these patients tends to extrapolate their social circle, and it is often present inside healthcare settings. Due to the assumption that there is a low likelihood of success in treatment, several professionals underestimate the obese patient's ability to achieve positive therapeutic results. Assuming those patients as less able to be properly treated, the healthcare team becomes less engaged, often indulging on procedures and/or attitudes that lack effectiveness or proven safety, creating burdens to – and actually delaying – the beginning of an adequate treatment [3]. In our experience, a significant part of health professionals still think and act (but not talk) as if obese patients were to blame for their condition despite the fast growing amount of evidences on obesity's multicausality.

J. Ettinger et al. (eds.), *Gastric Bypass*, https://doi.org/10.1007/978-3-030-28803-7_26

The negative stereotype of obese people is understandable (however indefensible) as the result of a prior lack of evidence on genetic, epigenetic, biological, metabolic, and environmental causation of the syndrome. However, historical issues have also played a significant role on the development of discrimination: examples are found in the Hebrew-Christian culture, which preaches gluttony as a capital sin, and in Buddhism, which, since the twelfth century, has linked obesity to a karmic consequence of moral failure. Those ideas survived and were reiterated on theories dating back to the end of the nineteenth and beginning of the twentieth century, though in less obviously moralistic influenced versions. These state that obesity is portrayed as an effect of an underlying psychological conflict occurring in people who are essentially incapable of solving it: excessive eating would be a form of mitigating that conflict [3].

On the other hand, if one analyzes obesity from the point of view of psychological theories, it is possible to argue that cognitive-behavioral theories present some substantial merits. Among them, there is the tendency to avoid moral value judgments and to use scientific approaching methods which tend to be more pragmatically oriented and tend to be more suitable in terms of evidence-providing methodology [3].

As obesity is progressively identified as a chronic, recurrent, and severe disease with biologic, genetic, and/or environmental foundations, the influence and controversial effect of less scientifically elaborated explanations tend to decrease. With that in mind, one could expect that treatments focused on effective techniques and grounded on proper scientific evidence will probably win this epistemological battle over anecdotal reports constantly heralded on the media, causing the latter to submerge in ostracism. In this scenario, techniques that used to be mainstream should be made suitable and have their roles redefined, if possible and proven to be effective.

The Relation Between PD and Obesity

The interface between PD and obesity is very complex. Below we highlight some associations of interest [4, 5]:

- Obesity is very common among patients with schizophrenia, mood disorders (MD), attention deficit hyperactivity disorder (ADHD), and some eating disorders (ED).
- These PDs are common among patients that seek treatment for obesity [6]. We must note that patients with ED have a higher rate of association with MD and substance abuse [7].
- MD, overweight, and obesity are highly associated with compulsive binge eating episodes (the symptom, not necessarily the ED). And yet binge eating disorder (BED) itself is present in 4–6% of obese people, in 30% of obese patients (obese people that seek anti-obesity treatment), and in about 45% of BS candidates [3, 6].
- Obesity, metabolic syndrome, depressive disorder (DD), bipolar disorder (BD), and schizophrenia are independently associated with high levels of morbidity and mortality of cardiovascular diseases and type 2 diabetes [4, 5].
- Epidemiological studies show a positive relation between the presence of obesity and DD and BD in both women and men, with a variation of the level of obesity and age of onset. Patients with BD have elevated rates of overweight, obesity, and abdominal obesity. On the other hand, the presence of overweight, obesity, and visceral fat are also associated with some PDs [4, 5].
- People with depressive episodes during childhood have double the chance of being overweight during adult life [4].

In addition to these data, there is also an iatrogenic factor, that is, psychiatric medication favors both weight gain and metabolic disturbances. Worth saying is that patients with BED and schizophrenia that are not undergoing drug treatment at onset also present with higher weight and metabolic disturbances than the overall population [4].

On the other hand, central nervous system-acting weight loss medications may induce, worsen, and sometimes improve psychiatric conditions.

As the reader can figure out, the complexity and depth of these associations would demand a much larger space to be properly discussed.

Preoperative Psychiatric Evaluation

There is an almost mystical expectation involving preoperative psychiatric and psychological evaluations for BS: some people implicitly believe that these professionals, i.e., psychiatrists and psychologists, can effectively read minds and/or predict the future. That is clearly and obviously not real. In our opinion, professionals in these areas should adopt a more humble attitude and make this fact clear to patients, to the patients' family, and to the rest of the multidisciplinary team.

However, there is a good reason to undertake preoperative psychiatric evaluation: the high rate of psychiatric disorders within this population. Among the candidates for BS, the prevalence of PDs is clearly higher in relation to the overall population [3, 5]. This should not constitute a potential technical constraint to the procedure in patients with psychiatric disorders, even though this could be the case (see ahead). Actually, an improvement in mental health in the majority of the patients is observed [8], but nevertheless that stresses the need of psychiatric evaluation and reevaluation along the treatment.

Marcus et al. [9] found that 66% of BS candidates presented at least one axis I diagnosis [1] throughout their lifetime: MD (15.6%), anxiety disorder, AD (24%), and BED (16.3%) were the most commonly found diagnoses.

Segal and Cardeal [10] and Sarwer et al. [11] found similar results, with only approximately 25% of patients completely devoid of psychiatric diseases.

More recently, another study found similar figures in a larger population, with approximately 50% of BS candidates having at least three PD [12].

What is also interesting is that this population presented a higher usage rate of psychiatric medication when compared to the overall population, varying from 34.3% to 41%. In terms of distribution of medication type, the majority was taking antidepressants (30%) followed by anxiolytics (6.6%) and antipsychotics (3.3%). Most of these medications were prescribed by professionals who didn't have a proper psychiatric background [9]. This fact strongly suggests a high incidence of under- or misdiagnosis in this population at the time of the preoperative evaluation. In our opinion, this aspect speaks in favor of the aforementioned prejudice and, still worse, could be the cause of some unwanted psychiatric outcomes, such as the possibly higher postoperative suicide rates (see specific chapter for a deeper discussion).

The Relation Between PD and BS

As mentioned before, there is a lot of discussion on whether a predictive psychiatric/psychological success factor in BS exists. To illustrate this controversy, in a totally anticlimactic fashion, Herpertz et al. [13] considered the presence of psychiatric diagnosis as a good prognosis factor for BS outcome, except in the cases with severe axis I and II diagnosis.

Other reviews and studies found that patients with DD lost more weight than their peers [14] and that BED in surgery candidates did not present a significant impact on BS outcome [15].

BED seems more compromising when its onset is during the postoperative period. However we cannot reliably predict the postoperative onset, maintenance, or remission of a PD in a given patient [16]. Therefore, one could reasonably conclude that a postoperative follow-up is much more important than the preoperative evaluations.

This data contradicts the common belief that psychiatric patients are likely to endure complications in the postoperative period. But as we know, common sense tends to have no direct relationship to veracity and not be based on evidence. On the contrary, it may be mainly guided by prejudice. It is important to always keep in mind the myriad of prejudices whose verisimilitude is debated, and remember to include these on the list.

PDs may be present during postoperative period, but this topic will be explored in further detail in a later chapter of this book.

To address the question on how to deal with PD in bariatric surgery candidates, many Brazilian associations joined together and published the 1st Brazilian Consensus in Bariatric Surgery, according to the best scientific evidence available at the time, to guide BS procedures [17].

The following associations were part of the consensus:

- Brazilian Society of Bariatric Surgery (SBCB)
- Brazilian College of Surgeons (CBC)
- Brazilian College of Digestive Surgery (CBCD)
- Brazilian Society of Laparoscopic Surgery (SOBRACIL)
- Brazilian Association of Obesity Studies (ABESO)
- Brazilian Society of Endocrinology and Metabolism (SBEM)

The consensus is an encompassing document in the specific area of multidisciplinary interventions. In psychiatric terms, the Consensus states that:

Adverse conditions: current surgical procedures are not recommended for obesity control in the following situations:

A. Severe uncontrolled depressive states
B. Current uncontrolled psychotic states
C. Current drug abuse/dependence
D. Significant irreversible cognitive/intellectual limitation in patients without adequate family support

Note: Severe psychiatric disorders, under proper control, do not contraindicate the procedures.

Items A and B are obviously important; however, once treated and in remission, they are not contraindications. However, these patients must undergo suitable psychiatric follow-up after remission.

In relation to item C, in view of current evidence, our opinion is that the case of alcohol use disorder (AUD) is the diagnosis with which the correlation to the majority of drug-related postoperative problems is higher [7, 18]. AUD, MD, and suicide will be further discussed in a specific chapter.

Special and individual attention must be given to patients that fall within item D, above. Diagnosis as Prader-Willi syndrome and neurocognitive disorders (formerly included dementias, a term abandoned in the DSM V [1]) must be discussed deeply with the family and team, carefully assessing the cost-benefit relation, given that there are not enough algorithms nor evidences for generalized conclusions.

At our public and private hospitals, we follow the guidelines above, in addition to the guidelines set forth in Ministerial Directive no. 492, dated August 31, 2007, available at http://www.sbcbm.org.br/legislacao.asp?menu=3.

Surgery on Teenagers

The psychiatric and psychological evaluations of teenagers candidates for BS is still a topic under discussion. At our hospital, the parents or caregivers are also evaluated.

For this age group, a major concern comes with getting information about AUD and pregnancy. Changes on alcohol metabolism are the main reasons for this concern [18, 19].

Other important issues are the impact of hormonal changes caused by weight loss and the potential increase of female fertility during a life stage when women are usually highly exposed to new stimuli.

In the AMOS study, part of the SOS study, results seem to match those seen in the adult population [20].

Conclusion

Despite not being as common and pervasive as psychological evaluation, preoperative psychiatric evaluation for BS is important and necessary. However, it should not be yet another source of prejudice against the patient. Arguably, psychiatric evaluation should be an item to be included on global treatments which will have as ultimate aim obtaining excellence in patient care.

Aside from the overwhelmingly high prevalence of PD among BS candidates, one important reason to advise psychiatric evaluation during the preoperative phase is that unknown diseases that are already present can be identified. Furthermore, a better multidisciplinary care can take place, strengthening the ties between the team and the patient. An additional role which we always portray at our hospital and the private clinic is to demystify BS, PDs, and the potential interrelations between them, not only for the patient and the family but also for other members of the team that are not familiar with PDs.

The psychiatric appointment provides an opportunity for reviewing expectations and motivation in addition to fostering the discussion of information of great value and reinforcing and completing the actions of psychology. BS patients with PD can benefit from having their disease addressed during the preoperative period and planning their follow-up after surgery. However this intervention cannot be deemed as a penalty for having an additional disease. Identifying preoperative PD may actually improve global outcome, not only in the weight loss field.

It is very important to stress out that psychiatric and psychological evaluations and treatments are not interchangeable. The use of psychopharmacological and other biological tools and changes in their efficacy after surgeries are central aspects of that difference, and, as shown before, this use is more a rule than an exception.

Cases in which BS are contraindicated are rare. The preoperative psychiatric preparation is also limited to exceptional situations. In relation to that, in accordance with what the Brazilian Consensus in BS advocates, all items (eventual exception made to item C, above) are readily identifiable by various team members. As soon as this identification is made, prompt psychiatric referral should take place.

The postoperative psychiatric follow-up, ideally implemented by psychiatrists, specialized in – or at least very familiar with – obesity and BS, is indicated for all patients that require it, but only for them. As already mentioned, obesity is not a psychiatric disorder, nor is it a psychosomatic disease. Based on the available data, to require that all patients systematically go through long interventions in the "Psy" areas as part of a comprehensive multidisciplinary protocol of preparation or even as follow-up is a waste of resources driven by prejudice or by aspects that are not directly linked to the diseases involved. More refined referrals should be the aim of properly designed interventions.

Acknowledgment The author would like to thank Rodrigo Rezende and Nathalie Gil for their English revision.

References

1. American Psychiatric Association. Diagnostic and statistical manual of mental disorders. 5th ed. Arlington: American Psychiatric Association; 2013.
2. The ICD-10 classification of mental and behavioural disorders. 1st ed. Geneva: World Health Organization; 1992.
3. Segal A. Obesidade e comorbidade psiquiátrica: caracterização e eficácia terapêutica de atendimento multidisciplinar na evolução de 34 pacientes. [Doutorado]. Universidade de São Paulo; 1999.
4. McElroy SL, Allison DB, Bray GA, editors. Obesity and mental disorders: Taylor & Francisco Group, many chapters; 2006.
5. Segal A, Kussunoki DK. Depressão e Síndrome Metabólica. In. Louzã Neto MR & Elkis H, editors. Psiquiatria Básica 2ª ed. Porto Alegre: Roca; 372–380, 2007.
6. Segal A, Kinoshita Kussunoki D, Aparecida Larino M. Post-surgical refusal to eat: anorexia nervosa, bulimia nervosa or a new eating disorder? A case series. Obes Surg. 2004;14(3):353–60.
7. Umberg E, Shader R, Hsu L, Greenblatt D. From disordered eating to addiction. J Clin Psychopharmacol. 2012;32(3):376–89.
8. Brandão I, Fernandes A, Osório E, Calhau M, Coelho R. A psychiatric perspective view of bariatric surgery patients. Arch Clin Psychiatry (São Paulo). 2015;42(5):122–8.
9. Marcus M, Kalarchian M, Courcoulas A. Psychiatric evaluation and follow-up of bariatric surgery patients. Am J Psychiatr. 2009;166(3):285–91.
10. Segal, A. e Cardeal, M.V. Psychiatric disorders among patients at the waiting list for bariatric surgery – HCFMUSP 1997. Non-published data.
11. Sarwer D, Cohn N, Gibbons L, Magee L, Crerand C, Raper S, et al. Psychiatric diagnoses and psychiatric treatment among bariatric surgery candidates. Obes Surg. 2004;14(9):1148–56.
12. Duarte-Guerra L, Coêlho B, Santo M, Wang Y. Psychiatric disorders among obese patients seeking bariatric surgery: results of structured clinical interviews. Obes Surg. 2014;25(5):830–7.
13. Herpertz S, Kielmann R, Wolf A, Hebebrand J, Senf W. Do psychosocial variables predict weight loss or mental health after obesity surgery? A systematic review. Obes Res. 2004;12(10):1554–69.

14. Averbukh Y, Heshka S, El-Shoreya H, Flancbaum L, Geliebter A, Kamel S, et al. Depression score predicts weight loss following roux-en-Y gastric bypass. Obes Surg. 2003;13(6):833–6.
15. Alger-Mayer S, Rosati C, Polimeni J, Malone M. Preoperative binge eating status and gastric bypass surgery: a long-term outcome study. Obes Surg. 2008;19(2):139–45.
16. Conceição E, Utzinger L, Pisetsky E. Eating disorders and problematic eating behaviours before and after bariatric surgery: characterization, assessment and association with treatment outcomes. Eur Eat Disord Rev. 2015;23(6):417–25.
17. Sociedade Brasileira de Cirurgia Bariátrica, Colégio Brasileiro de Cirurgiões, Colégio Brasileiro de Cirurgia Digestiva, Sociedade Brasileira de Cirurgia Laparoscópica, Associação Brasileira para o Estudo da Obesidade, Sociedade Brasileira de Endocrinologia e Metabologia. Consenso Brasileiro Multissocietário em Cirurgia da Obesidade. 2006. Available at: http://www.sbcbm.org.br/associados.asp?menu=2. Accessed in: July/2012.
18. Hagedorn J, Encarnacion B, Brat G, Morton J. Does gastric bypass alter alcohol metabolism? Surg Obes Relat Dis. 2007;3(5):543–8.
19. Woodard G, Downey J, Hernandez-Boussard T, Morton J. Impaired alcohol metabolism after gastric bypass surgery: a case-crossover trial. J Am Coll Surg. 2011;212(2):209–14.
20. Olbers T, Gronowitz E, Werling M, Mårlid S, Flodmark C, Peltonen M, et al. Two-year outcome of laparoscopic Roux-en-Y gastric bypass in adolescents with severe obesity: results from a Swedish Nationwide Study (AMOS). Int J Obes. 2012;36(11):1388–95.

Perioperative Complications

27

Juliana Henrique, Luis Felipe Okida, Rene Aleman, Emanuele Lo Menzo, Samuel Szomstein, and Raul J. Rosenthal

Introduction

Bariatric surgery (BS) remains the most effective treatment for severe obesity. Although BS has a very high safety profile, it still has both well-known and potential perioperative complications. The safety profile of such procedures has significantly increased over the years, particularly since the implementation of minimally invasive techniques. However, the substantial increase in the application of metabolic surgery procedures has also increased the overall number of complications. Some of them are common to any type of procedure and are mostly related to the underlying risk factors of this population.

Patients with Obesity in the Anesthesia Setting

In order to properly avoid and/or manage perioperative complications, a thorough knowledge of all the comorbidities of severely obese patients is indispensable. In fact, obesity is associated with many comorbidities, impairing several organ systems such as cardiovascular and respiratory, among others. Deleterious effects can be directly related to obesity or to one of the many associated comorbid conditions. In addition, peculiar anatomical features of severely obese patients (i.e., short and higher neck circumference, small oral cavity, restricted neck movements, short sternomental and thyromental distances) can be the reason for specific anesthetic-related complications. All of these features should be taken into consideration in the preoperative setting. As a result, taken as a whole, the severely obese patient represents a high-risk individual from the anesthesia standpoint. The main anesthetic complications in bariatric surgery are nerve injury, airway and ventilation problems, cardiovascular complications, potential issues related to drug pharmacodynamics, and venous thromboembolism (VTE) [1].

Nerve Injury

In super obese patients, especially those with diabetes, the occurrence of pressure sores and neural injuries is frequent. In a retrospective analysis comparing obese to nonobese patients undergoing surgery, it was shown that patients with obesity had a four times higher chance of presenting with peripheral nerve injury after a surgical procedure [2]. Placing pads under pressure points in order to avoid pressure sores and neurologic injury is an efficient alternative to avoid nerve damage [3].

J. Henrique · L. F. Okida · R. Aleman · E. L. Menzo
S. Szomstein · R. J. Rosenthal (✉)
Department of General Surgery and The Bariatric and Metabolic Institute, Cleveland Clinic Florida, Weston, FL, USA
e-mail: ROSENTR@CCF.ORG

J. Ettinger et al. (eds.), *Gastric Bypass*, https://doi.org/10.1007/978-3-030-28803-7_27

Airway Management

Airway management of bariatric surgical patients is considered a challenge for anesthesiologists. Several studies reported that increased body mass index (BMI) complicates mask ventilation in up to 8.8% of obese patients [4]. Additionally, BMI is associated with difficult intubation, and major airway complications may happen in 40% of obese patients undergoing surgery [5]. Based on these challenges and the higher likelihood of complications, it is recommended that alternative airway management devices be available at the time of anesthesia induction. According to Juvin et al., difficult or failed intubation is more usual in obese patients than in nonobese [6]. Moreover, obesity is associated with a 30% greater risk of challenging or failed intubation [7]. In a prospective cohort study performed by De Jong et al., 8.2% of 2103 obese patients undergoing surgery presented with difficult intubation, and the main predictors for this situation were Mallampati scores III or IV, history of obstructive sleep apnea syndrome, and reduced mobility of cervical spine [5]. Other factors potentially involved in adverse events associated with intubation are higher neck circumference, shorter neck, small oral cavity, abundance of intraoral soft tissue, restricted neck movements, and short sternomental and thyromental distance.

The evaluation of a potentially difficult intubation should be obtained in the preoperative setting in order to avoid life-threatening complications. The Mallampati score and the neck circumference are some of the most important airway parameters for risk assessment. Bahattin et al. reported that an increase in BMI and Mallampati scores significantly increased difficult mask ventilation and troublesome intubation [8]. In the previously cited study from De Jong et al., 38% of obese patients with difficult intubation required management with difficult airway techniques, including videolaryngoscopy, intubating laryngeal mask airway, and flexible fiber-optic intubation, awake or with light sedation [5]. Considering this high rate, anesthesiologists have to be aware of possible difficult intubation in a patient undergoing bariatric surgery and, therefore, may have to use more advanced techniques to achieve their goal. Even though less expected and rarely required in an elective scenario, cricothyrotomy would be another method to place a tube into the trachea if none of the previous techniques was successful. Nevertheless, excessive soft tissue in the anterior neck limits access to the cricothyroid membrane in obese patients, making it difficult to identify anatomic landmarks needed to perform a cricothyrotomy [9].

Ventilation

Based on the anatomical peculiarities of severely obese patients (heavy pannus, reduced chest cavity, relative muscular weakness, decreased chest excursion, and obstructing upper airway anatomy), respiratory drive and oxygenation are significantly affected. The functional residual capacity (FRC) and lung compliance are decreased, resulting in a higher resistance and work of breathing, thus impairing oxygenation.

Furthermore, difficult respiratory mechanics in the supine position increase the ventilation/perfusion mismatch. This is aggravated by the potential need for Trendelenburg position during the surgical procedure, which could lead to compression of the great vessels and reduced lung volume by abdominal weight, precipitating cardiorespiratory decompensation. On the other hand, the reverse Trendelenburg position is better tolerated and contributes to improved cardiovascular and respiratory dynamics.

During the preoxygenation phase of the obese patient, it is more difficult to build an oxygen reserve due to the decreased FRC. Also, morbidly obese patients run into hypoxia after only 3 minutes [10]. Moreover, a high inspiratory oxygen dose at the time of anesthesia induction can result in atelectasis, a predisposing condition for fever and pneumonia. Thus, in obese patients, using lung recruitment maneuvers and positive end-expiratory pressure (PEEP) $\geq$ 10 cm H_2O is beneficial for atelectasis avoidance, prevention of collapse of small airways, and improvement of ventilation/perfusion and oxygenation [11].

Cardiovascular Implications

Cardiovascular comorbidities may influence perioperative management and outcomes. Among these conditions are atherosclerotic cardiovascular disease, hypertension, arrhythmias, cardiomyopathy, and thromboembolic disease [12]. Thornqvist et al. analyzed the relationship between body mass index and the risk of perioperative cardiovascular adverse events in patients undergoing elective orthopedic surgery and concluded that underweight and extreme obesity were associated with a higher risk of major adverse cardiovascular events, such as ischemic stroke, acute myocardial infarction, and cardiovascular death [13]. Furthermore, 2% of obese patients undergoing surgery presented severe cardiovascular collapse and 1% presented supraventricular or ventricular arrhythmia in the perioperative period [5]. A retrospective review of postoperative complications comparing obese versus nonobese patients undergoing surgery concluded that patients with obesity presented a higher prevalence of myocardial infarction (0.5%) and morbidly obese patients had a higher prevalence of myocardial infarction and cardiac arrest, both complications with a statistically significant difference ($p < 0.05$) [2]. Considering the increased cardiovascular risk to bariatric patients, preoperative screening of comorbidities with appropriate therapy, combined with perioperative and postoperative hemodynamic optimization with close monitoring, is essential to limit cardiovascular complications [14].

Pharmacotherapy Considerations

Due to the physiological modifications of obesity, pharmacokinetics and pharmacodynamics are different in bariatric patients. For example, abnormal lung mechanics impair the absorption and elimination of inhaled drugs. The presence of higher amount of adipose tissue can alter the distribution of certain lipophilic drugs. Also, doses of the anesthetic drugs administered have to be carefully calculated and based mostly on ideal body weight as actual body weight cannot be used.

Venous Thromboembolism (VTE)

There is a known association between severe obesity and VTE. In fact, obese patients present several risk factors for VTE, such as diabetes, hypercholesterolemia, hypercoagulopathy, lower extremities venous stasis, and lymphedema [3].

Increased risk of venous thromboembolism includes patients with obesity and a history of smoking and those who are taking oral contraceptives, hormone replacement therapy, or antipsychotic medications. Overall, there is a fivefold increase in the incidence of pulmonary embolism (PE) during and after surgery [15]. However, when compared to orthopedic patients, laparoscopic procedures have been associated with a lower incidence of both nonfatal and fatal PE. This is probably due to less surgical trauma and a decreased prothrombotic state in laparoscopy than open surgical procedures.

Additionally, the anesthetic technique performed may play a role in the development of clots. Rodgers et al. compared epidural anesthesia (primary anesthetic or adjunct to general anesthesia) with general anesthesia alone, resulting in a 44% and 55% rate reduction of deep venous thrombosis and PE, respectively, for the epidural group [16]. Since general anesthesia is usually the standard method in bariatric surgery, the higher risk of venous thromboembolism should be considered [16, 17].

Following bariatric surgery, the reported rate of deep venous thrombosis and pulmonary embolism varies between 0.3% and 2.2% [18]. A systematic review of literature regarding this topic divided risk factors by patient-related and procedure-related conditions (Table 27.1) [18].

In order to prevent VTE, early ambulation reduces venous stasis and thereby reduces the odds of clot formation. Lower extremity compression also results in less venous stasis and varies from graduated compression stockings to intermittent pneumatic compression and sequential compression devices. Pharmacologic prophylaxis is a common approach to prevent VTE and includes unfractionated heparin, low-molecular-weight heparin, vitamin K antagonists, direct thrombin inhibitors, and factor Xa

Table 27.1 Risk factors for venous thromboembolism (VTE) following bariatric surgery

Patient-related risk factors
Increased age Gender: male Preoperative weight/body mass index Smoking History of VTE
Procedure-related risk factors
Operative time > 3 hours Open procedures Revision surgery Anastomotic leak

Adapted from Bartlett et al.

inhibitors. For patients with deep venous thrombosis, but with contraindication to anticoagulation, a vena cava filter is an option to prevent embolism to the lungs [18].

Esophageal Perforation

Some patients require a nasogastric tube (NGT) to empty the stomach and reduce the possibility of bronchoaspiration. Esophageal perforation is a high-mortality complication that, unfortunately, may happen during the perioperative period. Few studies reported that the incidence of this complication when placing a NGT varies from 3% to 5.7% and the most common site of iatrogenic esophageal perforation is the thoracic region, followed by cervical esophagus [19]. Another possible esophageal perforation occurs when inserting a bougie. This tube is usually placed into the stomach. Even though rare, there are some case reports of esophageal perforation after bougie insertion during bariatric procedures [20, 21]. Therefore, attention must be given when placing such tubes since obese patients have excessive fatty tissue in the neck, narrowing the trachea and esophagus. Occasionally, insertion through direct vision or even under fluoroscopic guidance may be recommended.

Other Complications in the Anesthetic Setting

Other possible anesthetic complications related to obese patients are esophageal intubation, dental injury, and aspiration of gastric content. The last condition can result in serious complications such as Mendelson's syndrome, progressing to systemic inflammatory condition and even death.

Laparoscopic Access and Safety

Debate exists on the best and safest initial trocar placement. Due to the considerable thickness of the abdominal wall, previous abdominal surgery, the presence of hepatomegaly or splenomegaly, and the relative paucity of intravisceral fat compared to the subcutaneous one, a more challenging first trocar access might ensue. Thus, complications due to trocar insertion, such as organ and vessel injuries, or development of subcutaneous emphysema, may occur, especially in the hands of an inexperienced surgeon.

There are three main techniques to insert the first trocar: insertion after establishment of the initial pneumoperitoneum with the Veress needle; insertion of the first trocar through a direct vision open approach (Hasson technique); or through the visualization of the abdominal wall different layers with an optical trocar, more often without previous pneumoperitoneum.

No technique is considered perfect and intra-abdominal injuries have been described with all three techniques [22]. Vascular and visceral injuries represent the most severe type of complication, whereas extraperitoneal insufflation and subcutaneous emphysema are considered minor complications [23].

One of the most feared complications and major cause of morbidity is the vascular injury, with an overall reported mortality rate of 15% [24]. However, injuries to great vessels in laparoscopic bariatric surgery are reported in much lower incidence with a calculated risk of 0.05% [22].

Vascular Injuries

Vascular injuries related to abdominal access can be grouped into major and minor vascular injuries. Major vascular injuries affect major vessels such as the aorta, inferior vena cava, and iliac vessels, while minor vascular injuries affect vessels of the abdominal wall (laceration of superior/inferior epigastric vessels during placement of lateral trocars), mesentery, omental (especially when adhesions are present), or other organs [25].

At Port Site

At the port site, a vascular injury is more likely to be tamponade while the cannula is in place. Delayed identification of the abdominal wall's bleeding can occur after the procedure is finished. Clinical manifestations include abdominal wall pain, abdominal wall or flank ecchymosis, and external bleeding from the trocar site. Patients can also present initially with hemodynamic instability due to significant blood loss from a port site that bleeds internally. Patients with an abdominal wall hematoma from laparoscopic access who are hemodynamically stable and with no signs of hematoma expansion can be managed conservatively by direct pressure, full-thickness abdominal wall suture ligation, or tamponade with Foley catheter balloon insertion through the trocar site. Intervention is indicated if the hematoma expands or the patient becomes hemodynamically unstable. For some patients, percutaneous embolization of the bleeding vessel may be an option [26].

Major Vascular Injury

Rarely, injury to major venous structures (i.e., inferior vena cava, iliac vein) can also occur, and massive air embolism has been reported due to unrecognized intravenous placement of a pneumoperitoneum needle and subsequent gas insufflation. Injury to the aorta or iliac vessels during abdominal access can lead to rapid exsanguination and death unless prompt vascular control and repair are undertaken [27]. Major vascular injuries may be recognized immediately by observing free blood in the abdominal cavity. However, vascular injury may not be appreciated right away as a result of bleeding into the mesentery or retroperitoneum rather than into the peritoneal cavity. The anesthesia team should be immediately notified that there is a problem. The bed should be placed into Trendelenburg position. If a vascular surgeon is not immediately available, a damage control approach can be performed as used in trauma surgery. To minimize ongoing blood loss, the abdomen should be rapidly opened with a midline incision, pressure should be applied directly to the bleeding site for initial control, and the abdominal cavity can be packed if the bleeding site is identified as a damaged large vein. These maneuvers allow for fluid resuscitation while awaiting the vascular surgeon, or arrangements for immediate transfer if subspecialty expertise is not available [27]. The supraceliac aortic clamping can be performed as a lifesaving maneuver to avoid massive blood loss when a large injury has occurred to a great caliber artery (aorta, iliac artery), although this approach claims for a rapid injury repair in the interest of its relevant ischemic impact in the abdominal viscera. Nonetheless, the dissection of the supraceliac aorta may be unfamiliar to novice surgeons [28].

Minor Vascular Injury

Compressive maneuvers can often be performed to control mild and moderate bleeding. Local compression allows a surgeon time to consider strategies for definitive hemostasis and may occasionally be a definitive treatment itself. Due to spasm, small-to-medium-caliber vessels are likely to slow and often stop bleeding with simple compression. In the laparoscopic setting, a gauze sponge can be passed through a 10 mm port. Under some circumstances, a piece of healthy and mobile omentum can be grasped and used to compress the area. Moreover, the vessel can be grasped directly (if possible) in order to prevent free blood spreading and darkening the visibility in the intra-abdominal site. This technique is useful for sudden, significant bleeding from division of the short gastric arteries during laparoscopy [27]. Dry hemostatic agents (i.e., sterile gelatin sponge, oxidized cellulose polymer) can easily be passed through a laparoscopic port and used in conjunction with mechanical compression. Fibrin glue (with the aid of a special laparoscopic applicator) has also been used to provide hemostasis during gastric bypass [29].

Once bleeding has slowed or ceased, the area is inspected to identify the bleeding point, which is isolated and controlled with a clip, suture, cautery, or any of the other methods described above. The field should then be irrigated carefully with saline. Irrigation should be used judiciously to minimize soiling of the tip of the laparoscope with blood and other fluids [27].

The need to convert to an open procedure is determined by the rate of bleeding, the amount of blood loss, the clinical status of the patient (tachycardia, hypotension, sepsis), the presence (or lack) of a clearly defined source, and the surgeon's ability to see and control the bleeding quickly using laparoscopic techniques. Patient factors such as advanced age or poor functional status and comorbidities should be taken into account when determining whether laparoscopic endeavors at hemostasis are likely to be successful and deciding how long to persist. If adequate visibility cannot be maintained, conversion to an open procedure will be needed. The decision to convert for bleeding is justifiable and prudent. An important source of patient morbidity results from the failure to convert to an open procedure in a timely fashion when bleeding is encountered [27].

Additional technical maneuvers in attempts to reduce intraperitoneal injury while placing the first trocar, such as temporarily lifting the abdominal wall with towel clamps, have been investigated. Still, these techniques apparently do not influence the frequency of failure entry. Another strategy is choosing a different anatomical entry site to avoid the midline and potential aortic or inferior vena cava injuries. Palmer's point is 3 cm below the left rib arch in the midclavicular line, and it is an area with less fat tissue than the umbilicus. This point in the left upper quadrant is away from the liver, spleen, and great vessels, and vascular damage is not likely to happen at this site [27, 30].

Bowel Injury

According to Krishnakumar et al., bowel injury is the third cause of death from laparoscopic surgeries after major vascular injury and anesthetic complications. Differently from injury to great vessels where the risk and complications are immediate, bowel injuries usually go unnoticed at the time of the procedure. In the postoperative period, thus, patients may present peritonitis, which is a significant cause of morbidity and mortality. If a bowel injury is noticed, immediate repair must be done [24].

Subcutaneous Emphysema

After laparoscopic procedures, asymptomatic subcutaneous emphysema is not uncommon. Clinically significant subcutaneous emphysema, however, is not frequent, and the incidence varies from 0.43% to 2.34% [31]. In obese patients, it can be difficult to identify by simple inspection or palpation. Cervical and facial emphysema can be more marked due to a thinner subcutaneous layer in these areas. Risk factors for developing subcutaneous emphysema in bariatric patients are higher insufflation pressure, use of six or more surgical ports, prolonged surgical procedures (longer than 200 minutes), and older age. This last risk factor is likely due to the reduced natural subcutaneous tissue resistance [31]. Kayaalp et al. state that the possible relationship between bariatric surgery and subcutaneous emphysema might be the frequent trocar displacement by virtue of the increased thickness of subcutaneous tissue in obese patients. Conservative management of the subcutaneous emphysema is the treatment of choice in most cases [31].

The presence of air in the subcutaneous tissue may indicate esophageal perforation, emphysema in that layer, pneumothorax, and pneumomediastinum can occur after dissection of the phrenoesophageal membrane. To dissect accurately the distal esophagus, the gastroesophageal junction, and the diaphragmatic crus, the membrane has to be taken down and the mediastinum exposed to carbon dioxide gas under pressure. In addition, dissection of the surrounding esophageal tissue can facilitate the gas inlet through the pleura, mediastinum, and neck, by anatomical planes. As the patient is usually positioned in the reverse Trendelenburg fashion, dissemination of the gas is a frequent consequence. Fortunately, the majority of cases are deemed as a mild accumulation of carbon dioxide, and its absorption takes place in a short period of time. If clinical manifestations as hypercarbia, desaturation, tachycardia, or hypotension arise during the procedure, a chest tube insertion must be considered and the insufflation pressure must be checked [32].

Complications During Pouch Creation

Transection

To create the gastric pouch, the omental bursa has to be exposed for placement of the stapler. This can be done by transecting the neurovascular bundle containing branches of the vagus nerve and the left gastric artery and vein [33]. Alternatively, this bundle can be preserved by creating an entry point via perigastric dissection. Transection of the lesser omentum is well tolerated and efficient because it does not influence clinical, functional, and laboratory results or even affect weight loss in an early stage and may technically alleviate gastric pouch formation [34–36]. Nonetheless, some studies have reported that vagus nerve preservation is associated with less postoperative dumping and reduced food intake [37, 38]. To elucidate the impact on the early postoperative course, Van Wezenbeek et al. prospectively collected data from 773 patients who underwent LRYGB. In 407 (52.7%) patients, the lesser omentum was transected, and in 366 (47.3%) patients, neurovascular bundle was preserved. The transection was an independent predictive factor for anastomotic leakage, postoperative bleeding, or intra-abdominal abscess formation after RYGB. A potential explanation may be the transection of both the left gastric artery and the left gastric vein. Hypothetically, transection of these vessels may compromise the blood supply to the newly created gastrojejunostomy, thereby increasing the risk of an anastomotic leakage. Furthermore, transection of these large blood vessels may hypothetically increase the chance of postoperative bleeding.

Additionally, dissection of the angle of His is one of the critical moments when the surgeon has to be fully aware of possible injury to short gastric vessels, spleen, and the diaphragmatic crus. Compression maneuvers and bleeding control regarding vascular injury described previously are necessary to avoid splenectomy. It is known that spleen extraction after incidental laceration significantly increases morbidity and mortality rates. These rates, elevated in patients with morbid obesity, prompt a spleen preservation policy during bariatric surgery [39]. Moreover, careless dissection or traction may lead to an organ perforation, either the esophagus or stomach. Primary suturing is required whenever an injury is perceived.

Staple Misfire

Many technical factors or elements related to the patient's condition can affect the outcomes of bariatric surgery. For the technical factors, Baker et al. warn that staple size must be selected appropriately for the tissue on which it is to be used to allow for proper staple formation while in turn achieving optimal staple line strength and tissue compression. Also, full-thickness oversewing past a fixed staple line may increase the risk of tearing at the point of suture penetration in the distended gastric pouch. Still, the author warns about firing the endocutters. Bunching of tissue at the crotch of the stapler must be avoided. This occurs after the first firing and often appears as the blade catches a staple in the crossover area and carries it to the newly formed crotch. Failure to note and remove this staple may result in a staple misfire. If left in place, the "crotch staple" causes the stapler to lock when firing is attempted. Besides, a wedge band bypass failure can occur when the staple driver hits the crotch staple secondary to excessive force and dislodges from its track. This results in staple formation on one side and the slicing open of the tissue on the opposite side. Finally, care must be taken while firing the stapler near the angle of

His. Migration of the stapler with incorporation of the esophagus can weaken the staple line because of the weaker nature of esophageal tissue. Bunching of fundus or a thick fundus can contribute to leaks if inadequate staple formation or tissue shearing occurs [40, 41].

Incidental Nasogastric Tube Transection

Employing the adequate stapler for the proper thickness of the organs/vessels may prevent bleeding and leakage. However, a complication seldom discussed in bariatric surgery is the incidental transection of nasogastric/orogastric tube, bougie, or thermometer probe. According to Sanchez et al., in a series of 727 patients who underwent LRYGB, the reported rate of tube transection was 1.2% [42]. In 2011, a multicenter retrospective analysis was performed by Abu-Gazala et al. describing a tube stapling rate of 0.5%. Interestingly, all of the complications occurred at the same part of the procedure: gastric pouch formation. No reported incidents were observed during sutures [43]. As stated by Higa et al., the management of this complication requires redo of the gastrojejunal anastomosis. Furthermore, under this circumstance an optional procedure would be a laparoscopic pouch trimming at two levels: the gastric and jejunal portions of the anastomosis, with retrieval of the tube under direct visualization. Conversion to open procedure may take place if the surgeon has difficulty in performing the repair laparoscopically and in a safe fashion. In the event there is not enough healthy tissue to be mobilized, oversewing of the defects and wide local drainage must be performed. A gastrostomy tube at the level of the gastric remnant would also be needed for postoperative nutrition [44].

Troublesome Anastomosis

The number of bariatric operations dramatically increased worldwide. Since the first case series of Roux-en-Y gastric bypass (RYGB) was published in 1994, multiple studies have demonstrated the feasibility and safety of the laparoscopic approach. Advantages of the laparoscopic technique include less blood loss, short length of stay, and faster recovery. Yet, some complications uncommonly reported in the open surgery started to rise with the minimally invasive procedure. Podnos et al. compared the frequency and type of postoperative complications after laparoscopic and open RYGB. A total of 3464 patients underwent a laparoscopic RYGB, and 2771 patients underwent open surgery, from 1994 to 2002. In this early series, the conversion to laparotomy rate was 2.2%, and it was related to hepatomegaly (48.7%), malfunction of the equipment (12.8%), short instruments or trocars (7.7%), inadequate exposure (7.7%), twisted retro colic limb (5.1%), injury to a vital structure such as the colon or the vena cava (5.1%), inability to safely insufflate the abdomen (5.1%), bleeding (2.6%), subcutaneous emphysema (2.6%), and gastrojejunal anastomotic leak (2.6%) [45].

After more than two decades of technical and technological advancement, anastomotic leak rates following gastric bypass slightly changed. According to Nguyen et al., rates vary from 0.6 to 4.4% in his 2007 published review article. Ghosh et al. found similar rates of anastomotic leak varying from 0.1 to 5.6% in 2016 [46, 47]. A search of the medical literature was conducted by the cited author to identify publications describing intraoperative bleeds, leaks, and interventions at the stapled line. Inclusion criteria were based on a positive intraoperative leak test and bleeding identified by the surgeon. Sixteen titles were included, but only four relevant articles provided information on those topics during laparoscopic RYGB (LRYGB). Madan et al. conducted a retrospective review of 752 patients who underwent LRYGB. The gastrojejunostomy (GJ) was created with a circular stapler in all of them. The total of patients was divided in two groups. Omental reinforcement was performed on gastrojejunostomies in which leaks were seen during the bariatric procedure. There were 387 patients in the first group, with 32 (8.2%) patients who had a staple line dehiscence or evidence of gastric pouch or gastrojejunostomy leak intraoperatively. Leaks/dehiscences were repaired with sutures and then reinforced with omentum. None of these patients developed anastomotic leaks postoperatively. Of the other 365 patients group, there were four (1.1%) leaks from the GJ and/or gastric pouch [48]. Lately, a systematic review addressed 15 published papers. Aiolfi et al. excluded studies with less than 100 patients per arm in an effort to control the effect of the learning curve. Results showed that there is not a statistically significant risk ratio when comparing LRYGB vs. open RYGB and comparing open approach vs. robotic RYGB. Although the variability in operative technique should be taken into account, the heterogeneity was low ($I^2 = 23.2\%$) adding consistency to the findings. Additionally, anastomotic leak rates ranged from 0.45 to 2.21% [49].

Alasfar et al. published a series of 290 patients who underwent LRYGB with a linear stapled technique for the gastrojejunostomy [50]. Endoscopy air leak test detected 11 leaks (3.79%), 10 located at the GJ site. All of the leaks were corrected with oversewing and passed the subsequent leak test. Intraoperative bleeding in the pouch was identified in ten patients. Endoscopic visualization of the blood vessel was possible in six of these, and suturing was performed. In four cases, the source of bleeding could not be seen, and conservative treatment with irrigation and removal of clots was successfully implemented [50].

In another retrospective study, 30 out of 933 patients (3.22%) developed upper gastrointestinal hemorrhage (UGIH) after LRYGB. Endoscopic examination revealed that in 27 cases (90%), the source of the bleeding was at the GJ staple line. A total of five patients had bleeding intraoperatively, and 16 developed UGIH within 4 hours of the operation. Blood transfusion was required in almost half of the patients, and a significant increase of length of stay was noticed [51].

More recently, Varban et al. assessed the relationship between technique and surgical devices on anastomotic and staple line leaks after LRYGB. For this case-control study, 16,258 patients were enrolled. Data collected from operative notes included type of gastrojejunal anastomosis, the use of buttressing material, buttressing manufacturer, location of buttressing, and the use of fibrin sealant. Leaks were identified in 71 patients (0.44%), and the leak rate decreased during the study period. After univariate analysis, cases with an increased blood transfusion requirement, conversions to open surgery, the use of buttressing material, and Covidien stapler brand were associated with a significantly higher rate of leak. After multivariate analysis, the use of buttressing material remained associated with a higher rate of leaks. Conversely, the use of fibrin sealant was related with a significantly lower rate, whether a univariate or multivariate analysis was utilized [52].

Despite some animal experiments with buttressing material in the gastrointestinal staple line suggesting better resistance under higher pressure than non-buttressed staple lines [53–55], medical literature has not yet shown clear evidence of those findings. Instead, most studies indicate that the use of buttressing material may decrease the likelihood of bleeding in the staple line. One of the hypotheses that may explain such finding is that the material itself may interfere in the healing process. Another theory is about adding material to the thickness of the tissue included in the anastomosis, impairing proper compression of the staples, enabling early staple line failure [52]. Regarding the efficacy of the fibrin sealant during gastric bypass, Silecchia et al., in a randomized multicenter trial, described a lower rate of overall reintervention in the group that used fibrin. The difference between the groups was not statistically significant, however [56].

Some other aspects about prevention of the staple line bleeding may be considered. Potentially, a shorter staple height may provide more compression of the tissues and better hemostasis. Regardless of that, a shorter staple height does not completely prevent bleeding, and it can increase the leak rate when tissue approximation is inadequate [57]. In addition, the hand-sewn gastrojejunostomy is associated with lower bleeding when compared with mechanical (linear/circular) stapler, according to Jiang et al.

Conversely, leakage rates and reoperation were similar in both groups (mechanical and hand-sewn anastomosis) [58].

Based on the Longitudinal Assessment of Bariatric Surgery study, roughly 0.1% of the patients undergoing LRYGB are at risk of bleeding from a major blood vessel [59]. According to the American Society for Metabolic and Bariatric Surgery (ASMBS), cases of bleeding requiring transfusion or reoperation are 1–4% of the patients undergoing RYGB [60–65]. The treatment of such complications will be ultimately dictated by the etiology and location of the bleeding site. Moreover, the therapy of LRYGB-associated bleeding may require a multimodal approach: surgical, endoscopic, interventional radiological, or a combination of them [66, 67].

Intra-abdominal bleeding may arise from within the gastrointestinal tract at the site of the anastomosis or the staple line. Clinical findings, such as abdominal tenderness, abdominal distension, hematemesis, or hematochezia, can be present and are highly suggestive of acute bleeding. Often, the bleeding will resolve without intervention soon after surgery. Nonetheless, bleeding can be problematic when present, significantly increasing associated morbidity and mortality. In the setting of an unstable patient, laparoscopic or open laparotomy should be performed to determine the bleeding source. Contrarily, in a stable patient, fluid resuscitation and blood transfusion should be the mainstay therapy.

The most likely sites of bleeding after LRYGB are the staple lines of the gastrojejunostomy, gastric pouch, excluded stomach, or jejunojejunostomy. A close and thorough clinical evaluation guides the surgeon to find the most likely location. Bleeding from the gastric pouch or gastrojejunostomy usually presents with hematemesis. On the other hand, melena often indicates a distal bleed at the site of the jejunojejunostomy or excluded stomach [67]. In the presence of evident or highly suggestive bleeding, the first clinical response should be aimed toward the cessation of anticoagulation, followed by a medical resuscitative therapy.

Early postoperative bleeding after LRYGB is a potentially life-threatening complication, as in other types of surgery. A rapid and appropriate response will undoubtedly reduce morbidity and mortality rates, as well as decrease the need of extensive and significantly invasive therapies. Usually, the progression leading to mortality is the following [68]:

1. Hemorrhage from the staple line
2. Development of an obstructing blood clot
3. Blood and fluid filling the biliary limb
4. Increase in the intragastric pressure
5. Staple line leakage at the gastric pouch or gastric remnant necrosis and perforation

Figure 27.1 represents a step-by-step approach to early postoperative GI bleeding in gastric bypass patients.

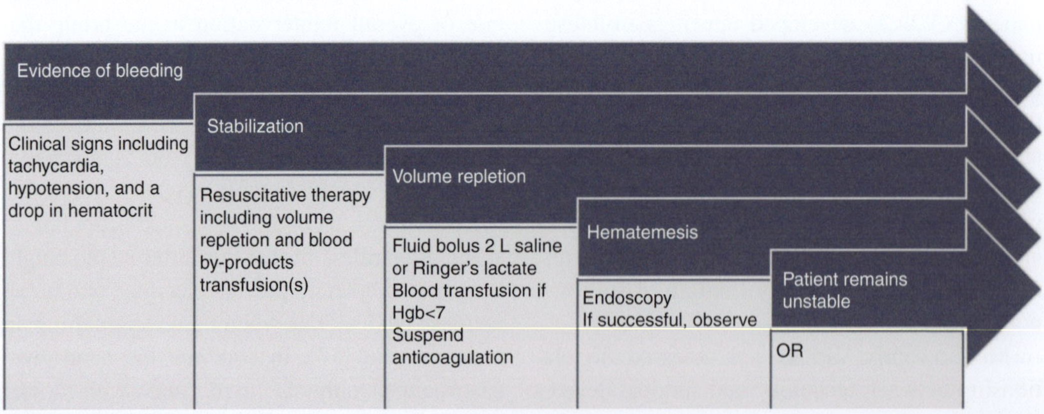

Fig. 27.1 Once the bleeding is first diagnosed, the patient need to be resuscitated and stabilized from an hemodynamic standpoint. Based on the hemodynamic status and the location of the bleeding, the definitive treatment can be done either endoscopically or surgically

As previously mentioned, the specific intervention is dictated by the type of bleeding, location, and patient's hemodynamics. Details of the operative technique (i.e., open vs. laparoscopic approach, technique of gastrojejunostomy, staple line reinforcement, Roux limb length, concomitant surgeries performed) have not been associated with the different rates of bleeding, and the therapy should be tailored to the suspected location of hemorrhage [66]. Intraluminal bleeding in anatomical areas accessible by endoscopy can be treated with such intervention. As shown in small series, staple line bleeding from the proximal gastric pouch has been effectively and safely managed with minimal dose epinephrine injections and electrocautery [51, 69, 70]. Overall, endoscopic therapies available have proven to be beneficial. However, the following findings, especially when multiple of them are present, might indicate the need for reoperation [69, 71, 72]:

- Heart rate > 100 beats/min
- Decrease in systolic blood pressure < 10 mmHg
- Persistent tachycardia
- More than 2 units of blood transfusions
- Presence of melena
- Presence of hematemesis

Ischemia of the tip on the alimentary limb involving the gastrojejunostomy is an unusual complication during Roux-en-Y gastric bypass. Revision of the anastomosis may be needed to manage this complication [73]. Recently, the increasing number of publications regarding indocyanine green (ICG) angiography favors this tool to be recognized as a relevant aid for the surgeon's naked eye when dealing with gastrointestinal anastomosis. After ICG intravenous injection, the surgeon switches the camera's white light to near-infrared light by clicking the pedal. A fluorescent image of the ICG traversing the vessels through the limb wall glows brightly when the organ is well-perfused. Both gastric and small bowel stumps can have real-time perfusion assessment by this simple technique. Further studies are necessary to evaluate if changes in the resection line after ICG fluorescence angiography are sufficient to prevent ischemia followed by leaks in the GJ anastomosis [74–76].

Recovery Room

Patients with obesity have a greater risk of hypoxia in the postoperative period, when compared to nonobese patients, due to physiologic changes. Therefore, following extubation, some measures may be used to main adequate oxygenation, such as administration of oxygen by face mask or nasal cannula; positioning patient in head up, which means sitting or semi-sitting, or lateral position; and the use of incentive spirometry as well as chest physiotherapy. These conditions improve pulmonary function, especially incentive spirometry, decreasing the rate of postoperative complications [77].

Conclusion

Scarce literature is found regarding perioperative complications during Roux-en-Y gastric bypass. To the best of our knowledge, this is the first attempt to divide the subject by anesthetic, access, transection, pouch creation, anastomosis, and recovery room complications. Here, we present a robust review pursuing assistance to surgeons for a better decision-making with respect to difficult situations and how to manage urgent issues in the perioperative period. The focus is to bring light to the most frequent complications and the rare ones for a skillful and accelerated resolution.

References

1. Adams JP, Murphy PG. Obesity in anaesthesia and intensive care. Br J Anaesth. 2000;85:91–108.
2. Bamgbade OA, Rutter TW, Nafiu OO, Dorje P. Postoperative complications in obese and nonobese patients. World J Surg. 2007;31:556–60.
3. Soleimanpour H, Safari S, Sanaie S, Nazari M, Alavian SM. Anesthetic considerations in patients undergoing bariatric surgery: a review article. Anesth Pain Med. 2017;7:e57568.

4. Leoni A, Arlati S, Ghisi D, et al. Difficult mask ventilation in obese patients: analysis of predictive factors. Minerva Anestesiol. 2014;80:149–57.
5. De Jong A, Molinari N, Pouzeratte Y, et al. Difficult intubation in obese patients: incidence, risk factors, and complications in the operating theatre and in intensive care units. Br J Anaesth. 2015;114:297–306.
6. Juvin P, Lavaut E, Dupont H, Lefevre P, Demetriou M, Dumoulin J-L, Desmonts J-M. Difficult tracheal intubation is more common in obese than in lean patients. Anesth Analg. 2003;97:595–600, table of contents.
7. Lundstrøm LH, Møller AM, Rosenstock C, Astrup G, Wetterslev J. High body mass index is a weak predictor for difficult and failed tracheal intubation: a cohort study of 91,332 consecutive patients scheduled for direct laryngoscopy registered in the Danish Anesthesia Database. Anesthesiology. 2009;110:266–74.
8. Tuncalı B, Pekcan YÖ, Ayhan A, Erol V, Yılmaz TH, Kayhan Z. Retrospective evaluation of patients who underwent laparoscopic bariatric surgery. Turk J Anaesthesiol Reanim. 2018;46:297–304.
9. Aslani A, Ng S-C, Hurley M, McCarthy KF, McNicholas M, McCaul CL. Accuracy of identification of the cricothyroid membrane in female subjects using palpation: an observational study. Anesth Analg. 2012;114:987–92.
10. Berthoud MC, Peacock JE, Reilly CS. Effectiveness of preoxygenation in morbidly obese patients. Br J Anaesth. 1991;67:464–6.
11. Hu XY. Effective ventilation strategies for obese patients undergoing bariatric surgery: a literature review. AANA J. 2016;84:35–45.
12. Lang LH, Parekh K, Tsui BYK, Maze M. Perioperative management of the obese surgical patient. Br Med Bull. 2017;124:135–55.
13. Thornqvist C, Gislason GH, Køber L, Jensen PF, Torp-Pedersen C, Andersson C. Body mass index and risk of perioperative cardiovascular adverse events and mortality in 34,744 Danish patients undergoing hip or knee replacement. Acta Orthop. 2014;85:456–62.
14. De Jong A, Verzilli D, Geniez M, Chanques G, Nocca D, Jaber S. Why is the morbidly obese patient at high risk of anesthetic complications? Presse Med. 2018;47:453–63.
15. Desciak MC, Martin DE. Perioperative pulmonary embolism: diagnosis and anesthetic management. J Clin Anesth. 2011;23:153–65.
16. Rodgers A (2000) Reduction of postoperative mortality and morbidity with epidural or spinal anaesthesia: results from overview of randomised. BMJ. 321:1493–1493.
17. Mao Y, Wen S, Chen G, Zhang W, Ai Y, Yuan J. Management of intra-operative acute pulmonary embolism during general anesthesia: a case report. BMC Anesthesiol. 2017;17:67.
18. Bartlett MA, Mauck KF, Daniels PR. Prevention of venous thromboembolism in patients undergoing bariatric surgery. Vasc Health Risk Manag. 2015;11:461–77.
19. Numata Y, Ishii K, Seki H, Yasui N, Sakata M, Shimada A, Matsumoto H. Perforation of abdominal esophagus following nasogastric feeding tube intubation: a case report. Int J Surg Case Rep. 2018;45:67–71.
20. Martines G, Digennaro R, De Fazio M, Capuano P. Endoscopic management of esophageal perforation caused by calibrating bougie during laparoscopic sleeve gastrectomy. Case Stud Surg. 2017;3:13.
21. Theodorou D, Doulami G, Larentzakis A, Almpanopoulos K, Stamou K, Zografos G, Menenakos E. Bougie insertion: a common practice with underestimated dangers. Int J Surg Case Rep. 2012;3:74–7.
22. Sundbom M, Hedberg J, Wanhainen A, Ottosson J. Aortic injuries during laparoscopic gastric bypass for morbid obesity in Sweden 2009-2010: a nationwide survey. Surg Obes Relat Dis. 2014;10:203–7.
23. Kosuta M, Palmisano S, Piccinni G, Guerrini J, Giuricin M, Nagliati C, Casagranda B, de Manzini N. Safety of Veress needle insertion in laparoscopic bariatric surgery. Surg Laparosc Endosc Percutan Tech. 2014;24:e1–4.
24. Krishnakumar S, Tambe P. Entry complications in laparoscopic surgery. J Gynecol Endosc Surg. 2009;1:4–11.
25. Shirk GJ, Johns A, Redwine DB. Complications of laparoscopic surgery: how to avoid them and how to repair them. J Minim Invasive Gynecol. 2006;13:352–9.
26. Fernández EML-T, Malagón AM, Arteaga I, Díaz H, Carrillo A. Conservative treatment of a huge abdominal wall hematoma after laparoscopic appendectomy. J Laparoendosc Adv Surg Tech A. 2005;15:634–7.
27. Sandadi S, Johannigman JA, Wong VL, Blebea J, Altose MD, Hurd WW. Recognition and management of major vessel injury during laparoscopy. J Minim Invasive Gynecol. 2010;17:692–702.
28. Twine CP, Lane IF, Williams IM. The retroperitoneal approach to the abdominal aorta in the endovascular era. J Vasc Surg. 2012;56:834–8.
29. Lee M-GM, Provost DA, Jones DB. Use of fibrin sealant in laparoscopic gastric bypass for the morbidly obese. Obes Surg. 2004;14:1321–6.
30. Abu-Amara M, Akle C, Adiseshiah M. Blind peritoneal access during laparoscopy: why is it still being used? Int Surg. 2009;94:201–4.
31. Kayaalp C, Yilmaz S, Aydin C, Piskin T. Massive subcutaneous emphysema involving the head and neck after laparoscopic Roux-en-Y gastric by-pass. Eur J Surg Sci. 2010;1:71–4.
32. Clements RH, Reddy S, Holzman MD, Sharp KW, Olsen D, Holcomb GW, Richards WO. Incidence and significance of pneumomediastinum after

laparoscopic esophageal surgery. Surg Endosc. 2000;14:553–5.
33. Berthoud HR, Neuhuber WL. Functional and chemical anatomy of the afferent vagal system. Auton Neurosci. 2000;85:1–17.
34. Wang Y, Liu J. Combination of bypassing stomach and vagus dissection in high-fat diet-induced obese rats-a long-term investigation. Obes Surg. 2010;20:375–9.
35. Perathoner A, Weiss H, Santner W, Brandacher G, Laimer E, Höller E, Aigner F, Klaus A. Vagal nerve dissection during pouch formation in laparoscopic Roux-Y-gastric bypass for technical simplification: does it matter? Obes Surg. 2009;19:412–7.
36. Kral JG, Görtz L, Hermansson G, Wallin GS. Gastroplasty for obesity: long-term weight loss improved by vagotomy. World J Surg. 1993;17:75–8. discussion 79
37. Bueter M, Löwenstein C, Ashrafian H, Hillebrand J, Bloom SR, Olbers T, Lutz T, le Roux CW. Vagal sparing surgical technique but not stoma size affects body weight loss in rodent model of gastric bypass. Obes Surg. 2010;20:616–22.
38. Frantzides CT, Carlson MA, Shostrom VK, Roberts J, Stavropoulos G, Ayiomamitis G, Frantzides A. A survey of dumping symptomatology after gastric bypass with or without lesser omental transection. Obes Surg. 2011;21:186–93.
39. Peters TG, Steinmetz SR, Cowan GS Jr. Splenic injury and repair during bariatric surgical procedures. South Med J. 1990;83:166–9.
40. Baker RS, Foote J, Kemmeter P, Brady R, Vroegop T, Serveld M. The science of stapling and leaks. Obes Surg. 2004;14:1290–8.
41. Silecchia G, Iossa A. Complications of staple line and anastomoses following laparoscopic bariatric surgery. Ann Gastroenterol Hepatol. 2018;31:56–64.
42. Sanchez BS, Safadi BY, Kieran JA, Hsu GP, Brodsky JB, Curet MJ, Morton JM. Orogastric tube complications in laparoscopic Roux-en-Y gastric bypass. Obes Surg. 2006;16:443–7.
43. Abu-Gazala S, Donchin Y, Keidar A. Nasogastric tube, temperature probe, and bougie stapling during bariatric surgery: a multicenter survey. Surg Obes Relat Dis. 2012;8:595–600. discussion 600–1.
44. Higa G, Szomstein S, Rosenthal R. Stapling of orogastric tube during gastrojejunal anastomosis: an unusual complication after conversion of sleeve gastrectomy to laparoscopic Roux-en-Y gastric bypass. Surg Obes Relat Dis. 2012;8:116–8.
45. Podnos YD, Jimenez JC, Wilson SE, Stevens CM, Nguyen NT. Complications after laparoscopic gastric bypass: a review of 3464 cases. Arch Surg. 2003;138:957–61.
46. Nguyen NT, Wilson SE. Complications of antiobesity surgery. Nat Clin Pract Gastroenterol Hepatol. 2007;4:138–47.
47. Ghosh SK, Roy S, Chekan E, Fegelman EJ. A narrative of intraoperative staple line leaks and bleeds during bariatric surgery. Obes Surg. 2016;26:1601–6.
48. Madan AK, Martinez JM, Lo Menzo E, Khan KA, Tichansky DS. Omental reinforcement for intraoperative leak repairs during laparoscopic Roux-en-Y gastric bypass. Am Surg. 2009;75:839–42.
49. Aiolfi A, Tornese S, Bonitta G, Rausa E, Micheletto G, Bona D. Roux-en-Y gastric bypass: systematic review and Bayesian network meta-analysis comparing open, laparoscopic, and robotic approach. Surg Obes Relat Dis. 2019; https://doi.org/10.1016/j.soard.2019.03.006.
50. Alasfar F, Chand B. Intraoperative endoscopy for laparoscopic Roux-en-Y gastric bypass: leak test and beyond. Surg Laparosc Endosc Percutan Tech. 2010;20:424–7.
51. Jamil LH, Krause KR, Chengelis DL, Jury RP, Jackson CM, Cannon ME, Duffy MC. Endoscopic management of early upper gastrointestinal hemorrhage following laparoscopic Roux-en-Y gastric bypass. Am J Gastroenterol. 2008;103:86–91.
52. Varban OA, Cassidy RB, Sheetz KH, Cain-Nielsen A, Carlin AM, Schram JL, Weiner MJ, Bacal D, Stricklen A, Finks JF. Technique or technology? Evaluating leaks after gastric bypass. Surg Obes Relat Dis. 2016;12:264–72.
53. Arnold W, Shikora SA. A comparison of burst pressure between buttressed versus non-buttressed staple-lines in an animal model. Obes Surg. 2005;15:164–71.
54. Mery CM, Shafi BM, Binyamin G, Morton JM, Gertner M. Profiling surgical staplers: effect of staple height, buttress, and overlap on staple line failure. Surg Obes Relat Dis. 2008;4:416–22.
55. Pinheiro JS, Correa JL, Cohen RV, Novaes JA, Schiavon CA. Staple line reinforcement with new biomaterial increased burst strength pressure: an animal study. Surg Obes Relat Dis. 2006;2:397–9.
56. Silecchia G, Boru CE, Mouiel J, et al. The use of fibrin sealant to prevent major complications following laparoscopic gastric bypass: results of a multicenter, randomized trial. Surg Endosc. 2008;22:2492–7.
57. Acquafresca PA, Palermo M, Rogula T, Duza GE, Serra E. Early surgical complications after gastric by-pass: a literature review. Arq Bras Cir Dig. 2015;28:74–80.
58. Jiang H-P, Lin L-L, Jiang X, Qiao H-Q. Meta-analysis of hand-sewn versus mechanical gastrojejunal anastomosis during laparoscopic Roux-en-Y gastric bypass for morbid obesity. Int J Surg. 2016;32:150–7.
59. Greenstein AJ, Wahed AS, Adeniji A, et al. Prevalence of adverse intraoperative events during obesity surgery and their sequelae. J Am Coll Surg. 2012;215:271–7.e3.
60. Schauer PR, Ikramuddin S, Gourash W, Ramanathan R, Luketich J. Outcomes after laparoscopic Roux-en-Y gastric bypass for morbid obesity. Ann Surg. 2000;232:515–29.
61. Nguyen NT, Longoria M, Chalifoux S, Wilson SE. Gastrointestinal hemorrhage after laparoscopic gastric bypass. Obes Surg. 2004;14:1308–12.

62. Website. Podnos YD, Jimenez JC, Wilson SE, et al. Complications after laparoscopic gastric bypass: a review of 3464 cases. ArchSurg 2003;138:957–961. Accessed 22 Mar 2019.
63. Dillemans B, Sakran N, Van Cauwenberge S, et al. Standardization of the fully stapled laparoscopic Roux-en-Y gastric bypass for obesity reduces early immediate postoperative morbidity and mortality: a single center study on 2606 patients. Obes Surg. 2009;19:1355–64.
64. Bellorin O, Abdemur A, Sucandy I, Szomstein S, Rosenthal RJ. Understanding the significance, reasons and patterns of abnormal vital signs after gastric bypass for morbid obesity. Obes Surg. 2011;21:707–13.
65. Abeles D, Kim JJ, Tarnoff ME, Shah S, Shikora SA. Primary laparoscopic gastric bypass can be performed safely in patients with BMI ≥ 60. J Am Coll Surg. 2009;208:236–40.
66. Rabl C, Peeva S, Prado K, James AW, Rogers SJ, Posselt A, Campos GM. Early and late abdominal bleeding after Roux-en-Y gastric bypass: sources and tailored therapeutic strategies. Obes Surg. 2011;21:413–20.
67. Dick A, Karl Byrne T, Baker M, Budak A, Morgan K. Gastrointestinal bleeding after gastric bypass surgery: nuisance or catastrophe? Surg Obes Relat Dis. 2010;6:643–7.
68. Nguyen NT, Rivers R, Wolfe BM. Early gastrointestinal hemorrhage after laparoscopic gastric bypass. Obes Surg. 2003;13:62–5.
69. Mehran A, Szomstein S, Zundel N, Rosenthal R. Management of acute bleeding after laparoscopic Roux-en-Y gastric bypass. Obes Surg. 2003;13:842–7.
70. Fernández-Esparrach G, Bordas JM, Pellisé M, et al. Endoscopic management of early GI hemorrhage after laparoscopic gastric bypass. Gastrointest Endosc. 2008;67:552–5.
71. Barkun AN, Bardou M, Kuipers EJ, Sung J, Hunt RH, Martel M, Sinclair P, International Consensus Upper Gastrointestinal Bleeding Conference Group. International consensus recommendations on the management of patients with nonvariceal upper gastrointestinal bleeding. Ann Intern Med. 2010;152:101–13.
72. García-Iglesias P, Villoria A, Suarez D, Brullet E, Gallach M, Feu F, Gisbert JP, Barkun A, Calvet X. Meta-analysis: predictors of rebleeding after endoscopic treatment for bleeding peptic ulcer. Aliment Pharmacol Ther. 2011;34:888–900.
73. Mittal T, Dey A, Nali A, Taha Mustafa SM, Malik VK. Alimentary limb ischemia during Roux-en-Y gastric bypass and its management. Obes Surg. 2018;28:1458.
74. Degett TH, Andersen HS, Gögenur I. Indocyanine green fluorescence angiography for intraoperative assessment of gastrointestinal anastomotic perfusion: a systematic review of clinical trials. Langenbeck's Arch Surg. 2016;401:767–75.
75. Ohi M, Toiyama Y, Mohri Y, et al. Prevalence of anastomotic leak and the impact of indocyanine green fluorescein imaging for evaluating blood flow in the gastric conduit following esophageal cancer surgery. Esophagus. 2017;14:351–9.
76. Alemanno G, Somigli R, Prosperi P, Bergamini C, Maltinti G, Giordano A, Valeri A. Combination of diagnostic laparoscopy and intraoperative indocyanine green fluorescence angiography for the early detection of intestinal ischemia not detectable at CT scan. Int J Surg Case Rep. 2016;26:77–80.
77. Thomas JA, McIntosh JM. Are incentive spirometry, intermittent positive pressure breathing, and deep breathing exercises effective in the prevention of postoperative pulmonary complications after upper abdominal surgery? A systematic overview and meta-analysis. Phys Ther. 1994;74:3–10. discussion 10–6.

Abdominal Pain After Gastric Bypass

28

Alexander Charles Morrell, André Luiz Gioia Morrell, Alexander Charles Morrell Jr., and Allan Gioia Morrell

Obesity is currently a worldwide public health problem, both in developed and emerging countries, especially in the Western world [1]. According to the World Health Organization, 600 million of obese adults around the world are estimated, besides a population of almost 2 billion people in overweight status. Nevertheless, obesity is not uncommonly accompanied by other comorbidities, such as type 2 diabetes mellitus, systemic arterial hypertension, cardiovascular disease, obstructive sleep apnea, and even some neoplasms, which in association with obesity almost always culminate in a drop in quality and a lower expectation of life [2–5].

Given the relevance of the topic and the ineffectiveness of the clinical treatment in some cases, bariatric surgery has gained space as a treatment option, proving to be a safe and reliable way for long-term weight loss and improvement or complete remission of comorbidities [6–9]. Among surgical options, RYGB currently represents approximately 47–49% of bariatric procedures [10] and morbidity and mortality at 30 days of 3–4% and 0.2–0.3%, respectively [8, 11].

Therefore, like any other surgery, the RYGB contemplates its risks and complications associated with the procedure, which we will discuss later. For a better understanding, the surgical complications of the procedure are divided between early and late, being the precocious occurring from the hospital discharge period to the surgical 30 postoperative (PO) and the late postoperative periods from 31 postoperative onward.

Not infrequently, the patients submitted to this type of surgery return to the hospital with complaints, which can reach up to 17.3% of the cases in 90 days. Match et al. [12] reported that PS complaints by patients previously submitted to bariatric surgery considered abdominal pain as the most prevalent symptom (24.4%) followed by nausea and vomiting (20.8%). In addition, it quotes as risk factors for hospital return the young patient, female sex, and associated comorbidities.

Thus, abdominal pain in patients previously submitted to RYGB is a frequent event, ranging from simple events to difficult and potentially life-threatening diagnoses [13–15].

Early Abdominal Pain

The picture of early abdominal pain in the patient after RYGB is one that occurs up to 30 PO. Among the most common affections, we have anastomosis dehiscence, portomesenteric

A. C. Morrell (✉)
General Surgery/Bariatric and Metabolic Surgery/Robotic Surgery, Sociedade Beneficente Israelita Brasileira Hospital Albert Einstein, São Paulo, SP, Brazil

A. L. G. Morrell · A. C. Morrell Jr. · A. G. Morrell
General Surgery/Bariatric and Metabolic Surgery, Sociedade Beneficente Israelita Brasileira Hospital Albert Einstein, São Paulo, SP, Brazil

J. Ettinger et al. (eds.), *Gastric Bypass*, https://doi.org/10.1007/978-3-030-28803-7_28

thrombosis, early intestinal obstruction, and hernia secondary to laparoscopic puncture site.

Fistula

Fistula is one of the most feared complications of bariatric surgeons, which, together with pulmonary thromboembolism, comprise the main causes of procedure-related mortality [21, 23]. It is estimated the occurrence of fistulas between 0.6 and 1% in the RYGB procedures, and most of them occur early, around the first week [29]. Regarding clinical factors, in a multivariate analysis cited by Fernandez et al. [22], high age, male gender, and multiple comorbidities were quoted as risk factors for fistula occurrence. However, the technique itself, conventional open surgery, as well as revision surgery are also risk factors for the appearance of this complication, while the use of linear or circular staplers for confection of the gastrojejunal anastomosis is still controversial [21, 24].

The clinical presentation is variable, which in initial and mild cases may present only by temperature increase, tachycardia>120 bpm, or respiratory discomfort, whereas in the more exuberant forms, they develop abdominal pain and rapid progression to sepsis [25]. The use of routine tests in the upper gastrointestinal tract in the recent postoperative period for the detection of fistulas has only 22% efficacy according to Hamilton et al. [25] and computed tomography about 56% of the diagnostic success [26].

In order to perform two anastomoses and stapling in this surgery, the fistula sites may be diverse. Gonzalez et al. [26] described 49% of them occurring in the gastrojejunal anastomosis, 25% in the excluded stomach, 13% in the jejunojejunal anastomosis, and 9% in the gastric pouch, while Ballesta et al. [27] cited up to 67.8% of them in the gastrojejunal anastomosis and only 3.4% in the excluded stomach.

The treatment of fistulas can be done both conservatively and surgically, depending mainly on the hemodynamic stability and absence of signs of sepsis of the patient. In nonsurgical management, fluid drainage and monitoring by drains in the anastomotic sites, intravenous broad-spectrum antibiotic and oral fasting, and optional enteral nutrition are the bases of treatment. Csendes et al. [28] in a study of conservative treatment of fistulas present in patients submitted to RYGB even quoted management without antibiotic therapy and described the closure of the fistula next to the 30th postoperative day. In selected cases, endoscopic prosthesis placement may be a conservative treatment option (Fig. 28.1a, b). If hemodynamic instability or clinical deterioration of the patient is present during conservative treatment, early surgical approach is indicated, with thorough washing

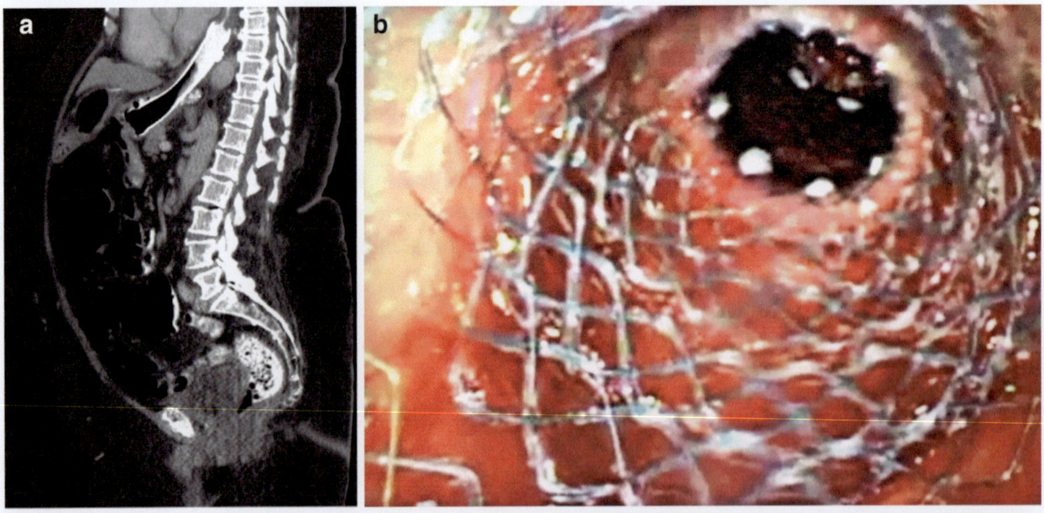

Fig. 28.1 (**a**) CT scan with endoscopic prosthesis inserted for fistula treatment. (**b**) Endoscopic aspect of metalic prosthesis

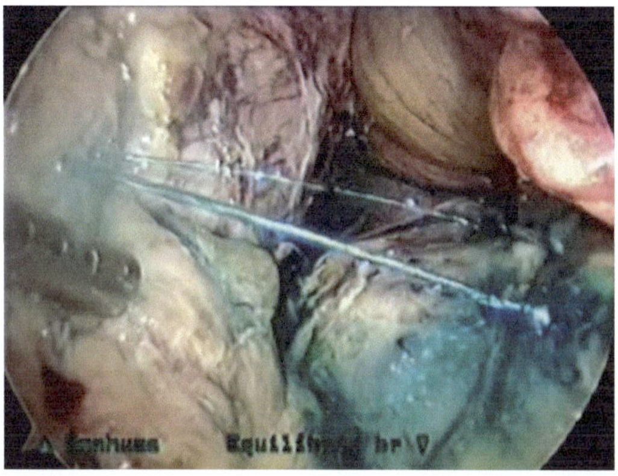

Fig. 28.2 Intraoperative aspect when perfoming positive methylene blue test aiming a better of fistulous area

of the abdominal cavity followed by drainage of the fistulous site or even possibly repair in anastomosis defects or clamp line (Fig. 28.2).

Portomesenteric Thrombosis

Portomesenteric thrombosis is a term referring to partial or total obstruction of the portal vein and/or mesenteric veins, being uncommon but potentially lethal and described after laparoscopic procedures [17]. In the scope of bariatric procedures, although more commonly found after vertical gastrectomies (sleeve gastrectomy), estimating their incidence by up to 1%, according to Salinas et al. [18], is a possible complication and present in the cases of RYGB, described by James et al. [19]. The clinical presentation is variable and can contemplate since abdominal pain issues are associated with nausea or even behave asymptomatic. Not infrequently, the condition occurs in patients with other predispositions to thromboembolic events other than obesity, such as protein S deficiency or presence of Leiden Factor V, mostly unknown before the procedure [19, 20]. The diagnosis can be made by computed tomography with oral and intravenous contrast, identifying the thrombosis in a portomesenteric region of variable extension. The treatment is performed through anticoagulation; however, the presence of peritoneal irritation or ischemia and intestinal necrosis demands an immediate surgical approach.

Early Intestinal Obstruction

Although it is an event that often presents later, intestinal obstruction can also occur in early PO. In a prospective study with more than 2000 patients, Shimizu et al. [16] described 0.5% of patients with obstructive symptoms in the first few days, with the mean of presenting them on the 5th postoperative day. The most frequent symptoms were nausea and vomiting (54%), followed by abdominal pain (45%). In the study, all cases were diagnosed by computed tomography with oral contrast, and the treatment was variable due to different obstructive etiologies (twisting of the jejunojejunal anastomosis, intraluminal clot next to jejunojejunal anastomosis, hematomas, previous pelvic adhesions), mostly performed by new surgical approach (Figs. 28.3 and 28.4).

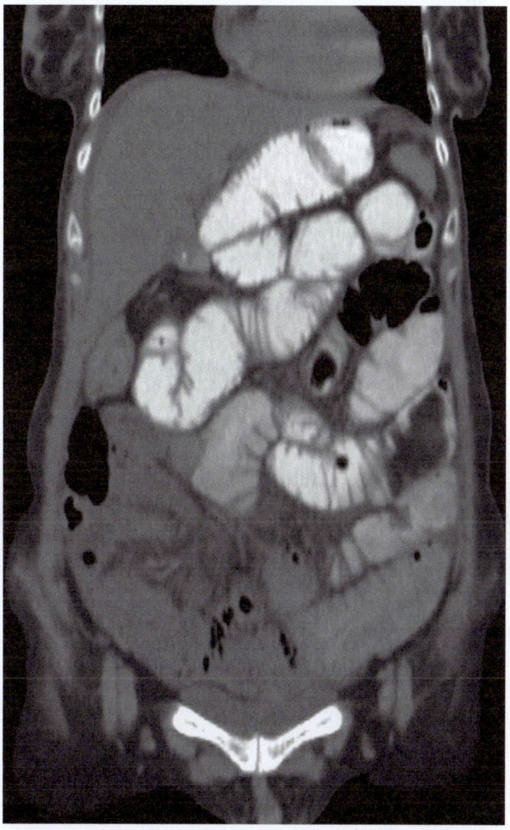

Fig. 28.3 Abdominal CT scan with small bowel obstruction, with orally administered contrast. Dilated bowel containing fluid associated to descompressed small bowel distal to the point of obstruction

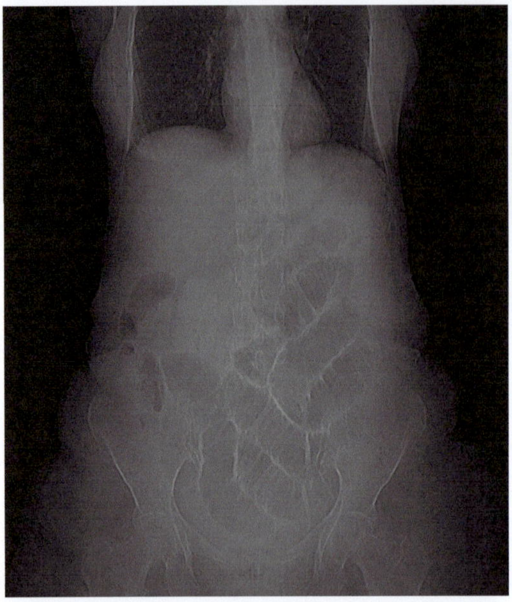

Fig. 28.4 Abdominal radiograph with predominantly centrally dilated loops of small bowel in an early postoperative patient

Early obstruction is associated with technical problems, especially in anastomosis confections, different from those presented late, which are mostly secondary to intra-abdominal adhesions or internal hernias.

Hernia in Trocar Sites

The hernias in place of puncture of trocars are possible complications in any laparoscopic procedure, and for that reason it is recommended by numerous studies the routine closure of these defects of the aponeurosis in punches equal or greater than 10 mm. In the obese patient, seen the fact greater intra-abdominal fat tissue, the aponeurotic closure is considerably more difficult and thus being sometimes ignored by surgeons [31]. An incidence of up to 0.5% of hernias at puncture sites is estimated in all laparoscopic procedures, and in a recent study, Coblijn et al. described 0.52% of their incidence in patients after bariatric procedures.

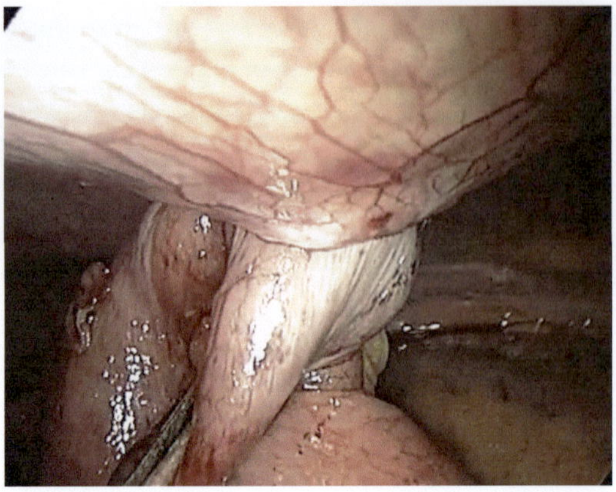

Fig. 28.5 Laparoscopic visualization of a small bowel herniating into the port trocar site

Clinically, these hernias may manifest early, and it is even described that half of them will occur up to the first postoperative month by Helgstrand et al. [31]. It frequently presents as mild abdominal pain, which can complicate with strangulation in 0.2–1% of procedures or even dramatic situations of gangrene and intestinal necrosis described by Losanoff et al. [32].

Another form of presentation is later in the course of abdominal discomfort and nausea and may even be a cause of intestinal obstruction; however, the strangulation of the hernia content in late forms is rare [33].

Although authors report the possibility of simple reduction of the hernia into the cavity under anesthesia [30], the laparoscopic approach to evaluation of the hernia content and its viability followed by correction of the aponeurotic defect contemplates a safer option as treatment (Fig. 28.5).

Late Abdominal Pain

The abdominal discomfort frames of the 30th postoperative day are set as late. Its causes may be diverse, and among them, we will discuss more about remnant gastric distension, anastomotic stenoses, marginal ulcer, cholelithiasis, intestinal obstructions, and internal hernias.

Remnant Gastric Distension

It is a rarer picture secondary to RYGB, however, with a high degree of morbidity if not diagnosed early. With the creation of the gastric pouch, much of the stomach becomes excluded from the food traffic, which constitutes a hollow viscus with a blind bottom. Thus, paralytic ileus or mechanical obstructions distal to the bile loop may result in distension to the excluded stomach, which progressively dilates and may progress to rupture, culminating in gastric secretion in the peritoneal cavity with severe peritonitis described by Papasavas et al. [34].

Clinically, the condition may present only with abdominal distension or discomfort in the upper abdomen; however, special care should be taken if an episode of sudden pain occurs, especially in the upper left quadrant, which may suggest perforation. The diagnosis can be suggested in abdominal radiographs with significant distension of the gastric bubble and better visualized on tomographic examination of the abdomen, already evaluating whether there is presence of pneumoperitoneum and possible perforation site in 86% of the exams [35].

Treatment consists primarily of decompression of the site, most often by performing percutaneous gastrostomy. In cases of suspected perforation or failure of percutaneous decompression, the early surgical approach is the best option [36].

Anastomotic Stenosis

Gastric stenosis in RYGB occurs in 3–27% of cases, and its pathophysiology is still not well defined [37]. It is believed that some factors, such as the use of staplers in the anastomosis and the type used, influence on its occurrence. It is estimated a greater chance of stenosis in the use of circular stapler <21 mm than linear or manual anastomosis [38]. In addition, other aspects such as anastomosis tension, hemodynamic stability, submucosal hematoma, or anastomosis fistula may influence its occurrence [39, 43].

Its appearance may be either early, associated with technical error or bleeding in the region most often, or later, around 8 weeks of PO; the latter is notoriously more frequent. It should be suspected mainly in patients who complain of abdominal discomfort, dysphagia or nausea, and vomiting associated with feeding and may even present symptoms of reflux [38].

Its diagnosis can be made more commonly by upper digestive endoscopy, defined as endoscopic resistance or inability to pass through the anastomotic region, which suggests a light <10 mm [40, 41], or by the use of routine tests in the upper gastrointestinal tract (Fig. 28.6a, b).

The treatment alternatives for stenosis are basically two: endoscopic dilatation and surgical re-boarding. Endoscopic dilatation is a procedure

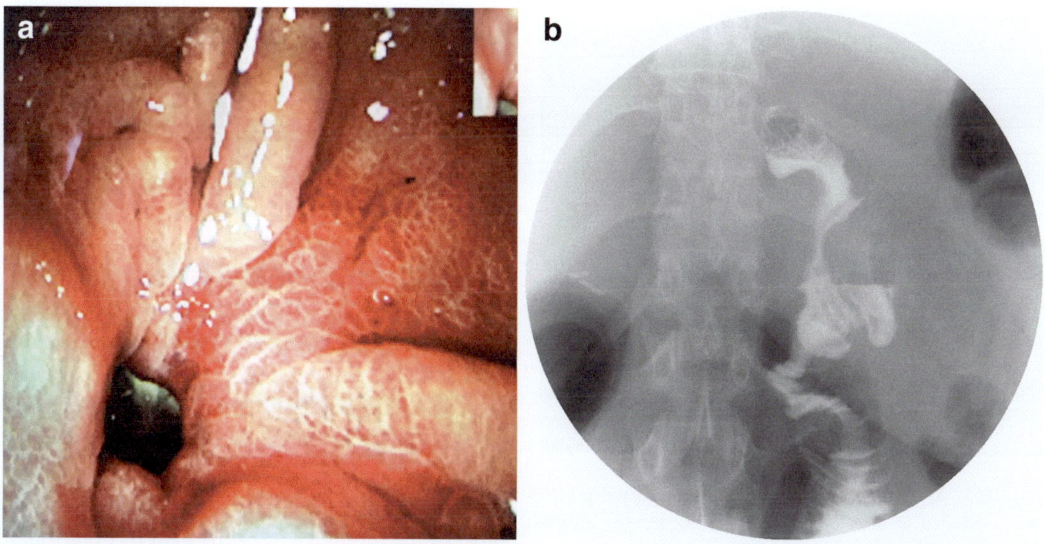

Fig. 28.6 (**a**) Endoscopic visualization of gastrojejunal stenosis (**b**) Contrast radiography revealing GJ stricture

known as safe, often requiring only one or two approaches, and there is no need for hospitalization [38]. Possible complication of dilatation is perforation; however, its incidence is small, ranging from 2 to 5% [37]. If the endoscopic procedure fails, the new surgical approach becomes an option, which can be done in a conventional or laparoscopic way (0.4%) [42].

Marginal Ulcer

Marginal ulcer or ischemic ulcer is a potentially fatal complication in RYGB postoperative, with incidence in the literature ranging from 0.6 to 16%. According to Sverden et al. [44], in a recent study, the presence of type 2 DM, previous history of peptic ulcer, and use of acetylsalicylic acid and NSAIDs are risk factors presenting it as complication in the PO. Its appearance is often close to the gastrojejunal anastomosis, and its pathophysiology is still not well defined; however, it is believed that jejunal lesion resulting from acid secretion is not uncommon presenting it concomitantly with gastro-gastric fistula [46] (Fig. 28.7). Some other causes that may be associated with ulcers are *H. pylori* infection, smoking, presence of foreign body in the site as unabsorbable wires, or tissue ischemia by tense anastomosis [45] (Fig. 28.8a, b).

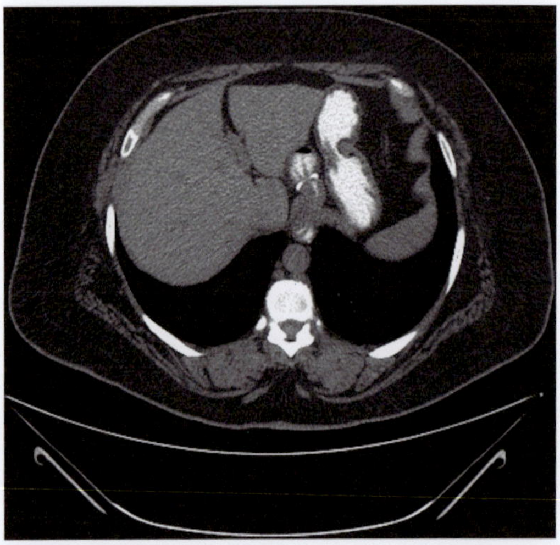

Fig. 28.7 Abdominal CT scan showing the gastric pouch and excluded stomach both enchanced by the orally administered contrast

The most common clinical features are abdominal pain, nausea, and vomiting [47], and bleeding in the gastrointestinal tract may be present [46]. Although a large portion of the patients exhibit the complaints previously described, a considerable portion of individuals remain asymptomatic to the condition [48]. Its definitive diagnosis is confirmed by digestive endoscopy, examination of choice in the suspected diagnosis.

Treatment of the marginal ulcer can be performed conservatively through gastric acid suppression and association of sucralfate, and it is successful in 95% of the patients [49]. In addition to drug therapy, it is recommended to suspend the use of NSAIDs and to encourage cessation of smoking in pertinent individuals. In patients positive for *H. pylori*, its eradication with antibiotic therapy and acid suppression is also recommended. In cases of urgency such as perforation or other associated complications such as gastrogastric fistula, persistent pain, or drug therapy fails, surgical treatment becomes indicated.

Cholelithiasis

Cholelithiasis is a common disease, especially in Western countries, often associated with obesity, through the formation of cholesterol stones [50]. Rapid weight loss is also strongly associated with the appearance of stones, especially in females [51]. Sugerman et al. [53] in a prospective multicenter study documented the reduction in the incidence of cholelithiasis after RYGB to 2% in the prophylactic use of UDCA (ursodeoxycholic acid) for 6 months after procedure.

It is estimated that cholelithiasis appearance in 30–36% of patients undergoing bariatric surgery in the first 6 months post-surgery and up to 41% of this group may be symptomatic [29, 52], being susceptible to choledocholithiasis, cholecystitis, cholangitis, and acute pancreatitis. In biliary colic presentations, there is abdominal pain, most commonly located in the upper abdomen or right hypochondrium, and may be associated with nausea and vomiting. Findings like jaundice or fever can be signs of complication. Most of the diagnosis is performed by abdominal

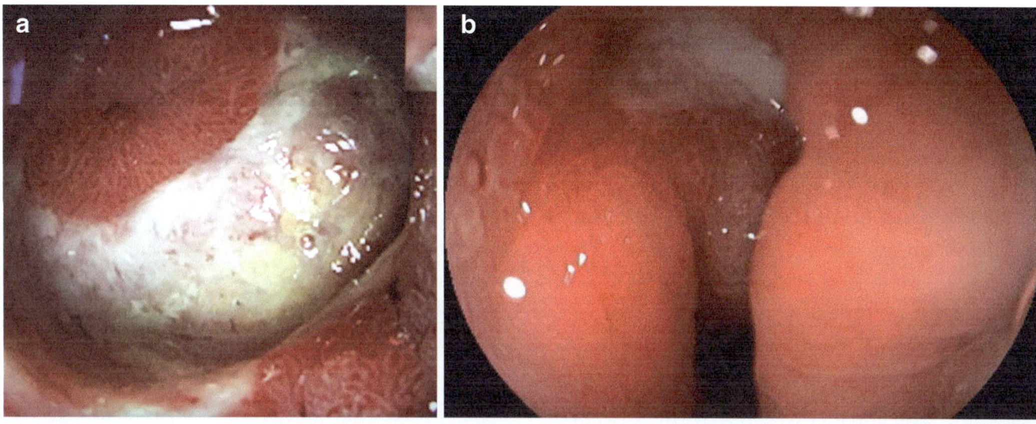

Fig. 28.8 Endoscopic aspects of a marginal ulcer

ultrasound examination with sensitivity of 84% and specificity of 99% [54]; in case of diagnostic doubt, one may choose MRCP (magnetic resonance cholangiopancreatography).

Treatment in the case of symptomatic cholelithiasis or cholecystitis is surgical, through laparoscopic cholecystectomy. Whether or not prophylactic cholecystectomy is performed during the bariatric procedure is controversial [29]. However, in cases of choledocholithiasis or cholangitis, altered digestive anatomy can turn the treatment into challenging cases, since they cannot access the biliary tract with endoscopic examination [55], needing it to be performed surgically or by transparetohepatic drainage.

Incisional Hernia

Incisional hernias in the RYGB range from 0 to 1.8% in laparoscopic procedures and up to 20% in the conventional open form, according to the literature [56, 57]. Their appearance often occurs with bulging in the region of the surgical incision, which worsens with cough or physical activity, associated with abdominal pain, and may or may not have obstructive symptoms.

The diagnosis is made clinically, through history and physical examination; however, in diagnosis doubt, especially in obese patients, the use of computed tomography can help (Fig. 28.9). There is no clinical treatment for incisional hernias.

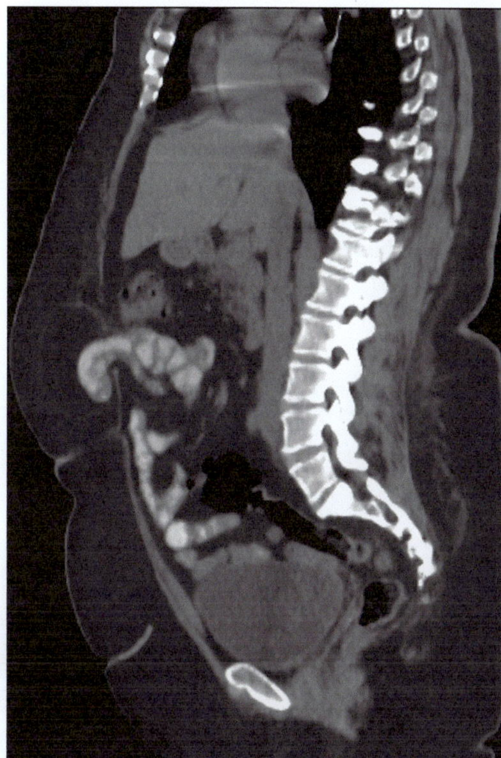

Fig. 28.9 Abdominal CT scan exhibiting a small bowel herniating through the abdominal wall defect

Internal Hernia

Internal hernias are extremely important occurrences in patients undergoing bariatric surgeries, especially in cases of RYGB. The incidence ranges from 1 to 6% in the literature [58, 61] and is the major cause responsible for intestinal obstruction in the postoperative period of RYGB [59, 60]. When making the anastomoses and creating both alimentary and biliopancreatic loops, the formation of three mesenteric defects will occur in the transmesocolic cases and two defects in the pre-colic cases. These defects are identified in the jejunojejunal anastomosis region, in the space between the transverse mesocolon and the mesentery of the loop taken for gastrojejunal anastomosis, and, in the cases of transmesocolic loops, in the open defect for transposition of the intestine to the upper abdomen region. It is believed that most cases of internal hernia occur in the region of the transverse mesocolon defect in the transmesocolic approaches, and thus, a pre-colic anastomosis could reduce this incidence [61, 62, 64]. Closure of the mesenteric defect and Petersen's space is intented to lower incidence of internal hernias and its mandatoriness is still debatable; however, Higa et al. [57], in a prospective study, discuss the importance of closure of defects with unabsorbable suture, and the incidence in these cases is significantly lower.

The clinical presentation is with acute abdominal discomfort in up to 75% of the cases; however, a large part of the patients have abdominal pain of intermittent or chronic course and may or may not be associated with obstructive conditions [65]. Computed tomography may be a diagnostic tool for some cases; however, it is estimated that up to 45% of them shows no significant changes. The presence of the "mesenteric swirl" sign is the most relevant finding, being a strong predictor of internal hernia [63]. In cases of significant clinical suspicion of internal hernia even without consistent radiographic findings, laparoscopy is extremely valuable and may be diagnostic and therapeutic (Fig. 28.10a, b).

The treatment of the cases is mostly surgical, and this will depend on the intraoperative findings. In the absence of alteration of the perfusion of the involved loops, the reduction of the hernia and closure of the mesenteric defect may be sufficient; however, if the viability of the involved loops is doubtful, segment resection followed by intestinal anastomosis should be performed.

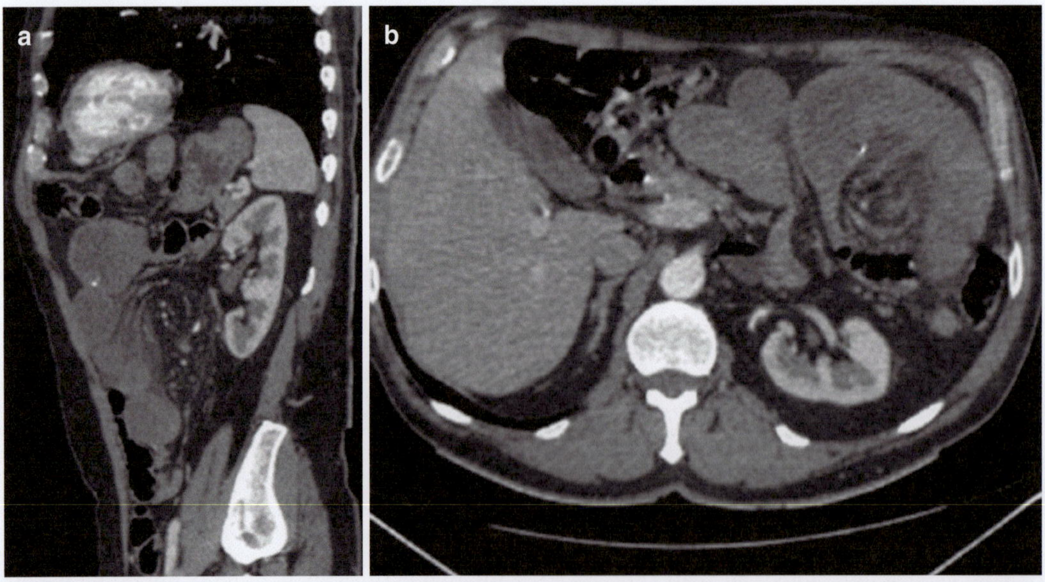

Fig. 28.10 Abdominal CT scan showing an anterior displacement of DJ flexure, in addition to rotation of the mesenteric vessels

Less Frequent Conditions Post-RYGB

Not only the events described above are likely to be seen as complications in patients undergoing RYGB. Other less frequent causes described in the literature may also present with abdominal discomfort, although they are of lesser relevance in usual medical practice.

Intestinal intussusception is described in up to 0.4% of patients and is often associated with pain in the upper abdomen region, which may or may not be accompanied by nausea and vomiting [66]. Computed tomography examination may be useful in diagnosis; however, in most cases diagnosis is performed intraoperatively. The reduction of the loop should be made and depending on its viability should be resected followed by an anastomosis.

In a case report, Sujka et al. [67] describe the occurrence of cecal volvulus as a cause of abdominal pain following patients after RYGB. In all cases the presentation was late, after 2 years of procedure, and presented significant weight loss after the procedure. Frederiksen et al. [14] also in a case report describe torsion of the mesentery as a cause of late abdominal pain in the follow-up of post-RYGB patients.

Nonsurgical conditions may also be responsible for the discomfort, such as the dumping syndrome, which diverges from its prevalence in the literature, from 16 to 34% [68, 69]. Symptoms are secondary to intestinal distension and vasoactive reflexes triggered by the osmotic mechanism and should be carefully evaluated to distinguish them from surgical etiologies.

References

1. Flegal KM, Carroll MD, Ogden CL, Johnson CL. Prevalence and trends in obesity among US adults, 1999-2000. JAMA. 2002;288:1723.
2. Ng M, Fleming T, Robinson M, et al. Global, regional, and national prevalence of overweight and obesity in children and adults during 1980-2013: a systematic analysis for the Global Burden of Disease Study 2013. Lancet. 2014;384:766.
3. Swinburn BA, Sacks G, Hall KD, et al. The global obesity pandemic: shaped by global drivers and local environments. Lancet. 2011;378:804.
4. http://www.who.int/mediacentre/factsheets/fs311/en/.
5. Bray GA, Bellanger T. Epidemiology, trends, and morbidities of obesity and the metabolic syndrome. Endocrine. 2006;29:109–17.
6. Karlsen TI, Lund RS, Roislien J, Tonstad S, Natvig GK, Sandbu R, Hjelmesaeth J. Health related quality of life after gastric bypass or intensive lifestyle intervention: a controlled clinical study. Health Qual Life Outcomes. 2013;11:17.
7. Sears D, Fillmore G, Bui M, Rodriguez J. Evaluation of gastric bypass patients 1 year after surgery: changes in quality of life and obesity-related conditions. Obes Surg. 2008;18:1522–5.
8. Flum DR, Belle SH, King WC, et al. Perioperative safety in the longitudinal assessment of bariatric surgery. N Engl J Med. 2009;361(5):445–54.
9. Shah M, Simha V, Garg A. Review: long-term impact of bariatric surgery on body weight, comorbidities, and nutritional status. J Clin Endocrinol Metab. 2006;91(11):4223–31.
10. Buchwald H, Oien DM. Metabolic/bariatric surgery worldwide 2011. Obes Surg. 2013;23:427.
11. Lancaster RT, Hutter MM. Bands and bypasses: 30-day morbidity and mortality of bariatric surgical procedures as assessed by prospective, multicenter, risk-adjusted ACS-NSQIP data. Surg Endosc. 2008;22(12):2554–63. https://doi.org/10.1007/s00464-008-0074-y. Epub 2008 Sep 20.
12. Macht R, George J, Ameli O, Hess D, Cabral H, Kazis L. Factors associated with bariatric postoperative emergency department visits. Surg Obes Relat Dis. 2016. pii: S1550-7289(16)00084-8. https://doi.org/10.1016/j.soard.2016.02.038.[Epub ahead of print].
13. Alsulaimy M, Dorsey A, Sethi S, Schauer PR, Aminian A. Encapsulated omental necrosis after Roux-en-Y gastric bypass. Surg Obes Relat Dis. 2016;12(4):919–20. https://doi.org/10.1016/j.soard.2016.02.011. Epub 2016 Feb 18.
14. Frederiksen SG, Ekelund M. Mesenteric torsion as a cause of late abdominal pain after gastric bypass surgery. Obes Surg. 2016;26(4):896–9. https://doi.org/10.1007/s11695-015-2042-7.
15. Sima E, Hedberg J, Sundbom M. Gastrointestinal symptoms, weight loss and patient satisfaction 5 years after gastric bypass: a study of three techniques for the gastrojejunal anastomosis. Surg Endosc. 2016;30(4):1553–8. https://doi.org/10.1007/s00464-015-4374-8. Epub 2015 Jul 11.
16. Shimizu H, Maia M, Kroh M, Schauer PR, Brethauer SA. Surgical management of early small bowel obstruction after laparoscopic Roux-en-Y gastric bypass. Surg Obes Relat Dis. 2013;9(5):718–24. https://doi.org/10.1016/j.soard.2012.05.009. Epub 2012 Jun 21
17. Noh KW, Wolfsen HC, Bridges MD, Hinder RA. Mesenteric vein thrombosis after laparoscopic anti reflux surgery. Dig Dis Sci. 2007;52(1):273–5.
18. Salinas J, Barros D, Salgado N, Viscido G, Funke R, Pe´rez G, Pimentel F, Boza C. Portomesenteric vein thrombosis after laparoscopic sleeve gastrectomy. Surg Endosc. 2014;28:1083–9.

19. James AW, Rabl C, Westphalen AC, Fogarty PF, Posselt AM, Campos GM. Portomesenteric venous thrombosis after laparoscopic surgery: a systematic literature review. Arch Surg. 2009;144(6):520–6. https://doi.org/10.1001/archsurg.2009.81.
20. El Lakis MA, Pozzi A, Chamieh J, Safadi B. Portomesenteric vein thrombosis after laparoscopic sleeve gastrectomy and laparoscopic Roux-en-Y gastric bypass: a 36-case series. Surg Endosc. 2016.[Epub ahead of print].
21. Smith MD, Adeniji A, Wahed AS, Patterson E, Chapman W, Courcoulas AP, Dakin G, Flum D, McCloskey C, Mitchell JE, Pomp A, Staten M, Wolfe B. Technical factors associated with anastomotic leak after Roux-en-Y gastric bypass. Surg Obes Relat Dis. 2015;11(2):313–20. https://doi.org/10.1016/j.soard.2014.05.036. Epub 2014 Nov 8.
22. Fernandez AZ Jr, EJ DM, Tichansky DS, Kellum JM, Wolfe LG, Meador J, Sugerman HJ. Experience with over 3,000 open and laparoscopic bariatric procedures: multivariate analysis of factors related to leak and resultant mortality. Surg Endosc. 2004;18(2):193–7. Epub 2003 Dec 29.
23. Melinek J, Livingston E, Cortina G, Fishbein MC. Autopsy findings following gastric bypass surgery for morbid obesity. Arch Pathol Lab Med. 2002;126(9):1091–5.
24. Sima E, Hedberg J, Ehrenborg A, Sundbom M. Differences in early complications between circular and linear stapled gastrojejunostomy in laparoscopic gastric bypass. Obes Surg. 2014;24(4):599–603. https://doi.org/10.1007/s11695-013-1139-0.
25. Hamilton EC, Sims TL, Hamilton TT, Mullican MA, Jones DB, Provost DA. Clinical predictors of leak after laparoscopic Roux-en-Y gastric bypass for morbid obesity. Surg Endosc. 2003;17(5):679–84. Epub 2003 Mar 7.
26. Gonzalez R, Sarr MG, Smith CD, Baghai M, Kendrick M, Szomstein S, Rosenthal R, Murr MM. Diagnosis and contemporary management of anastomotic leaks after gastric bypass for obesity. J Am Coll Surg. 2007;204(1):47–55. Epub 2006 Nov 17.
27. Ballesta C, Berindoague R, Cabrera M, Palau M, Gonzales M. Management of anastomotic leaks after laparoscopic Roux-en-Y gastric bypass. Obes Surg. 2008;18(6):623–30. https://doi.org/10.1007/s11695-007-9297-6. Epub 2008 Apr 8.
28. Csendes A, Burdiles P, Burgos AM, Maluenda F, Diaz JC. Conservative management of anastomotic leaks after 557 open gastric bypasses. Obes Surg. 2005;15(9):1252–6.
29. Monkhouse SJ, Morgan JD, Norton SA. Complications of bariatric surgery: presentation and emergency management--a review. Ann R Coll Surg Engl. 2009;91(4):280–6. https://doi.org/10.1308/003588409X392072. Epub 2009 Apr 2.
30. Coblijn UK, de Raaff CA, van Wagensveld BA, van Tets WF, de Castro SM. Trocar port hernias after bariatric surgery. Obes Surg. 2016;26(3):546–51. https://doi.org/10.1007/s11695-015-1779-3.
31. Helgstrand F, Rosenberg J, Bisgaard T. Trocar site hernia after laparoscopic surgery: a qualitative systematic review. Hernia. 2011;15(2):113–21. https://doi.org/10.1007/s10029-010-0757-x. Epub 2010 Dec 9.
32. Losanoff JE, Richman BW, Jones JW. Trocar-site hernia complicated by necrotizing fasciitis--case report and review of the literature. Hernia. 2003;7(4):220–3. Epub 2003 Apr 10.
33. Tonouchi H, Ohmori Y, Kobayashi M, Kusunoki M. Trocar site hernia. Arch Surg. 2004;139(11):1248–56.
34. Papasavas PK, Yeaney WW, Caushaj PF, Keenan RJ, Landreneau RJ, Gagné DJ. Perforation in the bypassed stomach following laparoscopic Roux-en-Y gastric bypass. Obes Surg. 2003;13(5):797–9.
35. Hainaux B, Agneessens E, Bertinotti R, De Maertelaer V, Rubesova E, Capelluto E, Moschopoulos C. Accuracy of MDCT in predicting site of gastrointestinal tract perforation. AJR Am J Roentgenol. 2006;187(5):1179–83.
36. Gagner M, Gentileschi P, de Csepel J, Kini S, Patterson E, Inabnet WB, Herron D, Pomp A. Laparoscopic reoperative bariatric surgery: experience from 27 consecutive patients. Obes Surg. 2002;12(2):254–60.
37. Kumbhari V, Tieu AH, Ngamruengphong S, Aguila G, Schweitzer MA, Khashab MA, Singh VK. Endoscopic management of stomal stenosis after Roux-en-Y gastric bypass. Gastrointest Endosc. 2015;82(4):747. https://doi.org/10.1016/j.gie.2015.05.032. Epub 2015 Jun 25.
38. Espinel J, Pinedo E. Stenosis in gastric bypass: endoscopic management. World J Gastrointest Endosc. 2012;4(7):290–5. https://doi.org/10.4253/wjge.v4.i7.290.
39. de-la-Cruz-Vigo F, de-la-Cruz-Vigo JL. Stenosis in gastric bypass for morbid obesity. [aArticle in English, Spanish]. Rev Esp Enferm Dig. 2010;102(3):151–8.
40. Wetter A. Role of endoscopy after Roux-en-Y gastric bypass surgery. Gastrointest Endosc. 2007;66(2):253–5.
41. Lee JK, Van Dam J, Morton JM, Curet M, Banerjee S. Endoscopy is accurate, safe, and effective in the assessment and management of complications following gastric bypass surgery. Am J Gastroenterol. 2009;104(3):575–82; quiz 583. Epub 2009 Feb 3. https://doi.org/10.1038/ajg.2008.102.
42. Rosenthal RJ. Dilating the stenotic gastrojejunostomy after laparoscopic Roux-en-Y gastric bypass for morbid obesity: when things go wrong. J Gastrointest Surg. 2009;13(9):1561–3. https://doi.org/10.1007/s11605-009-0860-4. Epub 2009 Mar 19.
43. Elder KA, Wolfe BM. Bariatric surgery: a review of procedures and outcomes. Gastroenterology. 2007;132(6):2253–71.
44. Sverdén E, Mattsson F, Sondén A, Leinsköld T, Tao W, Lu Y, Lagergren J. Risk factors for marginal ulcer after gastric bypass surgery for obesity: a population-based cohort study. Ann Surg. 2016;263(4):733–7. https://doi.org/10.1097/SLA.0000000000001300.

45. Sapala JA, Wood MH, Sapala MA, Flake TM Jr. Marginal ulcer after gastric bypass: a prospective 3-year study of 173 patients. Obes Surg. 1998;8(5):505–16.
46. Chau E, Youn H, Ren-Fielding CJ, Fielding GA, Schwack BF, Kurian MS. Surgical management and outcomes of patients with marginal ulcer after Roux-en-Y gastric bypass. Surg Obes Relat Dis. 2015;11(5):1071–5. https://doi.org/10.1016/j.soard.2014.12.011. Epub 2014 Dec 19.
47. Jordan JH, Hocking MP, Rout WR, Woodward ER. Marginal ulcer following gastric bypass for morbid obesity. Am Surg. 1991;57(5):286–8.
48. Gumbs AA, Duffy AJ, Bell RL. Incidence and management of marginal ulceration after laparoscopic Roux-Y gastric bypass. Surg Obes Relat Dis. 2006;2(4):460–3.
49. Sanyal AJ, Sugerman HJ, Kellum JM, Engle KM, Wolfe L. Stomal complications of gastric bypass: incidence and outcome of therapy. Am J Gastroenterol. 1992;87(9):1165–9.
50. Friedman GD, Kannel WB, Dawber TR. The epidemiology of gallbladder disease: observations in the Framingham Study. J Chronic Dis. 1966;19(3):273–92.
51. Liddle RA, Goldstein RB, Saxton J. Gallstone formation during weight-reduction dieting. Arch Intern Med. 1989;149(8):1750–3.
52. Shiffman ML, Sugerman HJ, Kellum JM, Brewer WH, Moore EW. Gallstone formation after rapid weight loss: a prospective study in patients undergoing gastric bypass surgery for treatment of morbid obesity. Am J Gastroenterol. 1991;86(8):1000–5.
53. Sugerman HJ, Brewer WH, Shiffman ML, Brolin RE, Fobi MA, Linner JH, MacDonald KG, MacGregor AM, Martin LF, Oram-Smith JC, et al. A multicenter, placebo-controlled, randomized, double-blind, prospective trial of prophylactic ursodiol for the prevention of gallstone formation following gastric-bypass-induced rapid weight loss. Am J Surg. 1995;169(1):91–6; discussion 96–7.
54. Shea JA, Berlin JA, Escarce JJ, Clarke JR, Kinosian BP, Cabana MD, Tsai WW, Horangic N, Malet PF, Schwartz JS, et al. Revised estimates of diagnostic test sensitivity and specificity in suspected biliary tract disease. Arch Intern Med. 1994;154(22):2573–81.
55. Wright BE, Cass OW, Freeman ML. ERCP in patients with long-limb Roux-en-Y gastrojejunostomy and intact papilla. Gastrointest Endosc. 2002;56(2):225–32.
56. Nguyen NT, Goldman C, Rosenquist CJ, Arango A, Cole CJ, Lee SJ, Wolfe BM. Laparoscopic versus open gastric bypass: a randomized study of outcomes, quality of life, and costs. Ann Surg. 2001;234(3):279–89. discussion 289-91.
57. Higa KD, Boone KB, Ho T. Complications of the laparoscopic Roux-en-Y gastric bypass: 1,040 patients--what have we learned? Obes Surg. 2000;10(6):509–13.
58. Steele KE, Prokopowicz GP, Magnuson T, Lidor A, Schweitzer M. Laparoscopic antecolic Roux-en-Y gastric bypass with closure of internal defects leads to fewer internal hernias than the retrocolic approach. Surg Endosc. 2008;22(9):2056–61. https://doi.org/10.1007/s00464-008-9749-7. Epub 2008 Feb 13.
59. Gunabushanam G, Shankar S, Czerniach DR, Kelly JJ, Perugini RA. Small-bowel obstruction after laparoscopic Roux-en-Y gastric bypass surgery. J Comput Assist Tomogr. 2009;33(3):369–75. https://doi.org/10.1097/RCT.0b013e31818803ac.
60. Husain S, Ahmed AR, Johnson J, Boss T, O'Malley W. Small-bowel obstruction after laparoscopic Roux-en-Y gastric bypass: etiology, diagnosis, and management. Arch Surg. 2007;142(10):988–93.
61. Higa KD, Ho T, Boone KB. Internal hernias after laparoscopic Roux-en-Y gastric bypass: incidence, treatment and prevention. Obes Surg. 2003;13(3):350–4.
62. Al Harakeh AB, Kallies KJ, Borgert AJ, Kothari SN. Bowel obstruction rates in antecolic/antegastric versus retrocolic/retrogastric Roux limb gastric bypass: a meta-analysis. Surg Obes Relat Dis. 2016;12(1):194–8. https://doi.org/10.1016/j.soard.2015.02.004. Epub 2015 Feb 11
63. Al-Saeed O, Fahmy D, Kombar O, Hasan A. Sixty-four-slice multidetector computerized tomography in the evaluation of transmesenteric internal hernias following Roux-en-Y bariatric surgery. Med Princ Pract. 2013;22:540–4. https://doi.org/10.1159/000351616. Epub 2013 Aug 8.
64. Iannelli A, Buratti MS, Novellas S, Dahman M, Amor IB, Sejor E, Facchiano E, Addeo P, Gugenheim J. Internal hernia as a complication of laparoscopic Roux-en-Y gastric bypass. Obes Surg. 2007;17(10):1283–6.
65. Al-Mansour MR, Mundy R, Canoy JM, Dulaimy K, Kuhn JN, Romanelli J. Internal hernia after laparoscopic antecolic Roux-en-Y gastric bypass. Obes Surg. 2015;25(11):2106–11. https://doi.org/10.1007/s11695-015-1672-0.
66. Stephenson D, Moon RC, Teixeira AF, Jawad MA. Intussusception after Roux-en-Y gastric bypass. Surg Obes Relat Dis. 2014;10(4):666–70. https://doi.org/10.1016/j.soard.2014.01.026. Epub 2014 Jan 30
67. Sujka J, Teixeira AF, Jawad MA. Suspected cecal volvulus as a reason for abdominal pain after gastric bypass: a case series. Surg Obes Relat Dis. 2015;11(4):978–9. https://doi.org/10.1016/j.soard.2015.04.010. Epub 2015 Apr 23.
68. Cawley J, Sweeney MJ, Kurian M, Beane S. New York State Bariatric Surgery Workgroup. Predicting complications after bariatric surgery using obesity-related co-morbidities. Obes Surg. 2007;17(11):1451–6.
69. Lee CJ, Clark JM, Schweitzer M, Magnuson T, Steele K, Koerner O, Brown TT. Prevalence of and risk factors for hypoglycemic symptoms after gastric bypass and sleeve gastrectomy. Obesity (Silver Spring). 2015;23(5):1079–84. https://doi.org/10.1002/oby.21042. Epub 2015 Apr 10.

Marginal Ulceration After (Laparoscopic) Roux-en-Y Gastric Bypass: Pathophysiology, Diagnostics, Treatment, and Prevention

29

U. K. Coblijn, B. A. van Wagensveld, S. M. Lagarde, and S. M. M. de Castro

Introduction

Marginal ulceration (MU) is defined as an ulcer at or next to the gastrojejunostomy occurring mostly after (laparoscopic) Roux-en-Y gastric bypass ((L) RYGB) (Fig. 29.1). In the medical literature, two other synonyms are frequently used to describe this ulcer: an ischemic ulcer and anastomotic ulcer. In this chapter we will refer to this type of ulcer as "marginal ulcer." A MU is a possible serious complication, which occurs in 0.6 till 16% of all patients after (L)RYGB [1–5]. Even though several new procedures such as sleeve gastrectomy are increasingly being performed, (L)RYGB remains one of the most frequent performed procedures worldwide, and this is not anticipated to change over time. As the number of performed procedures increases due to its successes [6] and the increase of patients with morbid obesity [7], a subsequent rise in the absolute number of patients with a MU will be expected. A MU can develop into a potentially severe and even lethal complication due to asymptomatic progression resulting in massive bleeding or a perforation [8–10]. The present chapter will focus on the present knowledge about the pathophysiology, diagnosis, and treatment of MU after (L)RYGB. The last part of the chapter will discuss the prevention of MU.

U. K. Coblijn (✉)
Department of Surgery, Vrije Universiteit Medical Center, Amsterdam, The Netherlands

B. A. van Wagensveld · S. M. M. de Castro
Department of Surgery, Onze Lieve Vrouwe Gasthuis, Amsterdam, The Netherlands

S. M. Lagarde
Department of Surgery, Erasmus Medical Center, Rotterdam, The Netherlands

Incidence

The incidence of MU is widespread through the literature and, as already mentioned, ranges from 0.6 till 16 percent in different studies [2, 5]. Most studies focus on the incidence of symptomatic MU, e.g., patients who present with complaints of MU such as epigastric burn and abdominal pain. However, two studies looked at the overall incidence of MU. One performed a gastroscopy 1 month and 2 years after surgery in all patients who underwent gastric bypass surgery. They found an incidence of 4.1% in the first month, which decreased to 0.5% after 2 years. The other study performed a gastroscopy at 3 months after surgery and found an incidence of 7.6% [3, 11].

On daily notice, symptoms are important to identify MU; however, in the previous cited study of Garrido et al., all patients with MU at endoscopy (7.6%) were asymptomatic [11]. It could be hypothesized that those ulcers were still more superficial due to the early detection by standard

J. Ettinger et al. (eds.), *Gastric Bypass*, https://doi.org/10.1007/978-3-030-28803-7_29

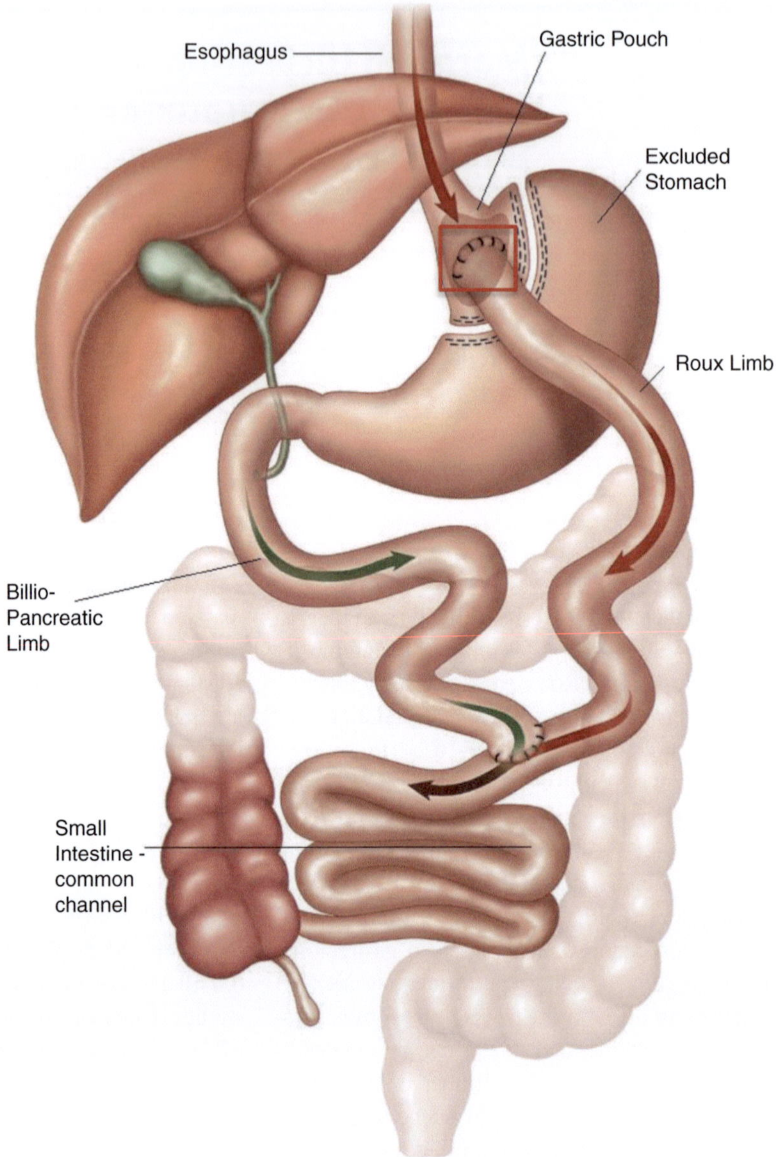

Fig. 29.1 Roux-en-Y gastric bypass and the marginal ulcer location. (Adapted from: [49])

endoscopy and therefore less prone to cause symptoms, but it does show the sometimes asymptomatic nature of MU.

A review published in 2013 found, with all studies combined, a mean incidence of MU around 4.6% throughout the years. Considering the time in which a MU is likely to develop, it can be shortly after surgery (within the first month) or even years after [12]. The mean time till development of a MU was around 14 months [13]. Due to the difference in development interval, it can be hypothesized that a different pathophysiology exists in early and late MUs.

Pathophysiology and Risk Factors

Most likely the pathophysiology of the development of MU is multifactorial and can be different per case.

Anatomy

In the early 1990s, Capella et al. discovered that the anatomic location of the pouch is associated with MU. The hypothesis is that the anatomic location corresponds with the concentration of the parietal cells in the stomach. The concentration of parietal cells is highest in the antrum of the stomach, whereas more proximal they virtually disappear. Therefore, patients with a large, less proximal pouch have a higher risk for MU because a part of the antrum, with the high incidence of parietal cells, is included [14]. In contrast, the more proximal the pouch, the lower the incidence of MU [15–17]. If a (L)RYGB is performed with a micropouch, the incidence of MU decreases [18, 19].

All the above and the introduction of the laparoscopic technique to perform a gastric bypass contributed to a standardized approach for pouch formation in (L)RYGB [19, 20].

However, the place and size of the pouch are not the only explanation as studies performing a 24 h pH measurement in the pouch show that around 10% of the time, the pH is still below 4 even though the pouch is oriented in the most proximal part of the stomach, causing exposure of the vulnerable jejunal mucosa to gastric acid [21, 22]. Furthermore, a dilated gastric pouch may be predisposed to late marginal ulceration because of the increased number of parietal cells [23, 24]. The low pH can be used as a potential target for prophylactic therapies such as a short course of proton pump inhibitors or H_2 antagonists [25, 26]. Some surgeons advocate prophylactic vagotomy in patients undergoing (L)RYGB in order to reduce the amount of acid in the pouch [4, 27].

Type of Procedure and Surgical Technique

As found in the earlier mentioned systematic review of 2013, no difference in the incidence of MU can be found in open versus laparoscopic RYGB. There are reports suggesting that the type of suture material and technique of creating the anastomosis could be of importance in the risk for developing a MU [25, 28]. Factors such as suture material and anatomic location could influence the incidence of a MU. Capella et al. found that using staples to create the anastomosis increased the risk on postoperative MU if this was compared to the use of absorbable suture materials [1, 29, 30]. Suture materials were found at endoscopy and performed to diagnose MU, in almost a third of the patients [2, 14].

Another hypothesis is that local ischemia at the anastomosis increases the risk of MU development as its synonym, ischemic ulcer, indicates. Therefore, tension at the gastrojejunal anastomosis is considered to increase the risk on MU apart from the risk on anastomotic leakage.

Some patients develop gastro-gastric fistulae (i.e., fistula between remnant stomach and pouch) as a complication, of which the first sign can be a MU, possibly caused by more acid in the pouch due to the fistulae [14]. However, the pathophysiology may also be the other way around in which a MU causes a fistula.

H. pylori

The contribution of *H. pylori* infection to the development of MU is questionable, as in contrast to its importance in the development of "normal" peptic ulcer disease. Even more, no evidence exists linking the presence of *H. pylori* to the development of MU. It seems that patients who developed MU after LRYGB were not infected with *H. pylori* at the time of their diagnosis as shown by Suggs et al. where all the 23 patients who developed a MU tested negative for *H. pylori* serology [31].

In some clinics, every patient who is scheduled for gastric bypass surgery is screened for the presence of *H. pylori*. The incidence of preoperative infection with MU is between 22% and 67% [32–34]. Even though MU might not be associated with *H. pylori*, it is advised to test for its presence prior to surgery due to the association of *H. pylori* with gastric cancer in the general population. After (L)RYGB the remnant stomach is left in situ without easy endoscopic access for early diagnosis of possible gastric cancer [19, 35].

Patient Demographics

Many studies have looked for potential modifiable patient associated risk factors associated with MU. Several studies looked into different medications and their influence on the development of MU. For nonsteroidal anti-inflammatory drugs (NSAIDS), it is known that by means of the inhibition of COX-2 in the general population, they increase the risk for peptic ulcer disease [36, 37]. The association between MU and NSAIDS is also seen in most studies with patients after (L)RYGB [12, 13, 38]. Also patients who use (inhalation) corticosteroids seem to have an increased risk for developing a MU [12, 13]. The presence of diabetes mellitus, hypertension, and obstructive sleep apnea does not seem to correlate with the development of MU [12, 27]. The use of tobacco predisposed for the development of MU as shown by Wilson et al. and different other studies [13, 38]. Some clinics require their patients to quit smoking prior to surgery. The pathogenesis of tobacco in the development of MU is unknown; it is thought that with the vasoconstriction caused by tobacco, local ischemia at the anastomosis increases which subsequently predisposes for MU.

Symptomatology and Diagnostics

Although the symptomatology of MU differs in every patient, most people suffer from abdominal pain or epigastric burn, especially prior to eating, and nausea [11, 27, 39]. However, some patients have no symptoms at all until they present with a sudden perforation or severe bleeding [8, 9]. NSAIDS or anticoagulation use increases the risks of severe bleeding from a marginal ulcer. In the general population, the use of anticoagulants (aspirin or vit. K antagonists) is usually combined with proton pump inhibitor (PPI) treatment, and this should also be done in bariatric surgery patients.

The incidence of perforated MU is around 1–2% of the total bariatric population, therefore around 6–7% of all the patients with MU [10, 13, 40]. Patients who present with a perforated MU can present with a septic profile and severe abdominal pain due to the leakage of stomach contents into the peritoneal cavity [9].

Diagnostics of choice in the elective setting is upper endoscopy, during which a corpus alienum, if applicable, can be removed [3, 38, 39]. When a perforation is suspected, an X-ray or CT scan can be the (easy accessible) diagnostics of choice as those patients might be septic and quick management is required.

Treatment

A MU can be treated conservatively with PPIs or needs invasive treatment with endoscopy and sometimes surgery. If possible, the treatment of choice is conservative therapy. When diagnosed with a MU without acute symptoms such as sepsis, severe pain, or bleeding, the initial treatment should start with PPIs (two times daily), combined with Sucralfate® for relief of symptoms such as epigastric burn. No evidence exists that intravenously proton pump inhibitor treatment is preferable compared to oral therapy. Cessation of risk factors such as smoking and using NSAIDs, corticosteroids, or anticoagulants is mandatory [13, 41]. The systematic review of 2013 indicates that over two thirds of the patients with MU can be successfully treated with PPIs, H_2 antagonists, Sucralfate®, or a combination of these [12, 42].

The other 1/3 patients often need treatment by endoscopic interventions or surgery. Especially patients with recurrent ulcers may benefit from endoscopic removal of a corpus alienum (e.g., suture material or staples) from the ulcer bed.

Some patients need surgery to be cured of their ulcers as conservative treatment fails or in an acute situation. Most of the patients who undergo surgery are those with a perforation (around 6.7% of all MU presentations), with significant bleeding which cannot be cured with a PPI, with gastro-gastric fistulae (to treat the fistulae, when the fistulae are resected, the pH of the pouch will increase and the MU will heal), or with retractable ulcers [10, 42–44]. Most revisions can be performed laparoscopically, which is equally effective and safe compared to the open procedures. During the revisional procedure, the (sometimes dilated) pouch is partially resected and reconstructed, and a new anastomosis is created (Fig. 29.2).

Prevention

Since Capella et al. showed the importance of preoperative pouch formation in preventing marginal ulceration [1], the procedure of pouch formation has been standardized. This pouch is created in the lesser curvature of the stomach using one horizontal and two vertical firings of a 45 mm linear stapler. Special attention should be paid to the posterior part of the pouch as this is easily left to large when posterior adhesions are

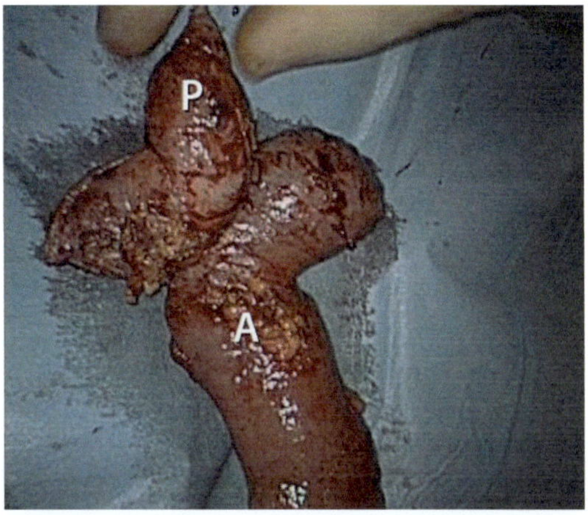

Fig. 29.2 The resected dilated part of the pouch (P) and alimentary limb (A) including anastomotic ulcer (not visible from the outside) after resection. (Ref. [24])

not properly removed. Guideline for pouch size is around 15 till 30 milliliters.

Some authors advocate a standard gastroscopy around 6 weeks to 3 months after surgery to inspect the pouch and remove any remnant sutures which could cause a MU [45]. Multiple studies found a decrease in ulcer formation if absorbable suture were used instead of staples [1, 28]. However, the large meta-analysis of Jiang et al., published in 2016, did not find an association. The study did show that a hand-sewn anastomosis was associated with less postoperative bleeding and wound infection compared to a stapled one [46]. Csendes et al. investigated the role of remnant stomach evacuation in prevention of MU and found that with the remnant stomach in situ, the incidence of MU was 12.3%, whereas with the remnant stomach removed, the incidence was 4.1%. However, up until now, this did not change the operative procedure since removal of the remnant stomach increases majority and thereby the risk of surgery. All patients in the study of Csendes et al. underwent postoperative endoscopy independent of the presence or absence of any symptoms [3]. This effect of removal of the remnant stomach is probably due to the subsequent absence of acid production in the remnant stomach, caused by the hormonal feedback mechanism, autonomous of usage of the (remnant) stomach.

All patients should be encouraged preoperatively to stop smoking [38]. Patients who use NSAIDs should stop using these, and alternatives should be prescribed if possible. The same should be done for patients who use corticosteroids or anticoagulants. If it is impossible to change the patient's medication, lifelong PPI use should be considered [25, 26].

Evidence exists that all patients should use a prophylactic course of PPIs for some time after surgery to prevent the development of MU. One study shows a decrease from 6.2 to 1.8% after the introduction of a 6-month course of prophylactic PPIs [26]. A recent study suggests that a longer duration of PPI usage is preferable compared to shorter duration [47, 48].

References

1. Capella JF, Capella RF. Staple disruption and marginal ulceration in gastric bypass procedures for weight reduction. Obes Surg. 1996;6(1):44–9.
2. Rasmussen JJ, Fuller W, Ali MR. Marginal ulceration after laparoscopic gastric bypass: an analysis of predisposing factors in 260 patients. Surg Endosc. 2007;21(7):1090–4.
3. Csendes A, Burgos AM, Altuve J, Bonacic S. Incidence of marginal ulcer 1 month and 1 to 2 years after gastric bypass: a prospective consecutive endoscopic evaluation of 442 patients with morbid obesity. Obes Surg. 2009;19(2):135–8.
4. Sapala JA, Wood MH, Sapala MA, Flakee TM Jr. Marginal ulcer after gastric bypass: a prospective 3-year study of 173 patients. Obes Surg. 1998;8(5):505–16.
5. Sanyal AJ, Sugerman HJ, Kellum JM, Engle KM, Wolfe L. Stomal complications of gastric bypass: incidence and outcome of therapy. Am J Gastroenterol. 1992;87(9):1165–9.
6. Buchwald H, Oien DM. Metabolic/bariatric surgery worldwide 2011. Obes Surg. 2013;23(4):427–36.
7. World Health Organisation. Obesity and overweight. https://www.who.int/news-room/fact-sheets/detail/obesity-and-overweight.
8. Caruana JA, McCabe MN, Smith AD, Panemanglore VP, Sette CD. Risk of massive upper gastrointestinal bleeding in gastric bypass patients taking clopidogrel. Surg Obes Relat Dis. 2007;3(4):443–5.
9. Felix EL, Kettelle J, Mobley E, Swartz D. Perforated marginal ulcers after laparoscopic gastric bypass. Surg Endosc. 2008;22(10):2128–32.
10. Kalaiselvan R, Exarchos G, Hamza N, Ammori BJ. Incidence of perforated gastrojejunal anastomotic ulcers after laparoscopic gastric bypass for morbid

obesity and role of laparoscopy in their management. Surg Obes Relat Dis. 2012;8(4):423–8.
11. Garrido AB Jr, Rossi M, Lima SE Jr, Brenner AS, Gomes CA Jr. Early marginal ulcer following Roux-en-Y gastric bypass under proton pump inhibitor treatment: prospective multicentric study. Arq Gastroenterol. 2010;47(2):130–4.
12. Coblijn UK, Goucham AB, Lagarde SM, Kuiken SD, van Wagensveld BA. Development of ulcer disease after Roux-en-Y gastric bypass, incidence, risk factors, and patient presentation: a systematic review. Obes Surg. 2014;24(2):299–309.
13. Coblijn UK, Lagarde SM, de Castro SM, Kuiken SD, van Wagensveld BA. Symptomatic marginal ulcer disease after Roux-en-Y gastric bypass: incidence, risk factors and management. Obes Surg. 2015;25:805–11.
14. Capella JF, Capella RF. Gastro-gastric fistulas and marginal ulcers in gastric bypass procedures for weight reduction. Obes Surg. 1999;9(1):22–7.
15. Siilin H, Wanders A, Gustavsson S, Sundbom M. The proximal gastric pouch invariably contains acid-producing parietal cells in Roux-en-Y gastric bypass. Obes Surg. 2005;15(6):771–7.
16. Mason EE, Printen KJ, Blommers TJ, Lewis JW, Scott DH. Gastric bypass in morbid obesity. Am J Clin Nutr. 1980;33(2 Suppl):395–405.
17. Printen KJ, Scott D, Mason EE. Stomal ulcers after gastric bypass. Arch Surg. 1980;115(4):525–7.
18. Sapala JA, Wood MH, Sapala MA, Schuhknecht MP, Flake TM Jr. The micropouch gastric bypass: technical considerations in primary and revisionary operations. Obes Surg. 2001;11(1):3–17.
19. Wittgrove AC, Clark GW, Tremblay LJ. Laparoscopic gastric bypass, Roux-en-Y: preliminary report of five cases. Obes Surg. 1994;4(4):353–7.
20. Wittgrove AC, Clark GW, Schubert KR. Laparoscopic gastric bypass, Roux-en-Y: technique and results in 75 patients with 3–30 months follow-up. Obes Surg. 1996;6(6):500–4.
21. Hedberg J, Hedenstrom H, Sundbom M. Wireless pH-metry at the gastrojejunostomy after Roux-en-Y gastric bypass: a novel use of the BRAVO system. Surg Endosc. 2011;25(7):2302–7.
22. Mason EE, Munns JR, Kealey GP, Wangler R, Clarke WR, Cheng HF, et al. Effect of gastric bypass on gastric secretion. Am J Surg. 1976;131(2):162–8.
23. Hedberg J, Hedenstrom H, Nilsson S, Sundbom M, Gustavsson S. Role of gastric acid in stomal ulcer after gastric bypass. Obes Surg. 2005;15(10):1375–8.
24. Coblijn UK, Lagarde SM, Tuynman JB, van Meyel JJ, van Wagensveld BA. Delayed massive bleeding two years after Roux-en-Y gastric bypass. JSLS. 2013;17(3):476–80.
25. D'Hondt MA, Pottel H, Devriendt D, Van RF, Vansteenkiste F. Can a short course of prophylactic low-dose proton pump inhibitor therapy prevent stomal ulceration after laparoscopic Roux-en-Y gastric bypass? Obes Surg. 2010;20(5):595–9.
26. Coblijn UK, Lagarde SM, de Castro SM, Kuiken SD, van Tets WF, van Wagensveld BA. The influence of prophylactic proton pump inhibitor treatment on the development of symptomatic marginal ulceration in Roux-en-Y gastric bypass patients: a historic cohort study. Surg Obes Relat Dis. 2016;12(2):246–52.
27. Azagury DE, Abu Dayyeh BK, Greenwalt IT, Thompson CC. Marginal ulceration after Roux-en-Y gastric bypass surgery: characteristics, risk factors, treatment, and outcomes. Endoscopy. 2011;43(11):950–4.
28. Bendewald FP, Choi JN, Blythe LS, Selzer DJ, Ditslear JH, Mattar SG. Comparison of hand-sewn, linear-stapled, and circular-stapled gastrojejunostomy in laparoscopic Roux-en-Y gastric bypass. Obes Surg. 2011;21(11):1671–5.
29. Sacks BC, Mattar SG, Qureshi FG, Eid GM, Collins JL, Barinas-Mitchell EJ, et al. Incidence of marginal ulcers and the use of absorbable anastomotic sutures in laparoscopic Roux-en-Y gastric bypass. Surg Obes Relat Dis. 2006;2(1):11–6.
30. Vasquez JC, Wayne OD, Farrell TM. Fewer gastrojejunostomy strictures and marginal ulcers with absorbable suture. Surg Endosc. 2009;23(9):2011–5.
31. Suggs WJ, Kouli W, Lupovici M, Chau WY, Brolin RE. Complications at gastrojejunostomy after laparoscopic Roux-en-Y gastric bypass: comparison between 21- and 25-mm circular staplers. Surg Obes Relat Dis. 2007;3(5):508–14.
32. Erim T, Cruz-Correa MR, Szomstein S, Velis E, Rosenthal R. Prevalence of Helicobacter pylori seropositivity among patients undergoing bariatric surgery: a preliminary study. World J Surg. 2008;32(9):2021–5.
33. Ramaswamy A, Lin E, Ramshaw BJ, Smith CD. Early effects of Helicobacter pylori infection in patients undergoing bariatric surgery. Arch Surg. 2004;139(10):1094–6.
34. Csendes A, Burgos AM, Smok G, Beltran M. Endoscopic and histologic findings of the foregut in 426 patients with morbid obesity. Obes Surg. 2007;17(1):28–34.
35. Clark GW, Wittgrove AC. Laparoscopic gastric bypass in a porcine model. J Laparoendosc Surg. 1996;6(3):197–8.
36. Hayllar J, Bjarnason I. NSAIDs, Cox-2 inhibitors, and the gut. Lancet. 1995;346(8990):1629.
37. Cashman JN. The mechanisms of action of NSAIDs in analgesia. Drugs. 1996;52(Suppl 5):13–23.
38. Wilson JA, Romagnuolo J, Byrne TK, Morgan K, Wilson FA. Predictors of endoscopic findings after Roux-en-Y gastric bypass. Am J Gastroenterol. 2006;101(10):2194–9.
39. Csendes A, Torres J, Burgos AM. Late marginal ulcers after gastric bypass for morbid obesity. Clinical and endoscopic findings and response to treatment. Obes Surg. 2011;21(9):1319–22.
40. Dallal RM, Bailey LA. Ulcer disease after gastric bypass surgery. Surg Obes Relat Dis. 2006;2(4):455–9.

41. ASMBS. Safety and effectiveness of newer bariatric and metabolic surgery procedures. asmbs org 2012 June 1 [cited 2015 Jan 15]. Available from: URL: https://asmbs.org/resources/studies-weigh-in-on-safety-and-effectiveness-of-newer-bariatric-and-metabolic-surgery-procedure.
42. Gumbs AA, Duffy AJ, Bell RL. Incidence and management of marginal ulceration after laparoscopic Roux-Y gastric bypass. Surg Obes Relat Dis. 2006;2(4):460–3.
43. Racu C, Dutson EP, Mehran A. Laparoscopic gastrojejunostomy revision: a novel approach to intractable marginal ulcer management. Surg Obes Relat Dis. 2010;6(5):557–8.
44. Madan AK, DeArmond G, Ternovits CA, Beech DJ, Tichansky DS. Laparoscopic revision of the gastrojejunostomy for recurrent bleeding ulcers after past open revision gastric bypass. Obes Surg. 2006;16(12):1662–8.
45. Frezza EE, Herbert H, Ford R, Wachtel MS. Endoscopic suture removal at gastrojejunal anastomosis after Roux-en-Y gastric bypass to prevent marginal ulceration. Surg Obes Relat Dis. 2007;3(6):619–22.
46. Jiang HP, Lin LL, Jiang X, Qiao HQ. Meta-analysis of hand-sewn versus mechanical gastrojejunal anastomosis during laparoscopic Roux-en-Y gastric bypass for morbid obesity. Int J Surg. 2016;32:150–7.
47. Kang X, Zurita-Macias L, Hong D, Cadeddu M, Anvari M, Gmora S. A comparison of 30-day versus 90-day proton pump inhibitor therapy in prevention of marginal ulcers after laparoscopic Roux-en-Y gastric bypass. Surg Obes Relat Dis. 2016;12(5):1003–7.
48. Ying VW, Kim SH, Khan KJ, Farrokhyar F, D'Souza J, Gmora S, et al. Prophylactic PPI help reduce marginal ulcers after gastric bypass surgery: a systematic review and meta-analysis of cohort studies. Surg Endosc. 2015;29(5):1018–23.
49. Weight loss surgery; Roux-en-Y gastric bypass. Ref Type: Generic. https://weightlosssurgery.ca/about-our-surgeries/comparison-chart-procedures/laparoscopic-roux-en-y-gastric-bypass/.

30 Rhabdomyolysis

João Ettinger, Paulo Vicente Filho, Euler Ázaro, and Paulo Benigno

Introduction

Morbid obesity is a global scourge. The worldwide prevalence of obesity has nearly doubled between 1980 and 2008. In 2008, 10% of men and 14% of women in the world were obese, compared with 5% for men and 8% for women in 1980. Given the absence of effective methods for conservative treatment of obesity, the number of bariatric surgery operations performed in growing every year. The most common complications of bariatric surgery include staple line leakage, suture line bleeding, episodes of pulmonary embolism, and infection of the surgical site. Another potentially life-threatening complication of bariatric surgery is rhabdomyolysis (RML) [1]. RML is a clinical and biochemical syndrome caused by skeletal muscle necrosis that results in extravasation of toxic intracellular contents from the myocytes into the circulatory system. The incidence of RML in bariatric surgery varies from 6% to 75% [2–4] (Table 30.1). Postoperative RML in morbidly obese patient occurs due to the prolonged muscle compression in many nonphysiological surgical positions, but mainly in procedures longer than 4–5 hours [4–6]. In bariatric surgery, the excessive weight, the presence of diabetes, an ASA physical status >II, and prolonged surgical time also lead to RML [5, 6]. Full recovery can be expected with early diagnosis and treatment of the many complications that can develop in patients with this syndrome [7]. If prevention of RML is not done, or the diagnosis is delayed, and appropriate treatment is not instituted, serious complications and even death can occur.

J. Ettinger (Deceased) · P. V. Filho (✉) · E. Ázaro
P. Benigno
Bahia School of Medicine and Public Health, Salvador, Bahia, Brazil
e-mail: andre.teixeira@orlandohealth.com

Pathophysiology

RML is the dissolution of striated muscle of any part of the human body which results in the release of muscle cell constituents into the extracellular fluid and circulation. Its consequence is the development of a nonspecific clinical and biochemical syndrome, harmful to the human organism [6–9, 12]. Myocytes in physiological form show a typical distribution of intra- and extracellular ions, which is critical to the maintenance of normal function. Ions in the body are either predominantly intracellular or extracellular; none of these have the same distribution [6]. Muscular injury leads to disruption of the internal cellular structures of muscle cells. Cells with damaged membranes allow the uncontrolled influx of sodium, chloride, calcium, and water down their electrochemical gradients. Large amounts of intravascular fluid (up to 12 liters) can leave the circulation and become sequestered as edematous fluid in damaged muscle tissue. This fluid shift produces an intravascular

J. Ettinger et al. (eds.), *Gastric Bypass*, https://doi.org/10.1007/978-3-030-28803-7_30

Table 30.1 Research articles about rhabdomyolysis in bariatric surgery

Author Journal	Year	*N*	Study type	Technique	Total RML	Mild RML CPK <4000 UI/L	Severe RML CPK >4000 UI/L	Operative time Mean – min	BMI Mean kg/m²
Khurana et al. *Arch Surg*	2004	353	Retrospective	Laparoscopic DS	–	Not studied	1.4% 5 patients	246	56 kg/m² Patients with RML
Mognol et al. *Obes Surg*	2004	66	Prospective	LAGB X LRYGBP	22.7% 15 patients	15.2% 10 patients	7.5% 5 patients	110 LAGB 390 LRYGBP	43.9 kg/m² 58.8 kg/m²
Carvalho et al. *Obes Surg*	2006	98	Prospective	ORYGBP	37.8% 38 patients	37.8% 38 patients	None	220	43.2 kg/m²
Faintuch et al. *Obes Surg*	2006	129	Retrospective	ORYGBP	12.9% 16 patients	8.5% 11 patients	3.8% 5 patients	320 mild RML 340 severe RML	50.8 kg/m² mild RML 54.6 kg/m² Severe RML
Lagandré et al. *Obes Surg*	2006	49	Prospective	LAGB X intestinal bypass X RYGBP	26.5% 13 patients	24.5% 12 pac	2.04% 1 patient	195 without RML 272 with RML	49.7 kg/m²
Ettinger et al. *Obes Surg*	2008	114	Retrospective	ORYGBP X LRYGBP	7% 8 patients	7% 8 patients	None	182 ORYGBP 171 LRYGBP 176 total	44.6 kg/m² ORYGBP 41.5 kg/m² LRYGBP 43.1 kg/m² Total

From Ettinger et al. [2]

ORYGBP open Roux-en-Y gastric bypass, *LRYGBP* laparoscopic Roux-en-Y gastric bypass, *LAGB* laparoscopic adjustable gastric banding, *DS* duodenal switch, *RML* rhabdomyolysis

hypovolemia and subsequently hemodynamic instability [13, 14]. The dramatic decrease in plasma volume leads to vasoconstriction, prerenal failure, and, eventually, acute intrarenal failure [12]. Chloride and calcium also enter the cells, causing serum hypocalcemia and calcium deposition in skeletal muscle and renal tissues [15]. Among the intracellular components that leak out of damaged skeletal muscle, the most immediately important one is potassium. Because this electrolyte is moving from an intracellular area of high concentration into the serum, where a low concentration is normal, lethal hyperkalemia can develop rapidly with cardiotoxic effects and dysrhythmias [16]. Phosphate also leaves the cells, producing hyperphosphatemia. Injured myocytes also leak lactic acid and other organic acids, promoting metabolic acidosis and aciduria. Purines released from disintegrating cells are metabolized to uric acid and can lead to hyperuricemia [6, 17]. Myoglobin is an oxygen-carrying molecule that gives muscles their red-brown color. Lysis of as little as 100 g of skeletal muscle results in myoglobinuria. Myoglobin is also nephrotoxic in patients with concomitant oliguria and aciduria [6, 18]. Thromboplastin and tissue plasminogen are released from injured muscle tissue, making patients with RML susceptible to disseminated intravascular coagulation, mainly when associated with sepsis [14, 17–21]. RML also produces extreme increases in serum levels of creatinine phosphokinase (CPK). CPK has no toxic effects, and elevated plasma CPK levels are simply a marker of increased permeability of muscle membranes. However, high values are pathognomonic for RML, because no other condition will lead to such extreme CPK elevations [22].

Rhabdomyolysis in Morbidly Obese

Rhabdomyolysis was initially described in patients injured in disasters such as the 1940 bombing of London during World War II and the 1908 earthquake in Sicily. RML has been seen following traumatic injury, and it is also seen in patients undergoing elective surgery. RML has been reported in a number of surgical disciplines including urology, neurosurgery, orthopedics, and cardiovascular and bariatric surgery [23]. RML in morbidly obese patients is caused by tissue compression with extended periods of immobilization. This leads to muscle ischemia which interferes with oxygen delivery to the cells, thereby limiting production of adenosine triphosphate (ATP) and function of sodium-potassium ATPase membrane pumps. This results in a loss of intracellular fluid and release of myoglobin, intracellular enzymes, and electrolytes into the bloodstream, which leads to electrolyte imbalance, hypovolemia, compartment syndrome, disseminated intravascular coagulation (DIC), cardiac disorders, and acute kidney injury. Renal failure may be seen in up to 33% of all RML cases, and patients who develop acute renal injury are at an increased risk of death (up to 50%) [23]. Animal studies have demonstrated myonecrosis when an intracompartmental pressure of 30 mmHg was applied for 4–8 hours [6]. Recognized risk factors for the development of postoperative RML are prolonged duration of operation, massive obesity, surgical compressive positioning, and endocrine or metabolic disorders such as diabetes and hypertension. Another cause is peripheral vascular disease which is a predisposing factor for compartmental syndrome [24]. Long duration of surgery promotes more tissue compression and ischemia. RML has occurred after operations in nonobese patients when the surgery was >7 hours. Obese patients are at risk during shorter operative procedures, longer than 230 minutes [25]. Obesity increases tissue compression [7], where the weight is >30% above ideal weight [4]. RML is a complication of various non-physiological positions, e.g., the seated, lateral decubitus, prone, exaggerated or high lithotomy, genupectoral, knee-chest or tucked, supine, and hyperlordotic positions [26–28]. Super-obese male patients (BMI >50) with hypertension, diabetes, and peripheral vascular disease are at greater risk for RML. Diabetic obese patients were found to be at an eight times increased risk of developing RML [25, 26]. These factors are not independent: super-obese male patients are more likely to be diabetic and hypertensive, and bariatric surgery in this population may be more difficult and likely to be associated with longer duration of operations and consequently more tissue compression. Other potential etiologic factors include family history of muscle disease and the consumption of certain drugs, notably anti-cholesterol statins [29]. Recent publications showed improved postoperative outcome and reduced incidence of myocardial damage at the first month following surgery on continuous statins, without clinical or laboratory evidence of rhabdomyolysis [30].

Anesthetic and perioperative medications such as propofol, barbiturates, salicylates, benzodiazepines, antihistamines, and opiates have been associated with an increased risk of RML [23], although Lehavi et al. suggest that propofol-based anesthesia is not related to increased incidence of RML in morbidly obese patients undergoing short, uncomplicated bariatric surgery [30].

Prevention of Rhabdomyolysis in Morbidly Obese

Prevention of RML avoids serious outcomes of this important complication (Table 30.2). Prevention is enhanced by careful padding at all pressure points during surgery mainly around the hips, shoulders, and buttocks (areas adjacent to bone prominences) to minimize the surface and deeper pressure, by distributing pressure over a greater surface area [3, 4, 31]. Some authors argue that this may be counterproductive as it increases the force per unit area and is reflected

Table 30.2 Methods to prevent rhabdomyolysis in morbidly obese submitted to surgical treatment

Padding pressure areas
Use of pneumatic beds during operation
Use of two combined surgical tables
Optimal position on surgical table
Limit surgical time:
Reduce weight before bariatric surgery or perform surgery in two stages
Avoid early in the learning curve operating super-obese patients
Changing patient position intra- and postoperatively
Aggressive fluid replacement perioperatively
Early ambulation
Discontinue statin therapy
Correct risk factors for RML after surgery (Table 30.2)

From Ettinger et al. [55]

by the continuing high incidence of RML where padding of pressure points has still been utilized during bariatric surgery [23]. The use of pneumatic beds during surgery is important to prevent the occurrence of RML [26]. Obese surgical patients can position themselves on the surgical table before induction of anesthesia, to the most appropriate position, avoiding positions that can increase muscle compression [27]. The use of two combined surgical tables to decrease the pressure on the back surface of the massively obese patient can prevent RML. Changing patient position, both intraoperatively (for operations lasting >2–3 hours) and postoperatively, is recommended to protect injured and uninjured muscle tissue in the morbidly obese patient [28]. The duration of immobilization is greater for very heavy patients. This is not only because the operation takes longer but also because other aspects of the operation including the placement of central lines or arterial lines are more likely to be difficult and time-consuming. The longer the immobilization, the greater is the RML risk, so one potential new solution proposed by some surgeons is to decrease the longer operative time by dividing the procedure into two stages, doing a gastric sleeve resection initially, and then when the patient has lost considerable weight performing the definitive bypass. Regan's group [32] concluded that laparoscopic sleeve gastrectomy with second-stage Roux-en-Y gastric bypass is feasible and effective. This two-stage approach is

Table 30.3 Intraoperative prevention of rhabdomyolysis in morbidly obese

Measures
Hydration >13 ml/kg/h
Maintain diuresis >2.3 ml/kg/h
Operative time <2 h

From Ettinger [54]

a reasonable alternative for surgical treatment of the high-risk super-super-obese (BMI >60) patient. Another way to limit the duration of surgery in high-risk patients is alerting surgeons early in their learning curve not to select patients who fall into this group, or to offer such patients a staged procedure. It is also important to have a hospital bed designed for morbidly obese patients to be used during the postoperative time.

Since RML was first described aggressive intraoperative (Table 30.3) and postoperative, fluid replacement was seen as a way to prevent and treat this patients. A high urine output should be instituted with the administration of IV fluids and diuretics, before, during, and after surgery [3, 12, 26]. So far, recently, Matlok et al. argued that decreasing intravenous fluid administration may reduce the risk of RML after bariatric surgery. The analysis of the volume of fluids administered intravenously from the induction of anesthesia, through surgery, perioperative period, to 24 hours after surgery showed that in the group of patients who developed RML, the median administered fluid volume was 3750 ml, compared with 3000 ml for the group who did not develop the condition. Every 500 ml above the median resulted in an increase in the OR of RML by 11%. More research must be done to confirm this finding [1].

Diagnosis of Rhabdomyolysis

Clinical Findings and Physical Evaluation

The initial expression of RML can be sudden, and an early diagnosis requires a high degree of suspicion [6]. In most cases, RML proceeds subclinically and is identified on the basis of increased blood levels of myoglobin and enzymes released by the injured muscles. The characteristic triad of complaints in rhabdomyolysis is muscle pain, weakness, and dark urine. However, more than half of patients may not report muscular symptoms. Usually, the first systemic clinical sign is the appearance of urine with altered color that can range from pink to brown and black [6, 7, 11]. Myoglobinuria is suspected with the presence of altered urine color [11] and requires differential diagnosis among several entities [28].

The syndrome has local and systemic features. Local signs and symptoms are nonspecific and may include muscle pain, tenderness, swelling, bruising, and weakness. Systemic features include tea-colored urine, fever, malaise, nausea, emesis, confusion, agitation, delirium, and anuria [7] (Table 30.4). Compartment syndrome is a potential complication of severe rhabdomyolysis that may develop after fluid resuscitation, with worsening edema of the limb and muscle.

Patients with an epidural in place may not complain of pain and surreptitiously develop renal failure from RML. In these patients, regular postoperative CK levels are essential in order to identify rhabdomyolysis early.

During the physical examination, decubitus ulcer and eruptions can be present in pressure zones, mainly at the hips, limbs, and buttocks. Muscle weakness may be present, depending upon the severity of muscle injury. Skin changes of ischemic tissue injury, such as discoloration or blisters, may also be seen but are present in less than 10 percent of patients [12, 28] (Tables 30.5 and 30.6).

Table 30.4 Clinical features of rhabdomyolysis

Local features	Systemic features
Muscle pain Tenderness Swelling Bruising Weakness	Tea-colored urine Fever Nausea Malaise Emesis Confusion Agitation Delirium Anuria

From Sauret et al. [7]

Table 30.5 Rhabdomyolysis complications

Early	Late
Hyperkalemia	Acute kidney injury (AKI)
Hypocalcemia	Disseminated intravascular coagulation
Hepatic inflammation	Compartment syndrome
Cardiac arrhythmia	
Compartment syndrome	

From Sauret et al. [7]

Table 30.6 Risk factors for acute renal failure from rhabdomyolysis after bariatric surgery

Hypoalbuminemia
Hyperkalemia or hypophosphatemia
Sepsis
CPK peak >6000 IU/l
Hypertension
Diabetes
Preexisting azotemia

From Mognol et al. [3]

Laboratory Findings

Although history and physical examination can provide clues, the actual diagnosis of RML is confirmed by laboratory studies [6, 10, 30]. CK testing should be performed in all patients after bariatric surgery to make an early diagnosis and properly start fluids and diuretics [25]. The diagnosis can be confirmed by identifying high levels of creatine phosphokinase (CPK). Serum CPK five times the normal value or >1000 IU/L is considered as a biochemical diagnosis of RML [3]. The elevation in CPK levels is the most sensitive diagnostic evidence of muscle injury and is present in 100% of RML cases [5–7]. CK >5000 U/L indicates serious muscle injury. When the RML syndrome is present, extreme quantities of CKMM are released into the blood system, and peak concentrations of 100,000 IU/ml or more are not unusual. No other condition will cause such extreme CPK elevations [6]. Small amounts of CKMB may also be present. The serum CK begins to rise within 2–12 hours following the onset of muscle injury, and peak values occur 4–7 days after injury and remain elevated for up to 12 days [28]. In patients whose CK does not decline as expected, continued muscle injury or the development of a compartment syndrome may be present. In some cases, the CPK isoenzymes MM and MB are measured to distinguish a cardiac from a skeletal source [11]. An electrocardiogram must also be done to differentiate RML from myocardial infarction [3].

Urinary myoglobin provokes a typical reddish brown color. Visible changes in the urine only occur once urine levels exceed from about 100 to 300 mg/dL [33]. Urine myoglobin concentration >300 ng/ml is associated with an increased risk of RML and ARF. Urinalysis in patients with RML will also reveal the presence of protein, brown casts in tubules, and uric acid crystals and may reflect electrolyte wasting consistent with renal failure [6].

When RML is present, there is generally an increase in blood urea nitrogen and creatinine due to prerenal causes of ARF from dehydration and myoglobinuria [34]. Both ARF and increased release of creatine from skeletal muscle cause the serum concentration of urea nitrogen and creatinine to increase in RML. Volume depletion resulting in renal ischemia, tubular obstruction due to heme pigment casts, and tubular injury from free chelatable iron all contribute to the development of renal dysfunction.

A classical pattern of changes in serum electrolytes occurs in RML. At the outset, serum levels of potassium and phosphate increase as these components are released from the cells, and then levels decrease as they are excreted in the urine. Serum concentration of calcium initially decreases as calcium moves into the damaged muscle cells and then gradually increases during the recovery phase due to the release of calcium from injured muscle and elevated 1,25-dihydroxyvitamin D levels [32]. Severe hyperuricemia may develop because of the release of purines from damaged muscle cells [33, 34]. High anion acidosis can also occur with RML [34]. Severe rhabdomyolysis may be associated with the development of disseminated intravascular coagulation due to the release of thromboplastin and other prothrombotic substances from the damaged muscle. Clotting studies are useful for detecting any indication of disseminated intravascular coagulation [6]. Serum aspartate aminotransferase (AST), alanine aminotransferase (ALT), aldolase, troponin I, and lactate dehydrogenase (LDH) enzymes can increase due to muscular injury [28, 34]. Serum carbonic anhydrase III has also been suggested as a marker for the diagnosis of RML [28]. Arterial blood gas analysis is helpful for detecting underlying hypoxia and metabolic acidosis and monitoring sodium bicarbonate therapy [6]. Muckart et al. concluded in a prospective study that venous bicarbonate (VBC) concentration has an important role as a predictive factor that allows identification of patients at risk of developing myoglobin-induced acute kidney injury (AKI). A VBC <17 mmol/L was significantly predictive of ARF development [35].

Image Examinations

Radiographic evaluation can also be valuable for diagnosing RML when clinical findings and physical examination are not elucidating (Table 30.7). Magnetic resonance imaging (MRI) and computed tomography (CT) are helpful in the diagnosis of RML [37]. MRI accurately identifies muscular edema in the affected muscle groups. In Lamminen et al.'s prospective study, MRI had a higher sensitivity in the detection of abnormal muscles than CT or ultrasound (US) (100%, 62%, and 42%, respectively) [38]. CT evaluation can reveal muscle necrosis and calcification that occur early in the course of RML [39]. CT for the diagnosis of RML must be non-contrast enhanced to avoid acute renal failure [40]. 111 In-labeled antimyosin monoclonal antibody and technetium-99m pyrophosphate (99mTc-PYP) scintigraphy have also been used to make the diagnosis of RML and evaluate

Table 30.7 Image examinations to detect RML and the findings

Magnetic resonance imaging	Muscular edema
Computed tomography	Muscle necrosis and calcification
Ultrasound	Hyperechoic areas
Technetium-99m scintigraphy	Accumulation of the radioactivity in the damaged skeletal muscle

From Ettinger et al. [56]

muscle injury [28]. Ultrasound has also been known to have some value in identifying injured musculature in RML by revealing hyperechoic areas within the muscles examined [41]. Plain muscle X-ray does not have value in RML [42]. A muscle biopsy in the affected site can be done if any doubt remains. Findings on biopsy include loss of normal cross-striations and cell nuclei and the absence of inflammatory cells [28].

Electromyographic (EMG) is an important diagnostic tool in the work-up of patients presenting acute or subacute severe muscle weakness and significantly elevated CPK when the differential diagnosis includes RML and inflammatory myopathies [36].

Rhabdomyolysis Treatment

The treatment of RML is geared toward preserving renal function, which is done by preventing factors that can lead to ARF, which are dehydration, hypovolemia, tubular obstruction, aciduria, and free radical release [43]. Early recognition allows the administration of fluid, bicarbonate, and mannitol [4, 6, 10, 44]. These measures help to prevent volume depletion, tubular obstruction, aciduria, and free radical release which is the mechanism for renal failure in rhabdomyolysis [4, 10]. Hypovolemia may result from sequestration of water by muscles and must be prevented by the early and aggressive administration of intravenous fluids [7, 45]. Expanding the intravascular volume maximizes renal excretion by flushing out the tubular debris and limiting the time that nephrotoxins are in contact with renal tissues [6, 45]. Treatment of RML requires aggressive administration of fluids to ensure urine output >1.5 ml/kg/h [46] or 150–300 ml/h until myoglobinuria has ceased [6, 7, 10, 13]. Maintaining a urine output this high may require intravenous infusion of fluids between 500 and 1000 ml/h [13], and all patients should have a urinary catheter placed in order to adequately monitor fluid output [47]. Increasing intraoperative fluids does not seem to prevent RML or progression to acute kidney injury; however, early fluid resuscitation within 6 h resulting in a forced diuresis may preserve renal function and prevent mortality [48].

Diuretics are also used, mainly mannitol and loop diuretics. The addition of mannitol to the fluid regimen serves several purposes: mannitol increases renal blood flow and glomerular filtration rate; mannitol is an osmotic agent that attracts fluids from the interstitial compartment, thus counterbalancing hypovolemia and reducing muscular swelling and nerve compression. Mannitol is an osmotic diuretic that increases urinary flow and prevents obstructive myoglobin casts, and mannitol scavenges free radicals. Many authors assert that loop diuretics (furosemide, bumetanide, and torsemide) must be used if fluids and mannitol are insufficient to maintain a brisk urine output [10, 13]. They increase tubular flow and calcium losses and decrease the risk of precipitation of myoglobin [49], although they may acidify the urine [49, 50]. However, there is no evidence that diuretics improve the final outcome [7]. These aggressive and successful measures were first described in trauma patients who had traumatic rhabdomyolysis [19], but to date no randomized controlled trial has shown unquestionable results in preventing acute kidney injury with the use of diuretics. Dialysis does not reduce myoglobin [51].

The use of sodium bicarbonate helps to correct the acidosis induced by the release of protons from damaged muscles to prevent precipitation of myoglobin in the tubules and reduce the risk of hyperkalemia [49]. Bicarbonate and acetazolamide are used for producing more alkaline urine when blood pH is >7.45 [46]. Some investigators assert that the urine must be alkalinized to pH 6.0, 6.5, 7.0, or even 7.53 to prevent the dissociation of myoglobin into its nephrotoxic components [5, 10, 17, 52]. On the other hand, there are also some concerns about the use of sodium bicarbonate because it may worsen hypocalcemia or precipitate calcium phosphate deposition in various tissues [7]. Allopurinol may be useful because it reduces the production of uric acid and also acts as a free radical scavenger. Another purine analog pentoxifylline has been considered in the management of RML because of its capacity to enhance capillary flow and decrease neutrophil adhesion and cytokine release [49]. Electrolyte disorders should be prevented or promptly treated [33]. Control of hyperkalemia is an important therapeutic goal. Calcium salts and calcium kayexalate (sodium polystyrene sulfonate and exchange resin) should be used with caution because they enhance the risk of intramuscular calcium deposition. Hypocalcemia usually does not require correction, particularly because this would increase the risk of intramuscular calcium deposition [49].

Dialysis is necessary if the kidneys no longer respond to the abovementioned supportive measures and severe renal dysfunction has set in [3, 46]. Dialysis is indicated not only in patients with overt hyperkalemia but also in patients whose serum potassium rises rapidly and those with acidosis [49].

Compartment syndrome may be an early or late complication that results mainly from direct muscle injury [6, 7, 33]. This complication occurs primarily in muscles whose expansion is limited by tight fascia. Peripheral pulses may still be palpable, and in these cases, nerve deficits (mainly sensory) are the more important finding. Compartment syndrome may develop or worsen during fluid resuscitation due to the development of edema of limbs and/or muscles. Decompressive fasciotomy, muscular debridement, and escharotomies should also be considered in patients with evidence of neurovascular compression and decubitus ulcer if the compartment pressure is >30 mmHg [6, 7, 31, 33].

References

1. Matłok M, Major P, Małczak P, Wysocki M, et al. Reduction of the risk of rhabdomyolysis after bariatric surgery with lower fluid administration in the perioperative period: a cohort study. Pol Arch Med Wewn. 2016;126(4):237–42.
2. Ettinger JEMT, Marcílio de Souza CA, Ázaro E, et al. Clinical features of rhabdomyolysis after open and laparoscopic Roux-en-Y gastric bypass. Obes Surg. 2008;18:635–43.
3. Mognol P, Vignes S, Chosidow D, et al. Rhabdomyolysis after laparoscopic bariatric surgery. Obes Surg. 2004;14:91–4.
4. Bostanjian D, Anthone GJ, Hamoui N, et al. Rhabdomyolysis of gluteal muscles leading to renal failure: a potentially fatal complication of surgery in the morbidly obese. Obes Surg. 2003;13:302–5.
5. Lagandré S, Arnalsteen L, Vallet B, et al. Predictive factors for rhabdomyolysis after bariatric surgery. Obes Surg. 2006;16:1365–70.
6. Criddle LM. Rhabdomyolysis. Pathophysiology, recognition, and management. Crit Care Nurse. 2003;23:14–22, 24–6, 28 passim; quiz 31–2.
7. Sauret JM, Marinides G, Wang GK. Rhabdomyolysis. Am Fam Physician. 2002;65:907–12.
8. Lane R, Phillips M. Rhabdomyolysis. BMJ. 2003;327(7413):115–6.
9. Criner JA, Appelt M, Coker C, et al. Rhabdomyolysis: the hidden killer. Medsurg Nurs. 2002;11:138–43.
10. Vanholder R, Sever M, Erek E, et al. Rhabdomyolysis. J Am Soc Nephrol. 2000;11:1553–61.
11. Torres-Villalobos G, Kimura E, Mosquedo JL, et al. Pressure-induced rhabdomyolysis after bariatric surgery. Obes Surg. 2003;13:306–13.
12. Collier B, Goreja MA, Duke BE III. Postoperative rhabdomyolysis with bariatric surgery. Obes Surg. 2003;13:941–3.
13. Abassi A, Hoffman A, Better O. Acute renal failure complicating muscle crush injury. Semin Nephrol. 1998;18:558–65.
14. Cheney P. Early management and physiologic changes in crush syndrome. Crit Care Nurs Q. 1994;17:62–73.
15. Russel TA, et al. Nephrol Nurs J. 2000;27:567–77.
16. Gronert GA. Cardiac arrest after succinylcholine: mortality greater with rhabdomyolysis than receptor upregulation. Anesthesiology. 2001;94:523–9.
17. Curry SC, Chang D, Connor D. Drug- and toxin-induced rhabdomyolysis. Ann Emerg Med. 1989;18:1068–84.
18. Haskins N. Rhabdomyolysis and acute renal failure in intensive care. Nurs Crit Care. 1998;3:283–8.
19. Slater MS, Mullins RJ. Rhabdomyolysis and myoglobinuric renal failure in trauma and surgical patients: a review. J Am Coll Surg. 1998;186:693–716.
20. Hollenstein U, Thalhammer F, Burgmann H. Disseminated intravascular coagulation (DIC) and rhabdomyolysis in fulminant varicella infection – case report and review of the literature. Infection. 1998;26:306–8.
21. Riggs JE, Schochet SS Jr, Parmar JP. Rhabdomyolysis with acute renal failure and disseminated intravascular coagulation: association with acetaminophen andethanol. Mil Med. 1996;161:708–9.
22. Dayer-Berenson L. Rhabdomyolysis: a comprehensive guide. Nephrol Nurs J. 1994;21:15–8.
23. Chakravartty S, Sarma DR, Patel AG. Rhabdomyolysis in bariatric surgery: a systematic review. Obes Surg. 2013;23(8):1333–40.
24. Gorecki PJ, Cottam D, Ger R, et al. Lower extremity compartment syndrome following a laparoscopic Roux-en-Y gastric bypass. Obes Surg. 2002;12:289–91.

25. Tolone S, Pilone V, Musella M, et al. Rhabdomyolysis after bariatric surgery: a multicenter, prospective study on incidence, risk factors, and therapeutic strategy in a cohort from South Italy. Surg Obes Relat Dis. 2016;12(2):384–90. Epub 2015 Nov 14.
26. Iseri C, Senkul T, Reddy PK. Major urologic surgery and rhabdomyolysis in two obese patients. Int J Urol. 2003;10:558–60.
27. Hofmann R, Stoller ML. Endoscopic and open stone surgery in morbidly obese patients. J Urol. 1992;148(3 Pt 2):1108–11.
28. Wiltshire JP, Custer T. Lumbar muscle rhabdomyolysis as a cause of acute renal failure after Roux-en-Y gastric bypass. Obes Surg. 2003;13:306–13.
29. Phillips PS, Haas RH. Statin myopathy as a metabolic muscle disease. Expert Rev Cardiovasc Ther. 2008;6(7):971–8. Review.
30. Lehavi A, Sandler O, Mahajna A, Weissman A, Katz YS. Comparison of rhabdomyolysis markers in patients undergoing bariatric surgery with propofol and inhalation-based anesthesia. Obes Surg. 2015;25(10):1923–7.
31. Khurana RN, Baudendistel TE, Morgan EF, et al. Postoperative rhabdomyolysis following laparoscopic gastric bypass in the morbidly obese. Arch Surg. 2004;139:73–6.
32. Regan JP, Inabnet WB, Gagner M, et al. Early experience with two-stage laparoscopic Roux-en-Y gastric bypass as an alternative in the super-super-obese patient. Obes Surg. 2003;13:861–4.
33. Milone L, Strong V, Gagner M. Laparoscopic sleeve gastrectomy is superior to endoscopic intragastric balloon as a first stage procedure for super-obese patients(BMI ≥50). Obes Surg. 2005;15:612–7.
34. Grover DS, Atta MG, Eustace JA, et al. Lack of clinical utility of urine myoglobin detection by microconcentrator ultrafiltration in the diagnosis of rhabdomyolysis. Nephrol Dial Transplant. 2004;19:2634–8.
35. Harriston S. A review of rhabdomyolysis. Dimens Crit Care Nurs. 2004;23:155–61.
36. Muckart DJ, Moodley M, Naidu AG, et al. Prediction of acute renal failure following soft-tissue injury using the venous bicarbonate concentration. J Trauma. 1992;33:813–7.
37. Al-Shekhlee A, Hachwi R, Jaberi MM, et al. The electromyographic features of acute rhabdomyolysis. J Clin Neuromuscul Dis. 2005;6:114–8.
38. Carvalho DAF, Valezi AC, Brito EM, et al. Rhabdomyolysis after bariatric surgery. Obes Surg. 2006;16:740–4.
39. Lamminen AE, Hekali PE, Tiula E, et al. Acute rhabdomyolysis: evaluation with magnetic resonance imaging compared with computed tomography and ultrasonography. Br J Radiol. 1989;62:326–30.
40. Messing ML, Feinzimer ET, Brosnan JJ, et al. CT of rhabdomyolysis associated with malignant hyperthermia and seizures. Clin Imaging. 1993;17:258–9.
41. Russ PD, Dillingham M. Demonstration of CT hyperdensity in patients with acute renal failure associated with rhabdomyolysis. J Comput Assist Tomogr. 1991;15:458–63.
42. Steeds RP, Alexander PJ, Muthusamy R, et al. Sonography in the diagnosis of rhabdomyolysis. J Clin Ultrasound. 1999;27:531–3.
43. Nakahara K, Tanaka H, Masutani K, et al. The value of computed tomography and magnetic resonance imaging to diagnose rhabdomyolysis in acute renal failure. Nephrol Dial Transplant. 1999;14:1564–7.
44. Sharon GC, et al. Orthop Nurs. 2005;24:443–7.
45. Pasnik K, Krupa J, Stanowski E, et al. Successful treatment of gastric fistula following rhabdomyolysis after vertical banded gastroplasty. Obes Surg. 2005;15:428–30.
46. Better OS, Stein JH. Early management of shock and prophylaxis of acute renal failure in traumatic rhabdomyolysis. N Engl J Med. 1990;322:825–9.
47. Filis D, Daskalakis M, Askoxylakis I, et al. Rhabdomyolysis following laparoscopic gastric bypass. Obes Surg. 2005;15:1496–500.
48. Moghtader J, Brady WJ, Bonadio W. Exertional rhabdomyolysis in an adolescent athlete. Pediatr Emerg Care. 1997;13:382–5.
49. Sinert R, Kohl L, Rainone T, et al. Exercise-induced rhabdomyolysis. Ann Emerg Med. 1994;23:1301–6.
50. Singh D, Chander V, Chopra K. Rhabdomyolysis. Methods Find Exp Clin Pharmacol. 2005;27:39–48.
51. Ron D, Taitelman U, Michaelson M, Bar-Joseph G, Bursztein S, Better OS. Prevention of acute renal failure in traumatic rhabdomyolysis. Arch Intern Med. 1984;144(2):277–80.
52. Wakabayashi Y, Kikuno T, Ohwada T, Kikawada R. Rapid fall in blood myoglobin in massive rhabdomyolysis and acute renal failure. Intensive Care Med. 1994;20(2):109–12.
53. Harper J. Rhabdomyolysis and myoglobinuric renal failure. Crit Care Nurse. 1990;10:32–6.
54. Ettinger JEMTM. Rhabdomyolysis in morbidly obese submitted to open and laparoscopic gastric bypass. PhD thesis. Escola Bahiana de Medicina e Saúde Pública. Salvador, Brazil 2007.
55. Ettinger JEMTM, dos Santos Filho PV, Azaro E, et al. Prevention of rhabdomyolysis in bariatric surgery. Obes Surg. 2005;15:874–9. (review).
56. Ettinger JEMTM, Marcílio de Souza CA, Santos-Filho PV, et al. Rhabdomyolysis: diagnosis and treatment in bariatric surgery. Obes Surg. 2007;17:525–32. (review).

31 Depressive Disorders, Alcohol Use Disorders, and Suicidality in Bariatric Surgery

Adriano Segal

Introduction

The link between obesity and mental health (or its absence) has been the focus of medical attention since ancient times, with several theories trying to make a cause-effect association ever since. Most of the time, obesity has been seen as a result of inappropriate personality features or as a result of poor coping mechanisms, implying it was a psychosomatic disorder [1].

During the final decade of the last century, the direction of this cause-effect view has somehow changed and obesity started to be viewed by some authors and clinicians as a cause of poor mental health due to its broad negative impact on quality of life (QoL) (not only in terms of psychosocial negative impact but also in terms on health negative impact) rather than its effect [1].

Through the last years, obesity and mental disorders started to be viewed as independent categories that shared common physiopathological pathways [2, 3]. Moreover, with voluntary weight loss in obesity, improvement in quality of life and positive impact in some psychiatric disorders are repeatedly described [4, 5]. Despite that, alcohol-related disorders and suicidality started to appear throughout the bariatric surgery literature [6–8].

Here we will summarize these topics, starting with depressive disorders and alcohol use disorders. Suicidality will end this chapter.

Due to the extension of this chapter's theme, each of the items that are of paramount relevance will be only briefly discussed, so we recommend further reading about those topics.

Depressive Disorders

Depressive Episode and Depressive Disorder

Along with bipolar disorders, depressive disorders (DD) are the most commonly diagnosed conditions in general psychiatry. Major DD represents the classic condition in this group of disorders. It is characterized by discrete episodes of at least 2 weeks' duration with clear-cut changes in affect, cognition, and neurovegetative functions and inter-episode remissions [9].

A depressive episode (DE) is a transversal diagnose and can be present in a variety of disorders and/or diseases. Depressive disorder (DD) as opposed to DE is a longitudinal diagnose, usually referring to a chronic recurrent disorder.

A. Segal (✉)
Obesity and Diabetes Center, German Hospital Oswaldo Cruz, São Paulo, Brazil

Obesity and Metabolic Syndrome Outpatient Clinic, Service of Endocrinology and Metabolism-HCFMUSP/SP, São Paulo, Brazil

Brazilian Society of Bariatric and Metabolic Surgery, São Paulo, Brazil

Brazilian Association for the Study of Obesity and Metabolic Syndrome, São Paulo, Brazil

Segal Clinic, São Paulo, Brazil

J. Ettinger et al. (eds.), *Gastric Bypass*, https://doi.org/10.1007/978-3-030-28803-7_31

The DSM V diagnostic criteria for DE and DD [9] are adapted in Table 31.1.

The differential diagnosis of a DE are shown in Table 31.2 [9].

Lifetime prevalence estimates of MDE ranged from 1.5% to 19.0%. One-year prevalence estimates ranged from 0.8% to 5.8% [10].

The 1-year prevalence of major depressive disorder is approximately 7%, with marked differences by age group such that the prevalence in 18- to 29-year-old individuals is threefold higher than the prevalence in individuals aged 60 years or older. Females experience 1.5- to 3-fold higher rates than males, beginning in early adolescence [9]. The median age of onset is around 25 years old and tends to be higher in high-income countries (around 30 years old) [10].

DD is associated with a wide variety of chronic physical disorders, like arthritis, asthma, cancer, cardiovascular disease, diabetes, hypertension, and chronic respiratory disorders, among other conditions. Also there are associations with numerous adverse outcomes, including but not limited to persistence and severity of a wide range of secondary disorders as well as increased risk of early mortality due to physical disorders and suicide [10]. DD is frequently associated to substance use disorders, panic disorder,

Table 31.2 DE differential diagnosis

Manic episodes with irritable mood or mixed episodes
Mood disorder due to another medical condition (e.g., multiple sclerosis, stroke, hypothyroidism)
Substance/medication-induced depressive or bipolar disorder
Attention-deficit hyperactivity disorder
Adjustment disorder with depressed mood
Sadness

Table 31.1 Adapted DSM V diagnostic criteria for depressive episode

A. Five (or more) of the following symptoms have been present during the same 2-week period and represent a change from previous functioning: at least one of the symptoms is either (1) depressed mood or (2) loss of interest or pleasure Note: Do not include symptoms that are clearly attributable to another medical condition 1. Depressed mood most of the day, nearly every day, as indicated by either subjective report or observation made by others. (Note: In children and adolescents, it can be irritable mood) 2. Markedly diminished interest or pleasure in all, or almost all, activities most of the day, nearly every day 3. Significant weight loss when not dieting or weight gain (e.g., a change of more than 5% of body weight in a month), or decrease or increase in appetite nearly every day (Note: In children, consider failure to make expected weight gain) 4. Insomnia or hypersomnia nearly every day 5. Psychomotor agitation or retardation nearly every day 6. Fatigue or loss of energy nearly every day 7. Feelings of worthlessness or excessive or inappropriate guilt nearly every day 8. Diminished ability to think or concentrate, or indecisiveness, nearly every day 9. Recurrent thoughts of death, recurrent suicidal ideation without a specific plan, or a suicide attempt or a specific plan for committing suicide
B. The symptoms cause clinically significant distress or impairment in social, occupational, or other important areas of functioning
C. The episode is not attributable to the physiological effects of a substance or to another medical condition Note: Criteria A to C represent a major depressive episode (MDE) Note: Responses to a significant loss (e.g., bereavement, financial ruin, losses from a natural disaster, a serious medical illness, or disability) may include the signs and symptoms noted in Criterion A, which may resemble a depressive episode. Although such symptoms may be understandable, the presence of a MDE in addition to the normal response to a significant loss should also be carefully considered. This decision requires clinical judgment based on the individual's history and the cultural norms for the expression of distress in the context of loss
D. The occurrence of the major depressive episode is not better explained by schizoaffective disorder, schizophrenia, schizophreniform disorder, delusional disorder, or other specified and unspecified schizophrenia spectrum and other psychotic disorders
E. There has never been a manic episode or a hypomanic episode Note: This exclusion does not apply if all the manic-like or hypomanic-like episodes are substance-induced or are attributable to the physiological effects of another medical condition

obsessive-compulsive disorder, anorexia nervosa, bulimia nervosa, and borderline personality disorder [9].

The pathophysiology of DD (and other psychiatric disorders) has a series of common pathways with obesity pathophysiology, and the amelioration of the weight and metabolic status that is consequent to any successful obesity treatment (behavioral, pharmacological, or surgical) tends to ameliorate those common pathways, leading to an improvement in a variety of neuropsychiatric markers [2, 3, 11, 12].

The treatment of both DD and DE includes biological and psychotherapeutic (notably, behavioral-cognitive psychotherapies) approaches. The association of both strategies seems more efficacious than any of them separately [13, 14].

It is important to stress out that after each DE, the odds of having a subsequent episode are progressively higher, emphasizing the need of continuous and proper psychiatric treatment in this population. On the other hand, the risk of recurrence becomes progressively lower over time as the duration of remission increases. The persistence of even mild depressive symptoms during remission is a predictor of recurrence [9], so full remission should be the goal of the treatment. Unfortunately, nonspecialized treatment providers may erroneously assess remission, favoring chronicity, recurrence, and possible disastrous outcomes.

Depressive Disorders Among Bariatric Surgery Patients

Prior to Surgery

There is a consensus in the literature about a high prevalence of psychopathology among bariatric surgery candidates. More interesting is the fact that obese patients, i.e., obese individuals seeking for treatment, have higher psychopathologies rates than obese persons who are not seeking obesity treatments, including having history of depressive and anxiety disorders [1, 15].

In a recent cross-sectional study [16], Duarte-Guerra et al. used the SCID I [17] to interview 393 treatment-seeking obese patients (79% women, mean age 43, mean BMI 47.8 kg/m^2) looking for DSM-IV-TR [18] axis I diagnosis. They have found that about 60% of patients had any given psychiatric disorder. Current anxiety disorders were the most frequent diagnosis (46.3%). Also, lifetime rate of any psychiatric disorder was of 80.9%, and lifetime affective disorders were the most frequent diagnosis (total 64.9%; bipolar disorders 35.6% and DD 29.3%). Roughly half of the patients presented three or more comorbid psychiatric disorders among those who had any lifetime psychiatric disorder.

In a meta-analysis published in 2016, Dawes et al. showed results from 59 studies reporting the prevalence of preoperative mental health conditions (65,363 patients). Among these, the most common psychiatric disorders were depression (19% ranging from 14% to 25%) and binge eating disorder (17% ranging from 13% to 21%) [19].

After Surgery

Rutledge et al. studied 55 patients for 5 years in terms of pre- to post-surgery involvement with antidepressants, anxiolytics, psychotherapies, and overall psychiatric treatment along with changes in weight and metabolic function. There was evidence of decreased antidepressant use and of depression therapies following bariatric surgery, but no improvements on rates of anxiolytic use and anxiety therapies or on overall psychiatric treatment involvement despite metabolic improvements [20].

Lier et al. studying 127 patients (94 women) with mean BMI = 45.3 ± 5.2 kg/m^2 and mean age 41.3 ± 10.3 found a substantive improvement in the prevalence of psychiatric disorders after 1 year of surgery (87 patients). Forty-eight percent of patients had a psychiatric disorder prior to surgery, and 18% had a comorbid psychiatric disorder 1 year after [21].

Brandão et al. published a review of the literature from 2002 to 2014 in PubMed. They have found improvements in the areas of eating behaviors, body image, and mood disorders. They also stress that those improvements may be circumscribed to first years of the postoperative period [22].

In the aforementioned meta-analysis [19], the authors conclude that there is no solid information on the correlation of preoperative mental health status and postoperative weight loss and that there are moderate-quality evidences supporting a link between bariatric surgeries and lower rates of depression postoperatively.

Alcohol-Related Disorders

A serious problem seen not only in the now abundant literature about the theme but also in the clinical setting is the appearance (or reappearance) of problematic alcohol consumption after surgery. This aspect may trigger a variety of unwanted outcomes, among which the failure in losing weight is the less disturbing. Although of interest, we will not go through each of the alcohol use disorders consequences due to the format of the chapter.

In the DSM V [9], alcohol-related disorders encompass *alcohol use disorder* (AUD), *alcohol intoxication*, *alcohol withdrawal*, *other alcohol-induced disorders*, and *unspecified alcohol-related disorder*. Here we will focus on AUD. Its diagnostic criteria are shown in Table 31.3.

Weight loss surgery candidates may have a higher lifetime rate of AUD, up to 32.6% compared to the 14.6% seen in the general population

Table 31.3 Adapted DSM V diagnostic criteria for AUD

A. A problematic pattern of alcohol use leading to clinically significant impairment or distress, as manifested by at least two of the following, occurring within a 12-month period: 1. Alcohol is often taken in larger amounts or over a longer period than was intended 2. There is a persistent desire or unsuccessful efforts to cut down or control alcohol use 3. A great deal of time is spent in activities necessary to obtain alcohol, use alcohol, or recover from its effects 4. Craving or a strong desire or urge to use alcohol 5. Recurrent alcohol use resulting in a failure to fulfill major role obligations at work, school, or home 6. Continued alcohol use despite having persistent or recurrent social or interpersonal problems caused or exacerbated by the effects of alcohol 7. Important social, occupational, or recreational activities are given up or reduced because of alcohol use 8. Recurrent alcohol use in situations in which it is physically hazardous 9. Alcohol use is continued despite knowledge of having a persistent or recurrent physical or psychological problem that is likely to have been caused or exacerbated by alcohol 10. Tolerance, as defined by either of the following: (a) A need for markedly increased amounts of alcohol to achieve intoxication or desired effect (b) A markedly diminished effect with continued use of the same amount of alcohol 11. Withdrawal, as manifested by either of the following: (a) The characteristic withdrawal syndrome for alcohol (refer to Criteria A and B of the criteria set for alcohol withdrawal, pp. 499–500) (b) Alcohol (or a closely related substance, such as a benzodiazepine) is taken to relieve or avoid withdrawal symptoms
Specify if: *In early remission:* After full criteria for AUD were previously met, none of the criteria for AUD have been met for at least 3 months but for less than 12 months (with the exception that Criterion A4 may be met) *In sustained remission:* After full criteria for AUD were previously met, none of the criteria for AUD have been met at any time during a period of 12 months or longer (with the exception that Criterion A4 may be met)
Specify if: *In a controlled environment:* This additional specifier is used if the individual is in an environment where access to alcohol is restricted
Code based on current severity: *Note for ICD-10-CM codes:* If any other alcohol-induced mental disorder is also present, do not use the codes below for alcohol use disorder. Instead, the comorbid alcohol use disorder is indicated in the fourth character of the alcohol-induced disorder code
Specify current severity: 305.00 (F 10.10) Mild: Presence of 2–3 symptoms 303.90 (F 10.20) Moderate: Presence of 4–5 symptoms 303.90 (F 10.20) Severe: Presence of 6 or more symptoms

[23]. At the same time, bariatric surgeries, especially Roux-en-Y gastric bypass (RYGB), alter alcohol pharmacokinetics as shown by shorter interval to reach maximum blood concentration, higher maximum alcohol concentration, and longer time needed to eliminate alcohol [7, 23].

King et al. studied 1945 participants (78% female) showed that preoperative prevalence of AUD is comparable to that present 1 year after the surgery (around 7.5%) but increased to 9.6% at 2 years of follow-up after surgery. The main isolated risk factors were male sex, younger age, smoking, regular alcohol consumption, recreational drug use, lower interpersonal support, and undergoing RYGB [7].

Another study, with 11,115 patients, comparing AUD-related outcomes in RYGB, vertical banded gastroplasty, and gastric banding showed that RYGB patients had twice the chance of being admitted to inpatient care for alcohol problems [24], a similar finding to those showed by Conason et al. in a prospective study in 2013 and by Mitchell et al. in 2015 [25, 26].

On the other hand, a retrospective study published in 2015 on 659 charts found a low prevalence of alcohol use as well as a decrease in the rate of alcohol use during the postoperative period, independent of surgical technique, clinical factors, and percentage of weight loss [27].

Padola et al. [28] stated that despite being at elevated risk, RYGB patients have a low prevalence of AUD. Risk factors for developing AUD were in line with those shown in the study by King et al. [7] but included symptoms of attention deficit and hyperactivity disorder.

Also in 2015, Steffen et al. published a review article in which they reinforce the previous findings, i.e., RYGB is associated with higher risk of AUD in a minority of patients. The authors also discuss the possible mechanisms for that outcome, i.e., pharmacokinetics changes and neurobiological pathways through dopamine release in the nucleus accumbens besides indicating the present lack of scientific robust basis for the concept of addiction transfer [29]. In the same line, Blackburn et al. discuss that the alterations in alcohol metabolism and pharmacokinetics are unlikely to be the sole or even the main mechanism for AUD after bariatric surgeries, implying the central reward system as another candidate to cause AUD in bariatric patients [30].

American Society for Metabolic and Bariatric Surgery Statement

ASMBS released a statement on alcohol use and bariatric surgery [31] whose conclusions are quoted below:

1. "*There is conflicting data as to the lifetime and current prevalence of AUD in patients seeking weight loss surgery. Most studies indicate that AUD affects a minority of bariatric surgery patients. Studies have shown that some individuals are at risk for AUD relapse or for developing new-onset AUD after weight loss surgery, especially after gastric bypass. Other studies have shown a decrease in high-risk drinking after surgery compared with baseline.*
2. *Based on current studies, gastric bypass surgery is associated with:*
   - *Accelerated alcohol absorption (shorter time to reach maximum concentration)*
   - *Higher maximum alcohol concentration*
   - *Longer time to eliminate alcohol in both men and women*
   - *Increased risk for development of AUD*
3. *The data are less clear regarding altered pharmacokinetics after sleeve gastrectomy and there is no evidence that alcohol absorption is affected by gastric banding. Given the recent increase in popularity of sleeve gastrectomy, more studies regarding the pharmacokinetic effects of sleeve gastrectomy on alcohol metabolism are needed.*
4. *Patients undergoing bariatric surgery should be screened and educated regarding alcohol intake both before and after surgery. Active AUD is considered a contraindication by most programs and in published guidelines. Adequate screening, assessment, and preoperative preparation may help decrease the risk of AUD in bariatric surgery patients. A period of sustained abstinence with treatment*

is indicated before weight loss surgery. A history of AUD is not a contraindication to bariatric surgery. However, patients should be made aware that AUD can occur in the long term after bariatric surgery."

We would like to finish this topic adding that special attention should be payed to adolescent bariatric patients. They represent a growing subpopulation undergoing bariatric surgeries who benefit from them in a comparable extent to that of adults [32] but may be at higher risks of AUD and other substance use disorders [33].

Suicidality During the Postoperative Period

This is a still poorly understood aspect that seems to be linked to bariatric surgeries long-term outcome.

For instance, in a 2005 case series [34], the characteristics of three cases of suicide following bariatric surgery were presented. In each of the cases, there was recurrent MDD before and after surgery, which means that those patients were at a higher risk even before the surgical procedure. That point precludes a simple cause-effect assumption.

In 2007, Omalu et al. found a substantial excess of death due to suicide and coronary heart disease in the long term. Interestingly, the authors acknowledge the absence of "psychological support" [35] but do not cite explicitly the higher psychiatric disorders prevalence in this population which can be, at least to some extent, responsible for such outcomes.

Tindle et al. found similar figures in 2010 in roughly the same period as the previous study and also acknowledge the lack of mental disorder proper treatment [8].

Adams et al. in a control matched outcome study showed that after a mean follow-up of 7.1 years, 171 deaths from specific disease were prevented per 10,000 operations. On the other hand, there was an increase of 35 non-disease-related deaths per 10,000 operations. That leads to a net prevention of 136 deaths. In the surgery group, deaths not caused by disease (these include suicide, accidents not related to drugs, poisonings of undetermined intent, and other deaths) were 1.58 times the number present at the control group. Unfortunately, the article does not cite if psychiatric treatment was offered for the bariatric surgery group [36].

Mitchell et al. stated that there is a higher than average rate of suicide among this group of patients [37]. The authors go through a number of possible explanatory causes such as persistence or recurrence of medical comorbidities after bariatric surgery, disinhibition/impulsivity secondary to alcohol kinetic changes, hypoglycemia, and changes in pharmacokinetics among others.

Morgan and Ho describe 110 patients hospitalized due to deliberate self-harm during the postoperative period in a cohort of 12,062 patients, studied for 5 years. Despite being a higher rate than in the general population, this number did not present an elevation of the preoperative rate of self-harm hospitalizations [38].

As a mean of comparison, we will show suicide data of some psychiatric disorders [9].

- Bipolar disorder: 36% (15 times the risk of general population and 25% of all suicide attempts).
- Bipolar II disorder: 32%.
- Specific phobia: 1.6 times the risk of general population.
- OCD: 50% have suicidal thoughts; 25% attempt suicide.
- Anorexia nervosa: 12/100000 /year.
- Bulimia nervosa: elevated suicide risk.
- AUD: important contributor to suicide risk during severe intoxication and in the context of a temporary alcohol-induced depressive and bipolar disorder. There is an increased rate of suicidal behavior as well as of completed suicide among individuals with the disorder.

As one can see, the suicide risk of psychiatric disorders commonly found amidst the bariatric population is considerably high. It is possible that rates seen in the postoperative population represent at least partially undiagnosed and/or untreated psychiatric disorders and not simply a complication of bariatric surgeries or of weight loss.

Final Remarks

The topics in this chapter are extremely relevant and impacting in the management of a great part of bariatric patients. Despite that, the data available in bariatric surgery x psychiatric disorders is not always sufficient in terms of generalization. Moreover, we do not observe psychiatrist in most of the clinical and/or research groups.

It is our opinion that this is a situation that is bound to change as neurosciences evolve, as the knowledge of intimate relations – such as those between gut and brain – becomes more abundant and comprehensive and as literature keeps on bringing to light psychiatric issues rather than just psychological aspects.

It is important to remember that many of the psychiatric disorders have proper treatments with adequate effectiveness and well-established algorithms. Not offering this option due to any reason is not adequate and is untenable.

References

1. Segal A. Obesidade e comorbidade psiquiátrica: caracterização e eficácia terapêutica de atendimento multidisciplinar na evolução de 34 pacientes. Doctorate Thesis. São Paulo: Faculdade de Medicina da Universidade de São Paulo; 1999.
2. Lopresti A, Drummond P. Obesity and psychiatric disorders: commonalities in dysregulated biological pathways and their implications for treatment. Prog Neuropsychopharmacol Biol Psychiatry. 2013;45:92–9.
3. Lopresti A, Hood S, Drummond P. A review of lifestyle factors that contribute to important pathways associated with major depression: diet, sleep and exercise. J Affect Disord. 2013;148(1):12–27.
4. Herpertz S, Kielmann R, Wolf A, Langkafel M, Senf W, Hebebrand J. Does obesity surgery improve psychosocial functioning? A systematic review. Int J Obes (Lond). 2003;27(11):1300–14.
5. Lasikiewicz N, Myrissa K, Hoyland A, Lawton C. Psychological benefits of weight loss following behavioural and/or dietary weight loss interventions. A systematic research review. Appetite. 2014;72:123–37.
6. Hagedorn J, Encarnacion B, Brat G, Morton J. Does gastric bypass alter alcohol metabolism? Surg Obes Relat Dis. 2007;3(5):543–8.
7. King W, Chen J, Mitchell J, Kalarchian M, Steffen K, Engel S, et al. Prevalence of alcohol use disorders before and after bariatric surgery. JAMA. 2012;307(23):2516.
8. Tindle H, Omalu B, Courcoulas A, Marcus M, Hammers J, Kuller L. Risk of suicide after long-term follow-up from bariatric surgery. Am J Med. 2010;123(11):1036–42.
9. American Psychiatric Association. Diagnostic and statistical manual of mental disorders. 5th ed. Arlington: American Psychiatric Association; 2013.
10. Kessler R, Bromet E. The epidemiology of depression across cultures. Annu Rev Public Health. 2013;34(1):119–38.
11. Purkayastha S, Cai D. Neuroinflammatory basis of metabolic syndrome. Mol Metab. 2013;2(4):356–63.
12. Gonnissen H, Hulshof T, Westerterp-Plantenga M. Chronobiology, endocrinology, and energy- and food-reward homeostasis. Obes Rev. 2013;14(5):405–16.
13. Parikh S, Quilty L, Ravitz P, Rosenbluth M, Pavlova B, Grigoriadis S, et al. Canadian Network for Mood and Anxiety Treatments (CANMAT) 2016 clinical guidelines for the management of adults with major depressive disorder: section 2. Psychological treatments. Can J Psychiatry. 2016;61(9):524–39.
14. Kennedy S, Lam R, McIntyre R, Tourjman S, Bhat V, Blier P, et al. Canadian Network for Mood and Anxiety Treatments (CANMAT) 2016 clinical guidelines for the management of adults with major depressive disorder: section 3. Pharmacological treatments. Can J Psychiatry. 2016;61(9):540–60.
15. Malik S, Mitchell J, Engel S, Crosby R, Wonderlich S. Psychopathology in bariatric surgery candidates: a review of studies using structured diagnostic interviews. Compr Psychiatry. 2014;55(2):248–59.
16. Duarte-Guerra L, Coêlho B, Santo M, Wang Y. Psychiatric disorders among obese patients seeking bariatric surgery: results of structured clinical interviews. Obes Surg. 2014;25(5):830–7.
17. First MB, Spitzer RL, Gibbon M, et al. Structured clinical interview for DSM-IV-TR axis I disorders, research version, patient edition. (SCID-I/P) New York: Biometrics Research, New York State Psychiatric Institute; November 2002.
18. American Psychiatric Association. Diagnostic and statistical manual of mental disorders. 4th ed. Text Revision (DSM-IV-TR). Washington, DC: American Psychiatric Association; 2000.
19. Dawes A, Maggard-Gibbons M, Maher A, Booth M, Miake-Lye I, Beroes J, et al. Mental health conditions among patients seeking and undergoing bariatric surgery. JAMA. 2016;315(2):150.
20. Rutledge T, Braden A, Woods G, Herbst K, Groesz L, Savu M. Five-year changes in psychiatric treatment status and weight-related comorbidities following bariatric surgery in a veteran population. Obes Surg. 2012;22(11):1734–41.
21. Lier HØ, Biringer E, Stubhaug B, Tangen T. Prevalence of psychiatric disorders before and 1 year after bariatric surgery: the role of shame in maintenance of psychiatric disorders in patients undergoing bariatric surgery. Nord J Psychiatry. 2012;67(2):89–96.

22. Brandão I, Fernandes A, Osório E, Calhau M, Coelho R. A psychiatric perspective view of bariatric surgery patients. Arch Clin Psychiatry (São Paulo). 2015;42(5):122–8.
23. Heinberg L, Ashton K, Coughlin J. Alcohol and bariatric surgery: review and suggested recommendations for assessment and management. Surg Obes Relat Dis. 2012;8(3):357–63.
24. Östlund M, Backman O, Marsk R, Stockeld D, Lagergren J, Rasmussen F, et al. Increased admission for alcohol dependence after gastric bypass surgery compared with restrictive bariatric surgery. JAMA Surg. 2013;148(4):374.
25. Conason A, Teixeira J, Hsu C, Puma L, Knafo D, Geliebter A. Substance use following bariatric weight loss surgery. JAMA Surg. 2013;148(2):145.
26. Mitchell J, Steffen K, Engel S, King W, Chen J, Winters K, et al. Addictive disorders after Roux-en-Y gastric bypass. Surg Obes Relat Dis. 2015;11(4):897–905.
27. de Araujo Burgos M, Cabral P, Maio R, Oliveira B, Dias M, de Figueiredo Melim D, et al. Prevalence of alcohol abuse before and after bariatric surgery associated with nutritional and lifestyle factors: a study involving a Portuguese population. Obes Surg. 2015;25(9):1716–22.
28. Spadola C, Wagner E, Dillon F, Trepka M, De La Cruz-Munoz N, Messiah S. Alcohol and drug use among postoperative bariatric patients: a systematic review of the emerging research and its implications. Alcohol Clin Exp Res. 2015;39(9):1582–601.
29. Steffen K, Engel S, Wonderlich J, Pollert G, Sondag C. Alcohol and other addictive disorders following bariatric surgery: prevalence, risk factors and possible etiologies. Eur Eat Disord Rev. 2015;23(6):442–50.
30. Blackburn A, Hajnal A, Leggio L. The gut in the brain: the effects of bariatric surgery on alcohol consumption. Addict Biol. 2017;22:1540–53.
31. Parikh M, Johnson J, Ballem N. ASMBS position statement on alcohol use before and after bariatric surgery. Surg Obes Relat Dis. 2016;12(2):225–30.
32. Olbers T, Gronowitz E, Werling M, Mårlid S, Flodmark C, Peltonen M, et al. Two-year outcome of laparoscopic Roux-en-Y gastric bypass in adolescents with severe obesity: results from a Swedish Nationwide Study (AMOS). Int J Obes (Lond). 2012;36(11):1388–95.
33. Zeller M, Washington G, Mitchell J, Sarwer D, Reiter-Purtill J, Jenkins T, et al. Alcohol use risk in adolescents 2 years after bariatric surgery. Surg Obes Relat Dis. 2017;13:85–94.
34. Omalu B, Cho P, Shakir A, Agumadu U, Rozin L, Kuller L, et al. Suicides following bariatric surgery for the treatment of obesity. Surg Obes Relat Dis. 2005;1(4):447–9.
35. Omalu B. Death rates and causes of death after bariatric surgery for Pennsylvania residents, 1995 to 2004. Arch Surg. 2007;142(10):923.
36. Adams T, Gress R, Smith S, Halverson R, Simper S, Rosamond W, et al. Long-term mortality after gastric bypass surgery. N Engl J Med. 2007;357(8):753–61.
37. Mitchell J, Crosby R, de Zwaan M, Engel S, Roerig J, Steffen K, et al. Possible risk factors for increased suicide following bariatric surgery. Obesity. 2013;21(4):665–72.
38. Morgan D, Ho K. Incidence and risk factors for deliberate self-harm, mental illness, and suicide following bariatric surgery. Ann Surg. 2017;265:244–52.

Nutritional Complications

32

Silvia Leite Faria, Orlando Pereira Faria, and Marina Kiyomi Ito

Introduction

In recent years, tremendous advances have occurred in the technology and knowledge involving bariatric and metabolic surgeries resulting in increased safety of the procedures, benefits to the patients, and decrease in patient morbidity. Perioperative complications related to the surgical procedure have decreased, as demonstrated in numerous studies [1].

However, postoperative complications, such as those related to nutritional deficiencies, due to hormonal changes and physiological functioning consequent to the surgeries, are well-known and, when detected, merit special attention [2, 3].

In addition, obese candidates for bariatric surgery (BS) show signs and symptoms of nutritional deficiency mainly caused by intake of high-calorie, low-nutrient food, use of "fad" diets, and use of medications which can interfere with vitamin status and the sense of satiety [4].

Indeed, anatomical changes that occur in BS result in lesser availability of nutrients, and the degree of nutritional deficiency will depend on the type of procedure performed [4].

Each type of procedure has its own nutritional consequences. We will focus on the most widely performed procedures, namely, adjusted gastric banding (AGB), duodenal switch (DS), sleeve gastrectomy (SG), and Roux-en-Y gastric bypass (RYGB), the last two of which are the most frequently performed [5].

As shown in Fig. 32.1, specific sites exist for absorption of vitamins and minerals. Altering these sites creates greater risk in developing nutritional deficiency and provokes higher patient demands for these nutrients [6].

Our concerns go beyond these causes. Patients show signs of food intolerance after BS and present low adherence to prescribed nutritional supplements. Table 32.1 shows the main causes of nutritional deficiencies relative to the procedures selected.

With specific concern for the nutritional complications of BS, we will divide them into two categories: short-term and long-term complications. The most common short-term complications are anemia and iron deficiency, thiamine deficiency (beriberi), vitamin B_{12} deficiency, dumping syndrome and/or hypoglycemia, and hair loss.

The long-term complications we will focus on are bone disease, lean tissue loss and sarcopenia, weight regain, and excessive weight loss [7–10].

S. L. Faria (✉)
Gastrocirurgia de Brasília & University of Brasília, Brasília, DF, Brazil

O. P. Faria
Bariatric and Metabolic Surgery, Gastrocirurgia de Brasília, Brasília, DF, Brazil

M. K. Ito
Department of Nutrition, University of Brasília, Brasília, DF, Brazil

J. Ettinger et al. (eds.), *Gastric Bypass*, https://doi.org/10.1007/978-3-030-28803-7_32

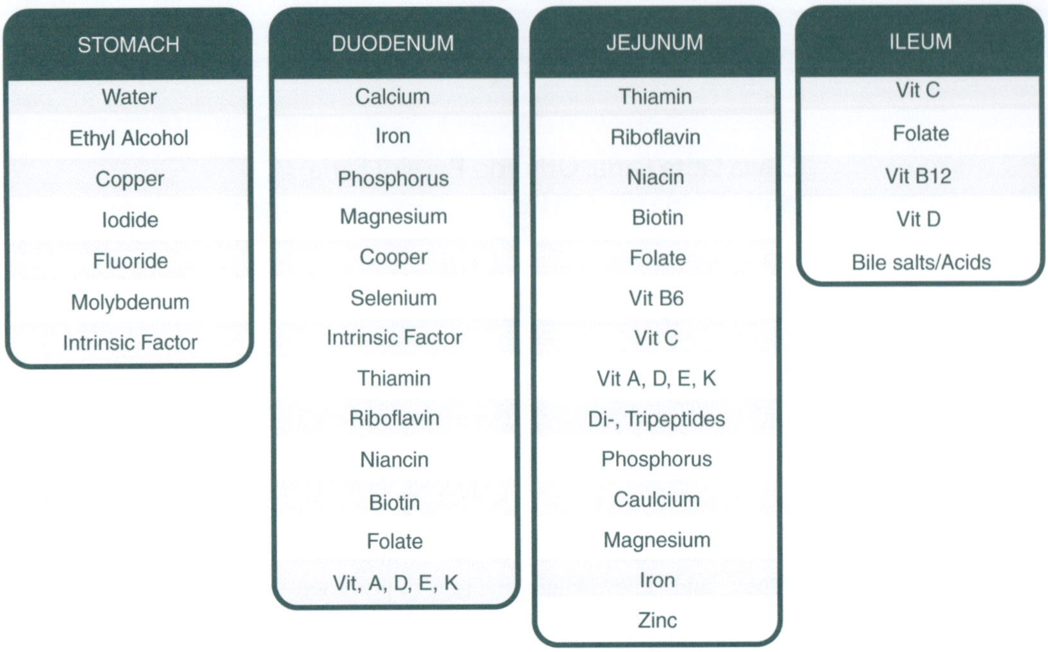

Fig. 32.1 Nutrients are absorbed in different places of the gastrointestinal tract

Table 32.1 The main causes for nutrient deficiencies among different bariatric procedures

Procedure	Causes for possible deficiency
SG	Low storage capacity, MVI[a] noncompliance and aversion to meat, low caloric intake
RYGB	Bypass active site, hypochlorhydria, reduced contact with intrinsic factor, low caloric intake, and MVI noncompliance
AGB	Vomiting, low caloric intake, low storage capacity, noncompliance MVI. Aversion to meat
BPD-DS	Malabsorption, delayed mixing fat with bile and pancreatic enzymes

SG sleeve gastrectomy, *RYGB* Roux-en-Y gastric bypass, *AGB* adjustable gastric banding, *BPD-DS* biliopancreatic diversion with duodenal switch

[a]MVI multivitamin

Anemia and Iron Deficiency

Anemia is defined as low blood hemoglobin concentration and is seen as a serious worldwide public health problem. According to the World Health Organization (WHO), hemoglobin (Hb) levels <12 g/dL in women (<11 g/dL in pregnant women) and <13 g/dL in men are cutoff values for the diagnosis of anemia [11]. In adults, depleted iron stores, with absence of inflammation, are indicated by serum ferritin levels below 15 ug/L [12]. Additionally, low transferrin saturation is indicative of iron deficiency. These conditions need to be treated adequately in order to minimize patient morbidity and optimize postoperative quality of life.

Although iron deficiency is the most common cause of anemia among bariatric patients, relevant nutritional causes involve folic acid, vitamin A, and B_{12} deficiencies.

The most recent and representative data available in the literature concerns anemia in RYGB patients [13]. Weng et al. systematically reviewed the prevalence of anemia in over 5000 RYGB patients and observed that a mean proportion of 12% of immediate postsurgical patients were anemic. This proportion grew even more over the long term, reaching postsurgical levels of 20.9%, 25.9%, and 23.1% at 12, 24, and 36 months, respectively [12].

Iron deficiency may occur as a result from limited exposure of food to gastric acid, bypass of the duodenum and proximal jejunum the region of optimal iron absorption, and reduction of meat intake.

Iron, ferritin, folic acid, and vitamin B_{12} status were also evaluated in the same study. Overall, ferritin levels were low in 7.9% of patients (pooled mean estimate of 87.6 ng/mL) following surgery, and it triplicated during the 36-month follow-up. Ferritin is the primary form of iron stores in the body, and, in the absence of inflammation, blood ferritin concentration is positively correlated with the size of the total body iron stores. Therefore, low serum ferritin seems consistent with depleted iron stores [11, 13]. The proportion of patients with low vitamin B_{12} also increased, from 2.3% to 6.5% at the 12-month follow-up, and continued until 36 months. In contrast, the proportion of patients with iron and folate deficiency did not change during the follow-up period [13]. As the absorption of folate occurs throughout the small intestine, whereas vitamin B_{12} absorption depends on the appropriate intrinsic factor and acid secretion in the stomach, RYGB patients may absorb less vitamin B_{12} due to insufficient levels of these two elements [14]. Accordingly, vitamin B_{12} deficiency, rather than folate, seems to better explain long-term iron deficiency anemia in those patients.

It is important to recognize that many preoperative patients are reported to be deficient in iron, folic acid, and vitamin B_{12} [15]. The mechanism that explains obesity-related anemia and vitamin A deficiency is the fact that inflammation, due to high adiposity and vitamin A deficiency, increases hepatic hepcidin production, which is a key regulator of iron homeostasis in the circulatory system. Increased hepcidin production blocks iron release from enterocytes and macrophages, thereby impairing iron homeostasis in obese individuals. The improvement in iron absorption after weight loss and decreased inflammation and higher hepcidin levels was elegantly shown in laparoscopic sleeve gastrectomy (LSG) patients monitored during 6 months post-surgery [16].

Similar to other essential nutrients, iron, folate, and vitamin B_{12} status and hematological parameters, such as hemoglobin, serum iron status, and ferritin, must be monitored in all bariatric patients to detect signs of nutritional deficiency anemia. Laboratory values must be observed considering age, gender, and, if relevant, stage of gestation. Long-term annual checkups are necessary because deficiencies were reported in patients 10 years after surgery [17].

Routine oral multivitamin/mineral supplementation of post-bariatric patients is necessary, although it is not sufficient to prevent iron deficiency in menstruating women. Indefinite long-term daily oral iron supplementation is necessary to prevent the development of iron deficiency in the majority of menstruating women. Iron deficiency should be treated. Daily supplementation of oral ferrous sulfate, ferrous fumarate, or ferrous gluconate to provide up to 150–200 mg of elemental iron and 1000 ug of vitamin B_{12} is recommended. Vitamin C may be added to improve iron absorption. Ferrous sulfates tend to present gastrointestinal effects (constipation), whereas other formulations seem to be better tolerated. Iron tablets can cause local irritation and erosion of gastric mucosa; a liquid preparation may be more appropriate. Lower doses reduce common gastrointestinal side effects. In case of oral iron intolerance, noncompliance or severe deficiency and with anemia present, intravenous infusion, with ferric gluconate or sucrose, may be necessary [18, 19].

Thiamine Deficiency

Thiamine deficiency, also recognized as beriberi, can occur in all bariatric procedures.

Thiamine is a water soluble vitamin absorbed in the proximal jejunum with support of an active transport system. Thiamine reserves in the body amount to only 30 mg and are depleted in as quickly as 20 days. Thiamine deficiency can cause devastating consequences, such as Wernicke encephalopathy and Korsakoff psychosis [2].

One of the causes for thiamine deficiency is related to decreased caloric ingestion. Besides that, more than 3 weeks of restrictive diet without thiamine supplementation, along with frequent vomiting, can lead to deficiency. Because it is primarily absorbed in the duodenum and proximal jejunum,

RYGB and BPD-DS patients are at increased risk for developing thiamine deficiency [2, 6, 19].

Thiamine is required for normal carbohydrate metabolism. Refeeding a malnourished patient with carbohydrate foodstuff can precipitate thiamine deficiency [20]. Intravenous glucose administration is a risk factor for triggering acute symptomatic vitamin B deficiency, leading to interruption of the citric acid cycle and lactate acidosis. Hence, prophylactic administration of thiamine 100 mg IV is recommended when starting intravenous fluids in high-risk patients [21].

The prevalence of thiamine deficiency among patients who adhere to multivitamin supplementation is lower than those who do not [20].

Thiamine deficiency is also common among bariatric candidates; the prevalence is between 15.5% and 33%, being higher among females [22].

The American Society for Metabolic and Bariatric Surgery (ASMBS) guidelines recommend that post-op RYGB patients take 3 mg of thiamine daily to prevent deficiency [7].

Thiamine deficiency is diagnosed based on signs and symptoms, along with serum thiamine levels, using an erythrocyte transketolase activity assay [7, 18, 22].

Any suspicion of this deficiency should be quickly treated, as its consequences can be irreversible. Sometimes, its signs and symptoms are quite common, so healthcare professionals should be aware and trained to diagnose and treat any clinical symptoms. It is better to overdose than to allow grave consequences to appear.

The early symptoms are neuritis, neuropathy – especially in the lower extremities – and muscle pain with atrophy and paraplegia. If not quickly recognized, it can lead to a cerebral beriberi. This attacks the central nervous system and the spinal cord and results in Wernicke-Korsakoff syndrome. Ataxia and oculomotor problems are further symptoms. If treated early, the prognosis of beriberi is positive, but mortality still ranges between 10% and 20%. Besides that, complete remission is rare as cognitive changes are not reversible in most cases [22].

Clinical manifestations of thiamine deficiency include Wernicke encephalopathy, peripheral neuropathies, nystagmus, and ocular palsies [22].

In order to prevent acute Wernicke encephalopathy, a daily prophylactic oral dose of 25–50 mg, in addition to multivitamins, starting as early as 6 weeks after surgery, might be recommended for malnourished patients [2, 6, 22].

Early symptoms of neuropathy can be treated with 20–30 mg oral doses of thiamine until symptoms disappear. For more advanced symptoms and for patients with protractile vomiting, 100 mg of thiamine parenterally for 5–7 days is recommended, followed by oral doses of 50 mg daily until complete recovery. During thiamine supplementation treatment, additional supplementation with specifically the B group or other vitamins is important [2, 6, 22].

B_{12}

The incidence of vitamin B_{12} deficiency may range from 26% to 70% [23–25]. RYGB is the procedure with higher levels of B_{12} deficiency. Among patients seeking bariatric surgery, the vitamin B_{12} assays that are currently used to diagnose clinical vitamin deficiency may reach a failure rate of 22–35%, and clinicians may not recognize this deficiency [25].

The American Academy of Family Physicians recommended a daily prophylactic dose of 1000 mcg to be used among post-bariatric patients. Vitamin B_{12} can be administered, either orally or sublingually, and is used to prevent nutritional deficiencies. Intramuscularly or parenterally, high doses, such as 1000 mcg or 3000 mcg, should be used in the case of deficiency or even as a preventive action before surgery.

Megaloblastic anemia is the disease that can occur among patients with chronic B_{12} deficiency. But prior to this anemia, patients usually present some of the following signs and symptoms, ataxia, optic atrophy, memory loss, mental status change, myeloneuropathy, megaloblastic anemia, and thrombocytopenia, but in most cases they are asymptomatic.

B_{12} blood levels below 400 pg/dL are accepted as indicators of possible deficiency of this vitamin. Levels below 100 pg/dL show a serious deficiency and should be treated with IM or IV supplementations [2, 6, 7, 19].

Dumping Syndrome and Hypoglycemia

Dumping syndrome (DS) is classified as either early or late. Its diagnosis can be facilitated by using Sigstad's scoring system. Points are given for each symptom experienced. A score over seven is indicative of dumping. A score of less than 4 suggests a different diagnosis [26].

Early DS occurs from 30 to 60 minutes after eating and includes symptoms of bloating, diarrhea, nausea, and lightheadedness. It occurs due to undigested calorie-dense liquids or solids which provoke hyperosmolarity of the intestinal content causing fluid to be drawn into the intestinal lumen leading to intestinal distention, fluid sequestration, decreased intravascular volume, and hypotension. Patients should be instructed to recognize the signs and symptoms and avoid high-calorie liquids and solids. Early DS is more frequent among RYGB patients. In general, 20–50% of all gastric surgery patients experience some of the symptoms of DS after their operation. Among RYGB patients, the incidence is 75% [26].

Postprandial DS, called hyperinsulinemic hypoglycemia, is a complication related to non-banding procedures. Symptoms can occur from 1 to 3 hours after meals, particularly meals rich in carbohydrates. In severe situations, DS may cause protein-wasting malnutrition. Studies from Salehi et al. reported evidence for the role of the incretin hormone glucagon-like peptide-1 (GLP-1) as a critical contributor to the inappropriate insulin secretion in this syndrome [27, 28].

Hypoglycemic symptoms can be broadly classified as autonomic (e.g., palpitations, lightheadedness, sweating) or neuroglycopenic (e.g., confusion, decreased attentiveness, seizure, loss of consciousness). More severe hypoglycemia associated with neuroglycopenia is rare, but can occur from 1 to 3 years post-RYGB [28].

Therapeutic approaches to post-hypoglycemia include diet and medication.

Dietary changes are the first-line treatment for DS. Patients should be advised to eat smaller and more frequent meals (about six per day). Patients should save fluids for after meals, separating their intake of "dry" from "wet" nutrients by more than 1 hour (because liquids accelerate gastric transit), lying down after meals, decreasing their carbohydrate intake, and preferentially eating complex carbohydrates rather than simple ones. Alcohol, coffee, and beverages with caffeine should be avoided. Patients may feel worse with milk and dairy products, so eliminating them has been helpful for many patients. Meals should be composed of carbohydrates (low-glycemic index), lipids, proteins, and fibers (mixed meals). Adding soluble fiber before or during the meals can help to slow the pace of the food through the gastrointestinal tract. Avoidance of sweets and simple carbohydrates is an essential element of the bariatric diet used to sidestep DS symptoms. Table 32.2 shows some important recommendation. To include fiber supplementation with meals to diminish the pace of food in the gastrointestinal tract is a good strategy (guar gum, glucomannan, and pectin, doses of 500 mg of each).

Table 32.2 Nutritional management of dumping syndrome (DS)

Dietary recommendations to prevent reactive hypoglycemia		
Include	Avoid	Example
Mixed meals	High-carbohydrate meals	Bagel with jelly Fruit salad
Artificial sweeteners	Simple sugars	Soda, juice, candy, cake
Soluble fiber	Caffeine (adrenaline)	Tea, coffee, Coke®
Three meals, plus up to three snacks	Alcohol	Wine, beer

If the dietetic intervention fails to cure these events, medications should be used for improvement. As a parallel treatment, physicians can use acarbose, octreotide, and diazoxide [26].

Very low levels of glucose should be treated with glucose infusion [28].

Hair Loss

Hair loss can seriously impact the lives of individuals and may lead to anxiety, low self-esteem, psychosocial problems, and depression. As a consequence, hair loss can be a stress factor for this population [29].

Hair loss among bariatric patients can occur within 3 months postsurgery. In most cases, hair loss occurring between 3 and 6 months postsurgery is related to rapid weight loss and low caloric intake. After 6 months, it can be related to nutritional deficiencies. Actually, patients with 6 months or more of surgery are supposed to adhere to vitamin, mineral, and protein supplements.

The causes for hair loss can also be related to age, sex, disease, and genetic factors. It is therefore important to investigate indications of any current illness, recent illnesses, autoimmune diseases, family history of hair loss, food intake, medications, as well as the use of cosmetics harmful to the hair [29, 30].

Hair follicles have two stages: the anagen (hair growth) stage and the telogen (inactive) phase. All hairs begin their cycle in the anagen phase, grow for a period of time, and move into the telogen phase, which lasts about 100–120 days. Then the hair falls out. This process, if accelerated, is called telogen effluvium, which is the cause of hair loss in bariatric patients [31, 32].

The causes for telogen effluvium are drugs, surgery, fever, childbirth, and diseases related to the thyroid, such as hyper- and hypothyroidism, rapid weight loss, anorexia, low protein intake, iron and zinc deficiency, and toxicity of heavy metals [29, 30, 33]. Among bariatric surgery patients, telogen effluvium may be associated with those patients not adhering to the supplement program or who have rapid weight loss, have difficulty in feeding themselves, or have poor dietary habits or food intolerances, especially with protein sources [33].

Hair loss after bariatric surgery often occurs between the third and sixth months after surgery and can last between 6 and 12 months or more. In the first 6 months, this framework can be reversed without intervention, although there is no consensus on treatment for these cases [23]. After 6 months postsurgery, nutritional causes are involved in hair loss [33]. In both cases, there is no harm to the follicle, so the hair can grow back [34].

The nutrients possibly related to hair loss are protein, iron, zinc, essential fatty acids, vitamin B_{12}, and biotin.

In order to prevent excessive hair loss, patients should be advised to increase protein intake (>60 grams per day) and also to adhere to vitamin and mineral supplementation [35]. Protein-energy deficiency is associated with increased hair loss [30, 33]. A protein deficiency can manifest itself through the reduction of hepatic proteins, including albumin, loss of muscle mass, asthenia, and alopecia [31].

It is believed that a reduction in the availability of protein can cause thinning of the hair, difficulty in the normal growth process, and diffuse alopecia. In relation to essential amino acids, their deficiency can affect growth and differentiation of hair, since they compose 27% of the protein content of hair [31]. Among all essential amino acids, a deficiency of L-lysine, in particular, can contribute to hair loss, while full-body supplies of L-lysine improve hair growth after periods of decline and improve the levels of iron in the body. Its bioavailable form is primarily found in fish, meat, and eggs, and a decrease in consumption of these foods may cause a negative balance of this amino acid affecting hair growth [32]. Thus, a supplementation of 1.5–2 g of L-lysine is recommended [33].

Iron deficiency is more prevalent among those who are in a fertile age, and serum ferritin levels below 40 μg are strongly associated with hair loss [33, 36]. Kantor related low concentrations of serum ferritin and hemoglobin with hair loss [37].

Observations have been made in treatments of telogen effluvium that a significant number of people respond well when treated with iron. In one study, which correlated low serum ferritin with hair loss among women, treatment for 6 months with daily supplementation of 72 mg of iron and 1.5 g of L-lysine decreased the percentage of hairs in the telogen phase, as well as the hair loss by 39% and increased levels of serum ferritin [32]. Iron supplementation recommended for patients with hair loss is 320 mg of ferrous fumarate or gluconate or 65 mg of elemental iron twice a day, with a volume of approximately 25% ingested being absorbed [19, 38]. For bariatric patients who are refractory to iron supplementation or have anemia related to iron deficiency or hemoglobin serum levels below 11 g/dL, parenteral infusion must be prescribed [39]. A study from Tovar-Ruiz found an association between a variable consisting in the addition of zinc and iron showing a significant association with hair loss. Sometimes, even with normal ranges, patients complain about hair loss. So, the variable addition (zinc + iron) is a good predictor of hair loss. Patients should keep the addition above 115 to improve hair loss. Zinc supplementation is necessary in some cases [40].

A biotin deficiency can cause depigmentation of hair and diffuse alopecia, since this vitamin plays an important role in the development of the hair follicles [31, 33]. It is believed that supplementation of biotin can prevent hair loss or accelerate growth after a period of decline [33].

Daily 1–2 mg doses of biotin may provide clinical support to cases of hair loss not responding to other types of treatment. Daily consumption of 2.5 mg was established as a safe limit of intake of biotin, the NOAEL (no-observed-adverse-effect level) [41].

Some studies have observed deficiency of essential fatty acids (linoleic and linolenic acids) in RYGB patients since this procedure alters the digestion of lipids and, as a consequence, the uptake of essential fatty acids [7, 40]. In relation to BPD and DS, only 28% of ingested fat is absorbed [41].

In patients with biotin deficiency, levels of linoleic acid lower than normal were observed, and, in cases of functional deficiency of biotin (due to lack of carboxylase) associated with hair loss, supplementation with polyunsaturated fatty acids may reduce this symptom, suggesting that hair loss can be caused by impairment of elongation of polyunsaturated fatty acids as a result of reduced activity of acetyl-CoA carboxylase [41].

For post-RYGB patients, among other supplements for hair loss, flaxseed oil (15 ml) is recommended. 15 The recommended dose of linolenic acid is from 0.5% to 1.0% of energy intake, and linoleic acid is from 3% to 5%. These amounts can be reached with two capsules of 1 g of linseed oil and 2.5 tablespoons of extra-virgin olive oil [19].

Brolin et al. observed deficiency of vitamin B_{12} in patients 6 months after bariatric surgery, becoming more common after a year [7]. As a consequence, it may alter the pigmentation of hair, which can be reversed with its supplementation. 16 The supplementation of vitamin B_{12} must be at least from 350 to 500 μg/day orally, but there may arise the need of a monthly intramuscular supplement of 1000 μg [10, 22].

In conclusion, patients who present hair loss after 6 months of surgery should follow this recommendation daily: consume 80 g of protein for women and 100 g for men (with sufficient amounts of L-lysine from 1.5 to 2 g/day); add 15 ml of flaxseed oil, 2.5 g of biotin, one or two multivitamin capsules with minerals (thus providing 200% of DRIs), 350–500 μg/day of B_{12}, and 320 mg of ferrous fumarate or gluconate or 65 mg of elemental iron twice daily.

Metabolic Bone Disease

Metabolic bone disease is a long-term adverse consequence of BS and is the most common among patients who have undergone RYGB and BPD [7]. Bone mineral metabolism is adversely affected by bariatric procedures, and the underlying mechanism is still not well-understood, but is largely related to changes in the absorption site, physiological and hormonal changes, low intake of calcium-rich foods, and low intake and absorption of vitamin D. These factors may lead the patient to an onset of secondary hyperparathyroidism and subsequently to osteopenia and osteoporosis. A comprehensive review on the multifactorial nature of the metabolic bone disease in post-bariatric patients has been published [43, 44], but evidences are still limited due to lack of robust longitudinal studies with evaluation of the various parameters involved in bone metabolism of this population. In addition, technical difficulties need to be considered. Bone mass and bone mineral density are often measured by dual-energy X-ray absorptiometry (DXA). Recent studies have pointed to the limitations of this method, in which the accuracy of DXA measurements is jeopardized by excess adiposity and the changes in body composition during the rapid weight loss following surgery, when compared to computed tomography (CT) measurements [44, 45]. Overall, current indicators of nutritional state concerning bone mineral density among BS patients include serum calcium, ionic calcium, serum phosphorus, alkaline phosphatase, 25-hydroxy-D-vitamin, parathyroid hormone (PTH), and bone density. At present, calcium and vitamin D supplements are recommended to all post-bariatric patients, with daily intake of 1700–2100 mg of elemental calcium in the form of calcium citrate and 800 International Units (IU) of vitamin D for patients who underwent RYGB and AGB [7, 19]. For the BPD patients, the recommendation is a daily intake of 2000 mg of elemental calcium and 2000 IU of vitamin D [45]. In treating vitamin D deficiency, a weekly dose of 50,000 IU of ergocalciferol taken orally for 8 weeks is suggested and can be administered in the preoperative period or immediately after surgery [7]. To note, suggested supplementation doses are currently highly discrepant and robust evidences are lacking concerning this nutritional treatment. Studies evaluating the efficacy of osteoporosis treatment in post-bariatric patients are still awaited [44, 47].

Loss of Fat-Free Mass (Lean Tissue Mass) and Sarcopenia

The loss of lean tissue mass during postoperative rapid weight loss and the risks it poses to the patient's health have been recognized as serious nutrition problems of bariatric patients. Although the intention of weight loss after BS is in the reduction of excess fat mass, fat-free mass (FFM) is also inevitably lost in the process. The loss of body weight following the surgery is due to not only loss of fat mass but also loss of FFM, composed of bone and lean tissue mass (LTM). FFM is important for the maintenance of body temperature, the skeletal integrity, and functionality of the body throughout life.

Factors that contribute to FFM loss in the post-bariatric period include the type of surgery, caloric restriction, low protein intake, inactivity, and magnitude of weight loss. Excessive loss of LTM is an adverse effect of weight loss because it has been associated with lower risk of post-BS mortality and morbidity [19, 48]. In addition, the resting energy expenditure and diet-induced energy expenditure seem to be directly associated with the amount of LTM, and therefore, its excessive loss may be one of the factors associated with late weight regain among post-BS patients [49].

Historically, the general understanding was that 25% of weight lost after BS would be in the form of FFM, but this rule has been criticized due to a lack of evidence. According to the systematic review by CHASTON et al. on weight loss-induced changes in FFM, BPD and RYGB patients lost significantly more FFM than the laparoscopic adjustable gastric banding (LAGB) patients. The median loss of FFM in relation to the lost weight was 25.6, 31.3, and 17.5% of following BPD, RYGB, and LAGB, respectively [49]. The follow-up period of these studies varied from 4 to 104 weeks (or 26 months). By prospectively comparing RYGB and SG patients, Moize et al. (2013) found no difference in LTM loss between these two types of surgeries, while according to our recent systematic review, the LTM loss of RYGB and SG patients ranged from 10.5% to 27.7% [51, 52].

The 2013 nutritional support guidelines for perioperative care of bariatric surgery patients [19] state that protein intake should be individualized and assessed and defined based on gender, age, and weight of the patient. It also recommends a minimal daily protein intake of 60 g and up to 1.5 g/kg ideal body weight per day (Grade D level of evidence). The main objective of sufficient protein intake is to avoid excessive loss of LTM. Despite these recommendations, postsurgery patients tend to ingest low amounts of food, especially protein foods, as a consequence of their reduced stomach capacity and changes in gut hormone that induce early satiety [19]. In a recent systematic review, most of the patients did not ingest the recommended 60 g/day of protein [52]. Of special note is the intolerance to certain foods, especially red meat and other fibrous protein sources [53], which contribute to low protein intake. Blood albumin and prealbumin levels have been used to monitor protein deficiencies, but these are not reliable markers for long-term protein status in this group of patients [52]. Low serum prealbumin levels shortly after the surgery have been reported to be consistent only with recent dietary energy and protein intake [54].

Thus, careful evaluation of body composition and daily protein ingestion is necessary to monitor protein status, and for those with low intake, supplementation may be necessary to avoid protein depletion states. Supplements, such as whey protein, soy isolate, and essential amino acids [55], have been used for the purpose.

Sarcopenia is defined as the presence of both low muscle mass and low muscle strength or performance (European Working Group on Sarcopenia in Older People – EWGSOP), and it has been applied to studies of frailty in the elderly population [55]. Sarcopenic obesity is becoming an important issue among the aging bariatric population. Long-term loss of LTM with decreased handgrip strength and a trend toward fat mass regain in a group of RYGB patients (9 years postsurgery) was observed [57]. The evidence accumulated to date indicates that avoiding the loss of LTM after BS is very important for the long-term success of the surgery. In order to maintain sufficient LTM and strength in the long run, an adequate protein intake, with or without the use of supplements, such as whey protein and physical activity, in order to maintain muscle strength, should be recommended, based on evidence still to be established. Information on dietary intake and patterns as well as physical activities are behavioral factors that are difficult to measure with accuracy. High-quality observational and interventional studies are necessary to better define these parameters.

Weight Regain

Bariatric surgery is the most efficient available tool to treat severe obesity. Most patients submitted to bariatric procedures achieve the objective, which is established as, besides the loss of at least 50% of excess weight (%EWL), the control of comorbidities and the achievement of a better quality of life. Recent cohort studies have shown that patients submitted to RYGB (10 years postsurgery) lost much more weight than nonsurgical matches and were able to sustain most of this weight in the long term [57]. RYGB weight loss was higher than SG and AGB weight loss. Recent data from the Longitudinal Assessment of Bariatric Surgery (LABS-2), the largest nonrandomized intervention trial study, showed that total body weight change was maximal at 1 year in the three subgroups (−38 ± 7% for RYGB, −26 ± 10% for vertical banded gastroplasty (VBG), and −13.2 ± 13% for AGB) [58].

However, as obesity is a chronic and serious disease, in some cases we can have recidivism of obesity after bariatric surgery. Long-term studies have demonstrated that weight regain (WR) occurs over time depending upon the procedure performed and duration of time since surgery. The SOS (Swish Obesity Study) study showed that at 10 years, patients who underwent RYGB experienced a mean WR of 12% total body weight. This translates into regaining 34% for the maximal weight loss at 1 year. It is observed that 20–50% of patients regain weight about 2 years after the procedure [59]. Behavioral, hormonal, and other factors related to the surgical procedure have been suggested as possible causes of this phenomenon. The importance is related to the risk of recurrence of all comorbidities that obesity favors, which in turn increases patient health risks and a return to a poor quality of life related to severe obesity [59].

Despite the occurrence of WR, there is no consensus about what is actually classified as a significant WR after bariatric surgery. Regaining more than 10% of the minimum weight has being used as one of the criteria [59].

In some ways weight regain may be physiological; two or more years after the bariatric procedure, patients continue suffering the influence of the environment and the influence of the aging which favors the increase of body fat.

Ongoing studies are trying to elucidate possible causes for WR. Until now it can be related to snacking-eating habit; low ingestion of protein and high ingestion of carbohydrates; increased fat mass and decreased fat-free mass (which leads to low basal metabolic rate); lower production of incretins, such as GLP1 and PYY; microbiota changes; lower diet-induced thermogenesis among this WR population; sedentary habits; excessive alcohol intake; and also the use of medications which lead to weight gain such as antidepressants, antidiabetics, mood stabilizers, and glucocorticoids, among others.

The treatment depends on the quantity of weight regained. In most cases, a low-calorie diet, rich in fiber and protein, excluding alcohol use and high glycemic meals, can help patients lose 5–10% of the weight regained. Figure 32.2 shows a food pyramid adapted for bariatric population, where 50% of total caloric intake should come from protein sources. Patients may be advised to increase low-glycemic index carbohydrates (three portions), fruits and vegetables, low quantity of mono- and polyunsaturated lipids, multivitamin and minerals daily, and a protein supplementation to achieve recommendations. High-protein meals lead to better satiety and higher levels of GLP1 and PYY, incretins related to satiety.

For WR patients who need to lose more than 10% of their weight, a concomitant use of medication can be prescribed.

Mechanisms related to WR among bariatric population are under investigation. Prospective studies should be done trying to create better strategies to avoid the recidivism of obesity and its comorbidities and also to treat WR in a long term.

Excessive Weight Loss

One undesirable side effect that is not well-established is excessive weight loss following bariatric surgery [57]. A very small number of patients become underweight (BMI <18.5 according to NIH criteria) and develop protein malnutrition. In most cases, besides the excessive weight loss, patients present sarcopenia and nutritional deficiencies.

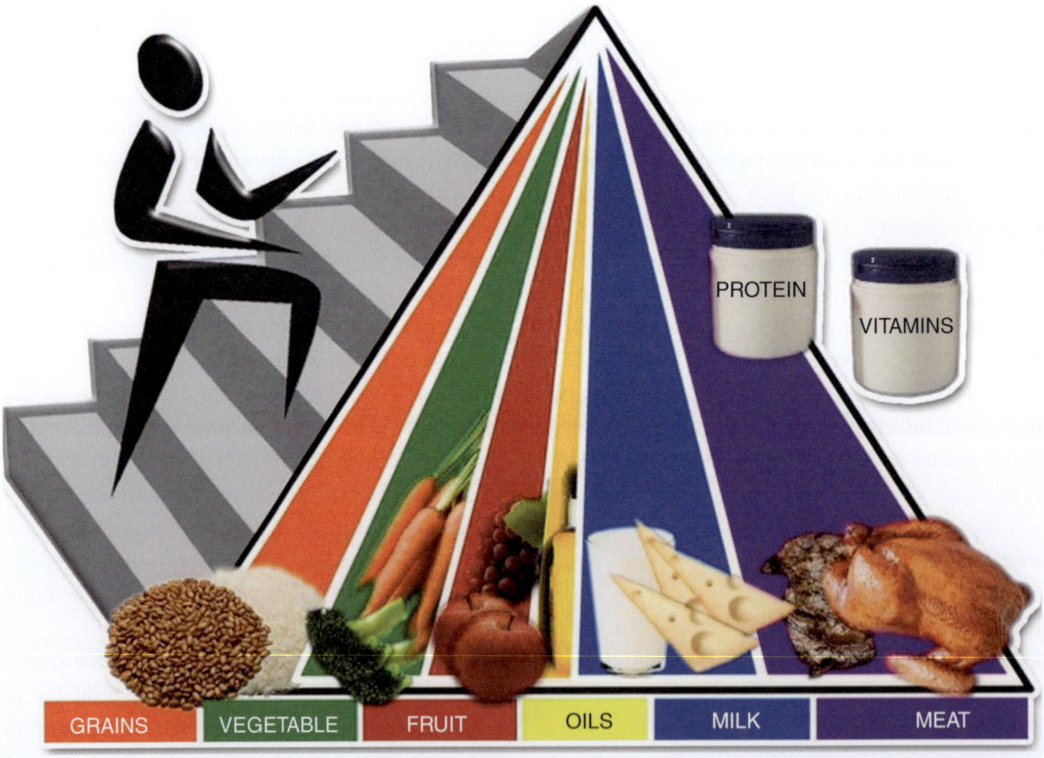

Fig. 32.2 Pyramid adapted for bariatric population

Protein calorie malnutrition has been reported following BPD-DS and RYGB long-limb (a distal gastric bypass performed in obese patients to induce greater amount of weight loss) procedures. The protein calorie malnutrition in these cases is thought to be secondary to severe malnutrition absorption and can result in total parenteral nutrition dependency [59].

Akusoba et al. suggested a clinical algorithm for excessive weight loss following RYGB. It is based on an initial evaluation of whether or not there is a gastrojejunal stricture or ulcer. If this complication is present, we should treat it. If it is not, the patient should be evaluated by the multidisciplinary team (made up of a primary care physician, dietician, gastroenterologist, psychologist, and nursing staff). These professionals should evaluate the occurrence of psychiatric disorders and adequate caloric intake. Each complication should be adequately treated. If no improvement is seen, a laparoscopic gastrostomy tube should be inserted into the remnant stomach. If there is improvement, the RYGB can be reversed to normal anatomy. If not, other etiologies should be investigated.

A high-calorie diet should be used including high-frequency meals, high-protein supplements, calorie-dense food, and an adequate amount of vitamins and minerals (200% of RDI),

Conclusion

The main objective of bariatric surgery is the improvement of the patient's quality of life, which includes the prevention and management of possible complications, among which are nutritional complications.

Although these deficiencies occur after all types of procedures, many studies have been carried out aiming to clarify how to manage nutritional complications. From what we know, these nutritional complications are detectable, preventable, and treatable. Healthcare professionals should be alerted about the signs and symptoms of these complications in order to diagnose and treat patients quickly.

Due to methodological limitations found in current literature, there is a need for well-designed observational and interventional studies that take into account the grave aspects and types of preoperative comorbidities and aim at fortifying a consensus related to the extent of postoperative supplementation. Such studies may provide findings that collaborate in the elaboration of future guidelines and the improvement of patient care. These studies, along with the engagement of multidisciplinary teams, could help healthcare professionals lessen the occurrence of nutritional complications among this patient population.

References

1. Carcore E, Chand P. Management and prevention of surgical and nutritional complications after bariatric surgery. Surg Clin North Am. 2016;96:843–56.
2. Levinson R, Silverman JB, Catella JG, Rybak I, Jolin H, Isom K. Pharmacotherapy prevention and management of nutritional deficiencies post Roux-en-Y-gastric bypass. Obes Surg. 2013;23:992–1000.
3. Kassir R, Debs T, Blanc P, Gugenhein J, Amor IB, Boutet C, Tiffet O. Complications of bariatric surgery: presentation and emergency management. Int J Surg. 2016;27:77–81. https://doi.org/10.1016/j.ijsu.2016.01.067.
4. Thibault R, Huber O, Azagury DE, Pichard C. Twelve key nutritional issues in bariatric surgery. Clin Nutr. 2016;35:12–7. https://doi.org/10.1016/j.jclnu.2015.02.012.
5. Neff KJ, Olbers T, le Roux CW. Bariatric surgery: the challenges with candidate selection, individualizing treatment and clinical outcomes. BMC Med. 2013;11:8.
6. Shikora SA, Kim JJ, Tarnoff ME. Nutritional and gastrointestinal complications after bariatric surgery. Nutr Clin Pract. 2007;40:22–9.
7. Aills L, et al. ASMBS allied health Nutritional guidelines for the surgical weight loss patient. Surg Obes Relat Dis. 2008;4:73S–108S.
8. Bordalo LA, Teixeira TF, Bressan J, et al. Bariatric surgery: how and why to supplement. Rev Assoc Med Bras. 2011;57:113–20.
9. Elliot K. Nutritional considerations after bariatric surgery. Crit Care Nurs Q. 2003;26(3):133–8.
10. Dind SA, McKenzie T, Vernon AH, Goldfine AB. Chapter 27, Bariatric surgery. In: Obesity, anorexia and nutrition. Endocrinology: Adult and Pediatric (Seventh Edition), 2016; p. 479–90.
11. WHO-1. Haemoglobin concentrations for the diagnosis of anaemia and assessment of severity. Vitamin and mineral nutrition information system. Geneva: World Health Organization; 2011 (WHO/NMH/NHD/MNM/11.1). http://www.who.int/vmnis/indicators/haemoglobin.pdf.

12. WHO-2. Serum ferritin concentrations for the assessment of iron status and iron deficiency in populations. Vitamin and mineral nutrition information system. Geneva: World Health Organization; 2011. http://www.who.int/vmnis/indicators/serum_ferritin.pdf.
13. Weng T-C, Chang C-H, Dong Y-H, et al. Anaemia and related nutrient deficiencies after Roux-en-Y gastric bypass surgery: a systematic review and meta-analysis. BMJ Open. 2015;5:e006964. https://doi.org/10.1136/bmjopen-2014-006964.
14. Rhode BM, Arseneau P, Cooper BA, et al. Vitamin B_{12} deficiency after gastric surgery for obesity. Am J Clin Nutr. 1996;63:103–9.
15. Lefebvre P, Letois F, Sultan A, et al. Nutrient deficiencies in patients with obesity considering bariatric surgery: a cross-sectional study. Surg Obes Relat Dis. 2014;10:540–6.
16. Cepeda-Lopez AC, Allende-Labastida J, Melse-Boonstra A, et al. The effects of fat loss after bariatric surgery on inflammation, serum hepcidin, and iron absorption: a prospective 6-month iron stable isotope study. Am J Clin Nutr. 2016;104:1030–8.
17. Obeid NR, Malick W, Concors SJ, et al. Long-term outcomes after Roux-en-Y gastric bypass: 10- to 13-year data. Surg Obes Relat Dis. 2016;12:11–20.
18. Levinson R, Silverman JB, Catella JG, et al. Pharmacotherapy: prevention and management of nutritional deficiencies post Roux-en-Y gastric bypass. Obes Surg. 2013;23:992–1000.
19. Mechanick JI, Youdim A, Jones DB, Garvey WT, Hurley DL, McMahon M, et al. Clinical practice guidelines for the perioperative nutritional, metabolic, and nonsurgical support of the bariatric surgery patient --2013 update: cosponsored by American Association of Clinical Endocrinologists, the Obesity Society, and American Society for Metabolic & Bariatric Surgery. Endocr Pract. 2013;19:337–72.
20. Sarker A, Meek CL, Park A. Biochemical consequences of bariatric surgery for extreme clinical obesity. Ann Clin Biochem. 2016;53:21–31. https://doi.org/10.1177/0004563215588116.
21. Tack J, Deloose E. Complications of bariatric surgery: dumping syndrome, reflux and vitamin deficiencies. Best Pract Res Clin Gastroenterol. 2014;28:741. https://doi.org/10.1016/j.bpg.2014.07.010.
22. Stroh C, Meyer F, Manger T. Beriberi, a severe complication after metabolic surgery – review of the literature. Obes Facts. 2014;7:246–52.
23. Fujioka K. Follow-up of nutritional and metabolic problems after bariatric surgery. Diabetes Care. 2005;28(2):481–4.
24. Vieira C, Cosmo C, Lucena R. The importance of methylmalonic acid dosage on the assessment of patients with neurological manifestation following bariatric surgery. Obes Surg. 2011;21(12):1971–4.
25. Vargaz-Ruiz AG, Hernandez-Rivera G, Herrera MF. Prevalence of iron, folate and vitamin B_{12} deficiency anemia after laparoscopic Roux-en-Y gastric bypass. Obes Surg. 2008;18(3):288–93.
26. Berg P, McCallum R. Dumping syndrome: a review of the current concepts of pathophysiology, diagnosis and treatment. Dig Dis Sci. 2016;61:11–8.
27. Salehi M, Gastaldelli A, D'Alessio DA. Blockade of glucagon-like peptide 1 receptor corrects post-prandial hypoglycemia after gastric bypass. Gastroenterology. 2014;146:669–680.e2.
28. Patti ME, Goldfine AB. Hypoglicemia after gastric bypass: the dark side of GLP-1. Gastroenterology. 2014;146:605–8.
29. Williamson D, Gonzalez M, Finlay AY. The effect of hair loss on quality of life. J Eur Acad Dermatol Venereol. 2001;15:137–9.
30. Beattie PE. The patient with hair loss. Practioner. 2003;247(1643):128–34.
31. Geiler CC, Blume-Peytavi U, Orfanos CE. Metabolic disorders involving the hair. In: Camacho FM, Randall VA, Price VH, editors. Hair and its disorders. Biology, pathology and management. London: Martin Dunitz; 2000. p. 275–82.
32. Rushton DH. Nutritional factors and hair loss. Clin Exp Dermatol. 2002;27:396–404.
33. Jacques J. Micronutrition for the weight loss surgery patient. Edgemont: Matrix Medical Communication; 2006. p. 146–7.
34. Innis SM, Allardyce DB. Possible biotin deficiency in adults receiving long-term total parenteral nutrition. Am J Clin Nutr. 1983;37:185–7.
35. Marcason W. What are the dietary guidelines following bariatric surgery? J Am Diet Assoc. 2004;104(3):487–8.
36. Kushner R. Managing the obese patient after bariatric surgery: a case report of severe malnutrition and review of the literature. J Parenter Enteral Nutr. 2000;24:126–32.
37. Kantor J, Kessler LJ, Brooks DG, et al. Decreased serum ferritin is associated with alopecia in women. J Invest Dermatol. 2003;121(5):985–8.
38. Trost LB, Berfeld WF, Calogeras E. The diagnosis and treatment of iron deficiency and its potencial relationship to hair loss. J Am Acad Dermatol. 2006;54(5):824–44.
39. Malinowski SS. Nutritional and metabolic complications of bariatric surgery. Am J Med Sci. 2006;331(4):219–25.
40. Ruiz-Tovar J, Oller I, Llavero C, Zubiaga L, Diez M, Arroyo A, et al. Hair loss in females after sleeve gastrectomy: predictive value of serum zinc and iron levels. Am Surg. 2014;80(5):466–71.
41. Vannucchi H, Chiarello PG. Biotina e Ácido Pantotênico. In: Cozzolino SM, editor. Biodisponibilidade de Nutrientes. 2nd ed. São Paulo: Manole; 2007. p. 411.
42. Scopinaro N, Adami GF, Marinari G, et al. Biliopancreatic diversion: two decades of experience. In: Deitel M, Cowan GSM, editors. Update: surgery for the morbidly obese patient. Toronto: FD Communications Inc; 2000. p. 227–58.
43. Folli F, Sabowitz BN, Schwesinger W, et al. Bariatric surgery and bone disease: from clinical

perspective to molecular insights. Int J Obes (Lond). 2012;36:1373–9.
44. Yu EW. Bone metabolism after bariatric surgery. J Bone Miner Res. 2014;29:1507–18.
45. Tan HC, Tan MZ, Tham KW, et al. One-year changes in QCT and DXA bone densities following bariatric surgery in a multiethnic Asian cohort. Osteoporos Sarcopenia. 2015;1:115–20.
46. Malinowsky SS. Nutritional and metabolic complications of bariatric surgery. Am J Med Sci. 2006;331(4):219–25.
47. Sakhaee K, Poindexter J, Aguirre C. The effects of bariatric surgery on bone and nephrolithiasis. Bone. 2016;84:1–8.
48. Puzziferri N, Roshek TB, Mayo HG, Gallagher R, Belle SH, Livingston EH. Long-term follow-up after bariatric surgery: a systematic review. JAMA. 2014;312(9):934–42.
49. Cardeal MA, Faria SL, Faria OP, Facundes M, Ito MK. Diet-induced thermogenesis in postoperatve Roux-en-Y gastric bypass patients with weight regain. Surg Obes Relat Dis. 2016;12(5):1098–107.
50. Chaston TB, Dixon JB, O'Brien PE. Changes in fat-free mass during significant weight loss: a systematic review. Int J Obes (Lond). 2007;31(5):743–50.
51. Moize V, Andreu A, Rodriguez L, Flores L, Ibarzabal A, Lacy A, et al. Protein intake and lean tissue mass retention following bariatric surgery. Clin Nutr. 2013;32(4):550–5.
52. Ito MK, Vivian Siqueira Santos Gonçalves VSG, Faria SLCM, Moizé V, Porporatti AL, Guerra ENS, De Luca Canto G, Carvalho KMB. Effect of protein intake on the protein status and lean mass of post-bariatric surgery patients: a systematic review. Obes Surg. 2017;27:502. https://doi.org/10.1007/s11695-016-2453-0.
53. Nicoletti CF, Oliveira BAP, Barbin R, Marchini JS, Salgado Junior W, Nonino CB. Red meat intolerance in patients submitted to gastric bypass: a 4-year follow-up study. Surg Obes Relat Dis. 2015;11(4):842–6.
54. Aron-Wisnewsky J, Verger EO, Bounaix C, Dao MC, Oppert JM, Bouillot JL, et al. Nutritional and protein deficiencies in the short term following both gastric bypass and gastric banding. PLoS One. 2016;11(2):e0149588.
55. Katsanos CS, Madura JA, Roust LR. Essential amino acid ingestion as an efficient nutritional strategy for the preservation of muscle mass following gastric bypass surgery. Nutrition. 2016;32:9–13.
56. Cruz-Jentoft AJ, Baeyens JP, Bauer JM, et al. Sarcopenia: European consensus on definition and diagnosis: report of the European working group on sarcopenia in older people. Age Ageing. 2010;39:412–23.
57. Cole AJ, Adam JK, Lauren MB, Cyrus J, Jennifer RM, Shalamar DS, Carrie PE. Long-term body composition changes in women following Roux-en-Y gastric bypass surgery. J Parenter Enteral Nutr. 2017;41:583–91. https://doi.org/10.1177/0148607115625621.
58. Maciejewski ML, Arterburn DE, Scoyoc VL, Smith AV, Yancy WS, Weidenbacher HJ, et al. Bariatric surgery and long-term durability of weight loss. JAMA Surg. 2016;151:1046.
59. Twells LK, Gregory DM, Midodzi WK, Dillon C, Kovacs CS, MacDonald D, et al. The newfoundland and labrador bariatric surgery cohort study: rational and study protocol. BMC Health Serv Res. 2016;16:618. https://doi.org/10.1186/s12913-016-1869-5.
60. Akusoba I, El Chaar M. Laparoscopic Roux-en-Y gastric bypass reversal. Surg Obes Relat Dis. 2015;12:441–2.

33 Eating Disorders

Debora Kinoshita Kussunoki

Eating Disorders

Eating disorders (ED) are characterized by a persistent disturbance of eating-related behavior and excessive distress or concern about body shape or weight [1]. The most commonly ED categories linked to current obesity and obesity surgery are binge eating disorder (BED) and bulimia nervosa (BN). Night eating syndrome (NES) is not a distinct category but included as other specified feeding or eating disorders (OSFED) in the DSM-V [1] and known to be associated with overweight and obesity.

Although bariatric surgery candidates do not present anorexia nervosa (AN), it may appear at some point in life of the weight loss treatment-seeking patient. The diagnostic flux from one ED presentation to another occurs between AN and BN, and crossover BED and BN and between other OSFED has been reported [2].

Bariatric surgery candidates have a higher prevalence of eating disorders than the general population mainly binge eating disorder (BED) and bulimia nervosa (BN). Furthermore, the prevalence of lifetime obesity in ED cases is reported to be 28.8% (ranging from 5% in AN to 87% in BED) with an increase of threefold in lifetime obesity in ED patients over the last years [3].

We also included grazing, pica, and compensatory purging behaviors which may occur and affect the outcome of patients undergoing bariatric surgery.

Binge Eating Disorder

The most prevalent ED associated with obesity and bariatric surgery was first defined by Stunkard in 1959 [4] as the consumption of an "enormous amount of food" in a relatively short period of time, and it was described as a "rapid consumption of a large amount of food in a discrete period of time", usually less than 2 hours [1, 4].

Binge eating disorder (BED) was only recently included in DSM-V [1] as a category of ED; up until then it was classified as part of EDNOS (eating disorders not otherwise specified) among the pathologies needing further studies [1, 6].

BED diagnostic criteria include recurrent episodes of binge eating (BE), defined as eating in a discrete period of time (within 2 hours) an

D. K. Kussunoki (✉)
Obesity and Diabetes Center, German Hospital Oswaldo Cruz, São Paulo, Brazil

Obesity and Metabolic Syndrome Outpatient Clinic, Service of Endocrinology and Metabolism-HCFMUSP/SP, São Paulo, Brazil

Brazilian Society of Bariatric and Metabolic Surgery, São Paulo, Brazil

Brazilian Association for the Study of Obesity and Metabolic Syndrome, São Paulo, Brazil

Segal Clinic, São Paulo, Brazil

J. Ettinger et al. (eds.), *Gastric Bypass*, https://doi.org/10.1007/978-3-030-28803-7_33

amount of food that is definitely larger than most people would eat in a similar period of time under similar circumstances and must be accompanied by a sense of lack of control [1].

BE is also associated with at least three of these features: eating much more rapidly than normal, eating until feeling uncomfortably full, eating large amounts of food when not feeling physically hungry, and eating alone because of feeling embarrassed by how much one is eating and feeling disgusted with oneself, depressed, or very guilty afterward [1].

Other frequent psychopathological features among patients with BED are an overvaluation of shape and weight (in about 60% of patients with BED), constant polarization of thoughts on weight control, diet and binge avoidance, more atypical eating distribution along the day, and peculiar food choices [7].

The necessary frequency for the diagnosis of BE was reduced from twice a week for 6 months in DSM-IV TR to at least once a week for 3 months [1, 6]. The impact of this modification on the prevalence and lifetime prevalence of BED is unknown, although some studies have shown small statistical differences.

The literature shows that the relationship between obesity and mental disorders is strong, and bariatric candidates are more likely to have a psychiatric diagnosis, ED, and thereby BED, than the general population [8, 9]. Welch et al. (2016) [2] also suggested a relationship between the extent of morbidity and comorbidity in BED and the presence of obesity.

Prevalence rates of BED vary widely according to the population studied and the assessment method, ranging from 0.7% to 4% in community samples, 1–30% in patients seeking weight loss treatment (nonsurgical treatment), and 2–49% in bariatric candidates [10].

According to Marek et al. (2014) [11], an additional 3,43% of bariatric surgery candidates met the diagnostic threshold for BED when using this new DSM-V criteria. Vinai et al. (2015) [13] found a total amount of 48,3% of the bariatric surgery candidates with BED per DSM-V criteria. They also reported in a subsequent publication that psychological characteristics found in patients with BED following the DSM IV criteria seem to be confirmed among BED patients diagnosed following DSM-V criteria and reassure that the less restrictive diagnostic criteria are useful in identifying obese patients affected by severe psychopathology [14].

Bariatric candidates with BED have more axis I comorbidities than non-BED patients, mainly current mood disorder (27,3% vs 4,9%, $p = 0.002$), lifetime history of mood (52,3% vs 23,0% $p = 0,003$), current anxiety disorder (27,3 vs 8,2%, $p = 0,0$ [14]), and lifetime anxiety disorder (36,4% vs 16,4%, $p = 0.019$). BED also was associated with greater symptoms of depression [15].

The impact of pre-existing BE on post-operative weight loss was the subject of studies with mixed results. Konttinen et al. (2014) [16] found that pre-surgery eating behavior measured by the Three-Factor Eating Questionnaire was unrelated to subsequent weight changes, and Morseth et al. (2016) [17] found an even greater weight loss among patients with BE before the bariatric surgery than the non-BE patients in a 5-year follow-up of gastric bypass and duodenal switch.

There is still no consensus about prevalence of BED after bariatric surgery. Researches have used various methods and criteria to assess BED and BE after surgery and different lengths of follow-up, resulting in wide ranges of rates and noncomparable data. Some authors even suggest that BE may manifest itself as grazing after the bariatric surgery [18, 19].

Binge Eating Treatment

The main goal of the treatment should be abstinence from BE and afterward weight loss. Although the body weight could influence the wellness perception and mood, an excessive restraint diet can trigger more episodes of BE [20].

Behavioral interventions, psychotherapies as cognitive behavioral therapies (CBT), and pharmacological treatment are the options currently used, combined or not.

Antidepressants can be used for impulsiveness and eating but also for depressive and/or anxiety symptoms presented by the patient. Fluoxetine, sertraline, fluvoxamine, and bupropion are shown to have positive effects on these cases. Topiramate and lamotrigine have shown some efficacy either [20].

Pretreatment eating behavior seems to be unrelated to subsequent weight changes in patients undergoing bariatric surgery [16].

Bulimia Nervosa (BN)

BN is defined as frequent episodes of BE followed by inappropriate compensatory behavior to avoid weight gain, such as self-induced vomiting, excessive exercise, fasting, misuse of laxatives or diuretics, or other medications [1].

The lifetime prevalence of BN among young females is 1–1,5% [1, 21], the frequency of lifetime BN among obese patients seeking bariatric surgery is 9,2% and current BN is of 3,6% [8]. The recent reduction of BE frequency for BN diagnosis in DSM-V might increase the lifetime prevalence from 1,2% to 1,6% [22].

Careful investigation of the underlying causes and cognitions relative to some behaviors after surgery, such as frequent diarrhea along with a dumping episode or vomiting caused by deliberately rapid ingestion of large amounts of food, is required. Although they are behaviors commonly found after the surgery, it is convenient to rule out the possibility of a bulimic purging behavior. de Zwaan et al. (2010) [23] found 11,9% of patients report self-vomiting as a mean to control weight or shape.

We should also be alert to the intentional insulin or oral hypoglycemic drug omission as a form of weight control (diabulimia) in patients with diabetes [1, 24] even if the patient denies the behavior but presents poor glycemic control, recurrent episodes of ketoacidosis, and hypoglycemia secondary to intentional overdose and dietary manipulation [24].

In BN, further medical consequences are due to the mode and frequency of purging. Electrolyte and acid-base alterations can be associated with excessive vomiting or abuse of laxatives. Perimolysis, mucositis, cheilitis, and parotid gland enlargement can also be found in patients with intentional vomiting. Another possible complication of laxative abuse is the cathartic colon syndrome. Abuse of diuretics may lead to metabolic alkalosis and hypokalemia and, if severe, sometimes results in cardiac arrhythmias [25].

The treatment of BN involves nutritional rehabilitation with normalization of nutritional and eating habits, pharmacotherapy, and psychotherapies. Cognitive behavioral therapy (CBT) is the most recommended intervention, and antidepressants, particularly selective serotonin reuptake inhibitors, are the most effective drugs. Other pharmaceutical agents, including topiramate, oxcarbazepine, aripiprazole, and baclofen, have been reported to be effective for BN [20].

Night Eating Syndrome

Night eating syndrome (NES) was first described by Stunkard in 1959 as combination of eating disorder, sleep disorder, and mood disorder characterized by morning anorexia, evening hyperphagia, and insomnia [4].

Currently NES is part of the category "other specified feeding or eating disorder" in the DSM-V [1] described as recurrent episodes of night eating, manifested by eating after awakening from sleep or by excessive food consumption after the evening meal. There is awareness and recall of the eating. The morning anorexia criterion is abandoned in this version of the DSM.

Some biological factors are suggested to contribute or maintain the NES as a dissociation of the circadian control of eating. Studies involving melatonin, cortisol, insulin, and leptin showed a delay from 1 to 3 hours in the usual circadian rhythm of these hormones and a complete inversion of the rhythm of glucose [26].

NES has been found in patients with type 2 diabetes mellitus and associated with poor glycemic control in these patients [27–29]. NES has also a positive correlation with BMI and mood disorders. Besides the fact that not every individual with NES is obese, the prevalence of NES is higher in obese population than in general population [28].

NES has a point prevalence of 1% in the general population, 6–14% in individuals seeking treatment related to obesity, and rates of NES vary from 2% to 31% in bariatric surgery candidates [10] depending on the diagnostic criteria and the time of assessment.

The presence of NES after bariatric surgery may impact negatively in weight loss maintenance [28], but the literature is limited and shows mixed results. There is no clear evidence that NES prior to bariatric surgery is a negative predictor of weight loss.

Colles et al. (2008) [18] did not found association between the presence of NES prior to the surgical procedure to post-surgical NES and found that more than a half of post-operative NES cases had newly developed night eating after surgery. Also, there was a reduction from 17,1% to 7,8% in 12 months in a population submitted to laparoscopic adjustable gastric banding (LAGB) procedure.

Most of the studies for the treatment of NES suggest pharmacotherapy, mainly SSRIs, and particularly sertraline to be effective. There has also been reported use of escitalopram, topiramate, cognitive behavioral therapy, progressive muscle relaxation, and bright light treatment [28].

Grazing

Although grazing, picking, nibbling, and snack eating have been increasingly described as similar maladaptive behaviors among post-surgical patients associated with less weight loss or weight regain, there is still a lack of consensus about the definition, course, and impact in bariatric patients' outcome after surgery.

Conceição et al. (2014) [30] suggested grazing to be defined as an eating behavior characterized by repetitive eating of small or modest amount of food in an unplanned manner and/or not in response to hunger/satiety sensations. Also, they proposed two subtypes: a compulsive subtype and a non-compulsive subtype, characterized by eating in a distracted way. Grazing should be distinguished from prescribed high-frequency meal diets, either for weight loss purposes or due to restriction of intake volume imposed by the bariatric surgery.

Grazing is frequently found in different populations with rates of 91% in nonclinical samples [31], up to 89,8% in clinical samples [32], and up to 59,8% in bariatric population [33]. For this reason there is some doubt as to its non-regular eating behavior status, yet with considerable implications in a specific subgroup given that the unplanned pattern of eating could lead to an high caloric intake [30].

An overlap between grazing and BED has been described. Some authors found that among bariatric surgery candidates with BED some might develop graze eating after surgery (as many as 61% of these patients in the LAGB population) [18, 19].

Morseth et al. (2015) [17] questioned whether binge eating criteria should be re-evaluated for patients undergoing bariatric surgery since many of them keep reporting lack of control even when the amount of food is small [34] and many patients who reported BE before surgery resort to grazing [18]. More studies about grazing and correlate eating behaviors are needed.

Pica and Pagophagia

The essential feature of pica is the eating of nonnutritive nonfood substances on a persistent basis over a period of at least 1 month [1].

Some specific vitamin or mineral (e.g., iron, zinc) deficiencies have been reported, but no other abnormalities are found. The prevalence is unknown. The substances ingested might include paper, soil, ash, charcoal, or ice.

Pagophagia (ice eating) has been often associated with pregnancy and iron deficiency anemia and recently has been described in post-bariatric surgery patients [35].

Cases of pica are given attention after medical complication such as bezoar, intestinal perforations, infections, or poisoning [1]. Differential diagnosis should be done with some presentations of anorexia or bulimia nervosa including ingestion of tissue paper or cotton balls aiming appetite control.

Anorexia Nervosa and PSEAD

Although anorexia nervosa cannot be comorbid with obesity, it may be present at some point in the life of the patient seeking treatment for weight loss due to diagnostic flux between EDs or de novo appearance.

AN is characterized primarily by low weight below a minimally normal level for age, sex, developmental trajectory, and physical health, associated with intense fear of gaining weight and disturbance in the way which one's body weight or shape is experienced and persistent lack of recognition of the seriousness of the current low body weight [1]. The fear of becoming fat or weight gain may even increase as weight falls. There are two types of AN:

- Restricting type: During the last 3 months, the individual has not engaged in recurrent episodes of binge eating or purging behavior. This subtype describes presentations in which weight loss is accomplished primarily through dieting, fasting, and/or excessive exercise [1].
- B–inge eating/purging type: During the last 3 months, the individual has engaged in recurrent episodes of binge eating or purging behavior [1].

Marino et al. (2012) [36] reviewed cases of ED after bariatric surgery and found a small but growing number of articles and case studies, and Conceição et al. (2013) [37] described a series of 12 patients hospitalized with AN, BN, and post-surgical eating avoidance disorder (PSEAD) [38].

Segal et al. (2004) [38] observed a combination of various phobic-like anxiety symptoms associated with altered eating behaviors in a post-surgical population and proposed the criteria for a post-surgical eating disorder shown below.

PSEAD Proposed Criteria

1. Previous history of obesity grade III followed by bariatric surgery over the last 2 years
2. Higher speed of weight loss than the average usually associated with the technique employed, upon the diagnosis of change in eating behavior
3. Use of purgative strategies or excessive reduction of food intake, related or not to binge eating episode
4. Reaction of extreme anxiety and/or an active negative attitude when nutritional correction is introduced, which can be evidenced by:
    a. Intense fear of going back to the preoperative weight
    b. The patient not accepting orientation to interrupt the weight loss
    c. The patient denying doing something exaggerated that accounts for this loss
    d. The patient perceiving a positive return in the loss of weight, in spite of evidence to the contrary
5. Body image dissatisfaction or distortion
6. Follow-up nutritional tests with significant alterations and/or not in-line with the surgical technique, maintained for more than 2 months after initial interventions
7. Exclude AN and BN
8. Exclude simple phobias (i.e., food chocking)
9. Exclude organic causes
10. Mandatory criteria 1 and 2 or 3, 4, 6, 7, and 9

Even considering losing more weight than expected for the technique as an inappropriate behavior, the BMI range of the patients described was normal or above. Moreover, the most clinical relevant characteristics were laboratory findings and signs of malnutrition rather than BMI.

The description adds in relevant changes in patient relation with food with intense fear of regaining weight. The food choices are high caloric, more palatable, and "easy to swallow." The cognitive reactions included a distortion of beliefs: gaining 1 kg is one step only from gaining 50 kg. Noncompliance is the rule accompanied by extreme anxiety symptoms and phobic avoidance reactions whenever a nutritional advice is introduced [38].

The consequences of avoidant eating behavior after the surgery may be the emergence of severe malnutrition. Fandiño et al. (2005) [39] described a Wernicke-Korsakoff syndrome in a patient with PSEAD features.

Laboratory abnormalities and sustained malnutrition signs should alert the team to AN or PSEAD. The crude mortality rate (CMR) for AN is approximately 5% per decade. Medical complications associated with excessive weight loss and malnutrition of AN and suicide are the most common causes [1].

Conclusion

Obesity and psychiatric disorders are strongly associated with about two thirds of the bariatric surgery candidates meeting the criteria for any current psychiatric disorder. Moreover, eating disorders (ED) and inadequate eating behaviors are frequently described among bariatric surgery candidates, especially binge eating disorder (BED) and loss of control (LOC) in eating [40, 41].

The prevalence of the EDs post-operatively may vary according to the time of assessment like other psychiatric disorders' distribution over time. The lowest rates are found in short term, with some increase after 24 months of follow-up [16]. Weight loss per se and its consequent reduction in the chronic inflammatory state due to obesity may help the prevalence reduction of many psychiatric disorders [42].

A possible flux between EDs and subthreshold EDs, before and after the surgery, highlights the need for further efforts to characterize and better understand their clinical evolution and relationship with the bariatric surgery.

Although the post-surgical presence of BED, NES, and grazing can negatively affect the results of weight loss, there is no supportive data to predict the impact of pre-surgical EDs in the post-surgical weight loss.

Attention to signals and symptoms of other classical EDs (AN, BN) when assessing the patient at follow-up appointments is indispensable not because of the insufficient weight loss but for the early detection of clinical, metabolic, and nutritional complications as consequences of purging or eating avoidance behaviors.

Some studies refer an unfavorable course of eating disorders or psychiatric disorders after obesity surgery, but most of these studies do not have a proper psychiatric care, worsening the prognosis of these disorders without a complete effective intervention.

In general, the prognosis of post-surgical EDs tends to be more benign if immediately diagnosed and if suitable treatment is installed, emphasizing the demand for a psychiatric assessment and follow-up with specific attention to eating disorders and the particularities of post-bariatric surgery eating behaviors.

Systematic psychiatric evaluation of patients prior to bariatric surgery is recommended, and further controlled studies, with appropriate assessment instruments, comparing different techniques and post-surgical follow-up times are required.

Acknowledgment The author would like to thank Rodrigo Rezende for his English revision.

References

1. American Psychiatric Association. Diagnostic and statistical manual of mental disorders. 5 th ed. Washington, DC: American Psychiatric Association; 2013.
2. Welch E, Jangmo A, Thornton L, Norring C, von Hausswolff-Juhlin Y, Herman B, et al. Treatment-seeking patients with binge-eating disorder in the Swedish national registers: clinical course and psychiatric comorbidity. BMC Psychiatry. 2016;16(1):163.
3. Villarejo C, Fernández-Aranda F, Jiménez-Murcia S, Peñas-Lledó E, Granero R, Penelo E, et al. Lifetime obesity in patients with eating disorders: increasing prevalence, clinical and personality correlates. Eur Eat Disord Rev. 2012;20(3):250–4.
4. Stunkard A. Eating patterns and obesity. Psychiatry Q. 1959;33(2):284–95.
5. American Psychiatric Association. Diagnostic and statistical manual of mental disorders. 3 rd ed. Washington, DC: American Psychiatric Association; 1987.
6. APA (American Psychiatric Association). DSM-IV-TR: diagnostic and statistical manual of men-

tal disorders (Revised 4th ed). Washington, DC: American Psychiatric Association; 2000.
7. Amianto F, Ottone L, Abbate Daga G, Fassino S. Binge-eating disorder diagnosis and treatment: a recap in front of DSM-5. BMC Psychiatry. 2015;15(1):70.
8. Duarte-Guerra L, Coêlho B, Santo M, Wang Y. Psychiatric disorders among obese patients seeking bariatric surgery: results of structured clinical interviews. Obes Surg. 2014;25(5):830–7.
9. Dawes A, Maggard-Gibbons M, Maher A, Booth M, Miake-Lye I, Beroes J, et al. Mental health conditions among patients seeking and undergoing bariatric surgery. JAMA. 2016;315(2):150.
10. Parker K, Brennan L. Measurement of disordered eating in bariatric surgery candidates: a systematic review of the literature. Obes Res Clin Pract. 2015;9(1):12–25.
11. Marek R, Ben-Porath Y, Ashton K, Heinberg L. Impact of using DSM-5 criteria for diagnosing binge eating disorder in bariatric surgery candidates: change in prevalence rate, demographic characteristics, and scores on the Minnesota multiphasic personality inventory – 2 restructured form (MMPI-2-RF). Int J Eat Disord. 2014;47(5):553–7.
12. Malik S, Mitchell J, Engel S, Crosby R, Wonderlich S. Psychopathology in bariatric surgery candidates: a review of studies using structured diagnostic interviews. Compr Psychiatry. 2014;55(2):248–59.
13. Vinai P, Da Ros A, Speciale M, Gentile N, Tagliabue A, Vinai P, et al. Psychopathological characteristics of patients seeking for bariatric surgery, either affected or not by binge eating disorder following the criteria of the DSM IV TR and of the DSM 5. Eat Behav. 2015;16:1–4.
14. Vinai P, Da Ros A, Cardetti S, Casey H, Studt S, Gentile N, et al. The DSM-5 effect: psychological characteristics of new patients affected by Binge Eating Disorder following the criteria of the DSM-5 in a sample of severe obese patients. Eat Weight Disord. 2015;21(1):107–13.
15. Jones-Corneille L, Wadden T, Sarwer D, Faulconbridge L, Fabricatore A, Stack R, et al. Axis I psychopathology in bariatric surgery candidates with and without binge eating disorder: results of structured clinical interviews. Obes Surg. 2010;22(3):389–97.
16. Konttinen H, Peltonen M, Sjostrom L, Carlsson L, Karlsson J. Psychological aspects of eating behavior as predictors of 10-y weight changes after surgical and conventional treatment of severe obesity: results from the Swedish Obese Subjects intervention study. Am J Clin Nutr. 2014;101(1):16–24.
17. Morseth M, Hanvold S, Rø Ø, Risstad H, Mala T, Benth J, et al. Self-reported eating disorder symptoms before and after gastric bypass and duodenal switch for super obesity—a 5-year follow-up study. Obes Surg. 2015;26(3):588–94.
18. Colles S, Dixon J, O'Brien P. Grazing and loss of control related to eating: two high-risk factors following bariatric surgery. Obesity. 2008;16(3):615–22.
19. Saunders R. "Grazing": a high-risk behavior. Obes Surg. 2004;14(1):98–102.
20. Yager J, Devlin M, Halmi K, Herzog D, Mitchell J, Powers P, et al. Guideline watch (August 2012): practice guideline for the treatment of patients with eating disorders, 3rd edition. Focus. 2014;12(4):416–31.
21. Smink F, van Hoeken D, Hoek H. Epidemiology of eating disorders: incidence, prevalence and mortality rates. Curr Psychiatry Rep. 2012;14(4):406–14.
22. Trace S, Thornton L, Root T, Mazzeo S, Lichtenstein P, Pedersen N, et al. Effects of reducing the frequency and duration criteria for binge eating on lifetime prevalence of bulimia nervosa and binge eating disorder: implications for DSM-5. Int J Eat Disord. 2012;45:531–6.
23. de Zwaan M, Hilbert A, Swan-Kremeier L, Simonich H, Lancaster K, Howell L, et al. Comprehensive interview assessment of eating behavior 18–35 months after gastric bypass surgery for morbid obesity. Surg Obes Relat Dis. 2010;6(1):79–85. 2011;45(4):531–6.
24. Pinhas-Hamiel O, Levy-Shraga Y. Eating disorders in adolescents with type 2 and type 1 diabetes. Curr Diab Rep. 2012;13(2):289–97.
25. Westmoreland P, Krantz M, Mehler P. Medical complications of anorexia nervosa and bulimia. Am J Med. 2016;129(1):30–7.
26. Goel N, Stunkard A, Rogers N, Van Dongen H, Allison K, O'Reardon J, et al. Circadian rhythm profiles in women with night eating syndrome. J Biol Rhythms. 2009;24(1):85–94.
27. Allison K, Engel S, Crosby R, de Zwaan M, O'Reardon J, Wonderlich S, et al. Evaluation of diagnostic criteria for night eating syndrome using item response theory analysis. Eat Behav. 2008;9(4):398–407.
28. de Zwaan M, Marschollek M, Allison K. The night eating syndrome (NES) in bariatric surgery patients. Eur Eat Disord Rev. 2015;23(6):426–34.
29. Hood M, Reutrakul S, Crowley S. Night eating in patients with type 2 diabetes. Associations with glycemic control, eating patterns, sleep, and mood. Appetite. 2014;79:91–6.
30. Conceição E, Mitchell J, Engel S, Machado P, Lancaster K, Wonderlich S. What is "grazing"? Reviewing its definition, frequency, clinical characteristics, and impact on bariatric surgery outcomes, and proposing a standardized definition. Surg Obes Relat Dis. 2014;10(5):973–82.
31. Reas D, Wisting L, Kapstad H, Lask B. Nibbling: frequency and relationship to BMI, pattern of eating, and shape, weight, and eating concerns among university women. Eat Behav. 2012;13(1):65–6.
32. Masheb R, Roberto C, White M. Nibbling and picking in obese patients with Binge Eating Disorder. Eat Behav. 2013;14(4):424–7.
33. Conceição E, Crosby R, Mitchell J, Engel S, Wonderlich S, Simonich H, et al. Picking or nibbling: frequency and associated clinical features in bulimia nervosa, anorexia nervosa, and binge eating disorder. Int J Eat Disord. 2013;46(8):815–8.

34. Niego S, Kofman M, Weiss J, Geliebter A. Binge eating in the bariatric surgery population: a review of the literature. Int J Eat Disord. 2007;40(4):349–59.
35. Tabaac B, Tabaac V. Pica patient, status post gastric bypass, improves with change in medication regimen. Ther Adv Psychopharmacol. 2014;5(1):38–42.
36. Marino J, Ertelt T, Lancaster K, Steffen K, Peterson L, de Zwaan M, et al. The emergence of eating pathology after bariatric surgery: a rare outcome with important clinical implications. Int J Eat Disord. 2012;45(2):179–84.
37. Conceição E, Orcutt M, Mitchell J, Engel S, LaHaise K, Jorgensen M, et al. Characterization of eating disorders after bariatric surgery: a case series. Int J Eat Disord. 2012;46(3):274–9.
38. Segal A, Kinoshita Kussunoki D, Larino MA. Post-surgical refusal to eat: anorexia nervosa, bulimia nervosa or a new eating disorder? A case series. Obes Surg. 2004;14(3):353–60.
39. Fandiño J, Benchimol A, Fandiño L, Barroso F, Coutinho W, Appolinário J. Eating avoidance disorder and Wernicke-Korsakoff syndrome following gastric bypass: an under-diagnosed association. Obes Surg. 2005;15(8):1207–10.
40. Opolski M, Chur-Hansen A, Wittert G. The eating-related behaviors, disorders and expectations of candidates for bariatric surgery. Clin Obes. 2015;5(4):165–97.
41. Kessler RC, Berglund PA, Chiu WT, Deitz AC, Hudson JI, Shahly V, et al. The prevalence and correlates of binge eating disorder in the World Health Organization World Mental Health Surveys. Biol Psychiatry. 2013;73(9):904–14.
42. Capuron L, Poitou C, Machaux-Tholliez D, Frochot V, Bouillot J, Basdevant A, et al. Relationship between adiposity, emotional status and eating behaviour in obese women: role of inflammation. Psychol Med. 2010;41(07):1517–28.

Gallbladder Stones and Choledocholitiasis

34

Pablo A. Acquafresca, Mariano Palermo, and Mariano E. Giménez

Cholelithiasis

It is known that the rapid weight loss is a predisposing factor to develop biliary lithiasis. The physiopathology is related with a supersaturation of bile with cholesterol, bile stasis, and increase in mucin concentration in bile. Therefore after any bariatric procedure (but gastric bypass specially), where a rapid weight loss occurs, this can become a threat. Furthermore the treatment can be a challenge due to anatomical changes caused by the bariatric procedure [1].

Diverse kinds of protocols exist: prophylactic (simultaneous cholecystectomy and gastric bypass in patients, whether they have or do not have cholelithiasis) [2, 3], elective (simultaneous cholecystectomy with conventional gastric bypass in the patients with asymptomatic cholelithiasis) [4, 5], and conventional (cholecystectomy only in the presence of cholelithiasis with symptoms) surgeries [6, 7].

The incidence of cholelithiasis post gastric bypass is estimated to be around 37%. Almost 50% developed disease in the first year of monitoring and 60% in the first 6 months. Meanwhile the patients undergoing sleeve gastrectomy have an incidence of cholelithiasis of 27%, being most of the cases developed in the first and a half year [8].

P. A. Acquafresca · M. Palermo (✉) · M. E. Giménez
Division of Bariatric Surgery Centro CIEN – DIAGNOMED, Affiliated Institution to the University of Buenos Aires and DAICIM Foundation, Buenos Aires, Argentina

Compared with the general population, the obese have high serum cholesterol levels, determining a higher incidence of lithiasis, which is further increased in the patient population undergoing a bariatric procedure. The latter is linked to several factors, among which stands out the large weight loss (especially in the first 6 months after surgery) which favors a significant mobilization of cholesterol from adipose tissue reservoir and reduced production of bile salts and phospholipids to the gallbladder.

Furthermore, after bariatric surgery occurs a decrease in the gallbladder motility due to nerve damage, a deficit in phospholipids and contraction stimulating proteins, and an increase of mucin secretion toward the gallbladder leading to an acceleration of the nucleation process. This predominance of cholesterol over the bile salt and phospholipids in bile promotes the formation of gallstones [9, 10].

Other factors that promote the formation of lithiasis post-surgery, such as decreased motility by altering vagal innervation derived from the surgical process, are present in some cases but are not constant. Instead, rapid weight loss (more than 50% of excess weight lost 3 months after laparoscopic RYGB) is the only predictor of gallbladder disease present in every study [11].

Regarding prophylactic surgery (cholecystectomy in patients without gallbladder stones), the majority of surgeons concur that a watchful waiting should be taken and only perform the bariatric procedure, because the number of

J. Ettinger et al. (eds.), *Gastric Bypass*, https://doi.org/10.1007/978-3-030-28803-7_34

patients that will develop symptomatic cholelithiasis is low (around 6–8% of them), and this leads to an elevated number of patients exposed to an unnecessary procedure with potential complications [4, 11]. Laparoscopic cholecystectomy in bariatric patients may be challenging due to suboptimal port placement and difficult body habitus. Furthermore, it is accompanied by potential risks such as lengthening of operative time, increased morbidity, and prolonged hospitalization. Serious complications have been reported as high as 2–3% of cases [12].

Some studies have shown that an elective approach (simultaneous cholecystectomy only in the patients with cholelithiasis) may be favored because of better short-term outcomes with significantly lower rates of mortality, morbidity, reinterventions, and shorter hospital when compared with patients that had concomitant cholecystectomy. However, the long-term biliary morbidity requiring subsequent cholecystectomy was not clear in these studies [6].

But other papers have shown that the rate of subsequent cholecystectomy after RYGB is low (6.8%), being the main cause for the subsequent cholecystectomy the uncomplicated biliary disease, while choledocholithiasis and biliary pancreatitis occurred very rarely. It's estimated that the rate of subsequent cholecystectomy due to biliary colic or gallbladder dyskinesia is 5.3%; cholecystitis, 1.0%; choledocholithiasis, 0.2%; and biliary pancreatitis, 0.2%.

Furthermore about 95% of the subsequent cholecystectomies are performed laparoscopically with a very low conversion rate, and the risk to suffer a complication from a subsequent cholecystectomy is extremely low (0.1%) for all patients without concomitant cholecystectomy during RYGB. Therefore, a routine concomitant cholecystectomy cannot be recommended when weighing the observed low long-term morbidity against the known potential detrimental effect on the short-term outcome [6, 7].

On the other hand, when talking about patients with asymptomatic gallbladder stone, currently there is no consensus in the treatment in patients undergoing weight loss surgery. Asymptomatic gallstones (silent gallstones) represent a dilemmatic approach. The natural history of asymptomatic gallstones suggests that many affected individuals will remain asymptomatic. Recent trend analysis in gastric bypass patients suggests that concomitant cholecystectomy should be considered only in symptomatic gallstones [7].

The use of ursodeoxycholic acid (UDCA) also has been proposed as a preventive measure for the gallstone formation. The UDCA is a bile acid that dissolves gallstones by decreasing biliary cholesterol secretion to lower bile cholesterol saturation and by decreasing biliary glycoprotein secretion to lower biliary nucleating factors. It was reported that the oral dose of 600 mg UDCA following gastric bypass for 6 months or even until gallstone formation was associated with decreased rate of gallstone formation [13, 14]. However, the cost-effectiveness of the treatment is a matter of debate because even though the use of UDCA lessened the costs of concurrent cholecystectomy and reduced the hospital stay along with logical cost raise in selective cholecystectomy, the prescription of UDCA tends to be unaffordable as an additional cost.

Due to the previously exposed, it is possible to conclude that cholecystectomy should be performed only in patients with cholelithiasis symptoms. Regarding patients with silent cholelithiasis, the surgeon must evaluate every case in particular, follow up the patient, and in case of developing symptoms, perform the cholecystectomy, but it's admissible to choose a conservative management.

Choledocholitiasis

The presence of gallstones in the common bile duct (CBD) although is a rare complication after RYGB (around 0.2% of the bariatric patients) [7] represents an important challenge due to the anatomical modifications of the gastrointestinal tract (Fig. 34.1). The duodenum remains adjacent to the surgically excluded stomach. Therefore, for the endoscopist, accessing the ampulla is technically very difficult. The endoscope must pass through the mouth, esophagus, gastric pouch, Roux limb, and then return retrograde through the afferent limb to reach the ampulla. This total length may easily exceed 300 cm, making almost impossible for traditional endoscopy access to

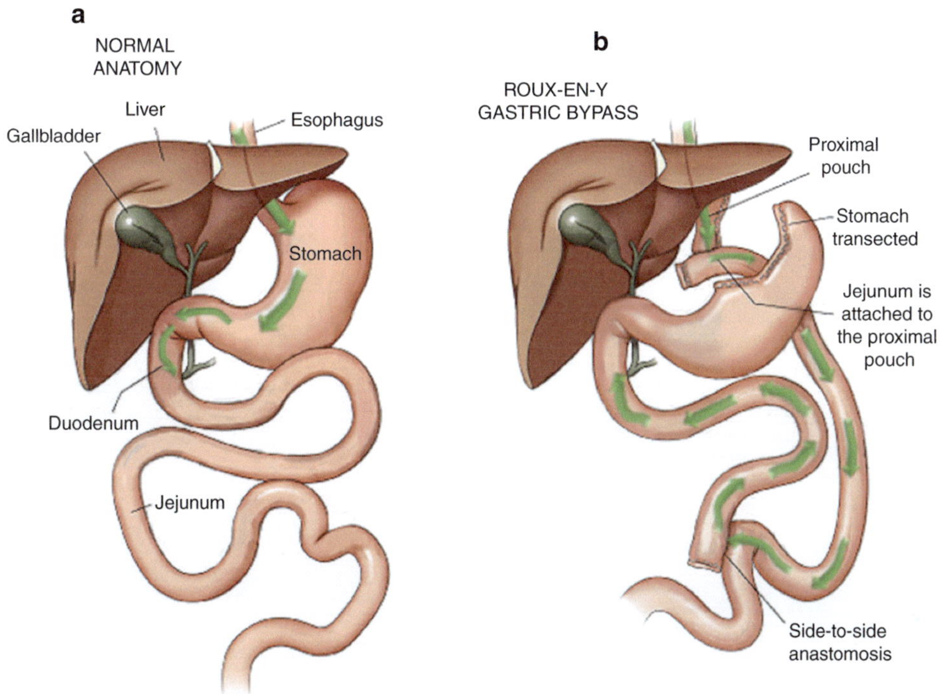

Fig. 34.1 (**a**) Green arrow showing the endoscopy path to the ampulla in normal anatomy. (**b**) Green arrow showing the endoscopy path to the ampulla in altered anatomy by gastric bypass

the papilla to perform an endoscopic retrograde cholangiopancreatography (ERCP).

This leads to having to pursue other methods to reach the papillae for the resolution of choledocholitiasis. Which of these methods should we choose must be based on the surgeon experience, the equipment available, and the location of the stone. But whatever the method, a special training is needed on endoscopy, percutaneous surgery, and laparoscopy.

The methods that have been described can be listed as follows:

- Laparoscopy-assisted transgastric ERCP (LAT-ERCP)
- Balloon enteroscopy-assisted ERCP (BEA-ERCP)
- Percutaneous biliary drainage with subsequent transfistula treatment
- Laparoscopic exploration of common bile duct

Due to the long anatomical route required to reach the biliopancreatic limb in patients with RYGB, a solution that has been found is to access the excluded stomach through laparoscopy and to insert the endoscope through a gastrotomy allowing to perform an ERCP like in a traditional way. The success rate of this procedure has been shown to be superior to BEA-ERCP; biliary cannulation rates up to 100% have been described and is associated with a significantly shorter endoscopic procedure time, but not a shorter total procedure time (laparoscopy plus ERCP) [15–17].

In this procedure a standard laparoscopic access to the abdominal cavity is performed with insertion of four trocars, then the greater curve of the antrum is mobilized, and a gastrotomy and purse-string suture are fashioned on the anterior side of the greater curvature of the gastric remnant near the antrum (Fig. 34.2). An additional 15 mm or 18 mm trocar must be placed in the left upper quadrant and inserted into the gastrotomy in the center of the purse-string suture (Fig. 34.3). This purse-string has to be tightly fixed around the trocar to prevent loss of insufflation pressure, and the gastrotomy should be made as lateral as possible along the greater curvature to permit smooth intu-

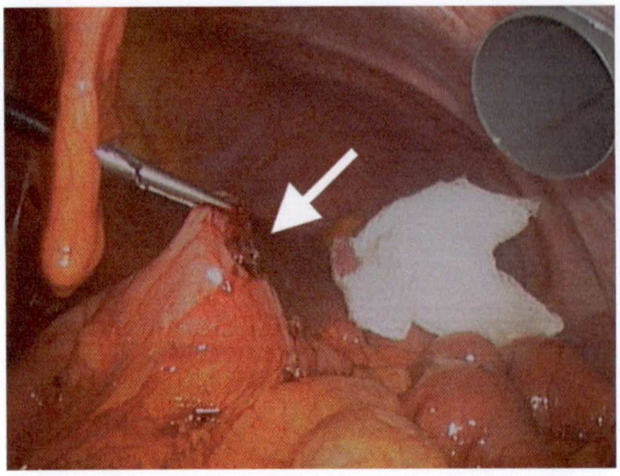

Fig. 34.2 Formation of a gastrotomy on the anterior wall of the greater curvature of the gastric remnant. (Courtesy M Falcao, J Campos Marins, M Galvao Neto, A Ramos)

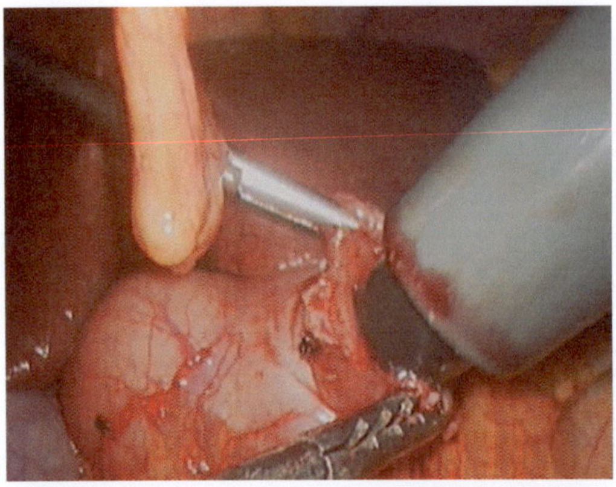

Fig. 34.3 Insertion of a 15 mm trocar into the gastric remnant through gastrotomy. (Courtesy M Falcao, J Campos Marins, M Galvao Neto, A Ramos)

bation of the pylorus. It's also recommended to occlude the biliopancreatic limb with an intestinal clamp to prevent over-insufflation of the small bowel that blocks the perioperative visualization.

Finally, a side-viewing endoscope is introduced through the 15 mm or 18 mm trocar secured into the gastrotomy, and ERCP can be performed under fluoroscopic guidance (Fig. 34.4). After the removal of the scope and the trocar, the purse-string is tied and the gastrotomy incision sutured (Fig. 34.5). Described By Manoel Galvao Neto from Brazil.

In case of patients with gallbladder in situ, delaying the definitive cholecystectomy until ERCP is performed is considered to be the safest option because in case of a difficult cannulation of the papilla, a guidewire can be inserted into the cystic duct to perform a *rendezvous* technique in order to achieve the cannulation. In this technique the guidewire that was inserted through the cystic duct is then moved into the main biliary duct and passed through the papilla. Therefore, the flexible wire is taken by the endoscopist and used as a guide to enter the papilla.

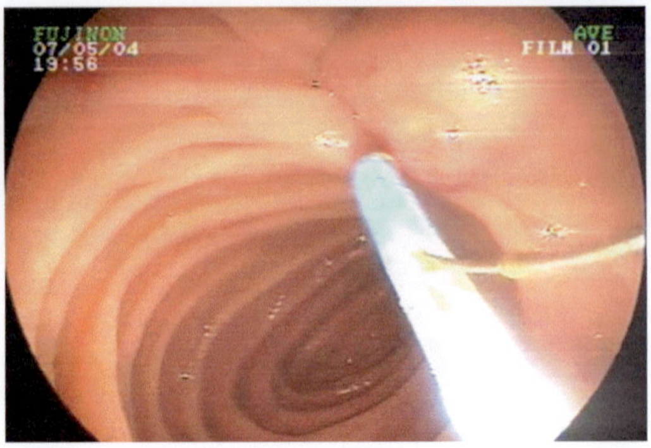

Fig. 34.4 ERCP with sphincterotomy and stone extraction. (Courtesy M Falcao, J Campos Marins, M Galvao Neto, A Ramos)

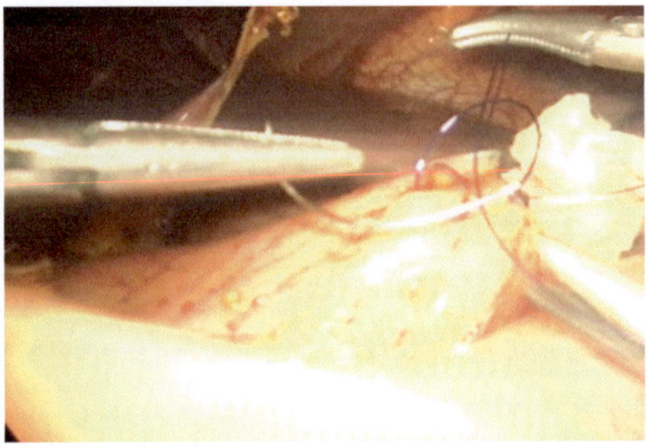

Fig. 34.5 Suture of the gastrotomy incision. (Courtesy M Falcao, J Campos Marins, M Galvao Neto, A Ramos)

Performance of the LAT-ERCP technique is influenced by the presence of postoperative adhesions which renders the transgastric access more difficult, sometimes being necessary to perform a minilaparotomy to achieve the transgastric access. This is expected in case of a history of open surgery, multiple laparoscopic interventions, and previous peritonitis or abscess formation.

When the need for repeat ERCP is anticipated during the first LAT-ERCP procedure, a gastrostomy tube can be inserted through the gastrotomy incision into the lumen of the stomach. Repeat ERCP can be performed percutaneously after the surgical gastrostomy tract has matured [18].

The LAT-ERCP, although is a complex procedure, in experimented hands allows to successfully treat choledocholitiasis with a biliary cannulation rates up to 100% and a low rate of complications like pancreatitis or post-sphincterotomy bleeding. In no case a leak of the gastrostomy suture was described [16–19].

The second option that we have to treat choledocholitiasis in patients with RYGB is the BEA-ERCP. The major advantage of balloon-assisted over conventional enteroscopy is the ability to reduce loops of small bowel which facilitates advancement of the endoscope in patients after Roux-en-Y reconstruction. In patients with Roux-en-Y anatomy, success rates varying from 60% to 90% for reaching the biliopancreatic limb and successful ERCP ranging from 46% tom 80% have been reported [20–29], clearly inferior to the success rate of the LAT-ERCP. The devices that are used for the BEA-ERCP can consist in a single- or double-balloon system (Figs. 34.6 and 34.7).

The system is composed of a 200-cm, thin endoscope, with a 145-cm soft overtube. Latex balloons are attached to the end of the endoscope and to the end of the overtube. By using a series of inflations and deflations of the balloons, along with reductions, the endoscopist may advance the scope through the lumen in an "accordion-like" fashion and reach the distal small bowel [30] (Figs. 34.8 and 34.9).

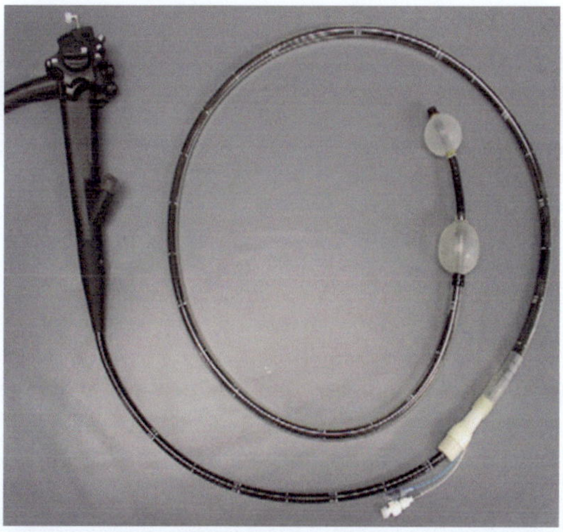

Fig. 34.6 Double-balloon endoscope

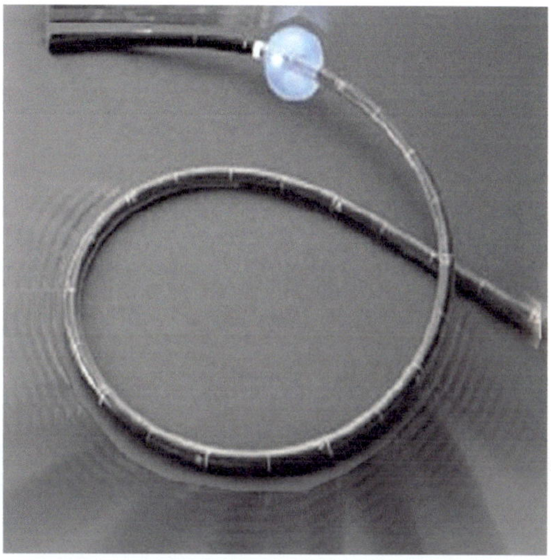

Fig. 34.7 Single-balloon endoscope

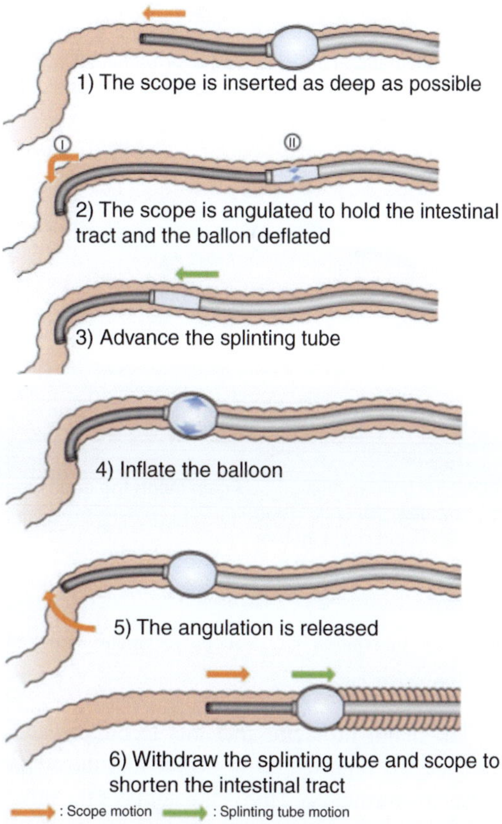

Fig. 34.8 Illustration of endoscopic technique with single balloon

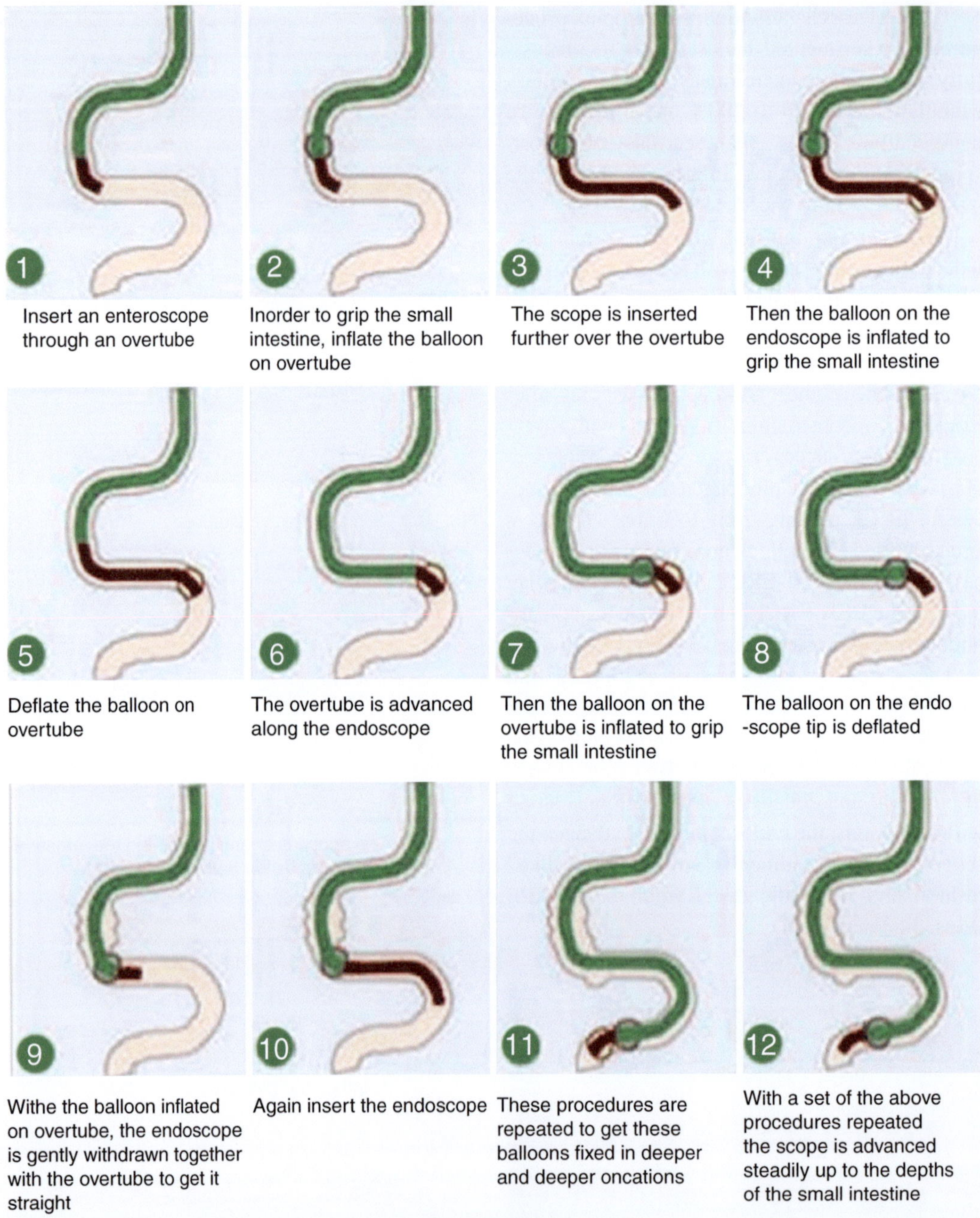

Fig. 34.9 Illustration of endoscopic technique with double balloon

The major problems that this technique must face are the long length of bowel that the scope must pass through and the acute angle of the afferent limb and Roux limb anastomosis which is also very difficult to navigate. Furthermore, attaching the balloon to the tip of the endoscope is often troublesome, and the balloon on the tip of the enteroscope can occasionally decrease the field of view if it becomes dislodged distally. It's an invasive and time-consuming procedure, but on the other hand, the morbidity rate is low, especially for diagnostic procedures, and the complication rate of diagnostic double-balloon endoscopies is 0.8% and that of therapeutic procedures 4.3% [31].

Another important drawback of this technique is that the highest success rate is described in patients with hepaticojejunostomy, while the success rate in patients with native papilla tend to be lower due to the fact that the endoscope is forward viewing and the straight angle with which accessories can be advanced [21]. The cannulation rates of intact papilla using double-balloon enteroscope have ranged from 25% to 80% [20, 22, 23].

There is also another problem; there is a limited availability of suitable equipment, as all accessories have to be of sufficient length. Unfortunately for double-balloon technique, there is a current trend in ERCP equipment to develop shorter rather than longer accessories. There is a lack of needle knifes, sphincterotomes, extraction balloons, lithotripsy devices, and retrieval baskets customized for the double-balloon system [32].

The previously described BEA-ERCP should not be considered as a first option when treating choledocholitiasis, especially if the physician is not an expert endoscopist. And if choledocholitiasis coexist with cholelithiasis, considering that the gallbladder will be removed, a laparoscopic approach is recommended (whether with a full laparoscopic resolution with CBD exploration or with a LAT-ERCP).

The third option available to treat the lithiasis of the CBD is the percutaneous approach. With this technique it is necessary first to perform a percutaneous biliary drainage, and later when the fistula between the biliary system and the skin is consolidated, a session to remove the stones can be performed.

The first step of the procedure consists of an ultrasound-guided puncture of the intrahepatic bile duct by using a 22G Chiba needle (Fig. 34.10), and then a percutaneous transhepatic cholangiogram should be performed to confirm the presence, location, number, and size of stones (Fig. 34.11). The choice whether to use a left-sided subxiphoid approach or a right-sided subcostal or intercostal approach must be based on individual and anatomic considerations, such as the position of the liver, bile duct anatomy (as seen on pre-procedural imaging), and number, position, and size of the bile duct stones.

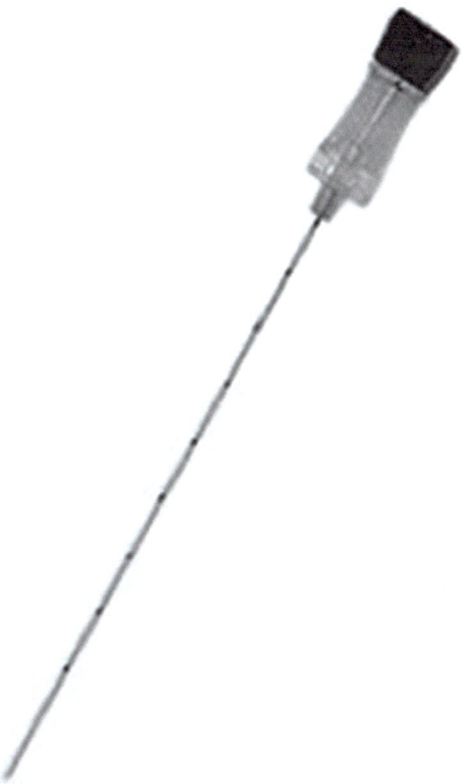

Fig. 34.10 22G Chiba needle

The percutaneous transhepatic cholangiogram can be achieved in 98% of the patients with dilatation of the bile ducts and in 90% of those without dilatation [33].

Once we gain access to the biliary system with the Chiba needle, a guide wire must be introduced, and by using Seldinger technique, an 8 or 10 Fr biliary drainage must be placed (Fig. 34.12).

After 7–10 days when the biliary system is decompressed, the symptoms of cholangitis (if were presents) are relieved and the fistula starts to consolidate; thus, it is possible to perform the treatment of the stones. By working through the biliary-cutaneous fistula, it is possible to push the stones into the duodenum or extract them through the skin's hole. In order to achieve this, a standard percutaneous transluminal angioplasty balloon catheter is advanced beyond the stones and positioned across the papilla. Then the sphincter

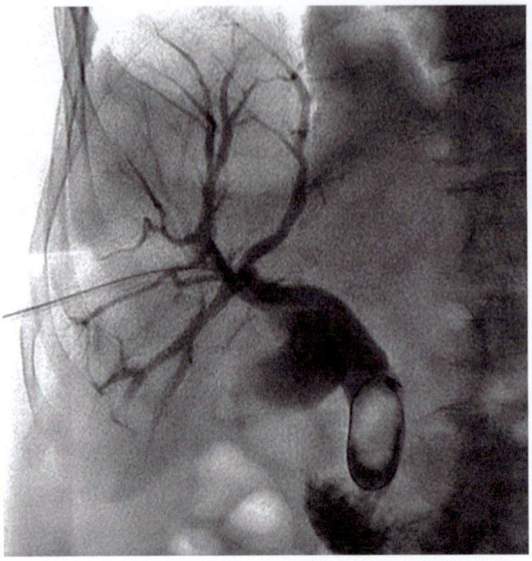

Fig. 34.11 Percutaneous transhepatic cholangiogram showing a big stone on distal common bile duct

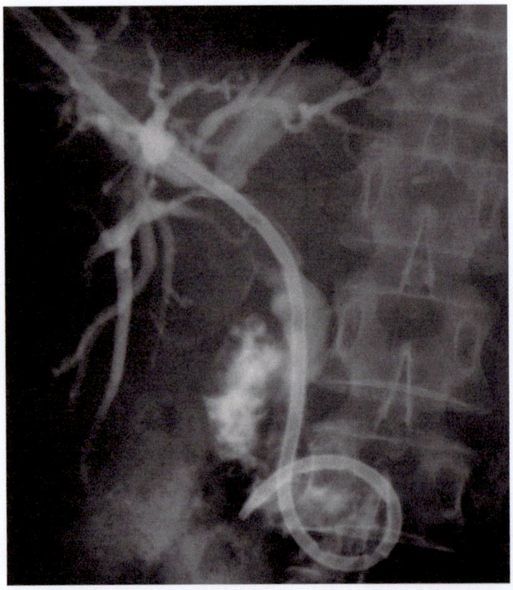

Fig. 34.12 Percutaneous biliary drainage with "pigtail" in duodenum

is dilated by an 8–12 mm balloon, depending on the size of the largest stone, until no waist could be seen in the balloon on fluoroscopy (Fig. 34.13). Once this is achieved, the balloon is deflated and the catheter withdrawn and positioned proximal to the stones. After reinflating the balloon, the stones are pushed forward through the dilated sphincter into the duodenum.

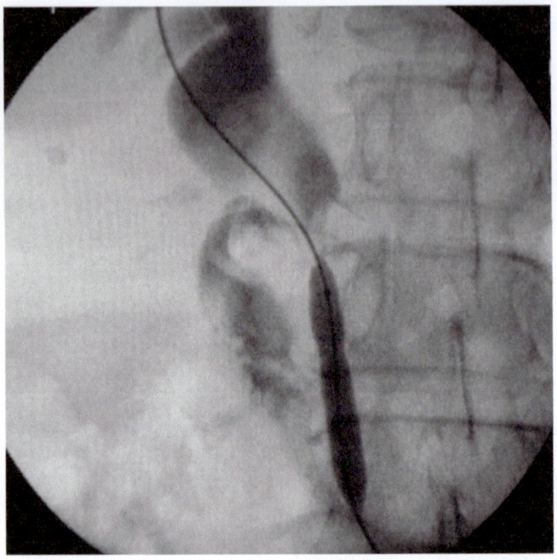

Fig. 34.13 Sphincter dilation with a 10 mm balloon. A waist can still be seen on the balloon

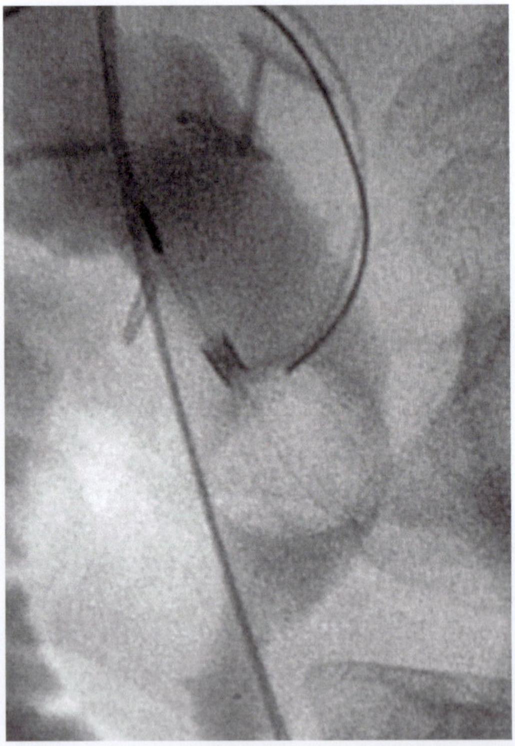

Fig. 34.14 A stone being grabbed with a Dormia basket

If the stone size exceeded 10 mm, mechanical lithotripsy with Dormia basket is recommended [34]. The stone fragments are then evacuated into the duodenum by using the balloon catheter or Dormia basket (Fig. 34.14).

If the stone's size is not too big, another option is to grab the stone with the Dormia basket and pull it out through the skin's hole. This maneuver could be dangerous if the stone is larger than the fistula diameter because the fistula could be damaged; thus it is recommended to place a second (safety) wire through the papilla in order to preserve the biliary access.

When all the stones seem to have been extracted, cholangiography must be performed to confirm complete stone clearance. Then a biliary drainage is placed in the CBD.

After approximately 24 hours later, a cholangiography must be performed to confirm CBD clearance, and if so, the external drain is removed. If residual stones are found, the procedure must be repeated until all stones are removed.

The success rate reported with this approach varies between 93% and 96% and the complications between 4.7% and 6.7% [34–37]. The complications described include hemobilia, pancreatitis, cholangitis, pleural effusion due to a transpleural biliary drainage, and bile peritonitis due to fistula disruption.

The last option available to treat choledocholitiasis is the laparoscopic approach with exploration of the CBD. In case we are treating a patient that has already been cholecistectomized, the laparoscopic approach should be considered as a second option, after the other minimal invasive approaches failed (endoscopic-percutaneous), as the patient's abdomen could be hostile due to adhesions which will make the CBD exploration difficult. But if the patient also has cholelithiasis and laparoscopic cholecystectomy must be performed, it is possible to do the treatment fully laparoscopic.

It is recommended to try first a transcystic approach to treat the stones. A technique similar to the percutaneous technique can be performed, and by introducing a percutaneous transluminal angioplasty balloon catheter through the cystic duct, the sphincter is dilated, and then, with the same balloon, the stone is pushed to the duodenum. It is also possible to do this maneuver with a Dormia basket through the cystic duct (Fig. 34.15). If this fails, one should consider to open the CBD and perform an exploration (Fig. 34.16).

If we decided to explore the CBD after stone extraction, we perform cholangiography, and if we are sure that there are no more stones, and the bile duct is dilated, we can perform a primary closure of the CBD. On the other hand, if the bile duct is thin, this measure is not so strongly recommended due to possible strictures at the suture site. In case we doubt the presence of more stones, we must place a T-tube in order to avoid a pressure increase inside the CBD and a bile leakage and, of course, to perform then a percutaneous approach through the T-tube to extract the remaining stones (Fig. 34.17).

In conclusion, with the set of therapeutic tools mentioned previously, one should be able to face

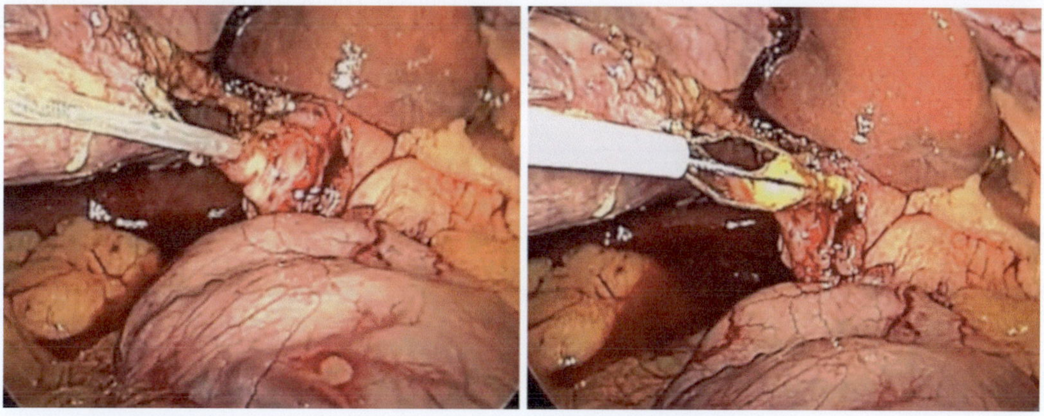

Fig. 34.15 A stone being pulled out with a Dormia basket through the cystic duct

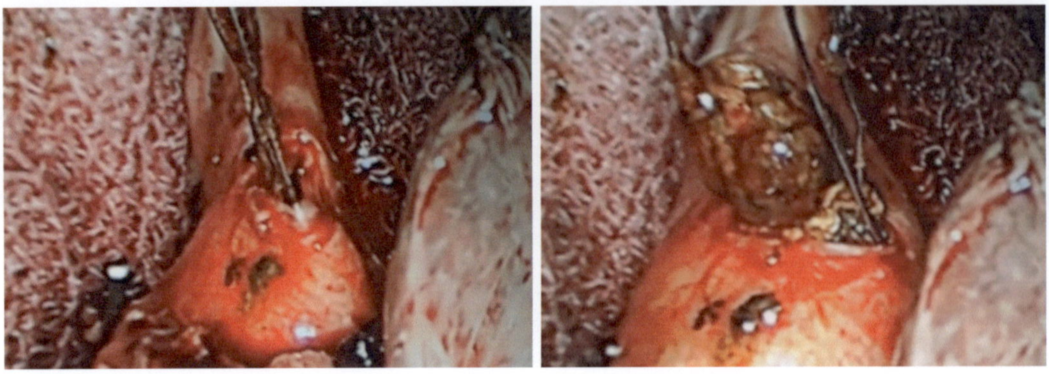

Fig. 34.16 A stone being pulled out with a Dormia basket through an incision on the CBD

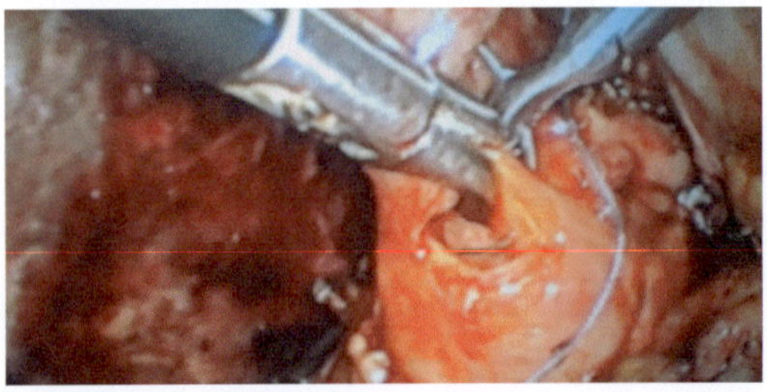

Fig. 34.17 Primary closure of the common bile duct after laparoscopic exploration

the problem of choledocholitiasis. A proper training is needed in laparoscopic surgery, endoscopy, and percutaneous surgery due to the high technical difficulty of treating CBD stones in patients with Roux-en-Y anatomy. Which path to follow should be based on details of every case and personal experience with every mentioned technique, and in case of lack of personal experience, it is strongly recommended to derivate these patients to a specialist.

References

1. Taha MIA, Freitas WR Jr, Puglia CR, Lacombe A, Malheiros CA. Fatores preditivos de colelitíase colelitíasem em obesos mórbidos após astroplastia em y de Roux. Trabalho realizado na Santa Casa de Misericórdia de São Paulo, SP. Rev Assoc Med Bras. 2006;52(6):430–4.
2. Nougou A, Suter M. Almost routine prophylactic cholecystectomy during laparoscopic gastric bypass is safe. Obes Surg. 2008;18:535–9.
3. Liem RK, Niloff PH. Prophylactic cholecystectomy with open gastric bypass operation. Obes Surg. 2004;14:763–5.
4. Tucker ON, Fajnwaks P, Szomstein S, Rosenthal RJ. Is concomitant cholecystectomy necessary in obese patients undergoing laparoscopic gastric bypass surgery? Surg Endosc. 2008;22:2450–4.
5. Escalona A, Boza C, Munoz R, Perez G, Rayo S, Crovari F, et al. Routine preoperative ultrasonography and selective cholecystectomy in laparoscopic Roux-en-Y gastric bypass. Why not? Obes Surg. 2008;18:47–51.
6. Worni M, Guller U, Shah A, Gandhi M, Shah J, Rajgor D, et al. Cholecystectomy concomitant with laparoscopic gastric bypass: a trend analysis of the nationwide inpatient sample from 2001 to 2008. Obes Surg. 2012;22:220–9.
7. Warschkow R, Tarantino I, Ukegjini K, Beutner U, Güller U, Schmied BM, Müller SA, Schultes B, Thurnheer M. Concomitant cholecystectomy during laparoscopic Roux-en-Y gastric bypass in obese patients is not justified: a meta-analysis. Obes Surg. 2013;23:397–407.
8. Ibarra E, Pascowsk M, Souza JM, Vega E, Duza G, Palermo M. Litiasis vesicular en pacientes sometidos a cirugía bariátrica: incidencia posquirúrgica según técnica. Pren Méd Argent. 2015;101(9):471–6.
9. Gustafsson U, Benthin L, Granstrom L, Groen AK, Sahlin S, Einarsson C. Changes in gallbladder bile composition and crystal detection time in morbidly obese subjects after bariatric surgery. Hepatology. 2005;41:1322–8.
10. Everhart JE. Contributions of obesity and weight loss to gallstone disease. Ann Intern Med. 1993;119:1029–35.
11. D'Hondt M, Sergeant G, Deylgat B, Devriendt D, Van Rooy F, Vansteenkiste F. Prophylactic cholecystectomy, a mandatory step in morbidly obese patients undergoing laparoscopic Roux-en-Y gastric bypass? J Gastrointest Surg. 2011;15:1532–6.
12. Strasberg SM, Hertl M, Soper NJ. An analysis of the problem of biliary injury during laparoscopic cholecystectomy. J Am Coll Surg. 1995;180:101–25.

13. Miller K, Hell E, Lang B, Lengauer E. Gallstone formation prophylaxis after gastric restrictive procedures for weight loss: a randomized double-blind placebo-controlled trial. Ann Surg. 2003;238:697–702.
14. Uy MC, Talingdan-Te MC, Espinosa WZ, Daez ML, Ong JP. Ursodeoxycholic acid in the prevention of gallstone formation after bariatric surgery: a meta-analysis. Obes Surg. 2008;18:1532–8.
15. Schreiner MA, Chang L, Gluck M, et al. Laparoscopy-assisted versus balloon enteroscopy-assisted ERCP in bariatric post-Roux-en-Y gastric bypass patients. Gastrointest Endosc. 2012;75:748–56.
16. Lopes TL, Clements RH, Wilcox CM. Laparoscopy-assisted ERCP: experience of a high-volume bariatric surgery center (with video). Gastrointest Endosc. 2009;70:1254–9.
17. Bertin PM, Singh K, Arregui ME. Laparoscopic transgastric endoscopic retrograde cholangiopancreatography (ERCP) after gastric bypass: case series and a description of technique. Surg Endosc. 2011;25:2592–6.
18. Tekola B, Wang AY, Ramanath M, et al. Percutaneous gastrostomy tube placement to perform transgastrostomy endoscopic retrograde cholangiopancreatography in patients with Roux-en-Y anatomy. Dig Dis Sci. 2011;56:3364–9.
19. Snauwaert C, Laukens P, Dillemans B, Himpens J, De Looze D, Deprez PH, Badaoui A. Laparoscopy-assisted transgastric endoscopic retrograde cholangiopancreatography in bariatric Roux-en-Y gastric bypass patients. Endosc Int Open. 2015;3:E458–63.
20. Chu YC, Yang CC, Yeh YH, et al. Double-balloon enteroscopy application in biliary tract disease-its therapeutic and diagnostic functions. Gastrointest Endosc. 2008;68:585–91.
21. Koornstra JJ. Double balloon enteroscopy for endoscopic retrograde cholangiopancreatography after Roux-en-Y reconstruction: case series and review of the literature. Neth J Med. 2008;66:275–9.
22. Aabakken L, Bretthauer M, Line PD. Double-balloon enteroscopy for endoscopic retrograde cholangiography in patients with a Roux-en-Y anastomosis. Endoscopy. 2007;39:1068–71.
23. Emmett DS, Mallat DB. Double-balloon ERCP in patients who have undergone Roux-en-Y surgery: a case series. Gastrointest Endosc. 2007;66:1038–41.
24. Moreels TG, Roth B, Vandervliet EJ, et al. The use of the double balloon enteroscope for endoscopic retrograde cholangiopancreatography and biliary stent placement after Roux-en-Y hepaticojejunostomy. Endoscopy. 2007;39:E196–7.
25. Spahn TW, Grosse-Thie W, Spies P, Mueller MK. Treatment of choledocholithiasis following Roux-en-Y hepaticojejunostomy using double-balloon endoscopy. Digestion. 2007;75:20–1.
26. Parlak E, Ciçek B, Dişibeyaz S, et al. Endoscopic retrograde cholangiography by double balloon enteroscopy in patients with Roux-en-Y hepaticojejunostomy. Surg Endosc. 2010;24:466–70.
27. Moreels TG, Hubens GJ, Ysebaert DK, Op de Beeck B, Pelckmans PA. Diagnostic and therapeutic double-balloon enteroscopy after small bowel Roux-en-Y reconstructive surgery. Digestion. 2009;80:141–7.
28. Kuga R, Furuya CK Jr, Hondo FY, Ide E, Ishioka S, Sakai P. ERCP using double-balloon enteroscopy in patients with Roux-en-Y anatomy. Dig Dis. 2008;26(4):330–5.
29. Wang AY, Sauer BG, Behm BW, et al. Single-balloon enteroscopy effectively enables diagnostic and therapeutic retrograde cholangiography in patients with surgically altered anatomy. Gastrointest Endosc. 2010;71:641–9.
30. Yamamoto H, Sekine Y, Sato Y, et al. Total enteroscopy with a nonsurgical steerable double-balloon method. Gastrointest Endosc. 2001;53:216–20.
31. Mensink PB, Haringsma J, Kucharzik T, et al. Complications of double balloon enteroscopy: a multicenter survey. Endoscopy. 2007;39:613–5.
32. Joyce AM, Ahmad NA, Beilstein MC, et al. Multicenter comparative trial of the V-scope system for therapeutic ERCP. Endoscopy. 2006;38:713–6.
33. Gimenez ME, Berkowski D, Cordoba P. Obstrucción biliar benigna. In: Gimenez M, Guimaraes M, Oleaga J, Sierre S, editors. Manual de técnicas intervencionistas guiadas por imágenes. Buenos Aires: Ediciones Journal; 2011. p. 119–38.
34. Kint JF, van den Bergh JE, van Gelder RE, Rauws EA, Gouma DJ, van Delden OM, Laméris JS. Percutaneous treatment of common bile duct stones: results and complications in 110 consecutive patients. Dig Surg. 2015;32:9–15. https://doi.org/10.1159/000370129.
35. García-García L, Lanciego C. Percutaneous treatment of biliary stones: sphincteroplasty and occlusion balloon for the clearance of bile duct calculi. AJR. 2004;182:663–70.
36. Szulman C, Giménez M, Sierre S. Antegrade papillary balloon dilation for extrahepatic bile duct stone clearance: lessons learned from treating 300 patients. J Vasc Interv Radiol. 2011;22(3):346–53.
37. Gil S, de la Iglesia P, Verdú JF, de España F, Arenas J, Irurzun J. Effectiveness and safety of balloon dilation of the papilla and the use of an occlusion balloon for clearance of bile duct calculi. AJR Am J Roentgenol. 2000;174(5):1455–60.

35 Hypoglycemia After Gastric Bypass

Glauco da Costa Alvarez

Along with the dramatic benefits that Roux-en-Y gastric bypass (RYGB) offers, this operation can have complications.

Postprandial hyperinsulinemic hypoglycemia is the least common and incompletely understood one. It is a metabolic complication that typically develops 6 or more months after RYGB, usually after a meal.

It can also occur after other types of bariatric operations, such as duodenal switch or sleeve gastrectomy [1, 2].

Some patients experience suggestive symptoms of hypoglycemia after RYGB, but whether these symptoms are always associated with low sugar blood glucose are unclear. Clinically significant hypoglycemia after RYGB has been estimated to occur in 0.2–0.36% of patients [3, 4].

Since RYGB is one of the most common bariatric procedures performed in the world, it is essential for patients to be aware of the true risk of this condition prior to surgery. The majority of patients experiencing hypoglycemia post-RYGB did not have abnormal glucose metabolism before RYGB (73%).

The mechanism of action of RYGB includes an increased postprandial gut hormone release, increased satiety [5, 6], reduced hunger [7], and alteration in food preference [8].

Dumping syndrome after gastric surgery is well recognized and refers to symptoms appearing shortly after food intake. Dumping is often categorized as either early or late, 10–30 minutes after food intake.

Symptoms and timing may vary [9]. Anna Laurenius has suggested that symptoms occurring within 30 minutes after food intake are referred to as dumping, while symptoms appearing 30 minutes after food intake are called hypoglycemia-like symptoms.

These hypoglycemia-associated symptoms are a warning for neuroglycopenia, which can lead to irrational behavior and, ultimately, to unconsciousness [10].

Most of the patients with RYGB have a marked decrease in blood glucose 1,5–3 hours after an oral carbohydrate load. This phenomenon is commonly called hyperinsulinemic or reactive hypoglycemia and can be explained as an overshoot in the secretion of insulin after rapid uptake of carbohydrates into the portal circulation. It is often caused by refined carbohydrate load [11].

A possible mechanism is the enhanced incretin effect (GLP1) that occurs after RYGB as ingested nutrients almost instantly are exposed to the small intestine [10].

Hypoglycemia awareness is a term defining patients not experiencing typical warning symp-

G. da Costa Alvarez (✉)
Department of Surgery, Federal University of Santa Maria, Santa Maria, Brazil

J. Ettinger et al. (eds.), *Gastric Bypass*, https://doi.org/10.1007/978-3-030-28803-7_35

toms, despite having plasma glucose level below 54 mg/dL.

Etiology

The primary etiologies of post-RYGB hypoglycemia are distinct and include dumping syndrome, factitious insulin/sulfonylurea administration, and nesidioblastosis; rare cases of insulinoma after RYGB have been reported [12].

Nesidioblastosis, defined as hyperinsulinemic hypoglycemia attributed to pancreatic β-cell hyperplasia, was thought to be a congenital disorder occurring in neonates and infants only. This was first described in adults in 1981 [13].

It is still considered a rare condition. There have been an increasing number of cases of non-insulinoma pancreatogenous hypoglycemia in obese patients who have undergone RYGB for morbid obesity [14, 15].

Pathophysiology

Post-RYGB hypoglycemia is most likely due to multifactorial alterations in hormonal and glycemic patterns that have not yet being fully elucidated.

RYGB patients can develop a severe dumping syndrome from rapid delivery of food into the small intestine, resulting in reactive hypoglycemia caused by an exaggerated release of insulin [16].

Various gut hormones, including glucagon-like polypeptide-1(GLP1), have been found to show increased expression in patients after RYGB, compared with nonsurgical obese patients [17].

L cells, located at the distal ileum, are stimulated to release GLP-1 after the rapid delivery of intraluminal nutrients.

GLP-1 functions on islet cell include increasing β-cell sensitivity to glucose, stimulating glucose-dependent insulin secretion, and inhibiting glucagon secretion on the alpha cell. On the other hand, GLP-1 is the initiator of the ileal brake phenomena, slowing small bowel motility in response to rapid delivery of food into the proximal small bowel.

This results in exaggerated secretion of GLP-1, resulting in the activation of the ileal brake at the consequence of deep insulin secretion and subsequent hypoglycemia.

Histopathologic examination of specimens from several patients undergoing partial pancreatectomy for postprandial hypoglycemia was initially proposed as demonstrating characteristics of nesidioblastosis. The condition is defined by β-cell hypertrophy and hyperfunction, islet cell hyperplasia, and neoformation of islets of Langerhans from pancreatic duct epithelium [14, 18, 19].

It has been further suggested that this findings are consistent with prolonged hypersecretion of GLP-1. However, this pathologic finding has been challenged by other groups, and clinical results are suboptimal [20, 21].

The physiologic counter-regulatory mechanism in response to hypoglycemia may also to be disrupted in post-RYGB hypoglycemic patients.

Kamvissi et al. proposed an anti-incretin theory suggesting that nutrient passage through the gastrointestinal tract after RYGB may also activate negative feedback mechanisms to balance the effects of incretins and to prevent postprandial hypoglycemia [22].

The failure of this counter-regulatory mechanism may accentuate hyperinsulinemic hypoglycemia.

Diagnosis

The diagnosis is made from the history (previous gastric surgery) and the constellation of symptoms, with few objective findings by examination.

Symptoms of postprandial hypoglycemia may develop months to years after surgery, 1–3 hours after carbohydrate ingestion [23].

Severe hypoglycemia symptoms, defined by Whipple's triad [24], include confusion, low plasma glucose concentration, and resolution of those symptoms after carbohydrate intake.

Specific symptoms of hypoglycemia are categorized as autonomic or neuroglycopenic. Autonomic symptoms include anxiety, sweating, tremors, and palpitation. Neuroglycopenic symptoms include confusion, weakness, lightheadedness, dizziness, blurred vision, disorientation, and eventually, loss of consciousness, coma, and even death [4].

When these patients are symptomatic, a fasting plasma glucose <50 mg/dl, a serum insulin level is the first step in the decision-making process to determine the etiology of the hypoglycemia.

Insulin is the central hormone in the body's regulation of carbohydrate and fat metabolism that originates from the β cells residing in the islets of Langerhans within the pancreas. Hyperinsulinemia is a condition in which the insulin level is >6 μU/ml.

Proinsulin is a precursor that resides within the β cells and is composed of insulin A and B chains linked together by C-peptide.

C-peptide is cleaved by an intracellular protease before being released into the circulation.

C-peptide elevated >5 ng/ml. A proinsulin level <5 pmol/L is highly sensitive toward eliminating insulinoma as a cause of endogenous hyperinsulinemia, leaving only nesidioblastosis as the diagnosis [25].

Continuous glucose monitoring (CGM) over the course of 3 days is more sensitive and allows for glucose monitoring while patients are eating as they would do normally [26].

A pattern of hyperglycemia within 30 minutes of a high glucose meal, followed significantly by hypoglycemia, is highly suggestive of the diagnosis [4].

These patients have a spontaneous return to euglycemia after the hypoglycemic episode.

The oral glucose tolerance test (OGTT) is primarily used owing to its simplicity to perform and ease of both administration and interpretation of results as an outpatient procedure. The mixed meal tolerance test (MMTT) is a preferred provocative test, in which a standardized carbohydrates, protein, and fat are given. Glucose and insulin levels are determined during the fasting state and at 30-minute intervals after the mixed meal. A positive MMTT demonstrates normal fasting glucose levels, hyperinsulinemia prior to hypoglycemia, hypoglycemia with plasma glucose levels <50–60 mg/dl, and symptoms of hypoglycemia.

Diagnostic imaging is necessary to distinguish nesidioblastosis of insulinoma after the biochemical evaluation (proinsulin level). Insulinoma can be identified using computed tomography and magnetic resonance imaging.

Selective intra-arterial calcium stimulation with hepatic venous sampling is a highly accurate and safe method for the preoperative localization of insulinomas.

Selective arterial calcium-stimulation tests were performed as a measure of the basal insulin level in the right hepatic vein in response to the sequential injection of calcium into the splenic, superior mesenteric, and gastroduodenal arteries.

The double gradient detected in the hepatic vein after sequential calcium injection in those arteries was considered to indicate hyperfunction of the B cells in the vascular distribution of the artery studied, which was identified in the angiographic findings [27].

This test might be more useful in localizing the B-cell mass in case of nesidioblastosis. Nevertheless, confirmation of the diagnosis cannot occur without histologic confirmation of a pancreatic surgical specimen.

Treatment

The reason not all RYGB patients develop symptoms might be from different diets. Meals with a high carbohydrate content and high glycemic index may provoke these hypoglycemic attacks, suggesting that the primary treatment of hyperinsulinemic hypoglycemia is related to the dumping syndrome. The primary goal is to change the patient's diet.

Carbohydrate restriction appears to be a good first-line approach in the management of post-RYGB postprandial hypoglycemia. A 30 g carb-restricted meal combined with a protein intake and consumption of fat and fiber, in a multiple small meals, may help to prevent postprandial hypoglycemia in patients with post-RYGB hypoglycemia [4, 28, 29].

Pharmacologic treatment for post-RYGB hypoglycemia has also been described.

Acarbose, an α-glycoside hydrolase inhibitor, decreases gastrointestinal absorption of carbohydrates. Acarbose has been found to attenuate the postprandial increase in glucose and insulin; its use by patients can be limited by the occurrence of flatulence and worsening diarrhea. Doses range from 100 mg to 300 mg [30, 31].

Nifedipine, a calcium channel blocker that reduces insulin secretion, has been used at a dose of 30 mg daily [32].

Diazoxide, an adenosine triphosphate-dependent potassium channel agonist of β cells, which reduces insulin release, has demonstrated moderate success in avoiding pancreatectomy in adults with postprandial hyperinsulinemic hypoglycemia after RYGB [33].

GLP-1 receptor antagonists have shown efficacy and are promising for long-term treatment.

The presumed pathophysiology of RYGB and their effects on GLP-1 expression with subsequent elevated insulin levels, blocking the action of GLP-1, can suppress postprandial insulin secretion. Infusions of GLP-1 receptor blockers correct the hypoglycemia and increase glucagon levels in individuals with recurrent hypoglycemia after RYGB [34–36].

Octreotide (somatostatin) has shown to improve symptoms in dumping syndrome by a combination of slowing small bowel motility, inhibition of insulin secretion, and inhibition splanchnic vasodilation.

Both short- and long-acting octreotides have been used, demonstrating beneficial effects on symptoms with the short-acting being better tolerated and more efficacious [37].

There are cases with no response to clinical treatment. With these exceptional cases, surgery may be considered.

Surgery should be evaluated in the context of the perioperative risk, long-term outcomes, potential weight regain, and its effect on obesity-related comorbidity and late complications such as diabetes, reflux, and diarrhea.

Different surgical approaches have been applied, but the physiology of the hypoglycemia was not adequately elucidated [38].

Different surgical techniques were applied including the placement of a gastric tube, gastric pouch restriction, reversal of the RYGB with and without sleeve gastrectomy, and pancreatic resection. In some series, several concomitant techniques were applied.

The placement of a gastrostomy tube was used in all patients before reversal in the two largest series of RYGB reversal for hypoglycemia [39, 40].

After nutritional delivery through the gastrostomy tube, no hypoglycemic symptoms were reported, and a marked normalization of the glucose tolerance test was defined. This is often considered a preferred early approach for patients who fail medical management.

Restoring restriction can be performed:

1. By adding a gastric pouch application in a dilated gastric pouch
2. With pouch revision using linear staplers to create a 30 ml pouch
3. With placement of a silastic ring or adjustable gastric band over small gastric pouch 1 cm above the gastrojejunal anastomosis [41, 42]

Restriction will lead to slower nutrient delivery to the jejunal limb. Long-term outcome, however, is not established [43].

Reversal of RYGB: some bariatric surgeons have suggested reversal of the gastric bypass by performing gastrogastrostomy, with or without resection of the Roux limb, on the assumption that this would also reverse the nesidioblastosis [39, 40].

Reversal of the gastric bypass does not ensure the resolution of pancreatogenous hypoglycemia [44–46]. Weight regain occurred in 4 of 11 patients.

At least in one case, there was almost complete weight regain. Two patients had pancreatic resection after reversal, both with a nesidioblastosis diagnosis, identified in the specimen.

In the largest series of nine patients, one had gastroesophageal reflux [40], two developed diarrhea, and one developed anastomotic stricture, which was endoscopically dilated.

Histologically, nesidioblastosis could not be evaluated, as resection was not made. Long-term data are lacking, and it is unclear whether these promising results are durable.

Pancreatic resection: distal, subtotal, and total pancreatectomies have been indicated for hypoglycemia after RYGB. Distal pancreatectomy, with or without splenectomy, was the most common finding in PubMed search.

Among the 51 (68%) patients identified, 6 (12%) were reoperated with extended resections due to recurrent or persistent hypoglycemia.

Three (6%) patients ended up with total pancreatectomy [43]. Two had RYGB reversal, and in one case pouch restriction was done, prior to pancreatic resection [42, 44, 47]. Two patients had concomitant banding of the gastric pouch [42].

In total, 34 of 51 (67%) patients had resolution of hypoglycemic symptoms after one or more pancreatic resections. In the group of 17 patients with persistent symptoms, 8 cases were classified as recurrent or ongoing symptoms, 5 as having occasional symptoms, 2 as frequent symptoms, 1 case had a good response to octreotide treatment, and 1 underwent RYGB reversal with minimal improvement of symptoms.

The duration of follow-up was short in most of the series [42, 44, 46–54]. Diabetes status was unknown in most of the patients.

Nesidioblastosis was confirmed from specimens in 47 patients. Subtotal pancreatic resection may not be the optimal treatment for hypoglycemia after RYGB in all patients, considering that the underlying cause for hyperinsulinemia may persist [55]. The adequate extent of resection is not defined, and symptoms may persist or recur.

Gastrostomy tube placement, the addition of restriction, or reversal of the RYGB have all been used as alternatives, with undefined effects in the long term. Partial pancreatectomy indications must be in exceptional cases.

Patients should be informed about the incomplete knowledge of post-RYGB hypoglycemia and the variability in treatment options, and outcomes should be reported.

References

1. Shantavasinkul PC, Torquati A, Corsino L. Post-gastric bypass hypoglycaemia: a review. Clin Endocrinol (Oxf). 2016;85:3–9.
2. Rariy CM, Rometo D, Korytkowski M. Post-gastric bypass hypoglycemia. Curr Diab Rep. 2016;16:19.
3. Marsk R, Jonas E, Rasmussen F, Naslund E. Nationwide cohort study of post-gastric bypass hypoglycaemia including 5,040 patients undergoing surgery for obesity in 1986–2006 in Sweden. Diabetologia. 2010;53:2307–11.
4. Kellogg TA, Bantle JP, Leslie DB, Redmond JB, Slusarek B, Swan T, et al. Postgastric bypass hyperinsulinemic hypoglycemia syndrome: characterization and response to a modified diet. Surg Obes Relat Dis. 2008;4:492–9.
5. Bueter M, Ashrafian H, le Roux CW. Mechanisms of weight loss after gastric by-pass and gastric banding. Obes Facts. 2009;2:325–31.
6. le Roux CW, Welbourn R, Werling M, et al. Gut hormones as mediators os appetite and weight loss after Roux-en-Y gastric by-pass. Ann Surg. 2007;246:780–5.
7. Schultes B, Ernst B, Wilms B, Thurnheer M, Hallschmid M. Hedonic hunger is increased in severely obese patients and is reduced after gastric by-pass surgery. Am J Clin Nutr. 2012;92:277–83.
8. Miras AD, le Roux CW. Bariatric surgery and taste: novel mechanisms of weight loss. Curr Opin Gastroenterol. 2010;26:140–5.
9. Tack J, Caenepeel P, De Wulf D, Bisschops R. Pathophysiology, diagnosis and management of postoperative dumping syndrome. Nat Rev Gastroenterol Hepatol. 2009;6:583–90.
10. Laurenius A, Werling M, le Roux CW, Fandriks L, Olbers T. More symptoms but similar blood glucose curve after oral carbohydrate provocation in patients with a history of hypoglycemia-like symptoms compared to asymptomatic patients after Roux-en-Y gastric by-pass. Surg Obes Relat Dis. 2014;10:1047–55.
11. Crapo PA, Scarlett JA, Kolterman OG, Sabders LR, Hofeldt FD, Olefsky JM. The effects of oral fructose, sucrose, and glucose in subjects with reactive hypoglycemia. Diabetes Care. 1982;5:512–7.
12. Zagury L, Moreira RO, Guedes EP, Coutinho WF, Appolinario JC. Insulinoma misdiagnosed as dumping syndrome after bariatric surgery. Obes Surg. 2004;14:120–3.
13. Harness JK, Geelhoed GW, Thompson NW, et al. Nesidioblastosis in adults. Arch Surg. 1981;116:575–80.
14. Service GJ, Thompson GB, Service JF, Andrews JC, Collazo-Clavell ML, Lloyd RV. Hyperinsulinemic hypoglycemia with nesidioblastosis after gastric bypass surgery. N Engl J Med. 2005;353:249–54.
15. Z'graggen K, Guwweidhi A, Steffen R, et al. Severe recurrent hypoglycemia after gastric by-pass surgery. Obes Surg. 2008;18:981–8.
16. Holst JJ. Glucagonlike peptide 1: a newly discovered gastrointestinal hormone. Gastroenterology. 1994;107:1848–55.
17. Goldfine AB, Mun EC, Devine E, et al. Patients with neuroglycopenia after gastric by-pass surgery have exaggerated incretin and insulin secretory responses to a mixed meal. J Clin Endocrinol Metab. 2007;92:4678–85.
18. Rabiee A, Magruder JT, Salas-Carrillo R, et al. Hyperinsulinemic hypoglycemia after Roux-en-Y gastric by-pass: unraveling the role of gut hormonal

and pancreatic endocrine dysfunction. J Surg Res. 2011;167:199–205.
19. Patti M, Goldfine AB. Hypoglycemia after gastric by-pass: the dark side of GLP-1. Gastroenterology. 2014;146:605–08. J Surg Res. 2011;167:199–205.
20. Meier JJ, Butler AE, Galasso R, Butler PC. Hyperinsulinemic hypoglycemia after gastric bypass surgery is not accompanied by islet hyperplasia or increased beta cell turnover. Diabetes Care. 2006;29:1554–9.
21. Butler PC, Meier JJ, Butler AE, Bhusshan A. The replication of beta cells in normal physiology, in disease and for therapy. Nat Clin Pract Endocrinol Metab. 2007;3:758–68.
22. Kamvissi V, Salerno A, Bornstein SR, Mingrone G, Rubino F. Incretins or -incretins? A new model for the ëntero-pancreatic axis. Horm Metab Res. 2015;47:84–7.
23. Tack J, Arts J, Caenepeel P, De Wulf D, Bisschops R. Pathophysiology, diagnosis and management of postoperative dumping syndrome. Nat Rev Gastroenterol Hepatol. 2009;6:583–56.
24. Cryer PE, Axelrod L, Grossman AB, et al. Evaluation and management of adult hypoglycemic disorders: an Endocrine Society clinical practice guideline. J Clin Endocrinol Metab. 2009;94:709–28.
25. Vezzosi D, Bennet A, Fauvel J, Caron P. Insulin, C-peptide and proinsulin for the biochemical diagnosis of hypoglycemia related to endogenous hyperinsulinism. Eur J Endocrinol. 2007;157:75–83.
26. Malik S, Mitchell JE, Steffen K, Engel S, Wiisanen R, Garcia L, et al. Recognition and management of hyperinsulinemic hypoglycemia after bariatric surgery. Obes Res Clin Pract. 2016;10:1–14.
27. Service FJ, Natt N, Thompson GB, et al. Noninsulinoma pancreatogenous hypoglycemia in adults independent of mutations in Kir6.2 and SURI genes. J Clin Endocrinol Metab. 1999;84:1582–9.
28. Bantle JP, Ilkramuddin S, Kellogg TA, Buchwald H. Hyperinsulinemic hypoglycemia developing later after gastric by-pass. Obes Surg. 2007;17:592–4.
29. Botros N, Rijnaarts I, Brandts H, Bleumink G, Janssen I, de Boer H. Effect of carbohydrate restriction in patients with hyperinsulinemic hypoglycemia after Roux-en Y gastric by-pass. Obes Surg. 2014;10:36–43.
30. Ritz P, Vaurs C, Bertrand M, Andruze Y, Guillaume E, Hanaire H. Usefulness of acarbose and dietery modifications to limit glycemic variability following Roux-en-Y gastric by-pass as assessed by continuous glucose monitoring. Diabetes Technol Ther. 2012;14:736–40.
31. Frankhouser SY, Ahmad AN, Peilli GA, Quintana BJ, Vengrove MA. Post-gastric-bypass hypoglycemia successfully treated with alpha-glucosidase inhibitor therapy. Endocr Pract. 2013;19:511–4.
32. Guseva N, Phillips D, Mordes JP. Successful treatment of persistent hyperinsulinemic hypoglycemia with nifedipine in an adult patient. Endocr Pract. 2010;16:107–11.
33. Spanakis E, Gragnoli C. Successful medical management of status post-Roux-en-Y-gastric bypass hyperinsulinemic hypoglycemia. Obes Surg. 2009;19:1333–4.
34. Salehi M, Progeon RL, D'Alessio DA. Gastric by-pass surgery enhances glucagon-like peptide 1-stimulated postprandial insulin secretion in humans. Diabetes. 2011;60:2308–14.
35. Salehi M, Gastaldelli A, D'Alessio DA. Altered islet function and insulin clearance cause hyperinsulinemia in gastric by-pass patients with symptoms of postprandial hypoglycemia. J Clin Endocrinol Metab. 2014;99:2008–17.
36. Salehi M, Gastaldelli A, D'Alessio DA. Blockade of glucagon-like peptide1 receptor corrects postprandial hypoglycemia after gastric by-pass. Gastroenterology. 2014;146:669–80.e2.
37. Didden P, Penning C, Masclee AA. Octreotide therapy in dumping syndrome: analysis of long term results. Aliment Pharmacol Ther. 2006;24:1367–75.
38. Cui Y, Elahi D, Anderson DK. Advances in the etiology and management of hyperinsulinemic hypoglycemia after Roux-en-Y gastric by-pass. J Gastrointest Surg. 2011;15:1879–88.
39. Campos GM, Ziemelis M, Paparodis R, Ahmed M, Davis DB. Laparoscopic reversal of Roux-en-Y gastric by-pass: technique and utility for treatment of endocrine complications. Surg Obes Relat Dis. 2014;10:36–43.
40. Vilallonga R, van de Vrande S, Himpens J. Laparoscopic reversal of Roux-en-Y gastric by-pass into normal anatomy with or without sleeve gastrectomy. Surg Endosc. 2013;27:4640–8.
41. de Heide LJ, Glaudemans AW, Oomen PH, Apers JA, Totté ER, van Beek AP. Functional imaging in hyperinsulinemic hypoglycemia after gastric bypass surgery for morbid obesity. J Clin Endroninol Metab. 2012;97:E963–7.
42. Z'graggen K, Guweidhi A, Steffen R, et al. Severe recurrent hypoglycemia after gastric by-pass surgery. Obes Surg. 2008;18:981–8.
43. Mala T. Postprandialhyperinsulinemic hypoglycemia after gastric by-pass surgical treatment. Surg Obes Relat Dis. 2014;10:1220–5.
44. Clancy TE, Moore FD Jr, Zimer MJ. Post-gastric by-pass hyperinsulinism with nesidioblastosis: subtotal or total pancreatectomy may be needed to prevent recurrent hypoglicemia. J Gastrointest Surg. 2006;10:1116–9.
45. Dapri G, Cadiere GB, Himpens J. Laparoscopic reconversion of Roux-en-Y gastric by-pass to original anatomy: technique and preliminary outcomes. Obes Surg. 2011;21:1289–95.
46. Lee CJ, Brown T, Magnuson TH, Egan JM, Carlson O, Elahi D. Hormonal response to a mixed-meal challenge after reversal of gastric by-pass for hypoglycemia. J Clin Endocrinol Metab. 2013;98:E1208–12.
47. Patti ME, McMahon G, Mun EC, et al. Severe hypoglycemia post-gastric by-pass requiring partial pancreatectomy: evidence for inappropriate

insulin secretion and pancreatic islet hyperplasia. Diabetologia. 2005;48:2236–40.

48. Ceppa EP, Ceppa DP, Omotosho PA, Dickerson JA 2nd, Park CW. Algorithm to diagnose etiology of hypoglycaemia after Roux-en-Y gastric by-pass for morbid obesity: case series and review of the literature. Surg Obes Relat Dis. 2012;8:641–7.
49. Qintar M, Sibai F, Taha M. Hypoglycemia due to an adult-onset nesidioblastosis, a diagnostic and management dilemma. Avicenna J Med. 2012;2:45–7.
50. Rabiee A, Magruder JT, Salas-Carrillo R, et al. Hyperinsulinemic hypoglycemia after Roux-en-Y gastric bypass: unraveling the role of the gut hormonal and pancreatic endocrine function. J Surg Res. 2011;167:199–205.
51. Alvarez GC, Faria EN, Beck M, Girardon DT, Machado AC. Laparoscopic spleen-reserving distal pancreatectomy as treatment for nesidioblastosis after gastric by-pass surgery. Obes Surg. 2007;17:550–2.
52. Barbour JR, Thomas BN, Morgan KA, Byrne TK, Adams DB. The practice of pancreatic resection after Roux-en-Y gastric by-pass. Am Surg. 2008;74:729–34.
53. Mathavan VK, Arregui M, Davis C, Singh K, Patel A, Meacham J. Management of postgastric by-pass noninsulinoma pancreatogenous hypoglycemia. Surg Endosc. 2010;24:2547–55.
54. Rumilla KM, Erickson LA, Service FJ, et al. Hyperinsulinemic hypoglycemia with nesidioblastosis: histological features and growth factor expression. Mod Pathol. 2009;22:239–45.
55. Ritz P, Hanaire H. Post-bypass hypoglycemia: a review of current findings. Diabetes Metab. 2011;37:274–81.

Dumping Syndrome

36

Christine Stier, Koschker Ann-Cathrin, and Sonja Chiappetta

Dumping syndrome is since long time well known as a postoperative complication of gastric surgery procedures. Due to increasing numbers of gastric surgery procedures resulting from bariatric surgery, the incidence of the dumping syndrome is on a dramatic rise and therefore has found back into the spotlight of therapeutical interest.

A Brief Historical Retrospection

Most likely the first publication regarding the topic in English language originates from 1913 and was written by A. Hertz [1]. It dealt with a symptom complex that may occur after gastric surgery the "post-gastrectomy-syndrome". The term "dumping syndrome" itself was created and therefore descends from C. Mix [2], who published an article in 1922 about the "dumping stomach following gastroenterostomy". Back then, "Dumping" described the assumed underlying reason of this syndrome – a speeded influx of chyme into the anastomosed jejunum. As early as 1935, dumping syndrome finds its way into the *Textbook of Gastroenterology* by Eusterman and Belfort, who described its occurrence after simple gastroenterostomy procedures as well as post-gastric resection [3]. They however stated that the dumping syndrome is as rare as barely deserves mention after a well-indicated and properly performed gastroenterostomy [3]. They already attributed its occurrence to the distension of the upper jejunum. Likewise, A. Snell [4] wrote in 1937 that it was found to be a rare complication and reported of just a "few cases". He stated the jejunum would most likely adapt and the symptoms would tend to disappear. In 1940, C. Glaessner [5] published nine cases. He attributed a "hyperglycaemic shock" as cause for the dumping syndrome relating to sudden increase of blood sugar as a direct result of rapid resorption in the jejunum. Schwartz [6] and his study group further investigated this theory, but could not find any correlation between glucose levels and appearing symptoms. They insisted, the underlying explanation must be due to the distention of the upper jejunum [5]. Firstly, they recommended frequent small meals as conservative therapy approach to improving symptoms. In 1941, Jordan [7] published in the JAMA that a quarter of all cases with unsatisfactory results of post partial gastrectomy account to anastomotic ulcer as well as dumping syndrome. In the printed discussion of Jordan's article by Mateer [8], he rated the incidence of the post-operative dumping syndrome to be as high as 14%.

C. Stier (✉)
Department of Surgical Endoscopy and Endocrinology, University Hospital Wuerzburg, Wuerzburg, Germany

K. Ann-Cathrin
Department of Endocrinology, University Hospital Wuerzburg, Wuerzburg, Germany

S. Chiappetta
Ospedale Evangelico Betania, Naples, Italy

J. Ettinger et al. (eds.), *Gastric Bypass*, https://doi.org/10.1007/978-3-030-28803-7_36

Thereupon, Custer [9] and his colleagues from the Mayo Clinic investigated 612 patients after subtotal gastrectomy and detected the post-gastrectomy dumping syndrome. A cohort of 500 patients represented group A. Retrospectively, they found an incidence of dumping syndrome in 5.6% of the cases. They categorized those patients according to the severity of their symptoms into three groups, from mild to severe to disabling. Subsequently, a second cohort of 112 patients, all operated by a single surgeon, were analysed prospectively. With particular focus on the dumping syndrome, the follow-up of group B revealed a considerable increased incidence of 12.5%. The Mayo studying group around Custer found that with tightening the diameter of the anastomosis, the syndrome could be influenced and recognized that with redo procedures an improvement or even the resolve the symptoms appears achievable. It was in 1970 that H. Sigstad developed and published a numeric scoring system for the evaluation of symptoms, which supports the establishment of the diagnosis of a dumping syndrome. The so-called Sigstad dumping score [10] still is implemented today and is a valuable and accepted diagnostic tool.

Current State of Knowledge

The dumping syndrome is a set of complex of symptoms, caused by accelerated gastric emptying of undigested chyme into the small bowel. It shows a wide range in the severity of its symptoms, from mild gastrointestinal discomfort, moderate vasomotor disturbance to severe hyperinsulinemic hypoglycaemia.

This is the valid definition of the dumping syndrome as we know it today, which shows that so far only marginal new insights into the pathophysiology of this phenomenon exist compared to the first half of the last century.

Other than the abovementioned early experiences with the post-gastrectomy syndrome, which was named "dumping syndrome" in 1922, today there is a classification into two different entities, based on the cause and timely appearance of the symptoms: the "early" and the "late" dumping syndrome. Due to the increasing number of bariatric surgery procedures being performed worldwide, it seems that bariatric surgery is the leading cause of the dumping syndrome [11]. The prevalence ranges from as high as 75% after proximal Roux-en-Y gastric bypass [11–17] to 33–45% after sleeve gastrectomy [19–21]. In clinical practice, however, symptoms vary greatly in severity. Due to the wide spectrum of the resulting impairment, therapy is not required in all cases.

Early Dumping Syndrome

Early dumping occurs within 30 minutes after ingestion. The underlying pathophysiology is fundamentally different from that of the late dumping. The union of both entities as the "dumping syndrome" originates from the preceding and triggering circumstance of previous gastric surgery. "Early dumping" as well as "late dumping" may occur as separate and stand-alone clinical picture, however, mixed disease patterns of both entities may also occur.

One of the functions of the stomach is that of a reservoir. Food is mixed and blended with gastric secretion, thereby initiating digestion through acid denaturation and enzymatic hydrolysis of proteins. Just as important is the allocation function of the pylorus. Chyme is delivered in small amounts to the duodenum. The remaining gastric content is forced back into the corpus of the stomach for further mixing. Thus, the amount of food reaching the intestine is constantly regulated. After a mixed meal, the regular emptying takes 3–4 hours. After alteration of the anatomy by creating a gastroenterostomy, this active allocation function of the pylorus is lost. Subsequently, exclusively the diameter and the thereby provided resistance of the gastroenterostomy determine gastric emptying. If the gastric emptying time shortens to just a few minutes as the anastomosis enlarges with time, chyme may "dump" into the small bowel. This "speedup influx" of hyperosmolar chyme may cause extensive bowel distention and therefore an intestinal volume shift. Hypersecretion of gastrointestinal hormones and autonomic dysregulation trigger this volume shift, which leads to symptoms of early dumping. Although these symptoms are nonspecific, they can basically be divided into systemic and abdominal manifestations. Abdominal symptoms include pain, gas bloat, fullness and an early satiety, borborygmi and diarrhoea. Very typical is the imperative desire to lie down after a meal. Systemic symptoms affect the circulation with tachycardia, palpitations, flushing, hypotension and sweating and may peak in a syncope.

Late Dumping Syndrome

Late dumping symptoms occur 1–3 hours after nutritional intake and are attributed to a reactive hyperinsulinemic hypoglycaemia. With an oral glucose tolerance test (OGTT) in 75% of the patients after proximal Roux-en-Y gastric bypass, symptoms of late dumping syndrome may be provoked. In clinical practice, however, the manifestations vary extremely in severity. As early as 1940, Glaessner reported an imbalance of the glucose metabolism as the cause of the dumping syndrome [6]. At that time, his theory was generally rejected. Other investigators did not retrace the relation between blood sugar and resulting symptoms. Today the pathogenesis of late dumping is still unclear: It has been suggested that the quicker influx of undigested carbohydrates into the small bowel leads to rapid absorption and therefore causes high blood sugar levels that cause an exagerrated insulin response. Retrospectively, Glaessner's theory on the pathophysiology of late dumping must be confirmed at least for the most parts. Further, this flood of glucose seems to trigger a surge in incretin secretion, thus additionally inducing a further insulin secretion. Consequently, blood glucose falls to hypoglycaemic levels [22–25] at times to the point of loss of consciousness or even cerebral cramps in extreme cases. Symptoms include perspiration, palpitations, hunger, weakness, confusion, tremor and syncope. The hypoglycaemia-induced graving for sweets explains at least in parts the often observable weight regain in bariatric patients with late dumping syndrome.

Interestingly, the symptoms do not occur immediately after surgery, but appear mostly after a few years. In our overall collective of patients suffering from late dumping syndrome over the last 2 years (n = 88), the time elapse from primary surgery to appearance of symptoms is 50.15 ± 26.77 (range 15–106) months. Again, this timely inhomogeneity represents the wide spectrum of this entity (Table 36.1).

Table 36.1 Symptoms of the dumping syndrome

Early dumping		Late dumping
Vaso-motorical disturbances	Vasovagal disturbances	Hyperinsulinemic hypoglycaemia
Gastrointestinal symptoms	Systemic symptoms	Perspiration
Abdominal pain, cramps	Desire to lie down after a meal	Hunger
Gas bloat	Tachycardia	Weakness
Early satiety; feeling full	Palpitations	Confusion
Borborygmi	Hypotension	Tremor
Diarrhoea	Perspiration; flushing	Syncope

Diagnosis

Sigstad Dumping Score [10]

The "Sigstad Score" is an important and evaluated diagnostic tool. Patients have to answer 16 questions about their present symptoms. Each symptom has a numeric rating, which is calculated as score at the end. A dumping syndrome is likely if the score is above 7, and very unlikely if it is below 4 (Table 36.2).

Oral Glucose Tolerance Testing (OGTT)

In the here pesented own results the OGTT is performed with 75 g of glucose. Within the last 2 years we have discovered 72 patients with resulting hypoglycaemia during OGTT out of 88 patients with a previous elevated Sigstad Score (87.8%). Serum insulin was measured simulanteously with the glucose samples at 0, 30, 60, 90, 120, 150 and 180 minutes. After oral glucose challege, hypoglycaemia had occurred mostly between 90 and 180 minutes and often lasted more than 30 minutes, so that individual patients might have presented with more than one documented hypoglycaemic value during

Table 36.2 Numeric rating with the Sigstadt score

Symptoms	Numeric rating
Shock	+5
Fainting, syncope, unconsciousness	+4
Desire to lie or sit down	+4
Breathlessness, dyspnoea	+3
Weakness, exhaustion	+3
Sleepiness, drowsiness, apathy, falling asleep	+3
Palpitation	+3
Restlessness	+2
Dizziness	+2
Headaches	+1
Feeling of warmth, sweating, pallor, clammy skin	+1
Nausea	+1
Abdominal fullness, meteorism	+1
Borborygmus	+1
Eructation	−1
Vomiting	−4

measurement. (n=35 at 90 minutes/n=42 at 120 minutes). A peak was observable at 120 minutes. With a lower frequency hypoglycaemia did not occur until after 150 or 180 minutes (n=19 at 150 minutes/n=12 at 180 minutes). Prior to OGTT, the HOMA-IR (homeostatic model assessment), which (HOMA-IR) is a marker of insulin resistance was determined in all patients [26–28]. The medium value was 1.23 ± 0.61 (range 0.3–2.9). This demonstrated that an obscure insulin resistance does not appear to cause the resulting exaggerated insulin output after oral carbohydrate intake. Only 9 patients showed a HOMA-IR above 2.0 (12.5%), whereas in 32 patients, the HOMA-IR was ≤1.0 (44.45%). Almost none of the patients had diabetes before the bariatric surgery (6/88).

HOMA-IR Valuation (According to the Local Lab) (Table 36.3)

- HOMA-IR = insulin (fasting insulin, μU/ml) × blood glucose (fasting glucose, mg/dl)/405 or
- HOMA-IR = insulin (fasting insulin, μU/ml) × blood glucose (fasting glucose, mmol/l)/22.5

Table 36.3 Valuation of HOMA-IR

Stage	HOMA-IR	Conclusion
1	<2	Insulin resistance unlikely
2	2.0–2.5	Clue to insulin resistance
3	2.5–5.0	Very likely insulin resistance
4	>5.0	Average value in diabetic individuals

Medium fasting glucose was 79.03 ± 6.56 mg/dl and therefore represents a value in regular ranges. According to the AWMF guidelines, the 120 minutes value is crucial in determining the diagnosis of diabetes. In case this value is above 140 mg/dl, there is a suspicion of diabetes. In the collective shown, the average value after 120 minutes was 47.63 ± 19.03 (range 14–113) mg/dl, and non of the individual values was in diabetic ranges. Medium fasting insulin was 6.91 ± 4.14 μU/ml (norm range: 5–30 μU/ml). From this normal level insulin exaggerated to a medium of 144.23 ± 101.55 (range 17.76–430.2) μU/ml after 30 minutes and 174.71 ± 147.86 (range 19.65–635.3) μU/ml after 60 minutes. An insulin value above 100 μU/ml was classified hyperinsulinaemic. After 30 minutes 43 patients showed elevated insulin values, and after 60 minutes 47 patients were hyperinsulinemic, whereas after 90 minutes only 10 of 72 insulin values were above 100 μU/ml (Fig. 36.1). The evaluation of this case series shows that diabetes seems not to play a role in the development of hyperinsulinaemia and the late dumping syndrome.

Continuous Glucose Monitoring (CGM)

The CGM continuously measures and displays interstitial glucose levels over several days under "real-life" conditions. It has been shown to be a useful tool for the establishment of diagnosis and the management of exceptional glycaemic fluctuations in patients with diabetes and diabetic comorbidities, as well as in patients with blood sugar abnormalities after gastric and bariatric surgery. CGM reveals hypoglycaemic episodes in real-time and can also be used to monitor treatment success [29–33]. Firstly in 2010, Hanaire et al. described the

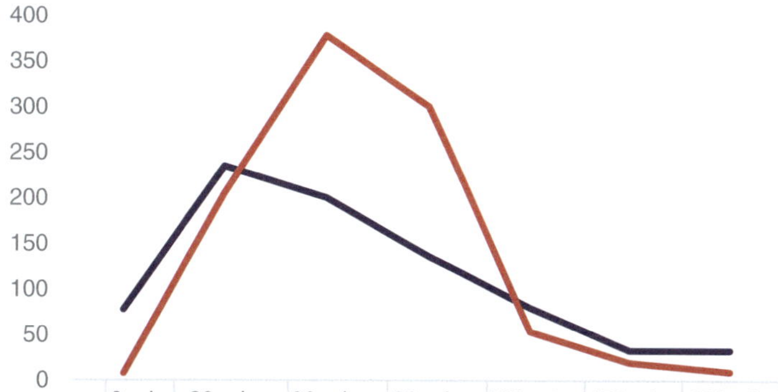

	0 min	30 min	60 min	90 min	120 min	150 min	180 min
Glucose	78	235	200	136	80	33	33
Insulin µU/ml	7.49	205.5	378.1	300.5	53.51	19.64	9.57

Fig. 36.1 Graph of an OGTT, demonstrating late dumping syndrome: female patient, 50 years, Roux-en-Y gastric bypass (RYGB) 2012, became symptomatic with late dumping since 2 months (03/16). If projected one over the other, the insulin curve is crossing and overshots the glucose curve. This seems to be characteristic for late dumping syndrome

use of the CGM to diagnose a hypoglycaemia originating from a late dumping syndrome after bariatric surgery, which was not detectable during a 72-hour fasting test [34]. As postprandial glycaemic fluctuations occure rapid and show large deviations, they can go undetected, if blood glucose is not measured during the episode itself [34]. Halperin et al. reported a 90% sensitivity and 50% specificity of CGM for the detection of clinically significant hypoglycaemia, compared to 33% sensitivity and 40% specificity for mixed meal tolerance test (MMTT), proved in ten patients with a history of post-gastric bypass neuroglycopenia [35]. CGM is also a valuable diagnostic test not only for symptomatic hypoglycaemic patients, but also for the identification of those patients who remain asymptomatic at low glucose levels. Vidal et al. reported that 12.5% of asymptomatic patients on CGM had hypoglycaemia (glucose <50 mg/dl) [36]. Additionally, Hanaire et al. revealed important pathophysiological mechanisms with CGM: The time to the postprandial peak of maximal interstitial glucose (IG) was significantly shorter in operated patients (42.8 ± 6.0 min) than in diabetic controls (82.2 ± 11.1 min, $P = 0.0002$), as were the rates of glucose increase to the peak (2.4 ± 1.6 vs. 1.2 ± 0.3 mg/mL/min; $P = 0.041$). True hypoglycaemia (glucose <60 mg/dL) was rare in this trial: the symptoms were probably more related to the speed of IG decrease than to the glucose level achieved [37]. Nielsen et al. reported that CGM was a valuable method for demonstrating increased glycaemic variability among 13 Roux-en-Y gastric bypass individuals, and for displaying the resulting dietary effects on reducing this glycaemic variability, including real hypoglycaemic events. In RYGB individuals, CGM-measured interstitial fluid glucose (IGF) overestimated the real glucose value by about 1 mmol/l in the hypoglycaemic range. This should be taken into consideration if CGM is used to diagnose hypoglycaemia after RYGB [31].

In the collective presented here, the CGM was useful to identify those patients who had an pathological altered OGTT and were in need of a further treatment. During the 7-day CGM measurement, 59 of these patients showed a treatment-requiring hypoglycemia.

Mixed Meal Tolerance Test (MMTT)

In 1982, Buss et al. reasoned that the OGTT has its limitations for the diagnosis of reactive hypoglycaemia. They stated that except under the conditions of an OGTT, a pure nutritional carbohydrate intake is rare [38]. The MMTT is the gold standard in paediatrics to measure the residual insulin production in patients with type 1 diabetes mellitus. However, a full MMTT is predominantly used in research and rarely performed in routine clinical practice, due to the intensity of sampling [39]. The question was and still is, whether the MMTT provides a more realistic clinical picture of the risk of post-surgery hypoglycaemia than the OGTT, which may overestimate the hypoglycaemic reaction during examination. The answer came last year from an Austrian working group that compared results of the MMTT with the CGM [40]. It

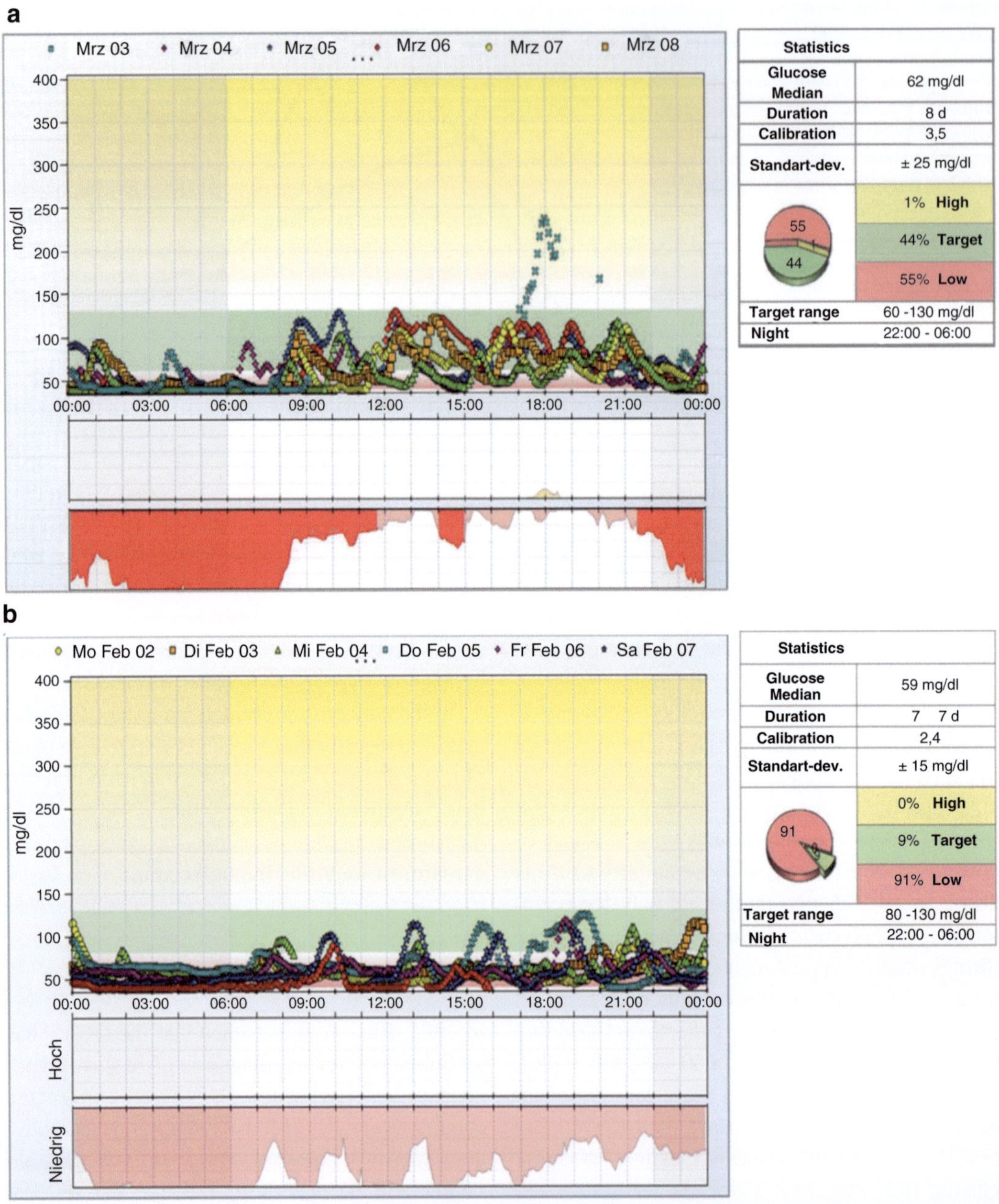

Fig. 36.2 (**a**) CGM, which pictures a late dumping syndrome with 55% of the values in hypoglycaemic levels: same female patient as demonstrated above, 50 years, RYGB 2012, became symptomatic with late dumping since 2 months (03/16). (**b**) CGM of a late dumping syndrome with 91% of hypoglycaemic values: female patient, 45 years, RYGB 2013, became symptomatic with late dumping since 9 months (11/15), fainted frequently

has been shown that the CGM can reliably and significantly detect more hypoglycemic episodes than MMTT, even without oral stimulation or a carbohydrate challange. This working group stated that assessed under real-life conditions, post-RYGB hypoglycaemia was found more frequently than expected by CGM. The CGM revealed hypoglycaemic episodes in a staggering 75% of the patients, while MMTT had a much lower detection rate of only 29% [40]. CGM also detected nocturnal hypoglycaemic episodes in 15 (38%) of the patients. Consistend with this are Halperin et al. findings, which demonstrated a very low sensitivity of 33% and low specificity of 40% for the MMTT [35]. This clarified that a MMTT definetily and significantly underestimates the presence of hypoglycaemia, although there is a monitored oral nutrition intake during examination.

Scintigraphy

In comparison to gastric emptying of the physiological stomach, pouch-emptying scintigraphy has no defined clearing rates yet. With our interventional group a pouch-emptying scintigraphy was implemented prior to the invasive revision of the gastroenterostomy. A correlation between the rapid pouch emptying within a few minutes and the symptoms of dumping could be demonstrated. For this examination, a semisolid test meal, enriched with Tc99, was used. This examination was performed not only prior to sheduled revisional surgery, but as well as 4 weeks after the surgical or endoluminal revision of the anastomosis to objectify a post-interventional delay of the influx into the alimentary limb. So far these data have not yet been published (Fig. 36.3).

Differential Diagnosis

Since dumping syndrome is a well-known complication after gastric surgery, the diagnostic approach must still exclude other causes for the abovementioned symptoms. Especially in the case of late dumping syndrome with recurrent hypoglycaemia, differential diagnosis includes carcinoid syndrome, VIPoma and insulinoma. In suspected carcinoid syndrome, an initial test is the 24-hour urine levels of 5-hydroxyindoleacetic acid. Further MR imaging of the pancreas and evaluation of serum chromogranin A is mandatory to exclude insulinoma.

Cardiovascular disease, diabetes mellitus, vitamin deficiency and neurological disease may be other causes for tachycardia, dizziness or syncope, which may also occur in early dumping. Gastrointestinal differential diagnosis include abnormal contractions of the duct (tract spasms), afferent loop syndromes, bowel obstruction, lactose intolerance, celiac disease, gastroenteric fistula, bacterial or viral colitis and inflammatory bowel disease, pancreatic insufficiency (steatorrhea) and small intestinal bacterial overgrowth.

Therapy

Since current data offer little scientific evidence for existing therapeutic algorithms, there is no established consensus for these guidelines yet.

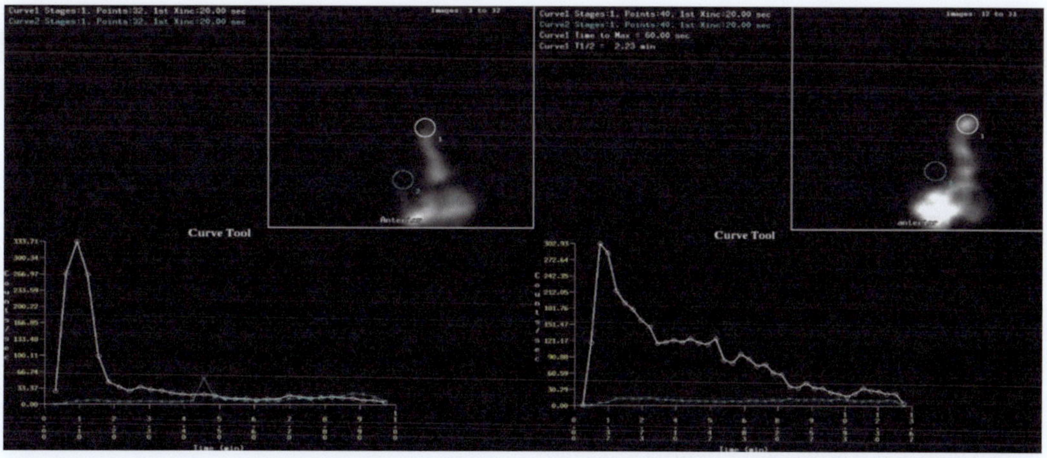

Fig. 36.3 Scintigraphy of the pouch emptying. Male patient, 32 years, RYGB 5/07, suffering from dumping since 8 months, pouch emptying prior and after endoluminal revision of the dilated pouch outlet. The scintigraphy showed a decelerated pouch emptying after intervention. Post-interventional, the patient was free of symptoms

Nutritional Amendment

Currently, a gradual conservative therapy is recommended. Diet changes should be made towards more frequent meals, with reduced carbohydrates and increased protein and fiber content [25, 41]. Patients are advised to eat smaller dishes up to six times per day. Food and drink must be strictly seperated to avoid fast washing out of the food from the pouch toward the small bowel. A further general recommendation is the use of viscous food additives to increase consistency of the nutrition, such as psyllium, guar gum or pectin. This may additionally delay gastric emptying. If dietary measures prove unsuccessful, drug therapy should be initiated.

Drug Therapy

Acarbose

Acarbose, an alpha-glucosidase inhibitor, that diminishes the indigestion and resorption of carbohydrates and is therefore actully the first step treatment of choice in late dumping syndrome [42–44]. Its efficacy in hyperinsulinemic hypoglycaemia has been confirmed in several studies. The downside of this drug remains the occurrence of troublesome and hampering side effects, some of which can lead to extensive flatulence and diarrhoea, due to the maldigestion of carbohydrates. The permanent use of this drug mostly requires supernatural adherence of the patients.

Calcium Antagonists

The effect of calcium antagonists such as verapamil has been proven in patients with insulinoma and could be a treatment option in late dumping syndrome [43].

Potassium Channel Activator

Another possible treatment option could be the potassium channel activator diazoxide [45, 46]. Diazoxide activates adenosine triphosphate (ATP)-sensitive potassium channels (KATP channel) in the pancreatic beta cells, which results in the inhibition of the calcium-dependent insulin release. It is used in hypoglycaemic states of diverse aetiologies, including islet cell tumours and glycogen storage disorders. As well as that, it is also an important therapeutic modality in malignant and metastatic insulinoma, in non-localizable tumours, when surgery is out of option. Thondam et al. described the effectiveness of diazoxide in three patients [45]. Other case reports can be found [46].

Somatostatin Analogs

Somatostatin analogs [47–50] are applied as treatment option of choice for severe early and late dumping syndrome. It is known, when administered to delay gastric emptying, to extend bowel transit, to diminish postprandial vasodilatation as well as to reduce the release of peptide hormones such as insulin. The short-acting drug octreotide is well known in its use after pancreatic surgery and can be used for the treatment of late dumping sndrome as well. With its half-life of 2–3 hours, it has to be administered subcutaneously 3–4 times a day (50–100 μg). Long-acting somatostatin analogs, such as pasireotide (half-life 11 h), may be more promising and lead to a better adherence of the patients [51]. Mild side effects of somatostatin analogs include pain, redness, and swelling at the injection site. Major side effects are fast, slow or irregular heartbeat, fruit-like breath odour, muscle cramps and stiffness, and in 10–50% development of gallstones.

GLP-1 Analogs

Due to treatment failure and side effects of currently used drugs, Abrahamson et al. already published a novel treatment option of postprandial hypoglycaemia following RYGB with glucagon-like peptide 1 (GLP-1) analogs and reported a protective effect of GLP-1 analogs on pronounced symptoms of postprandial hypoglycaemic episodes in five patients [52]. We have used GLP-1 analogs for the last 2 years in patients with confirmed late dumping syndrome instead of octreotide, with amazing success. 60–70% of patients improved significantly or were even completely free of symptoms after application. Figure 36.4 a, b: CGM prior, and with GLP-1therapy).

Surgical Therapy

For patients who do not respomd to diet or drug therapy, surgery should be considered.

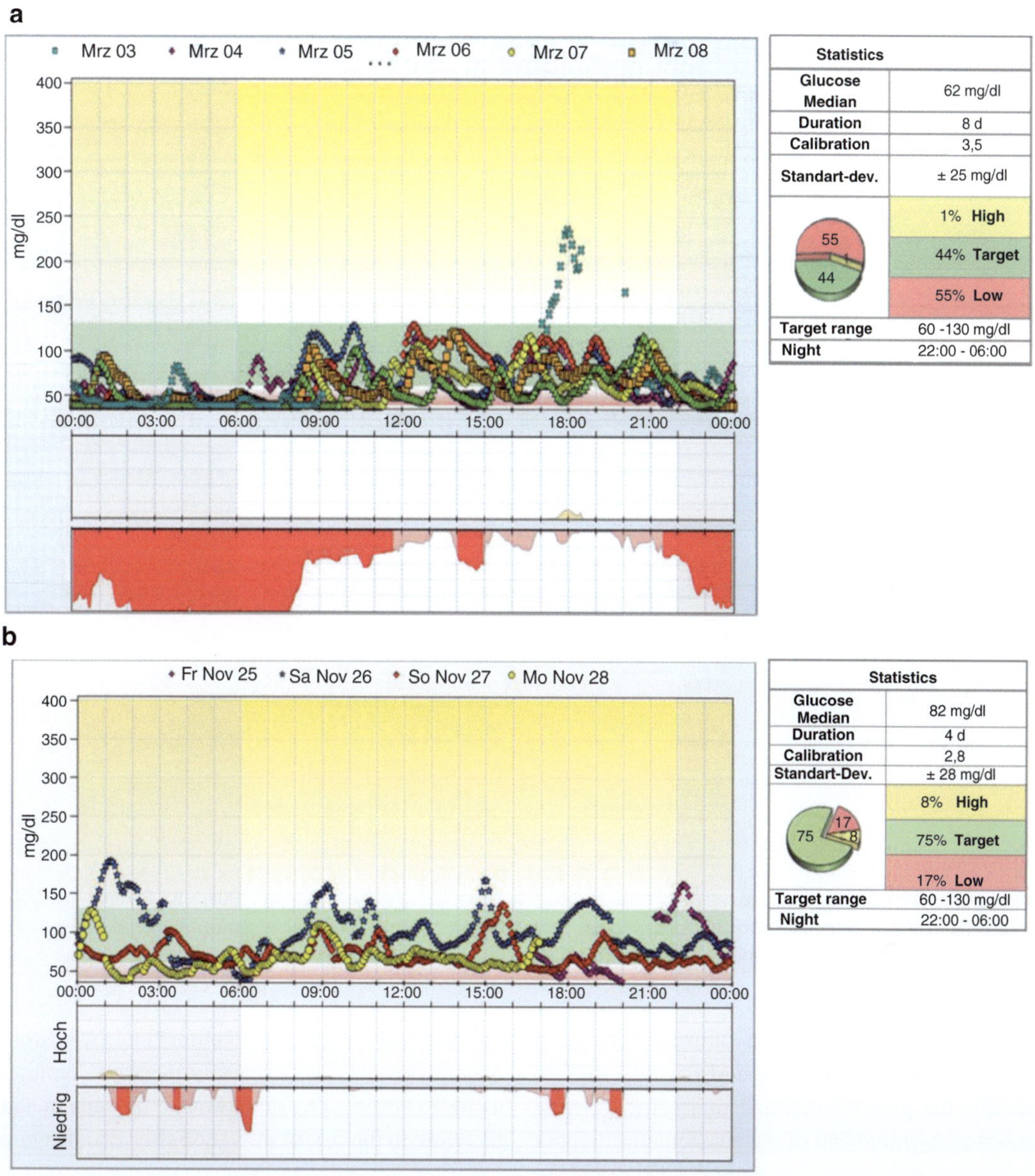

Fig. 36.4 (**a**, **b**) Baseline CGM and after 0.6 mg of daily GLP-1 analog injection. Target range improved from 44% to 75%, and hypoglycaemic values reduced from 55% to 17%. The corresponding control OGTT showed the lowest glucose value at 63 mg/dl.

Endoluminal Revision of the Gastroenterostomy

Following the idea that a tighter pouch outlet diminishes pouch emptying with effect on the umping syndrome, a constriction of the gastroenterostomy (outlet reduction) may be performed. Today, the endoluminale suture of a dilated outlet remains the procedure of first choice with promising results. With this technique, initially the gastral musosa near the anastomosis is ablated circular from a proximal position with an argon plasma coagulator. The actual tool is a double-lumen endoscope, armed with a round-needle (overstitch) and a Prolene thread, thus enabling

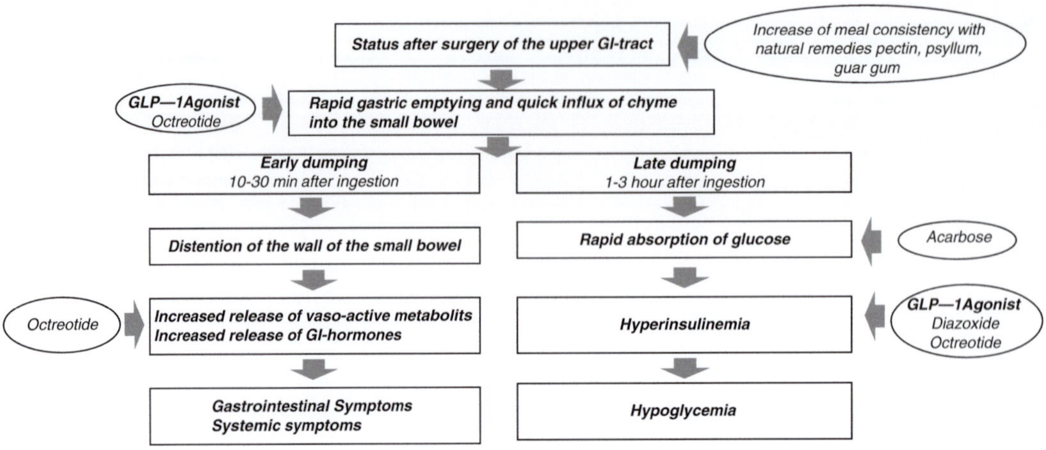

Fig. 36.5 Pathophysiology and medical treatment options [24]. (Modified according to a figure of "Pathophysiology, diagnosis and management of postoperative dumping syndrome", Tack J et al.)

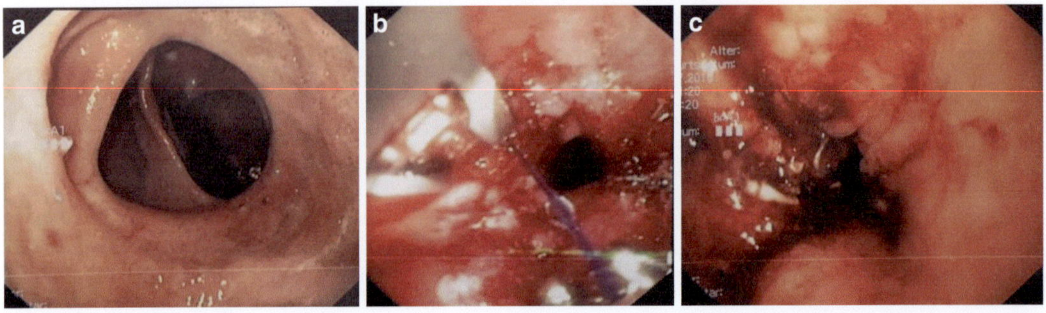

Fig. 36.6 (**a**–**c**) Endoluminal revision of the enlarged gastroenterostomy, female patient with confirmed late dumping syndrome, who responded neither to diet nor to drug therapy; 46y, RYGB 2008. (**a**) Preoperative. (**b**) During surgery. (**c**) Result with remnant swelling from APC application

endoluminale full-thickness suturing. The anastomosis is sutured above the alimentary limb to tighten the pouch outlet and redirect the chyme towards the blind end of the anastomatised upper jejunum during pouch emptying. This procedure is less invasive than the laparoscopic approach. A trial revealed a postoperative pain level of 0.46 out of 10 possible point of the visual pain scale [53] (Fig. 36.6).

Laparoscopic Restoration of Gastric Restriction with Implants

Aiming the same goal – the restoration of gastric restriction – band-like implants or a silastic ring may be applied [54, 55]. Extraluminal restriction with a band-like implant limits the pouch extension and diameter during ingestion and therefore confines nutrition intake and retards influx into the alimentary limb. With band-like implants, overeating is unfavourable. This leads to imperative vomiting as well as excess pressure towards the implant and therefore to the risk of migration (Fig. 36.7).

Laparoscopic Reversal of Roux-en-Y Gastric Bypass with Reinstallation of Pyloric Function

In some desperate cases without response to any treatment, some surgeons perform a reversal-RYGB. This restoration of the natural anatomy intents the re-installation of the pyloric allocation function to avoid the impeded passage into the small bowel. The possible simultaneous conversion to sleeve gastrectomy should prevent weight regain, but is coupled with a higher peri-operative risk [56]. However, proper pyloric function is not guaranteed after previous gastric surgery (Fig. 36.8).

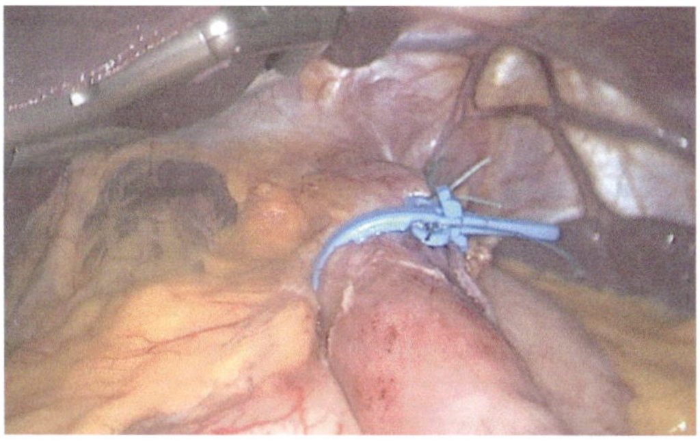

Fig. 36.7 Minimizer in situ, female patient, 32 years, RYGB 2011, became symptomatic with dumping since 8 months (09/14), fainted frequently during hypoglycemic episodes prior to intervention

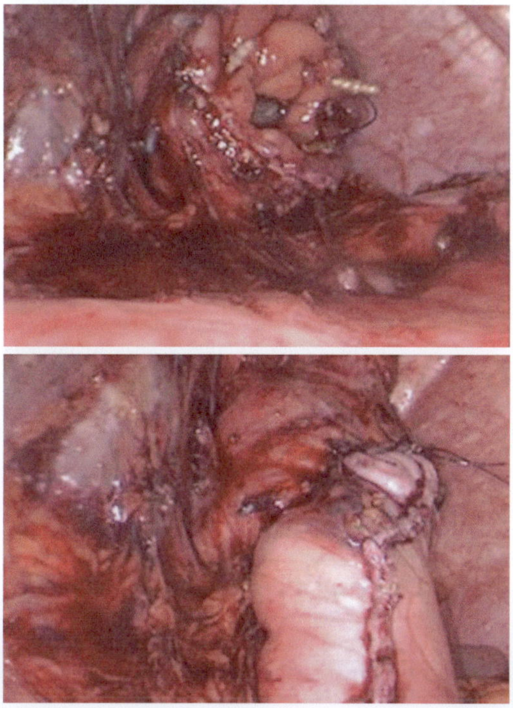

Fig. 36.8 Reversal Roux-en-Y gastric bypass with simultaneous sleeve gastrectomy, female patient, 27 years, RYGB 2010, became symptomatic with dumping since 14 months (02/14), fainted frequently, responded neither to diet nor to drug therapy and also endoluminal outlet repair failed complete remission. But also after reversal-RYGB, recurrent late dumping persisted, even much worse than after previous endoluminal revision

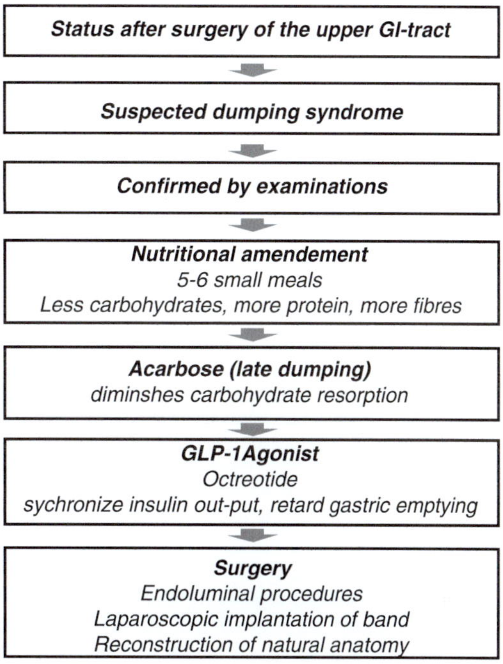

Fig. 36.9 Diagnosis and treatment algorithm. (Modified according to a figure of "Pathophysiology, diagnosis and management of postoperative dumping syndrome", Tack J. et al. [24])

In isolated cases of persistent treatment failure, even partial and total pancreatectomy has been described in the literature [57]. Only few individual surgeons attempted this disintegrating therapeutic approach. It is hoped that these reports remain isolated narratives of the past (Fig. 36.9).

The dumping syndrome, especially manifested late dumping, was and remains a treatment challenge. Due to the increasing incidence, more attention has to be paid to that entity.

References

1. Herzt AF. The cause and treatment of certain unfavourable after-effects of gastro-enterostomy. Ann Surg. 1913;58:466–72.
2. Mix CL. "Dumping stomach" following gastrojejunostomy. Surg Clin North Am. 1922;3:617–22.
3. Eusterman GB, Balfour DC. The stomach and duodenum, vol. 958. Philadelphia: W. B. Saunders Company; 1935.
4. Snell AM. Behavior of stomach after operation for duodenal ulcer. Am J Surg. 1937;33:451–66.
5. Glaessner CL. Hyperglycemic shock. Rev Gestroenterol. 1940;7:528–33.
6. Schwartz A, Reingold I, Necheles H. Investigation of the relationship between blood sugar and general complaints following subtotal gastric resection. Am J Dig Dis. 1942;9:151–4.

7. Jordan SM. End results of radical surgery of the gastrointestinal tract as seen by the gastroenterologist. JAMA. 1941;116:586–90.
8. Mateer JG. Discussion. JAMA. 1941;116:590.
9. Custer MD, Butt HR, Waugh JM. The so called "dumping syndrome" after subtotal gastrectomy. Ann Sug. 1946;123(3):410–8.
10. Sigstadt H. A clinical diagnostic index in the diagnosis of dumping syndrome. Changes in plasma volume and blood sugar after a test meal. Acta Med Scand. 1970;188(6):479–86.
11. Abell TL, Minocha A. Gastrointestinal complications of bariatric surgery: diagnosis and therapy. Am J Med Sci. 2006;331(4):214–8.
12. Abellán P, Cámera R, Merino-Torres JF, et al. Severe hypoglycemia after gastric bypass surgery for morbid obesity. Diabetes Res Clin Pract. 2008;79(1):e7–9.
13. Ceppa EP, Ceppa DP, Omotosho PA, et al. Algorithm to diagnose etiology of hypoglycemia after Roux-en-Y gastric bypass for morbid obesity: case series and literature. Surg Obes Relat Dis. 2012;8(5):641–7.
14. Tack J, Deloose E. Complications of bariatric surgery: dumping syndrome, reflux and vitamin deficiencies. Best Pract Res Clin Gastroenterol. 2014;28(4):741–9.
15. Dirksen C, Jorgensen NB, Bojsen-Moller KN, et al. Gut hormones, early dumping and resting energy expenditure in patients with good and poor weight loss response after Roux-en-Y gastric bypass. Int J Obes (Lond). 2013;37(11):1452–9.
16. Z'graggen K, Guweidhi A, Steffen R, et al. Severe recurrent hypoglycemia after gastric bypass surgery. Obes Surg. 2008;18(8):981–8.
17. Frantides CT, Carlson MA, Shostrom VK, et al. A survey of dumping symptomatology after gastric bypass with or without lesser omental transcetion. Obes Surg. 2011;21(2):186–93.
18. Banerjee A. The role of dumping syndrome in weight loss after gastric bypass surgery for morbid obesity. Diabetes Res Clin Pract. 2008;79(1):7–9.
19. Papamargaritis D, Koukoulis G, Sioka E, et al. Dumping symptoms and incidence of hypoglycemia after provocation test at 6 and 12 months after laparoscopic sleeve gastrectomy. Obes Surg. 2012;22(10):1600–6.
20. Tzovaras G, Papamargaritis D, Sioka E, et al. Symptoms suggestive of dumping syndrome after provocation in patients after laparoscopic sleeve gastrectomy. Obes Surg. 2012;22(1):23–8.
21. Natoudi M, Panousopoulos SG, Nemos N, et al. Laparoscopic sleeve gastrectomy for morbid obesity and glucose metabolism: a new perspective. Surg Endosc. 2014;28(3):1027–33.
22. Vecht J, Masclee AA, Lamers CB. The dumping syndrome. Current insights into pathophysiology, diagnosis and treatment. Scand J Gastroenterol Suppl. 1997;223:21–7.
23. Marsk R, Jonas E, Rasmussen F, et al. Nationwide cohort study of post-gastric bypass hypoglycaemia including 5,040 patients undergoing surgery for obesity in 1986 – 2006 in Sweden. Diabetologia. 2010;53:2307–11.
24. Tack J, Arts J, Caenepeel P, et al. Pathophysiology, diagnosis and management of postoperative dumping syndrome. Nat Rev Gastroenterol Hepatol. 2009;6(10):583–90.
25. Ukleja A. Dumping syndrome: pathophysiology and treatment. Nutr Clin Pract. 2005;20(5):517–25.
26. Gayoso-Diz P, Otero-González A, Rodriguez-Alvarez MX, et al. Insulin resistance (HOMA-IR) cut off values and the metabolic syndrome in a general adult population: effect of gender and age: EPIRCE cross-sectional study. BMC Endocr Disord. 2013;13:47.
27. Miccoli R, Biamchi C, Odoguardi L. Prevalence of the metabolic syndrome among Italian adults according to ATPII definition. Nutr Metab Cardiovasc Dis. 2005;13:250–4.
28. Ascaso JF, Romero P, Real JT, Priego A, Valdecabres C, Carmena R. Insulin resistance quantification by fasting insulin plasma values and HOMA index in a non-diabetic population. Med Clin (Barc). 2001;13:530–3.
29. Toft-Nielsen M, Madsbad S, Holst JJ. Exaggerated secretion of glucagon-like peptide-1 (GLP-1) could cause reactive hypoglycaemia. Diabetologia. 1998;41(10):1180–6.
30. Vaceou A. Continuous glucose monitoring in diabetes treatment. Diabetes Res Sci Technol. 2011;93(Suppl 1):S125–30.
31. Nielsen JB, Abild CB, Pedersen AM, et al. Continuous glucose monitoring after gastric bypass to evaluate the glucose variability after a low-carbohydrate diet and to determinate hypoglycemia. Obes Surg. 2016;26:2111–8.
32. Liebl A, Henrichs HR, Heinemann L, et al. Continuous glucose monitoring: evidence and consensus statement for clinical use. J Diabetes Sci Technol. 2013;7(2):500–19.
33. Mashist SK. Continuous glucose monitoring systems: a review. Diagnostics. 2013;3(4):385–412.
34. Hanaire H, Dubet A, Chauveau ME, et al. Usefulness of continuous glucose monitoring for the diagnosis of hypoglycemia after a gastric bypass in a patient previously treated for type 2 diabetes. Obes Surg. 2010;20(1):126–9.
35. Halperin F, Patti ME, Snow M, et al. Continuous glucose monitoring for evaluation of glycemic excursions after gastric bypass. J Obes. 2011;2011:869536; published online Feb. 2011.
36. Vidal J, Nicolau J, Romero F, et al. Long-term effects of Roux-en-Y gastric bypass surgery on plasma glucagon-like-peptide-1 and islet function in morbid obese subjects. J Clin Endocrinol Metab. 2009;94(39):884–91.
37. Hanaire H, Bertrand M, Guerci B, et al. High glycemic variability assessed by continuous glucose monitoring after surgical treatment of obesity by gastric bypass. Diabetes Technol Ther. 2011;13(6):625–30.
38. Buss RW, Kansal PC, Roddam RF, et al. Mixed meal tolerance test and reactive hypoglycemia. Horm Metab Res. 1982;14:281–3.

39. Besser RE, Shields BM, Casas R, et al. Lessons from the mixed-meal tolerance test. Diabetes Care. 2013;36:195–201.
40. Kehrfurt R, Langer FB, Schindeler K, et al. Hypoglycemia after Roux-en-Y gastric bypass: detection rates of continuous glucose monitoring (CGM) versus mixed meal test. Surg Obes Relat Dis. 2015;11(3):564–9.
41. Kellogg TA, et al. Postgastric bypass hyperinsulinemic hypoglycemia syndrome: characterization and response to a modified diet. Surg Obes Relat Dis. 2008;4(4):492–9.
42. Valderas JP, Ahuad J, Rubio L, et al. Acarbose improves hypoglycaemia following gastric bypass surgery without increasing glucagon-like peptide 1 levels. Obes Surg. 2012;22(4):582–6. https://doi.org/10.1007/s11695-011-0581-0.
43. Moreira RO, Moreira RB, Machado NA, et al. Postprandial hypoglycemia after bariatric surgery: pharmacological treatment with verapamil and acarbose. Obes Surg. 2008;18(12):1618–21.
44. Ritz P, Vaurs C, Bertrand M, et al. Usefulness of acarbose and dietary modifications to limit glycemic variability following Roux-en-Y gastric bypass as assessed by continuous glucose monitoring. Diabetes Technol Ther. 2012;14(8):736–40.
45. Thondam SK, Nair S, Wile D, Gill GV. Diazoxide for the treatment of hypoglycaemic dumping syndrome. QJM. 2013;106(9):855–8. https://doi.org/10.1093/qjmed/hcr234.
46. Spanakis E, Gragnoli C. Successful medical management of status post-Roux-en-Y-gastric-bypass hyperinsulinemic hypoglycemia. Obes Surg. 2009;19(9):1333–4. https://doi.org/10.1007/s11695-009-9888-5.
47. Hopman WP, Wolberink RG, Lamers CB, et al. Treatment of the dumping syndrome with the somatostatin analogue SMS 201-995. Ann Surg. 1988;207(2):155–9.
48. Nelson-Piercy C, Hammond PJ, Gwilliam ME, et al. Effect of a new oral somatostatin analog (SDZ CO 611) on gastric emptying, mouth to cecum transit time, and pancreatic and gut hormone release in normal male subjects. J Clin Endocrinol Metab. 1994;78(2):329–36.
49. Parkinson C, Drake WM, Roberts ME, et al. A comparison of the effects of pegvisomant and octreotide on glucose, insulin, gastrin, cholecystokinin, and pancreatic polypeptide responses to oral glucose and a standard mixed meal. J Clin Endocrinol Metab. 2002;87(4):1797–804.
50. van Berge Henegouwen MI, van Gulik TM, Akkermans LM, et al. The effect of octreotide on gastric emptying at a dosage used to prevent complications after pancreatic surgery: a randomised, placebo controlled study in volunteers. Gut. 1994;41(6):758–62.
51. Deloose E, Bisschops R, Holvoet L, et al. A pilot study of the effects of the somatostatin analog pasireotide in postoperative dumping syndrome. Neurogastroenterol Motil. 2014;26(6):803–9.
52. Abrahamsson N, Engström BE, Sundbom M, et al. GLP1 analogs as treatment of postprandial hypoglycemia following gastric bypass surgery: a potential new indication? Eur J Endocrinol. 2013;169(6):885–9. https://doi.org/10.1530/EJE-13-0504.
53. Stier C, Chiappetta S. Endoluminal revision (OverStitch (TM), Apollo Endosurgery) of the dilated gastroenterostomy in patients with late dumping syndrome after proximal Roux-en-Y gastric bypass. Obes Surg. 2016;26(8):1978–84. https://doi.org/10.1007/s11695-016-2266-1.
54. Rasera I Jr, Coehlo TH, Raveli MN, et al. A comparative, prospective and randomized evaluation of Roux-en-Y gastric bypass with and without the silastic ring: a 2-year follow up preliminary report on weight loss and quality of life. Obes Surg. 2016;26:762–8.
55. Bessler M, Daud A, Kim T, et al. Prospective randomized trial of banded versus nonbanded gastric bypass for the super obese: early results. Surg Obes Relat Dis. 2007;3(4):480–4.
56. Carter CO, Fernandez AZ, McNatt SS, Powell MS. Conversion from gastric bypass to sleeve gastrectomy for complications of gastric bypass. Surg Obes Relat Dis. 2016;12:572. pii: S1550-7289(15)00286-5. https://doi.org/10.1016/j.soard.2015.07.001.
57. Clancy TE, Moore FD Jr, Zinner MJ. Post-gastric bypass hyperinsulinism with nesidioblastosis: subtotal or total pancreatectomy may be needed to prevent recurrent hypoglycemia. J Gastrointest Surg. 2006;10(8):1116–9.

Endoscopic Treatment of Roux-en-Y Gastric Bypass Complications

37

Lyz Bezerra Silva, Gabriel Tavares Xavier Simplicio, and Josemberg Marins Campos

Introduction

The increasing prevalence of obesity leads to a rise of bariatric surgery procedures. Although bariatric surgery has been associated with a low morbidity, some outcomes are still of concern. Revisional surgery and reoperations increase incidence of adverse events after bariatric surgery. Therefore, bariatric endoscopy aims to treat these complications with endoluminal minimally invasive procedures.

Literature about devices like dilation balloons, clips, endoluminal suture, endoscopic scissors, and stents has been growing in the last years. This chapter aims to describe the role of bariatric endoscopy in diagnostics and treatment of complications after Roux-en-Y gastric bypass (RYGB).

Anastomotic Stricture

Gastrojejunal anastomotic stricture is one of the most common complications after RYGB and is diagnosed when the anastomotic lumen diameter is <10 mm, making it difficult for a standard endoscope (9.8 mm) to pass through. The main presenting symptom is dysphagia, usually occurring after solid food introduction. The suggested etiologies include ischemia, gastric hypersecretion, foreign body reaction to staples, and anastomotic surgical technique [1].

Upper gastrointestinal endoscopy is the diagnostic and therapeutic method of choice. In cases of early stenosis, occurring within the first week after surgery, initial administration of corticosteroids can reduce anastomotic edema and obstructive symptoms; when this approach fails, endoscopic therapy is indicated. Balloon dilation should be performed with caution, using low inflation pressure to reduce perforation risk [1, 2].

Initial treatment can be performed using TTS (through the scope) hydrostatic balloons, with increasing diameters up to a maximum of 15 mm when inflated [1]. Subsequent balloon dilation sessions up to 20 mm should be used as needed. This approach reaches success in 98% of cases, in a mean of 1.7 sessions per patient, with complication rate of 2.5%, mostly perforations and bleeding [1, 3]. In cases of failure associated with fibrotic tissue, an endoscopic stricturotomy can be performed using needle knife, followed by balloon dilation [4].

Food Impaction

Food impaction may occur after RYGB; it may be associated with the use of surgically implanted restrictive ring due to its slippage or erosion,

L. B. Silva · G. T. X. Simplicio
Department of Surgery, Federal University of Pernambuco, Recife, Brazil

J. M. Campos (✉)
Surgery Department, University Hospital, Pernambuco Federal University, Recife, Brazil

J. Ettinger et al. (eds.), *Gastric Bypass*, https://doi.org/10.1007/978-3-030-28803-7_37

dietary noncompliance, gastric pouch, or gastrojejunostomy stenosis. Clinical presentation is consistent with upper gastrointestinal obstruction, involving nausea, retrosternal pain, epigastric discomfort, and postprandial vomiting. Endoscopy can be used for diagnosis and immediate treatment [5].

An endoscopic retrieval basket is the most commonly used accessory for foreign body removal. When it is difficult to remove the fragments orally, retained residues can be gently pushed into the distal jejunal loop, passing the restriction point. It is advised to use minimal sedation during the procedure, due to a potentially increased risk of aspiration of gastric contents. This risk can be prevented by undertaking the procedure under general anesthesia after endotracheal intubation with or without the use of an overtube. It is also strongly advised that after resolution of symptoms, the etiology of the narrowing is investigated and resolved [5].

Marginal Ulcer

Marginal ulcer may occur either early or late in the postoperative period of RYGB, and the incidence rate is up to 16%. The pathophysiology is associated with mechanic and ischemic factors and seems to have a multifactorial etiology, including tobacco and alcohol consumption, nonsteroidal anti-inflammatory drug (NSAID) usage, *H. pylori* infection, leaks, and foreign bodies. Ulcers are more common at the jejunal side of the GJA, with varying size and depth [6–9]. The patients are commonly asymptomatic, but the main symptoms include epigastric pain, nausea, chest complaints, and obstructive symptoms caused by the inflammatory edema [6–9].

The upper GI endoscopy investigation confirms the diagnosis. Any foreign bodies, such as visible sutures and staples, should be removed to improve ulcer healing and treatment should include proton pump inhibitor and sucralfate prescription [6–9]. Gastroscopy should be repeated to ensure healing [9]. Ulcers can cause strictures due to fibrotic scar formation, and these can be treated through stenotomy and balloon dilation [3]. Prophylaxis with acid suppression after surgery is being increasingly used with the aim to prevent marginal ulcer. However, no consensus exist about the duration of the prophylaxis, usually varying from 30 days to 2 years, with some recommending lifelong usage [10].

Ring Complications

Intragastric Erosion

The incidence of intragastric ring erosion varies from 0.9% to 7%, occurring slowly with an inflammatory capsule formation that prevents leakage of gastric contents into the peritoneal cavity. Most common symptoms are nausea, vomiting, bleeding, and weight regain, and 15% of patients are asymptomatic [9].

Endoscopic evaluation should be performed and may show the ring inside the gastric pouch. The eroded ring should be removed using endoscopic scissors to section the ring. In cases of failure in cutting the ring, a gastric band cutter or lithotripter may be used. However, in early stages, an ulcer at the erosion site can be the only visible sign. In this case, PPIs should be prescribed until complete ring erosion, with endoscopy surveillance performed. In cases of early migration, if the ring has only a small area of intragastric erosion and is adherent to the gastric pouch wall, a dual channel device can also be used. This allows the introduction of a foreign body grasping forceps for traction, for better ring exposure. The other channel can then be utilized to pass an argon ablation catheter to divide the ring, or even scissors. Treatment should be scheduled as soon as possible, due to the risk of gastric wall bleeding or food impaction [10].

Ring Slippage

Ring distal displacement is a rare complication associated with a gastric pouch longitudinal axis angulation and proximal gastric dilation, leading to progressive obstructive symptoms, including vomiting, eructation, weight loss, malnutrition, and dehydration [10].

Diagnosis can be elucidated with contrast x-ray, showing an area of contrast retention, and endoscopy, which may show food stasis and mucosal folds convergence, caused by the jejunal obstruction just beneath the anastomosis [10]. Surgical approach in this situation increases the risk of perforation and bleeding, due to gastric pouch peritoneal adherences [11].

Management can be done through endoscopic 30 mm achalasia balloon dilation that promotes stretching or rupture of the ring and fibrotic bands, relieving symptoms with low morbimortality and complication rate; however, weight regain may be an important complication [10]. Stent placement can also be used, especially if symptoms persist, in order to induce an inflammatory/ischemic reaction around the ring, leading to intragastric erosion, with stent and ring removal after approximately 2 weeks. A fibrotic scar tissue forms in the ring erosion area, restricting the pouch diameter, with better weight control when compared to dilation [12–14].

Leaks after RYGB

The incidence of leaks after bariatric surgery has been decreasing in the last years, but the high morbimortality associated with this complication still concerns bariatric surgeons. After RYGB, most leaks occur at the gastrojejunostomy and angle of his. Ischemia, excessive tension, and technical factors are associated with the pathophysiology. Fistulas can be formed to the gastric remnant, resulting in a gastrogastric fistula that is associated with weight regain [15].

Leaks are classified according to the time of onset (acute <7 days; early <6 weeks; late 6–12 weeks; chronic >3 months) [16]. In acute/early leaks, the clinical presentation includes tachycardia, abdominal pain, fever, leukocytosis, and SIRS criteria [17]. The chronic inflammatory response leads to development of distal stenosis and a fibrotic septum between the perigastric fluid collection and intraluminal cavity, factors associated with perpetuation of leaks [12, 18, 19].

Endoscopic initial exam allows early diagnosis, evaluation of leak anatomy and associated strictures, and can be a therapeutic option. Clinical approach includes broad-spectrum antibiotic therapy and fluid resuscitation; after that, specific measures are taken. Revisional surgery is usually associated with elevated morbidity and mortality. The endoscopic management should be considered the first-line therapeutic option in hemodynamically stable patients due to decreased invasiveness [4, 15, 18, 20–27].

Endoscopic therapy has the aim of solving the three main issues perpetuating the leak: distal gastric stricture, increased intragastric pressure, and fistulous tract persistence [19]. Several procedures have been reported in the literature, including closure (stenting, clips, glues, and endoluminal suture) and internal drainage methods (septotomy with balloon dilation, endoscopic vacuum therapy (EVT), and pigtail drain) [20–24, 26–35].

Treatment choice is made according to time of onset, divided in four phases (Table 37.1).

In acute and late leaks, self-expandable metallic stents (SEMS) promote leak orifice occlusion and correction of axis deviation and distal strictures, decreasing intraluminal pressure, which leads to leak closure [15, 26, 28–30, 36, 37]. Stents should be removed in up to 6 weeks, which is usually enough to correct strictures and deviations, with lower migration and easier removal [18] (Fig. 37.1). After initial leak control, stent is

Table 37.1 Endoscopic algorithm approach of bariatric surgery leaks according to the time of development

Onset time	Treatment
Acute (<07 days)	*"Stent"* (or EVT[a])
Early (7–45 days)	*"Stent"* or *"pigtail"* (or EVT[a] or septotomy + balloon dilation[b])
Late (1.5–03 months)	*Septotomy + balloon dilation* (*"stent"*[c] *or "pigtail"* or EVT[a])
Chronic (>03 months)	*Septotomy + balloon dilation* (or EVT[a])

[a]Endoscopic vacuum therapy can be done in centers without advanced bariatric endoscopy services

[b]Septotomy + balloon dilation should be performed in early fistulas with fibrotic septum

[c]SEMS should be used in late fistulas associated with leakage of gastric content

removed even if complete orifice closure is not achieved. When needed, endoscopic treatment continues through septotomy, stenotomy, and balloon dilations, which will usually lead to complete fistula closure [18].

The placement of a double pigtail stent through the fistulous tract, communicating the perigastric collection and intraluminal cavity, creates an internal drainage system (Fig. 37.2a, b). The foreign body reaction also induces tissue reepithelization. This therapy has been described with high success and low complication rate in some series, especially in cases of smaller leaks (<10 mm) [22, 25, 38].

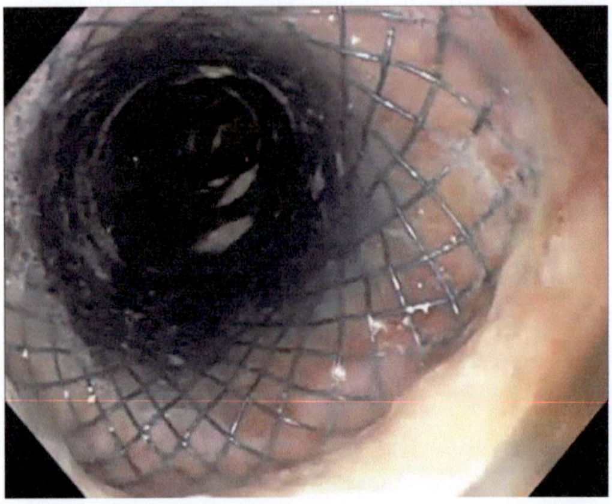

Fig. 37.1 Endoscopic view of a partially covered self-expandable stent at time of removal. In this image it is possible to see the mucosal ingrowth that makes removal of this kind of stent more difficult

Other endoscopic approaches include usage of endoscopic clips, biologic glue, and tissue sealants, with controversial results [35, 36]. Endoscopic vacuum therapy has also been described [21, 35, 39].

For *late and chronic leaks*, endoscopic multimodal treatment is usually done through multiple sessions using different techniques. When there is a septum adjacent to the fistulous orifice, septotomy is performed, decreasing flow of gastric contents through the fistula [27] (Fig. 37.3). Septotomy is done with needle knife or argon plasma coagulation (associated to less bleeding), followed by balloon dilation, that reduces the intraluminal pressure and facilitates the internal drainage. This therapy has been associated with high success rate in cases of late and chronic fistulas [20, 33, 34]. When there is stenosis and fibrotic tissue associated, stenotomy associated to balloon dilation may be used. This endoscopic

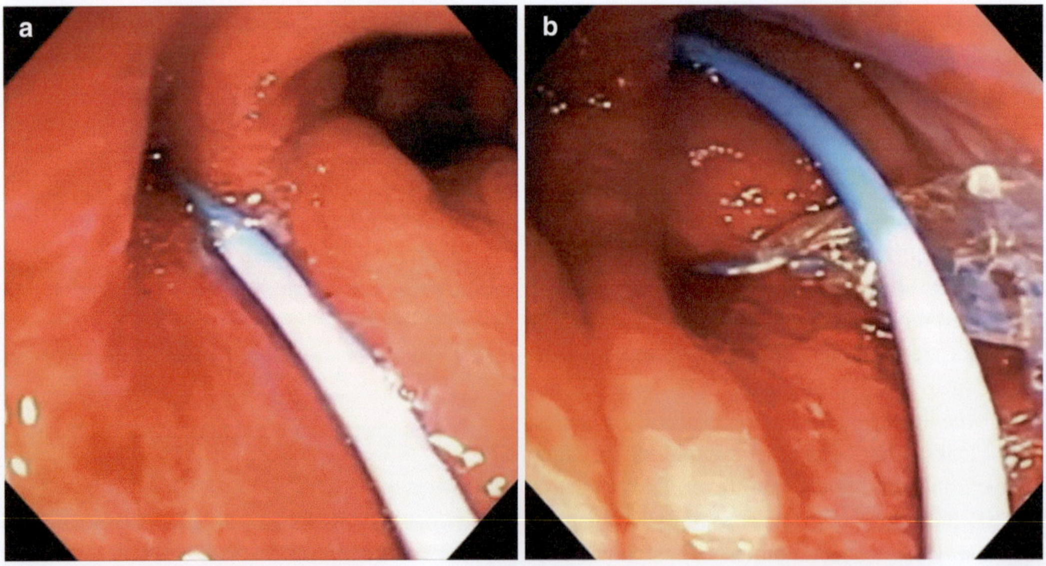

Fig. 37.2 (**a**) Endoscopic view of a double pigtail stent placed in a RYGB fistula. To the right of the image, it is possible to see the septum and the gastric pouch. (**b**) Endoscopic view of balloon dilation of gastric pouch aiming to reduce intragastric pressure and lead flow of gastric contents away from the fistula

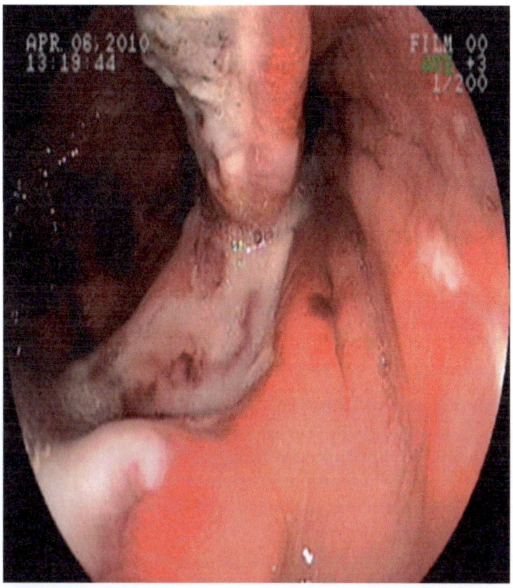

Fig. 37.3 Endoscopic view of leak orifice (left), septum, and gastric pouch (right), before septotomy

therapy can be performed on an outpatient basis, with low morbidity and mortality and better quality of life. The correction in flow of digestive contents will eventually lead to leak closure [20, 33, 34]. Stents can be used in selected cases, especially when there are anatomical defects or gastric content leakage. Internal drainage with double pigtail stent can be performed in late fistulas associated with long fistulous tract and perigastric abscess [25, 38].

Endoscopic vacuum therapy has also been described, with a high success rate. However, the EVT is associated with an elevated number of procedures to exchange the device [21, 35, 39].

Endoscopic Treatment of Weight Regain

Weight regain is a long-term complication of RYGB that involves genetic, psychologic, and behavioral factors. The gastrojejunostomy and gastric pouch enlargement have been shown to contribute to weight regain [40, 41]. Ramos et al. showed that in a 2-year follow-up, gastrojejunostomy diameter of 15 mm presented better weight loss outcomes when compared with 45 mm gastrojejunal anastomosis [42]. Traditionally, revisional surgery is the treatment of weight regain, which itself increases postoperative complication rates and 13% require an additional surgical intervention, with an even greater adverse outcome rate. In this context, bariatric endoscopy has been demonstrated as a viable approach for weight regain with fewer complications [41].

The most relevant aspects of weight regain after RYGB treated by endoscopy are large gastric pouch and gastrojejunal anastomosis dilation. However, other complications may be inducing the patient to gain weight, such as gastrogastric leaks, ring slippage or stricture, and stenosis [43]. Chronic stenosis causes food intolerance and leads to patient selection of most appealing foods, which are usually carbohydrates, sweets, and caloric liquids, which pass easily through the stricture.

The necessity of less invasive and morbid procedures to approach weight regain led to development of transoral outlet reduction techniques that include sclerotherapy, clipping, ablation, and suturing.

Argon plasma coagulation (APC) is a noncontact electrocoagulation method that results in superficial thermal coagulation and induces an inflammatory and fibrotic response. This fibrotic response can reduce the diameter of anastomosis when applied at dilated gastrojejunostomy [44, 45].

APC can only be employed to narrow the anastomosis, and it is not indicated in cases of enlarged pouch. To produce the desired effect, the argonium should be passed circumferentially at the gastrojejunostomy (Fig. 37.4). The procedure duration is approximately 5–10 min and hospital stay 30–60 min [45]. The cost is low and doesn't require an advanced center to perform the procedure, with sedation being the means of anesthesia [45].

The initial edema and inflammatory response cause immediate gastric restriction. This effect decreases over the time and fibrosis replaces the edema. More than one session is usually necessary to achieve long-lasting effects. The diameter reduction delays gastric emptying and may cause early satiety, improving weight reduction. A recent multicentric study showed that patients

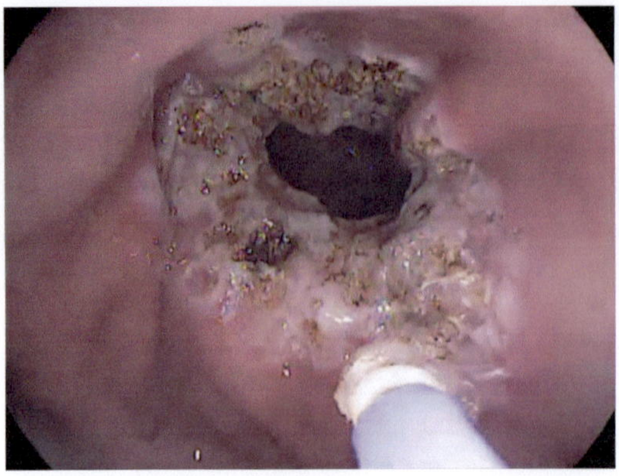

Fig. 37.4 Circumferential argon plasma coagulation in a dilated gastric bypass anastomosis

with weight regain after RYGB submitted to APC therapy can present 6–10% of total weight loss at 12 months, and this therapy achieves a significantly gastrojejunostomy diameter decrease [45]. However, complications can occur after APC therapy. One of the possible complications is anastomotic stricture that can reduce by itself or be treated with endoscopic balloon dilation. GJ ulcer, melena, and vomiting have also been reported [44, 45].

The use of endoluminal sutures allows concomitant reduction of dilated anastomosis and large pouch, performed using an endoscopic suture system. Argon plasma coagulation, when associated with procedure, leads to better weight loss outcomes and can achieve an EWL% of 24.9 +/− 2.6% after 1 year with a low complication rate that includes bleeding, abdominal pain, and nausea [41, 46]. The purse-string pattern is a recently described technique that results in better outcomes when compared to interrupted endoluminal stiches [43, 47, 48]. Schulman et al. compared TORe with purse-sting and interrupted technique and demonstrated that purse-string technique achieves a significantly greater outcomes in terms of percent total weight loss (TWL%) and percent regained weight loss (RWL%) [43]. The systolic blood pressure, glycated hemoglobin levels, and ALT levels in patients submitted to TORe also show significant improvement after 1 year [47]. Adverse events following endoluminal stiches include marginal ulcer, stricture, and bleeding [43, 47].

References

1. Campos JM, de Mello FST, Ferraz ÁAB, de Brito JN, Nassif PAN, dos Passos Galvão-Neto M. Dilatação endoscópica de anastomose gastrojejunal após bypass gástrico. ABCD Arquivos Brasileiros de Cirurgia Digestiva (São Paulo). 2012;25(4):283–9.
2. Espinel J. Stenosis in gastric bypass: endoscopic management. World J Gastrointest Endosc. 2012;4(7):290.
3. De Moura EGH, Orso IRB, Aurélio EF, De Moura ETH, De Moura DTH, Santo MA. Factors associated with complications or failure of endoscopic balloon dilation of anastomotic stricture secondary to Roux-en-Y gastric bypass surgery. Surg Obes Relat Dis. 2016;12(3):582–6.
4. Campos JM, Pereira EF, Evangelista LF, Siqueira L, Neto MG, Dib V, et al. Gastrobronchial fistula after sleeve gastrectomy and gastric bypass: endoscopic management and prevention. Obes Surg. 2011;21(10):1520–9.
5. Ferraz Á, Campos J, Dib V, Silva LB, De Paula PS, Gordejuela A, et al. Food intolerance after banded gastric bypass without stenosis: aggressive endoscopic dilation avoids reoperation. Obes Surg. 2013;23(7):959–64.
6. Coblijn UK, Lagarde SM, De Castro SMM, Kuiken SD, Van Tets WF, Van Wagensveld BA. The influence of prophylactic proton pump inhibitor treatment on the development of symptomatic marginal ulceration in Roux-en-Y gastric bypass patients: a historic cohort study. Surg Obes Relat Dis. 2016;12(2):246–52.
7. Kang X, Zurita-Macias L, Hong D, Cadeddu M, Anvari M, Gmora S. A comparison of 30-day versus 90-day proton pump inhibitor therapy in prevention of marginal ulcers after laparoscopic Roux-en-Y gastric bypass. Surg Obes Relat Dis. 2016;12(5):1003–7.
8. Moon RC, Teixeira AF, Goldbach M, Jawad MA. Management and treatment outcomes of marginal ulcers after Roux-en-Y gastric bypass at a single high volume bariatric center. Surg Obes Relat Dis. 2014;10(2):229–34.
9. Garrido AB, Rossi M, Lima SE, Brenner AS, Gomes CAR. Early marginal ulcer following Roux-en-Y gastric bypass under proton pump inhibitor treatment – prospective multicentric study. Arq Gastroenterol. 2010;47(2):130–4.
10. Campos JM, Evangelista LF, Ferraz ÁAB, Galvao Neto MP, De Moura EGH, Sakai P, et al. Treatment of ring slippage after gastric bypass: long-term results after endoscopic dilation with an achalasia balloon (with videos). Gastrointest Endosc. 2010;72(1):44–9.
11. Taddeucci RJ, Madan AK, Ternovits CA, Tichansky DS. Laparoscopic re-operations for band removal

after open banded gastric bypass. Obes Surg. 2007;17(1):35–8.
12. Marins Campos J, Moon RC, Magalhães Neto GEJ, Teixeira AF, Jawad MA, Bezerra Silva L, et al. Endoscopic treatment of food intolerance after a banded gastric bypass: inducing band erosion for removal using a plastic stent. Endoscopy. 2016;48(6):516–20.
13. Blero D, Eisendrath P, Vandermeeren A, Closset J, Mehdi A, Le Moine O, et al. Endoscopic removal of dysfunctioning bands or rings after restrictive bariatric procedures. Gastrointest Endosc. 2010;71(3):468–74.
14. Wilson TD, Miller N, Brown N, Snyder BE, Wilson EB. Stent induced gastric wall erosion and endoscopic retrieval of nonadjustable gastric band: a new technique. Surg Endosc. 2013;27(5):1617–21.
15. Bhayani NH, Swanström LL. Endoscopic therapies for leaks and fistulas after bariatric surgery. Surg Innov. 2014;21(1):90–7.
16. Rosenthal RJ, International Sleeve Gastrectomy Expert Panel, Diaz AA, Arvidsson D, Baker RS, Basso N, et al. International Sleeve Gastrectomy Expert Panel Consensus Statement: best practice guidelines based on experience of 12,000 cases. Surg Obes Relat Dis 2012;8(1):8–19.
17. Iossa A, Abdelgawad M, Watkins BM, Silecchia G. Leaks after laparoscopic sleeve gastrectomy: overview of pathogenesis and risk factors. Langenbecks Arch Surg. 2016;401(6):757–66.
18. Campos JM, Siqueira LT, Ferraz ÁAB, Ferraz EM. Gastrobronchial fistula after obesity surgery. J Am Coll Surg. 2007;204(4):711.
19. Zundel N, Hernandez JD. Strictures after laparoscopic sleeve gastrectomy. Surg Laparosc Endosc Percutan Tech. 2010;20(3):154–8.
20. Baretta G, Campos J, Correia S, Alhinho H, Marchesini JB, Lima JH, et al. Bariatric postoperative fistula: a life-saving endoscopic procedure. Surg Endosc Other Interv Tech. 2015;29(7):1714–20.
21. Schmidt F, Mennigen R, Vowinkel T, Neumann PA, Senninger N, Palmes D, et al. Endoscopic Vacuum Therapy (EVT)—a new concept for complication management in bariatric surgery. Obes Surg. 2017;27(9):2499–505.
22. Rebibo L, Hakim S, Brazier F, Dhahri A, Cosse C, Regimbeau JM. New endoscopic technique for the treatment of large gastric fistula or gastric stenosis associated with gastric leaks after sleeve gastrectomy. Surg Obes Relat Dis. 2016;12(8):1577–84.
23. Quezada N, Maiz C, Daroch D, Funke R, Sharp A, Boza C, et al. Effect of early use of covered self-expandable endoscopic stent on the treatment of postoperative stapler line leaks. Obes Surg. 2015;25(10):1816–21.
24. Puig CA, Waked TM, Baron TH, Wong Kee Song LM, Gutierrez J, Sarr MG. The role of endoscopic stents in the management of chronic anastomotic and staple line leaks and chronic strictures after bariatric surgery. Surg Obes Relat Dis. 2014;10(4):613–9.
25. Donatelli G, Dumont J, Cereatti F, Dhumane P, Tuszynski T, Vergeau B, et al. Endoscopic internal drainage as first-line treatment for fistula following gastrointestinal surgery: a case series. Endosc Int Open. 2016;04(06):E647–51.
26. Christophorou D, Valats J, Funakoshi N, Duflos C, Picot M, Vedrenne B, et al. Endoscopic treatment of fistula after sleeve gastrectomy: results of a multicenter retrospective study. Endoscopy. 2015;47:988–96.
27. Campos JM, Ferreira FC, Teixeira AF, Lima JS, Moon RC, D'Assunção MA, et al. Septotomy and balloon dilation to treat chronic leak after sleeve gastrectomy: technical principles. Obes Surg. 2016;26(8):1992–3.
28. Shehab H, Abdallah E, Gawdat K, Elattar I. Large bariatric-specific stents and over-the-scope clips in the management of post-bariatric surgery leaks. Obes Surg. 2018;28(1):15–24.
29. Southwell T, Lim TH, Ogra R. Endoscopic therapy for treatment of staple line leaks post-laparoscopic sleeve gastrectomy (LSG): experience from a Large Bariatric Surgery Centre in new Zealand. Obes Surg. 2016;26(6):1155–62.
30. Tringali A, Bove V, Perri V, Landi R, Familiari P, Boškoski I, et al. Endoscopic treatment of post-laparoscopic sleeve gastrectomy leaks using a specifically designed metal stent. Endoscopy. 2017;49(1):64–8.
31. Klimczak T, Klimczak J, Szewczyk T, Janczak P, Jurałowicz P. Endoscopic treatment of leaks after laparoscopic sleeve gastrectomy using MEGA esophageal covered stents. Surg Endosc Other Interv Tech. 2017;32(4):1–8.
32. Donatelli G, Ferretti S, Vergeau BM, Dhumane P, Dumont JL, Derhy S, et al. Endoscopic internal drainage with enteral nutrition (EDEN) for treatment of leaks following sleeve gastrectomy. Obes Surg. 2014;24(8):1400–7.
33. Mahadev S, Kumbhari V, Campos JM, Galvao Neto M, Khashab MA, Chavez YH, et al. Endoscopic septotomy: an effective approach for internal drainage of sleeve gastrectomy-associated collections. Endoscopy. 2017;49(5):504–8.
34. Shnell M, Gluck N, Abu-Abeid S, Santo E, Fishman S. Use of endoscopic septotomy for the treatment of late staple-line leaks after laparoscopic sleeve gastrectomy. Endoscopy. 2017;49(1):59–63.
35. Leeds SG, Burdick JS. Management of gastric leaks after sleeve gastrectomy with endoluminal vacuum (E-Vac) therapy. Surg Obes Relat Dis. 2016;12(7):1278–85.
36. Vix M, Marx L, Diana M, Perretta S, Donatelli G, Callari C, et al. Management of staple line leaks after sleeve gastrectomy in a consecutive series of 378 patients. Surg Endosc Other Interv Tech. 2012;26(1):S207.
37. Simon F, Siciliano I, Gillet A, Castel B, Coffin B, Msika S. Gastric leak after laparoscopic sleeve gastrectomy: early covered self-expandable stent reduces healing time. Obes Surg. 2013;23(5):687–92.

38. Lorenzo D, Guilbaud T, Gonzalez JM, Benezech A, Dutour A, Boullu S, et al. Endoscopic treatment of fistulas after sleeve gastrectomy: a comparison of internal drainage versus closure. Gastrointest Endosc. 2017;87(2):429–37.
39. Seyfried F, Reimer S, Miras AD, Kenn W, Germer CT, Scheurlen M, et al. Successful treatment of a gastric leak after bariatric surgery using endoluminal vacuum therapy. Endoscopy. 2013;45(SUPPL2):267–9.
40. Dayyeh BKA, Lautz DB, Thompson CC. Gastrojejunal stoma diameter predicts weight regain after Roux-en-Y gastric bypass. YJCGH. 2011;9(3):228–33.
41. Brunaldi VO, Jirapinyo P, De MDTH, Okazaki O, Bernardo WM, Neto MG, et al. Endoscopic treatment of weight regain following Roux-en-Y gastric bypass: a systematic review and meta-analysis. Obes Surg. 2017;28(1):266–76.
42. Ramos AC, Marchesini JC, de Souza Bastos EL, Ramos MG, de Souza MDG, Campos JM, et al. The role of gastrojejunostomy size on gastric bypass weight loss. Obes Surg. 2017;27(9):2317–23.
43. Schulman AR, Kumar N, Thompson CC. Transoral outlet reduction: a comparison of purse-string with interrupted stitch technique. Gastrointest Endosc. 2018;87(5):1222–8.
44. Baretta GAP, Alhinho HCAW, Matias JEF. Argon plasma coagulation of gastrojejunal anastomosis for weight regain after gastric bypass. Obes Surg. 2014;25(1):72–9.
45. Moon RC, Teixeira AF, Neto MG, Zundel N, Sander BQ, Ramos FM, et al. Efficacy of utilizing argon plasma coagulation for weight regain in Roux-en-Y gastric bypass patients: a Multi-center Study. Obes Surg. 2018;28(9):2737–44.
46. Kumar N, Thompson CC. Transoral outlet reduction for weight regain after gastric bypass: long-term follow-up. Gastrointest Endosc. 2016;83(4):776–9.
47. Jirapinyo P, Kröner PT, Thompson CC. Purse-string transoral outlet reduction (TORe) is effective at inducing weight loss and improvement in metabolic comorbidities after Roux-en-Y gastric bypass. Endoscopy. 2018;50(4):371–7.
48. Patel LY, Lapin B, Brown CS, Stringer T, Gitelis ME, Linn JG, et al. Outcomes following 50 consecutive endoscopic gastrojejunal revisions for weight gain following Roux-en-Y gastric bypass: a comparison of endoscopic suturing techniques for stoma reduction. Surg Endosc. 2017;31(6):2667–77.

Endoscopic Treatment of Weight Regain After Gastric Bypass

38

Luiz Gustavo de Quadros, Manoel Galvão Neto, Eduardo Grecco, Thiago Ferreira de Souza, Idiberto José Zotarelli Filho, and Andre Fernandes Teixeira

Introduction

According to the report issued by the International Federation for the Surgery of Obesity and Metabolic Disorders (IFSO) in 2015, approximately 86 thousand bariatric surgeries have been performed in Brazil, the second most frequent of which is laparoscopic gastric bypass. This technique promotes as much as an 80% loss of excess weight in the initial period (18 to 24 months), but the long-term failure rate ranges from 10.0% to 35.0% [1, 2]. The number of bariatric surgeries has increased exponentially throughout the world, with approximately 40 thousand procedures performed in 1997 and 468,609 performed in 2013 [3, 4]. According to the Brazilian Society of Bariatric and Metabolic Surgery, 100 thousand procedures are currently performed per year in the country.

The most common late-onset complication of bariatric surgery is the return of obesity, the main factors of which are poor eating habits and a sedentary lifestyle, which often lead to an increase in gastric reserve and dilation of the anastomosis [5–8]. An anastomosis less than 10.0 mm causes dietary selection due to intolerance or even vomiting and requires endoscopic treatment with dilation in most cases. However, a wide anastomosis has been associated with the return of obesity and may be associated with diminished satiety [5–8].

Approximately 52.0% of bariatric patients have psychiatric disorders associated with eating behavior in the preoperative period [3]. The reduction in the restriction due to a dilated anastomosis may serve as an additional factor to these eating disorders, exerting a direct influence on the result of the weight loss. Current discussions center on the efficacy and safety of the narrowing of the gastrojejunal anastomosis using fulguration with argon plasma, suturing, and surgical procedures in cases of the recurrence of obesity after bariatric surgery [3]. The main endoscopic procedures to reduce the diameter of the gastrojejunal anastomosis are overstitch (Apollo Endosurgery) and fulguration with argon plasma, as described by Aly in 2009 [9].

L. G. de Quadros
Department of Bariatric Endoscopy, Kaiser Day Hospital, São José do Rio Preto, Brazil

M. Galvão Neto (✉)
Faculty of Medicine of ABC – FMABC, Santo André, Brazil

Florida International University – FIU, Miami, FL, USA

EndoVitta Institute, São Paulo, Brazil

E. Grecco
ABC Medical School (FMABC), São Paulo, Brazil

T. F. de Souza
ABC Medical School (FMABC), São Paulo, Brazil

Faculty of Medicine of ABC – FMABC, Santo André, Brazil

EndoVitta Institute, São Paulo, Brazil

University of São Paulo – USP, São Paulo, Brazil

I. J. Z. Filho
São José do Rio Preto, Brazil

A. F. Teixeira
Bariatric and Laparoscopy Center, Orlando Health, Orlando, FL, USA

J. Ettinger et al. (eds.), *Gastric Bypass*, https://doi.org/10.1007/978-3-030-28803-7_38

Main Findings and Justification

The return of obesity is associated with a reduction in quality of life and the recurrence of comorbidities [7, 8, 10]. Endoscopic techniques have been developed in an attempt to reduce the diameter of the anastomosis and consequently promote weight loss.

As a consequence of weight regain, abnormal anatomic findings are encountered in 71.2% of patients: 58.9% with dilation of the gastrojejunal anastomosis, 28.8% with dilation of the pouch, and 12.3% with both types of dilation [9]. Several methods have been proposed to reduce regained weight after gastric bypass, such as the endoluminal reduction of the gastrojejunal anastomosis [endocinch (Bard®, Billerica, Massachusetts, USA); restorative obesity surgery endoluminal (ROSE) (USGI®, San Clemente, CA, USA); StomaphyX (EndoGastric Solutions®, Redmond, Washington, USA); OTSC Clip (Ovesco AG®, Tubingen, Germany); and Overstitch (Apollo Endosurgery® Inc., Austin, TX, USA)] and fulguration of the gastrojejunal anastomosis with argon plasma [9]. Surgical treatment is performed but is associated with a greater occurrence of complications and a higher morbimortality rate in comparison to endoscopic techniques [3, 11, 12].

Influence of the Pouch and Dilated Anastomosis on Weight Regain

The aim of endoscopic methods for the treatment of the anastomosis and pouch is not to exert an influence on postoperative weight loss, but rather on weight regain after the initial loss when such regain is significant [3]. Heneghan et al. (2012) [13] concluded that patients with a "normal" postoperative anatomy regain less weight than those with an altered surgical anatomy, such as an increase in the diameter of the gastrojejunal anastomosis. After evaluating 165 patients, Abu Dayyeh et al. (2015) [1] concluded that the diameter of the anastomosis is a risk factor for weight regain after Roux-en-Y gastric bypass (RYGB) and should be considered a predictor of weight regain.

In a prospective study involving 130 patients submitted to endoscopic exams in the preoperative and postoperative phases for the estimation of the size of the gastric pouch and diameter of the anastomosis using the diameter of endoscope as reference, the authors found no significant increase in the gastric pouch or dilation of the gastrojejunal anastomosis [14].

Ramos et al. (2017) [15] evaluated the size of the gastrojejunal anastomosis and its influence on weight loss. This was an elegant, balanced study performed in which an anastomosis calibrated at 15.0 mm demonstrated better results in comparison to 45.0 mm in 2 years of follow-up (18), since the diameter after endoscopic treatment should be between 10.0 and 15.0 mm.

Thompson et al. (2013) [16] demonstrated the effectiveness of treatment on the anastomosis in cases of the post-bypass recurrence of obesity in a controlled prospective study. Several other studies have confirmed the efficacy of the treatment of a dilated anastomosis regarding weight loss after the return of obesity.

Flanagan (1996) [17] evaluated the influence of the size of the gastric pouch and anastomosis on weight loss after RYGB during a 49-month period. Three hundred eighty patients having undergone surgery more than 1 year earlier were submitted to upper digestive endoscopy and divided into two groups: one with successful weight loss (Group A, n = 175) and one with weight regain (Group B, n = 205). Group B had a significantly greater occurrence of abnormal anatomy than Group A. Moreover, an increase in pouch size (length and width) was found in Group B, although the difference between the two groups was nonsignificant. No difference was found in the percentage of weight lost among those with a dilated pouch, those with an enlarged anastomosis and those with both conditions. The author found that there was a step-by-step progression in the increase in functional pouch volume, with statistically significant differences between time intervals. However, the difference in excess weight loss between patients with a larger pouch and those with a smaller pouch was nonsignificant.

Endoscopic Treatment of Pouch and/or Anastomosis

Weight recidivism recurs in approximately 20.0% of patients submitted to gastric bypass. The main factors involved in this recurrence are the interruption of follow-up with the multidisciplinary team and failure on the part of the patient to maintain adequate nutritional and lifestyle behaviors [1, 3]. Therefore, it is important to establish a balance in terms of diet, behavior, physical activity, and the control of anxiety as the basis of treating obesity. This is the first goal of treatment, especially for patients submitted to surgical procedures for the control of obesity [3].

Surgery is currently the best treatment option for morbid obesity. Therefore, the first criterion evaluated for the inclusion of a patient to undergo endoscopic treatment of the anastomosis is follow-up with a specialized multidisciplinary team [1]. Other important aspects include the time elapsed since surgery and endoscopic changes in the pouch and anastomosis. The weight loss curve after gastric bypass occurs in the first 2 years, with an acceptable variation of up to 5.0%. Therefore, weight regain after surgery is considered beginning at 10.0% of the nadir (surgery weight – minimum weight = nadir) [3, 14].

The most important aspects for the indication of endoscopic treatment are a large gastric pouch and gastrojejunal anastomosis. However, other concomitant findings may lead the patient to inadequate food intake [18]. Gastrogastric fistulas may promote the recurrence of the disease due to the reconnection with the excluded portion of the stomach.

Another important condition to consider is stenosis of the anastomosis or due to the presence of a containment ring, which is currently in disuse, but was widely employed in past, and many patients have such rings [19–21]. Chronic stenosis causes a condition of dietary intolerance in which the patient avoids particular foods [22]. As such patients have difficulty ingesting solid foods due to the obstruction mechanism, they tend to select carbohydrates, sweets, and fluids, which are poor in terms of nutrition and calories [14]. Thus, treatment in cases of a containment ring with symptoms of food intolerance is the removal of this foreign body. In the case of stenosis of the anastomosis, dilatation with a balloon or stenostomy should be performed, and in cases of slippage or food intolerance due to the ring, the use of an achalasia balloon or prosthetic should be the endoscopic treatment of choice [3].

It is imperative to know the standards of normality and the figures that are considered ideal for the size of the pouch and gastrojejunal anastomosis. A normal postoperative pouch size is 4.0 to 7.0 cm in length and <4.0 cm in width [15]. A long, narrow pouch provides a greater sensation of satiety compared to a short, wide pouch of the same capacity, at least in theory [15]. Therefore, a pouch with length of 4.0 to 7.0 cm would be a condition for endoscopic treatment using either endosuturing or argon plasma. As a wider pouch can hold a larger amount of food, even with the ideal anastomosis, the goal in such cases is a reduction in its volume, which can be achieved with endosuturing, as argon plasma alone cannot be used in such cases [15].

As the ideal gastrojejunal anastomosis is between 10.0 and 14.0 mm in maximum diameter, an anastomosis less than 10.0 mm leads to the patient to select foods that go down easily, and an anastomosis larger than 15.0 mm can lead to a reduction in satiety and the possibility of ingesting any type and amount of food [14]. A large variety of treatments have been used with the aim of narrowing the gastric passage, but the most widely employed are endosuturing and argon plasma coagulation [14].

Diagnosis Under Endoscopy

Prior endoscopic analysis is as important as the treatment itself [1, 3, 14]. This should be complete and delineate the important endoscopic aspects so that the team and patient can decide on the best form of treatment [1]. Endoscopic analysis enables the determination of the main possibilities and cues to perform the endoscopic diagnosis of a large pouch and anastomosis.

For such, we divide this section of the text into two subitems: measurement of the pouch measurement and measurement of the gastrojejunal anastomosis.

Measurement of the Pouch

Although reliable, this procedure should not take so long that its use is unviable at a reference service that performs a large number of exams per day. The length of the pouch can be determined through a simple measurement taken by the endoscope through the maxillary dental arch and measured by the small curve from the anastomosis to the esophagogastric transition. If a band is present, one should give the distance from it to the anastomosis (e.g., band to 2.0 cm from the anastomosis or band juxtaposed to the anastomosis, etc.). Pouch width is a more complicated task, but it is not possible to perform the back view maneuver easily on a narrow pouch. Therefore, in a practical manner, a wide pouch is that on which this maneuver can be performed easily.

Measurement of the Anastomosis

The gastrojejunal anastomosis should be measured along it largest axis with adequate distension of the pouch. Different methods are used (Figs. 38.1 and 38.2), such as a direct view, which is a less precise method; the use of endoscopic rulers, which are more precise; and the use of tweezers with known diameters. One must take into consideration the diverse situations throughout the world regarding access to materials as well as the economic factors of each country and each healthcare service. Therefore, the best method is that which is available and offers the most precision.

As relevant cutoff points, the measurement or description of some points is of the utmost importance. Stating that an anastomosis is 12.0 mm when it is actually 13.0 mm has little relevance. Stating that an anastomosis is 12.0 mm when it is actually 20.0 mm can make a large difference regarding the indication or non-indication of a method. Therefore, the following cutoff points should be described in the report: anastomosis <10.0 mm, from 10.0 to 15.0 mm, from 15.0 to 20.0 mm, or >20.0 mm [3]. Purely visual methods are only reliable with the device passing next to the anastomosis, at which point knowing the diameter of the device enables estimating with relative accuracy. However, this method is of little use for estimating other sizes of anastomosis [14].

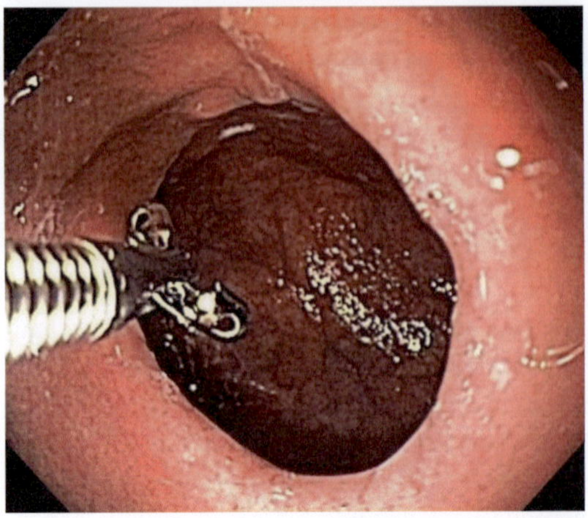

Fig. 38.1 Measurement of the anastomosis using forceps

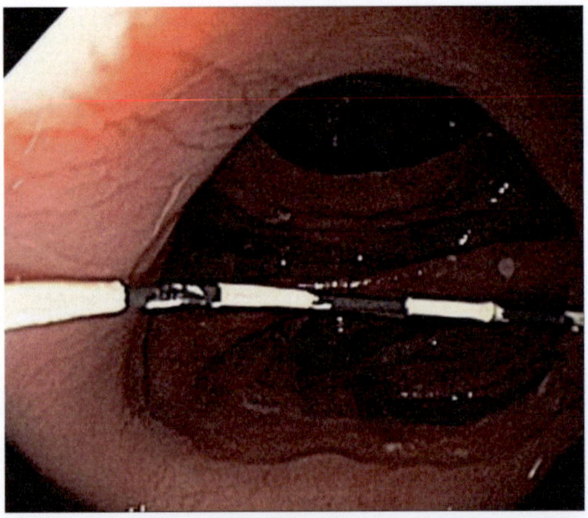

Fig. 38.2 Measurement of the anastomosis using ruler

A widely used method in endoscopic practice is the use of tweezers of known diameters. For instance, we can measure or see on the specifications the diameter of certain foreign body tweezers and then open the tweezers on top of the anastomosis. If the tweezers have a diameter of 20.0 mm, we could state whether the anastomosis is less than 20 mm, equal to 20 mm or greater than 20.0 mm, and so forth [14].

The most precise manner is the use of endoscopic rulers with different markings. The most widely used ruler in the USA is marked at 2.0-mm intervals with black and gray colors and is adjustable [14]. Once fabricated by Olympus, this ruler is no longer manufactured and is not available for sale in countries other than the USA. A simple, inexpensive manner to measure an anastomosis is to place marks on a cholangiography catheter or make rulers using cholangiography guide wires [14]. Besides the low cost, the black and white colors offer visual contrast that facilitates the measurement through the endoscope.

Endoscopic Technique: Treatment

After the selection and indication, treatment method is chosen. We can choose endoscopic suturing methods or the use of argon plasma coagulation isolated [5, 6]. Suturing enables the concomitant treatment of the dilated anastomosis and large pouch as well as the isolated treatment of one or the other. The cost and need for a high-complexity service are the main negative points and may be determinants in some places. In contrast, the fact that the procedures can be performed in a single session weighs in favor of this method [6]. Argon plasma can be used only to narrow the anastomosis and is not indicated for a large pouch [3]. This method is inexpensive, more available, and does not require a high-complexity service, and sedation is the means of anesthesia employed (Figs. 38.3 and 38.4) [3].

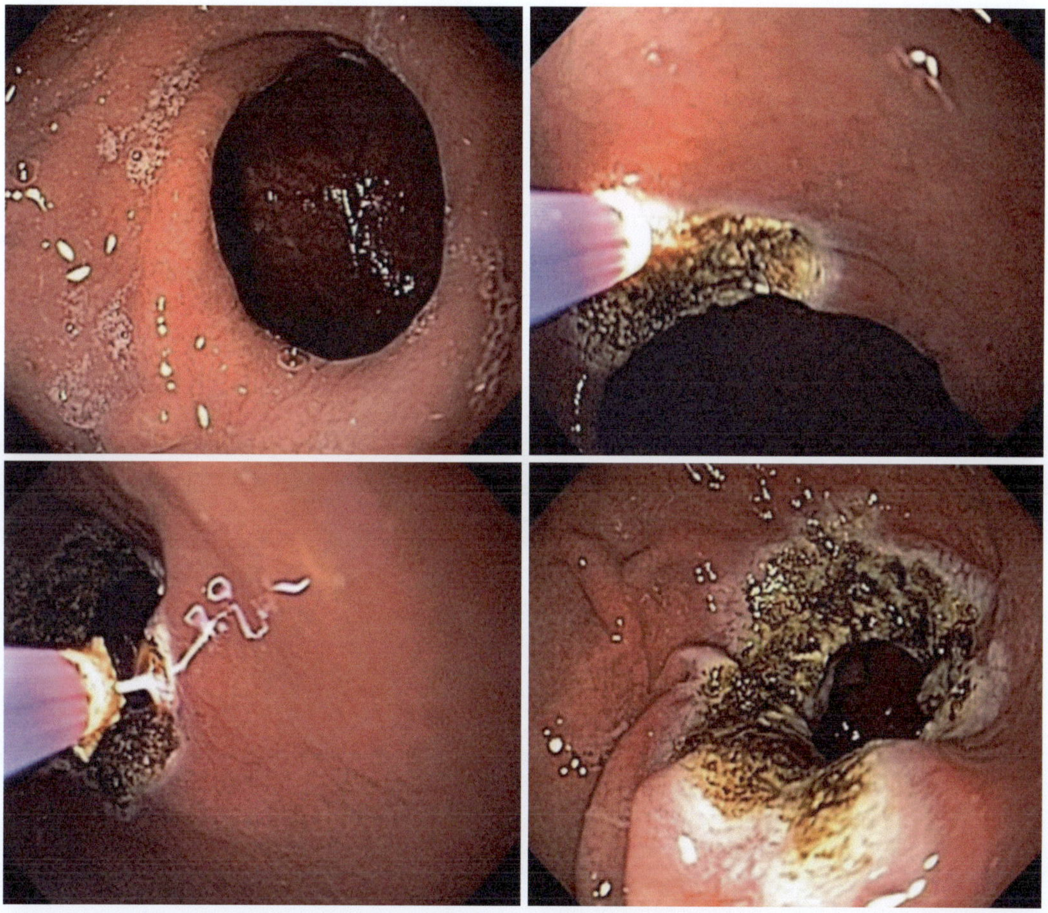

Fig. 38.3 Using of argon plasma coagulation alone

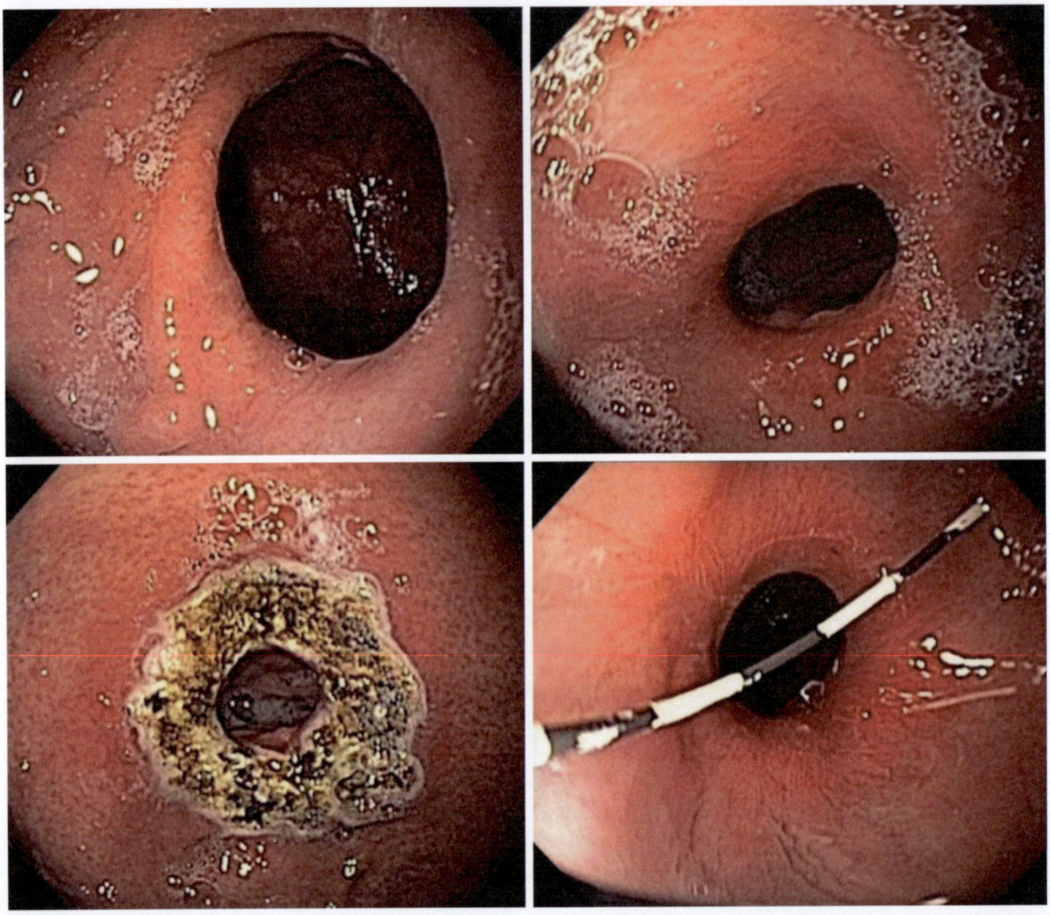

Fig. 38.4 Treatment using APC. This sequence shows an anastomosis after two sessions with the final diameter 10 mm

However, an average of three sessions at 2-month intervals is required to achieve the desired result, meaning that the patient must visit the medical office more often, which intensifies the follow-up care with the team [3].

Discussion

The return of obesity after bariatric surgery is associated with a reduction in quality of life and the recurrence of comorbidities [1, 3]. Therefore, endoscopic techniques have been developed in an attempt to reduce the diameter of the anastomosis and consequently promote weight loss [3].

Abnormal anatomic findings are encountered in 71.2% of patients with the recurrence of obesity: 58.9% with dilation of the gastrojejunal anastomosis, 28.8% with dilation of the pouch, and 12.3% with both types of dilation [9]. Thus, several methods have emerged to reduce the weight regained by patients having been submitted to gastric bypass, such as the endoluminal reduction of the gastrojejunal anastomosis [endocinch (Bard®, Billerica, Massachusetts, USA); restorative obesity surgery endoluminal (ROSE) (USGI®, San Clemente, CA, USA); StomaphyX (Endogastric Solutions®, Redmond, Washington, USA); OTSC Clip (Ovesco AG®, Tubingen, Germany); and Overstitch (Apollo Endosurgery® Inc., Austin, TX, USA)] and fulguration of the gastrojejunal anastomosis with argon plasma [3, 5, 7, 9, 10, 12, 14, 16, 20, 22–24].

Endosuturing in the gastrojejunal tract has been employed to manage complications in clinical practice over the years. Thompson et al. (2006) [10] demonstrated the applicability of this method in eight patients with a dilated gastrojejunal anastomosis and weight regain after gastric bypass. The mean diameter of the anastomosis was 25.0 mm and a 68% reduction occurred after the procedure (mean final diameter: 10 mm), with a 23.4% reduction in excess weight.

The over-the-scope clip (OTSC clip (Ovesco AG)) endoscopic system has also been used to reduce the diameter of the gastrojejunal anastomosis in patients with weight regain after gastric bypass. Heylen et al. (2011) [25] performed this procedure on 94 patients after gastric bypass who had a mean dilated gastrojejunal anastomosis of 35 mm in diameter and 10% weight regain. An average of one to two clips is employed, and the final diameter of the anastomosis was 8.0 mm (mean reduction of 80%). The body mass index at the 1-year follow-up reduced from a mean of 32.8 kg m^{-2} to 27.4 kg m^{-2}.

The use of plasma on the anastomosis is considered a safe, effective method for the treatment of the recurrence of obesity. Fulguration with argon promotes a reduction in the diameter of the anastomosis and consequent delay in gastric emptying, leading to early satiety and weight loss [3, 21]. The reduction in the diameter of a dilated anastomosis can lead to a 23.0% reduction in excess weight [26]. From the endoscopic standpoint, information such as the diameter of the anastomosis, complications after bariatric surgery, follow-up with a specialized team, and physical activity contribute to the determination of the method to be adopted in patients with weight regain after gastric bypass [27, 28].

One study compared the relative effectiveness of transoral outlet reduction (TORe) and the use of argon plasma coagulation at 3 and 6 months for the treatment of weight regain after RYGB [26]. The study involved 10 consecutive patients submitted to TORe using a plicature of interrupted tissue and 20 patients submitted to argon plasma coagulation. Mean age was 50.9 ± 1.7 years. The mean pre-RYGB body mass index was 46.7 ± 1.1 kg m^{-2}, and the nadir body mass index was 28.8 ± 0.8 kg m^{-2} [26]. TORe was performed 10.5 ± 0.9 years after RYGB, with a pre-TORe body mass index of 36.6 ± 1.0 kg m^{-2}. The mean opening of the gastrojejunal anastomosis was 18.5 ± 0.7 mm. The mean number of treatments with AP coagulation was 1.3 (range: 1 to 4). No important adverse events occurred. The weight loss results were better for the patents submitted to application at both 3 and 6 months. Larger studies with a longer follow-up are needed to evaluate differences in the durability of the results.

Baretta et al. (2015) [3] studied 30 patients submitted to treatment with argon plasma after gastric bypass (an average of three endoscopic sessions of AP coagulation with an intensity of 70 W at 2.0 L/min with 8 weeks between sessions) and found a mean weight loss of 15.0 kg.

In a retrospective study with 37 participants without the exclusion of eaters of sweets and snacks, De Souza et al. (2015) [28] used argon plasma and obtained a 50.0% success rate (100.0% in the group with adequate nutritional follow-up) and a 24.0% reduction in regained weight. In a prospective, controlled, longitudinal study involving argon plasma, Cambi et al. (2015) [29] report a 90.0% success rate and up to a 41% reduction in regained weight. A recent meta-analysis published by Brunaldi VO et al. demonstrated that full-thickness suture was efficient to treat this patients and that suture plus APC is more effective than suture alone [30].

The long-term results remain undefined. There is no scientific knowledge regarding the possibility of "new" weight regain and "new" dilation of the anastomosis. Fulguration of the anastomosis with endoscopic argon can be performed as many times as necessary. Endoscopic control should be performed frequently with the aim of preventing this probable dilation and consequent weight regain [3].

Conclusion

The present systematic review of the main national and international periodicals reveals good results regarding weight regain after narrowing of the gastrojejunal anastomosis using fulguration with argon plasma or suturing (with or without APC).

References

1. Abu Dayyed BK, Acosta A, Camilleri M, Mundi MS, Rajan E, Topazian MD, Gostout CJ. Endoscopic sleeve gastroplasty alters gastric physiology and induces loss of body weight in obese individuals. Clin Gastroenterol Hepatol. 2017;15(1):37–43.e1.
2. IBGE- Instituto Brasileiro de Geografia e Estatística. Disponível em: http://www.ibge.gov.br. Acesso em março de 2016.
3. Baretta GA, Alhinho HC, Matias JE, Marchesini JB, de Lima JH, Empinotti C, et al. Argon plasma coagulation of gastrojejunal anastomosis for weight regain after gastric bypass. Obes Surg. 2015;25(1):72–9.
4. OMS- Organização Mundial de Saúde. Disponível em: https://www.sbcbm.org.br/endoscopia-e-obesidade/. Acesso em: 25 de setembro de 2018.
5. Angrisani L, Santonicola A, Iovino P, Vitiello A, Zundel N, Buchwald H, et al. Bariatric surgery and endoluminal procedures: IFSO worldwide survey 2014. Obes Surg. 2017;27(9):2279–89.
6. Angrisani L, Santonicola A, Iovino P, Formisano G, Buchwald H, Scopinaro N. Bariatric surgery worldwide 2013. Obes Surg. 2015;25(10):1822–32.
7. Malik VS, Willett WC, Hu FB. Global obesity: trends, risk factors and policy implications. Nat Rev Endocrinol. 2013;9(1):13–27.
8. Malick KJ. Clinical applications of argon plasma coagulation in endoscopy. Gastroenterol Nurs. 2006;29(5):386–91; quiz 92–3
9. Aly A. Argon plasma coagulation and gastric bypass–a novel solution to stomal dilation. Obes Surg. 2009;19(6):788–90.
10. Thompson CC, Slattery J, Bundga ME, Lautz DB. Peroral endoscopic reduction of dilated gastrojejunal anastomosis after Roux-en-Y gastric bypass: a possible new option for patients with weight regain. Surg Endosc. 2006;20(11):1744–8.
11. Miranda da Rocha LC, Ayub Perez OA, Arantes V. Endoscopic management of bariatric surgery complications: what the gastroenterologist should know. Rev Gastroenterol Mex. 2016;81(1):35–47.
12. Galvao Neto M, Marins Campos J. Therapeutic flexible endoscopy after bariatric surgery: a solution for complex clinical scenarios. Cir Esp. 2015;93(1):1–3.
13. Heneghan HM, Yimcharoen P, Brethauer SA, Kroh M, Chand B. Influence of pouch and stoma size on weight loss after gastric bypass. Surg Obes Relat Dis. 2012;8(4):408–15.
14. De Quadros LG, Galvao Neto MD, Campos JM, Kaiser Junior RL, Grecco E, Flamini Junior M, et al. Validation of a new method for the endoscopic measurement of post-bariatric gastric outlet using a standard guidewire: an observer agreement study. BMC Res Notes. 2017;10(1):13.
15. Ramos AC, Marchesini JC, de Souza Bastos EL, Ramos MG, de Souza MDG, Campos JM, et al. The role of gastrojejunostomy size on gastric bypass weight loss. Obes Surg. 2017;27:2317.
16. Thompson CC, Chand B, Chen YK, Demarco DC, Miller L, Schweitzer M, et al. Endoscopic suturing for transoral outlet reduction increases weight loss after Roux-en-Y gastric bypass surgery. Gastroenterology. 2013;145(1):129–37.e3.
17. Flanagan L. Measurement of functional pouch volume following the gastric bypass procedure. Obes Surg, Oxford. 1996;6:38–43.
18. Yimcharoen P, Heneghan HM, Singh M, Brethauer S, Schauer P, Rogula T, et al. Endoscopic findings and outcomes of revisional procedures for patients with weight recidivism after gastric bypass. Surg Endosc. 2011;25(10):3345–52.
19. Trindade EM, Gebara T, Cambi MPC, Baretta GAP. Nutritional aspects and the use of nutritional supplements by women who underwent gastric bypass. Arq Bras Cir Dig. 2017;30(1):11–3.
20. Bege T, Emungania O, Vitton V, Ah-Soune P, Nocca D, Noel P, et al. An endoscopic strategy for management of anastomotic complications from bariatric surgery: a prospective study. Gastrointest Endosc. 2011;73(2):238–44.
21. Boules M, Chang J, Haskins IN, Sharma G, Froylich D, El-Hayek K, et al. Endoscopic management of post-bariatric surgery complications. World J Gastrointest Endosc. 2016;8(17):591–9.
22. Dakin GF, Eid G, Mikami D, Pryor A, Chand B, American Society for M, et al. Endoluminal revision of gastric bypass for weight regain–a systematic review. Surg Obes Relat Dis. 2013;9(3):335–42.
23. Jirapinyo P, Slattery J, Ryan MB, Abu Dayyeh BK, Lautz DB, Thompson CC. Evaluation of an endoscopic suturing device for transoral outlet reduction in patients with weight regain following Roux-en-Y gastric bypass. Endoscopy. 2013;45(7):532–6.
24. Kumar N, Thompson CC. Transoral outlet reduction for weight regain after gastric bypass: long-term follow-up. Gastrointest Endosc. 2016;83(4):776–9.
25. Heylen AM, Jacobs A, Lybeer M, Prosst RL. The OTSC(R)-clip in revisional endoscopy against weight gain after bariatric gastric bypass surgery. Obes Surg. 2011;21(10):1629–33.
26. Schulman A, Chan WW, Thompson CC. Endoscopic suturing for failed gastric by-pass: predictors of success. AGA. 2013;abstracts S–827 Mo1958.
27. Grund KE, Storek D, Farin G. Endoscopic argon plasma coagulation (APC) first clinical experiences in flexible endoscopy. Endosc Surg Allied Technol. 1994;2:42–6.
28. De Souza LM, de Quadros LG, Kaiser RL, Campos JM, Zotarelli IJ, et al. Argon plasma effect about anastomosis was significant to inhibit the weight regained in patients undergoing gastric bypass. J Obes Weight Loss Ther. 2015;5:264.

29. Cambi MP, Marchesini SD, Baretta GA. Post-bariatric surgery weight regain: evaluation of nutritional profile of candidate patients for endoscopic argon plasma coagulation. Arq Bras Cir Dig. 2015;28(1):40–3.
30. Brunaldi VO, Jirapynio P, Moura DTH, Okazaki O, Bernardo WM, Neto MG, et al. Endoscopic treatment of eight regain following Roux-en-Y Gastric Bypass: a systematic review and meta-analysis. Obes Surg. 2018;28(1):266–76.

Laparoscopic Bariatric Surgery Training and the Credentialing Process

39

Kais A. Rona, Angela S. Volk, James R. Pellechi, Daniel H. Shin, and Christopher G. DuCoin

Introduction

Bariatric surgery has been shown to be the most effective and sustainable intervention for morbid obesity and the treatment of obesity-related conditions [1–3]. Current evidence has reported significant mortality reduction by undergoing surgical weight loss procedures [4, 5]. With the advent of minimally invasive techniques, bariatric surgery has been proven to be safe and effective [1, 6–9]. Bariatric surgery consists of operations affecting malabsorption, the restriction of food intake, or a combination of these two [10]. The following operations are the current validated laparoscopic bariatric procedures: laparoscopic Roux-en-Y gastric bypass (RGB), laparoscopic gastric banding by vertical banded gastroplasty (VBG) or adjustable gastric band (AGB), laparoscopic biliopancreatic diversion (BPD) ± duodenal switch (DS), and laparoscopic sleeve gastrectomy (LSG) [10].

K. A. Rona · A. S. Volk
Department of Surgery, Tulane Medical Center, New Orleans, LA, USA

J. R. Pellechi
School of Medicine, Tulane Medical Center, New Orleans, LA, USA

D. H. Shin
Tulane School of Medicine, New Orleans, LA, USA

C. G. DuCoin (✉)
Department of Surgery, University of South Florida, Tampa, FL, USA
e-mail: CDucoin@health.usf.edu

According to the American Society for Metabolic and Bariatric Surgery (ASMBS), bariatric procedures performed in the United States have increased by 44% between 2011 and 2017 [11]. An estimated 228,000 operations were performed in 2017, with almost 60% being the laparoscopic sleeve gastrectomy [11]. The sleeve gastrectomy surpassed the Roux-en-Y gastric bypass (RGB) procedure in 2013 as the most commonly performed bariatric operation, and there has been a downward trend in RGB and gastric banding procedures since 2012 [11]. Notably, however, is the increase in revision surgeries since 2014, indicating the need for improvements in surgical training and education. With the rise in surgical weight loss procedures, and an overwhelming emphasis on laparoscopic techniques, it is important that surgeons performing bariatric operations are well versed in laparoscopy. Bariatric surgery fellowships or training programs must provide trainees with the knowledge and technical skill to master these complex laparoscopic operations.

How to Train a Fellow

The Fellowship Council (FC) is the accrediting body that oversees the quality of bariatric training and provides accreditation to programs meeting their requirements. In addition to providing oversight on accreditation and curriculum development, the FC provides a standardized application

J. Ettinger et al. (eds.), *Gastric Bypass*, https://doi.org/10.1007/978-3-030-28803-7_39

process for matching surgical residents with advanced surgery fellowships across the United States [12]. There are currently 80 accredited fellowship positions available in bariatric surgery per year in the United States. Among these, 31 are classified as "bariatric," 48 are classified as "advanced GI minimally invasive surgery/bariatric," and 1 program is classified as an "advanced GI minimally invasive surgery/bariatric/flexible endoscopy" [13].

The FC provides curriculum guidelines for bariatric training following the Accreditation Council for Graduate Medical Education (ACGME) core competencies. These include teaching the basic principles of patient care, meeting medical knowledge competencies, professionalism and practice-based competencies, and interpersonal and communications skills competencies, among others [14]. The current curriculum guidelines for bariatric surgery consist of five units, each with three subunits: objectives, content, and clinical skills. Table 39.1 summarizes Fellowship Council curriculum guidelines for an accredited program in bariatric surgery [15].

Although there is often an emphasis on case volume, bariatric fellowship training must be multifaceted and provide the necessary tools to cultivate a proficient and well-rounded bariatric surgeon. In addition to technical skill competencies, there should be an emphasis on patient care, didactic educational conferences, professionalism/leadership building, and research experience [16].

ASMBS guidelines list a variety of nonclinical endeavors that fellows should engage in. These include didactic educational sessions encompassing all aspects of bariatric surgery from patient care and medical knowledge to understanding how to organize and lead a bariatric practice [16]. These critical topics are available in *The ASMBS Textbook of Bariatric Surgery* and should be discussed at weekly didactic sessions. It is important to engage and involve all members of the bariatric team including residents, students, and staff. Additionally, these didactic sessions provide a valuable opportunity to present and discuss new and relevant scientific studies in the field of bariatric surgery.

Leadership building and research experience should be a critical component to any bariatric fellowship. Leadership should be emphasized on an institutional and national basis. Specifically, if the trainee has an interest in academic surgery, opportunities to build leadership skills such as resident education and leading bariatric seminars should be provided. On a larger scale, the trainee should pursue membership in key organizations such as the American Society for Metabolic and Bariatric Surgery (ASMBS), the American College of Surgeons (ACS), and the Society of American Gastrointestinal and Endoscopic Surgeons (SAGES). Not only will this allow collaboration with leaders in the field but will also provide the foundation and resources to build a bariatric practice. Involvement in research is also essential in enrichment of a trainee's education. Understanding the background process, organization, and implementation of research protocols can aid in preparing an individual for a career in academic surgery. Furthermore, participation in research is a measure to promote advancement within the surgical field.

Although the previously mentioned qualities of bariatric training are essential, the ability to teach the technical skills to perform safe bariatric surgery is the basis of any fellowship. In terms of operative experience, guidelines established by the American Society for Metabolic and Bariatric Surgery (ASMBS) suggest a minimum of 100 cases with 51 as primary surgeon to achieve technical competency [16, 17]. These include exposure to more than one type of weight loss operation, including 50 intestinal bypass operations (Roux-en-Y gastric bypass, one anastomosis gastric bypass, biliopancreatic diversion ± duodenal switch, or single anastomosis duodenal switch variants), 10 restrictive operations (gastric banding by vertical banded gastroplasty or sleeve gastrectomy), and 5 revision procedures [16, 17].

Bariatric trainees begin fellowship with variable experience in laparoscopic surgery. Despite this, most surgeons understand basic laparoscopic techniques. Therefore, the goal of fellowship is to enhance these skills to the level of proficiency. This should be achieved in a controlled fashion with both instruction from a bariatric expert and

Table 39.1 Summary of curriculum guidelines

Unit	Objectives	Content	Clinical skills
1. Understanding morbid obesity	Fellows will obtain an in-depth understanding of obesity and its related diseases, including surgical and nonsurgical treatment of these modalities	A. The epidemiology of obesity, including adolescent and geriatric obesity B. The physiologic and interactive mechanisms of morbid obesity C. The psychological issues associated with morbid obesity D. Identification and management of nutritional deficiencies related to surgery	A. Fellows will apply such knowledge in evaluating obese patients for appropriate management[a]
2. Nonoperative management of obesity	Fellows will obtain and apply a comprehensive knowledge of management options for obesity without surgery	A. Caloric management B. Exercise physiology C. Pharmacologic management	A. Fellows will develop an understanding of various diet and caloric management systems including how they work and short- and long-term outcomes. They will understand the potential complications of low-calorie diets and ability to monitor for adverse outcomes[a]
3. Primary operative management of morbid obesity	Fellows will develop surgical competence through experience with bariatric operations. Fellows will develop the skills and knowledge to evaluate and care for patients preoperatively and postoperatively	A. Fellows must be exposed to more than one type of weight loss operation: (a) Laparoscopic and open surgical access (b) Restrictive operations (c) Gastric bypass (d) Malabsorptive procedures[a]	A. Fellows will participate in weight loss operations B. The fellow should have assumed the role of primary surgeon in the majority of cases (at least 51%), defined as having performed key components of the operation[a]
4. Revisional operative management of morbid obesity	Fellows will develop understanding of revision options, including the benefits and risks of each. Fellows will develop surgical competence through experience with revisional bariatric procedures. Fellows will develop the skills and knowledge to evaluate and care for patients preoperatively and postoperatively	A. Fellows will have experience with procedures for revision to treat complications or failure of previous bariatric surgery	A. Fellows will participate in preoperative evaluations for surgical revision: (i) Order and interpret appropriate testing (ii) Consult with nonsurgical specialists when needed (iii) Evaluate most appropriate surgical options (iv) Educate patient on benefits and risks of each option
5. Management of complications of bariatric surgery	Fellows will gain a comprehensive understanding of the management of complications and obesity-related conditions	A. Early complications (a) Identification (b) Management B. Late complications (a) Identification (b) Management	A. Fellows will demonstrate the ability to detect postoperative complications through history and clinical examination B. Fellows will demonstrate an understanding of the physiologic impact of delaying diagnosis or treatment of postoperative complications[a]

[a]Denotes partial omission. A complete listing can be found by visiting https://fellowshipcouncil.org/wp-content/uploads/2012/02/Bariatric-Surgery1.pdf [15]

self-learning from the perspective of the trainee. Skills education should begin with the simplest procedures and advance to the most technically complex. In the case of bariatric surgery, the skills curriculum should begin with instruction on basic endoscopic skills. Focus should be placed on safe entry and maneuvering of the endoscope, evaluation of endoscopic anatomy, and therapeutic endoscopic procedures. Simultaneously, the trainee should partake in an intensive video review of the various bariatric procedures performed by the trainer's group. It is important that trainers provide videos of his/her procedures with the purpose of allowing the trainee to learn his/her exact technique as techniques may vary considerably among bariatric surgeons. Following video review, the trainee should observe the procedures intraoperatively and take detailed notes to help reinforce the information obtained from video review. Subsequently, the learner assumes the role of the assistant. Once the fellow has become a proficient assistant, opportunity should be given to perform the simpler tasks of the surgery. In the case of a sleeve gastrectomy, the trainee can begin with mobilization of the greater curvature of the stomach and through subsequent cases advance to mobilization of the cardia and finally performance of the entire sleeve gastrectomy. There should be emphasis on technique, economy of motion, and methods to avoid common complications. With respect to a gastric bypass, the less complex steps such as splitting the omentum and measuring the roux limb should be perfected before allowing the trainee to perform the more difficult aspects of the procedure including the retrogastric dissection, creating the jejunojejunal anastomosis, and creating the gastrojejunal anastomosis. Once the trainee has proved that he or she can perform all the required steps in a safe and efficient manner, then there should be transition to performing the entire operation with the trainer acting as an assistant and providing constructive feedback. Ideally, if the surgical procedures are recorded, the trainee can review their own performance and identify areas of possible improvement. This would optimize the learning potential for the training surgeon.

Learning Curve for Lap Roux-en-Y Gastric Bypass

In recent years, the prevalence of morbid obesity has grown exponentially, with the gastric bypass operation now being the most commonly performed procedure in the United States [18]. As surgical treatment remains the only effective method to achieve long-term weight loss, and to lower the burden of comorbid conditions of the morbidly obese patient, there is currently a great demand for experienced bariatric surgeons [19]. With the increasing utilization of laparoscopic techniques over the past decade, the annual number of laparoscopic Roux-en-Y gastric bypass (LRYGB) operations has risen considerably [20, 21]. While LRYGB offers several advantages over the open approach—including lower incidence of wound infections, fewer incisional hernias, decreased blood loss, decreased postoperative pain, and shorter hospital stays—it is a technically challenging operation requiring advanced laparoscopic skills [22, 23]. As such, LRYGB has been associated with a steep learning curve, which can be defined as the average number of cases performed by a surgeon before his or her outcomes are comparable to established benchmarks. The outcome parameters most commonly used to establish this learning curve include operative time, postoperative complications, and mortality.

Several studies have aimed to quantify the LRYGB learning curve, with estimates ranging from as few as 75 cases to as many as 500 [19, 20, 23, 24]. Oliak et al. showed that complication rates stabilized after completion of approximately 75 cases, with operative times decreasing significantly during the initial 75 cases and at a reduced rate thereafter [25]. Schauer et al. found that both complication rates and operative times approached those reported for open gastric bypass after an experience of 100 cases [23]. El-Kadre et al. proposed a learning curve of 500 cases, significantly longer than had been previously described; however, the most drastic reduction in both operative times and postoperative complication rates occurred during the first 100 cases [26]. Most likely, the practical learning curve for LRYGB is somewhere between 75 and 150 cases—a similar conclusion to that reached by Sánchez-Santos et al., who determined the average learning curve to range from 75 and 152 cases based on a systematic review of 14 reports describing 18 learning curves [27].

Completion of a 1-year fellowship in bariatric and minimally invasive surgery has been shown to substantially lessen the learning curve burden for LRYGB, as demonstrated by decreased operative times, lower postoperative complication rates, and diminished mortality during a surgeon's early experience as an independent practitioner [21, 27, 28]. While there remains other methods for obtaining training in laparoscopic bariatric surgery—such as a 2-day weekend course or mini-fellowships of various durations—these modalities do not provide sufficient training to begin performing bariatric surgery independently [20, 29]. Oliak et al. demonstrated fellowship training reduced operative times by 35% and major complications by 38% over a surgeon's initial 75 LRYGB procedures [28]. Sánchez-Santos et al. likewise showed that formal training with mentoring by an experienced bariatric surgeon reduces the learning curve of LRYGB by more than ten cases [27]. Of note, even though formal bariatric training can improve the learning curve for LRYGB, the number of cases required to master the operation may exceed the 50 case threshold for hospital credentialing, as recommended by the ASMBS [30]. While this result could be interpreted as evidence that a higher case volume is required to achieve benchmark outcomes, it is clear that the completion of a 1-year fellowship in bariatric and minimally invasive surgery was sufficient to allow recent fellowship graduates to achieve quality outcomes in independent surgical practice.

Minimum Requirements for Credentialing

In 2013, with the role of laparoscopy continuing to grow within the field of bariatric surgery, three national surgery associations—the American Society for Metabolic and Bariatric Surgery (ASMBS), the Society of American Gastrointestinal and Endoscopic Surgeons (SAGES), and the American College of Surgeons (ACS)—collaborated to create credentialing guidelines to assist institutions in the credentialing process for bariatric and minimally invasive surgery [31]. These guidelines have been widely endorsed by the ASMBS, SAGES, ACS, and the Society for Surgery of the Alimentary Tract (SSAT). Beyond defining the general credentialing requirements for bariatric surgeons, the joint task force additionally recommended the following criteria (taken directly from the joint task force's recommendations) for surgeons with no or limited experience in bariatric surgery or advanced laparoscopic surgery [31]:

1. The applicant surgeon must complete a structured training curriculum in bariatric surgery and advanced laparoscopic surgery as reviewed and approved by the bariatric medical director.
2. The applicant surgeon must have completed a general surgery residency.
3. The applicant surgeon's initial cases should be performed with a co-surgeon who is a fully credentialed bariatric surgeon.
4. The absolute number of cases is left up to the local credentialing committee. However, the local credentialing committees may wish to delineate separate requirements for those procedures that require gastrointestinal stapling versus those that do not.
5. It is advisable that the first cases be of lower technical difficulty with carefully determined lower risk patients as determined by the bariatric medical director.
6. The surgeon will actively participate with the MBSAQIP program and adhere to its standards by implementing changes in practice in accordance with feedback from the MBSAQIP or an equivalent regional/national quality improvement program.

Under these credentialing guidelines, the following procedures qualify as bariatric procedures (open or laparoscopic): adjustable gastric banding, biliopancreatic diversion with duodenal switch, revisional bariatric surgery, Roux-en-Y gastric bypass, sleeve gastrectomy, and vertical banded gastroplasty [31]. Local credentialing committees, however, may wish to create separate requirements for those procedures that require gastrointestinal stapling versus those that do not. For example, the ASMBS recommends that surgeons with privileges to perform open and advanced laparoscopic surgery must document 50 cases with satisfactory outcomes during their surgical residency or post-residency training in order to obtain privileges for procedures involving stapling or division of the GI tract [30]. This compares to just ten documented procedures with satisfactory outcomes, without requiring privileges to perform open bariatric procedures, if obtaining credentials to perform bariatric operations does not involve stapling or the division of the GI tract [30].

Of note, the guidelines established by the joint task force do not cover endoluminal bariatric procedures. Endoluminal procedures should be credentialed under endoscopic privileges [31]. The joint task force recommends that practitioners performing endoluminal bariatric procedures should be credentialed to perform bariatric surgery at that institution and, if not, that they should be an active member of an accredited, structured bariatric program [31]. In 2009, SAGES released a more algorithmic set of guidelines detailing the minimum requirements for granting laparoscopic privileges based on the candidate's previous experience with bariatric and laparoscopic procedures [29]. Mandatory for all candidates are the completion of formal residency training in general surgery as well as being part of a team that is dedicated to the long-term follow-up of the bariatric surgical patient.

When training a bariatric surgery fellow, institutions must adhere to nationally developed guidelines. With laparoscopic and minimally invasive procedures on the rise, the bariatric trainee must master surgical techniques and patient management. Trainees must be involved in non-operative patient management including preoperative evaluations and workups as well as postoperative management. The ASMBS requires that trainees perform a minimum of 100 cases. The trainee must lead the operation for 51 cases as the primary surgeon. Surgical exposure is required for both restrictive and malabsorptive procedures with at least 80% performed laparoscopic or robotic; 10 must be the sleeve gastrectomy, and at least 50 procedures must require an anastomosis [31].

Once bariatric privileges (open or laparoscopic) have been granted, the joint task force provided the following criteria (taken directly from the joint task force's recommendations) for maintenance and renewal of privileges [31]:

1. Privileges to perform bariatric surgery should be renewed at a minimum of every 2 years.
2. Maintenance of certification by the American Board of Surgery or its equivalent.
3. Continued active participation within a structured bariatric surgery program.
4. Ongoing participation with the MBSAQIP program or an equivalent regional/national quality improvement program.
5. The surgeon must demonstrate continued critical assessment of his/her outcomes as determined by periodic review of outcomes from an acceptable regional or national registry.
6. The chief of surgery or his/her designee should verify that these criteria have been met.

Reviewing outcomes is of utmost importance to ensure one is maintaining high-quality care. Created in 2012, the Metabolic and Bariatric Surgery Accreditation and Quality Improvement Program (MBSAQIP) encourages institutions to maintain the close surveillance of surgical outcomes to decrease morbidity and mortality rates after bariatric operations. It is recommended that surgeons practicing bariatric surgery are affiliated with institutions utilizing MBSAQIP or an additional national data registry to monitor and track outcomes [32]. SAGES recommends that the institution review the surgeon's outcome data within 6 months of initiation of a new program and at regular intervals thereafter, to ensure that patient safety is comparable to published outcome benchmarks. ASMBS also recommends reviewing the surgeon's outcome data after

6 months but with an additional review after the surgeon's first 50 procedures performed independently. Maintaining a data registry in the setting of bariatric surgery has been shown to decrease mortality and improve outcomes [31].

References

1. Fact Sheet. American Society for Metabolic and Bariatric Surgery. Available at: https://asmbs.org/app/uploads/2014/05/Metabolic+Bariatric-Surgery.pdf. Accessed 9 Oct 2018.
2. Weiner RA. Indications and principles of metabolic surgery. Chirurg. 2010;81(4):379–94.
3. Kaplan LM. Body weight regulation and obesity. J Gastrointest Surg. 2003;7(4):443–51.
4. Sjöström L, Narbro K, Sjöström CD, et al. Effects of bariatric surgery on mortality in Swedish obese subjects. N Engl J Med. 2007;357(8):741–52.
5. Adams TD, Gress RE, Smith SC, et al. Long-term mortality after gastric bypass surgery. N Engl J Med. 2007;357(8):753–61.
6. Poirier P, Cornier MA, Mazzone T, et al. Bariatric surgery and cardiovascular risk factors: a scientific statement from the American Heart Association. Circulation. 2011;123(15):1683–701.
7. Encinosa WE, Bernard DM, Du D, Steiner CA. Recent improvements in bariatric surgery outcomes. Med Care. 2009;47(5):531–5.
8. Flum DR, Belle SH, King WC, et al. Perioperative safety in the longitudinal assessment of bariatric surgery. N Engl J Med. 2009;361(5):445–54.
9. Zhao Y, Encinosa W. Bariatric Surgery Utilization and Outcomes in 1998 and 2004. Agency for Healthcare Research and Quality. Available at: https://www.hcup-us.ahrq.gov/reports/statbriefs/sb23.jsp. Published January, 2007. Accessed 9 Oct 2018.
10. Guidelines for Clinical Application of Laparoscopic Bariatric Surgery. SAGES. Available at: https://www.sages.org/publications/guidelines/guidelines-for-clinical-application-of-laparoscopic-bariatric-surgery/. Published March, 2008. Accessed 9 Oct 2018.
11. Estimate of Bariatric Surgery Numbers, 2011–2017. American Society for Metabolic and Bariatric Surgery. Available at: https://asmbs.org/app/uploads/2014/05/Metabolic+Bariatric-Surgery.pdf Accessed 9 Oct 2018.
12. Fowler DL, Hogle NJ. The fellowship council: a decade of impact on surgical training. Surg Endosc. 2013;27(10):3548–54.
13. Directory of Fellowships. The Fellowship Council. Available at: https://fellowshipcouncil.org/directory-of-fellowships/. Accessed 9 Oct 2018.
14. The Fellowship Council Core Curriculum for Advanced GI Surgery. The Fellowship Council. Available at: https://fellowshipcouncil.org/wp-content/uploads/2012/02/Core-Curriculum1.pdf. Accessed 9 Oct 2018.
15. Advanced GI. Surgery Curriculum for Bariatric Surgery Fellowship. The Fellowship Council and The American Society for Metabolic and Bariatric Surgery. Available at: https://fellowshipcouncil.org/wp-content/uploads/2012/02/Bariatric-Surgery1.pdf. Accessed 9 Oct 2018.
16. Core Curriculum for the American Society for Metabolic and Bariatric Surgery: Fellowship Training Requirements. ASMBS. Available at: https://asmbs.org/app/uploads/2018/07/2018-Curriculum-Final.pdf.
17. Fellowship Council Accreditation Guidelines and Definitions (2016). The Fellowship Council. Available at: https://fellowshipcouncil.org/wp-content/uploads/2012/02/FC-Accreditation-Guidelines-and-Definitions-4-2016-Web.pdf. Accessed 9 Oct 2018.
18. Cottam DR, Mattar SG, Schauer PR. Laparoscopic era of operations for morbid obesity. Arch Surg. 2003;138(11):367–75.
19. Sundbom M. Laparoscopic revolution in bariatric surgery. World J Gastroenterol. 2014;20(41):15135–43.
20. Schirmer BD, Schauer PR, Flum DR, Ellsmere J, Jones DB. Bariatric surgery training: getting your ticket punched. J Gastrointest Surg. 2007;11(7):807–12.
21. Ali MR, Tichansky DS, Kothari SN, et al. Validation that a 1-year fellowship in minimally invasive and bariatric surgery can eliminate the learning curve for laparoscopic gastric bypass. Surg Endosc. 2009;24(1):138–44.
22. Kothari SN, Boyd WC, Larson CA, Gustafson HL, Lambert PJ, Mathiason MA. Training of a minimally invasive bariatric surgeon: are laparoscopic fellowships the answer? Obes Surg. 2005;15(3):323–9.
23. Schauer P, Ikramuddin S, Hamad G, Gourash W. The learning curve for laparoscopic Roux-en-Y gastric bypass is 100 cases. Surg Endosc. 2003;17(2):212–5.
24. Ballantyne GH, Ewing D, Capella RF, et al. The learning curve measured by operating times for laparoscopic and open gastric bypass: roles of surgeon's experience, institutional experience, body mass index and fellowship training. Obes Surg. 2005;15(2):172–82.
25. Oliak D, Ballantyne GH, Weber P, Wasielewski A, Davies RJ, Schmidt HJ. Laparoscopic roux-en-Y gastric bypass: defining the learning curve. Surg Endosc. 2003;17(3):405–8.
26. El-Kadre L, Tinoco AC, Tinoco RC, Aguiar L, Santos T. Overcoming the learning curve of laparoscopic Roux-en-Y gastric bypass: a 12-year experience. Surg Obes Relat Dis. 2013;9(6):867–72.
27. Sánchez-Santos R, Estévez S, Tomé C, et al. Training programs influence in the learning curve of laparoscopic gastric bypass for morbid obesity: a systematic review. Obes Surg. 2011;22(1):34–41.
28. Oliak D, Owens M, Schmidt HJ. Impact of fellowship rraining on the learning curve for laparoscopic gastric bypass. Obes Surg. 2004;14(2):197–200.

29. Guideline for Institutions Granting Bariatric Privileges Utilizing Laparoscopic Techniques. SAGES. Available at: https://www.sages.org/publications/guidelines/guidelines-for-institutions-granting-bariatric-privileges-utilizing-laparoscopic-techniques/. Published July, 2009. Accessed 12 Oct 2018.
30. Granting Privileges in Bariatric Surgery. ASMBS. Available at: https://asmbs.org/resources/granting-privileges-in-bariatric-surgery. Published January, 2006. Accessed 12 Oct 2018.
31. Joint Task Force Recommendations for Credentialing of Bariatric Surgeons. ASMBS. Available at: https://asmbs.org/resources/joint-task-force-recommendations-for-credentialing-of-bariatric-surgeons. Published June, 2013. Accessed 12 Oct 2018.
32. Metabolic and Bariatric Surgery Accreditation and Quality Improvement Program. American College of Surgeons. Available at: https://www.facs.org/quality-programs/mbsaqip. Accessed 12 Oct 2018.

Training and Credentialing the Robotic Bariatric Surgeon

40

Kais A. Rona, Matthew N. Marturano,
Leland P. Chan, and Christopher G. DuCoin

Introduction

Robotic surgery debuted in medical literature in 1985 with the use of the Programmable Universal Machine for Assembly 560 for a neurosurgical biopsy. Since its debut, robotic surgery has transformed multiple aspects of patient care and become a significant contribution to the technical toolkit available to surgeons, finding traction in fields like bariatric surgery, orthopedic surgery, urology, and otolaryngology. Between 2000 and 2013 alone, there were over 1.745 million documented robotic surgical cases in the United States. Robotic surgery, as identified by the Society of American Gastrointestinal and Endoscopic Surgeons (SAGES), is any surgical technology that places a computer-assisted electromechanical device between surgeon and patient and that assumes at least a degree of partial control of the operation that was previously reserved explicitly for the surgeon. The US Food and Drug Administration (FDA) currently approve Intuitive Surgical's da Vinci robotic system, TransEnterix's Senhance Laparoscopy System, and Stryker's (formerly Mako's) RIO Robotic Surgery System.

In the past decade, bariatric surgery has steadily grown. Though the incidence of bariatric surgery appeared to have plateaued between 2003 and 2010 at 113,000 cases per year, the American Society for Metabolic and Bariatric Surgery (ASMBS) estimates that between 2011 and 2017 the incidence has increased to over 191,000 cases per year. Bariatric surgery has increasingly utilized robotic systems due to their comparative or lower adverse events rates and a shorter learning curve when compared to laparoscopic surgical techniques. As robotic surgery has gained popularity and utility, a growing need for credentialing and training surgeons in the use of such devices presented itself. The FDA currently places the responsibility of training development and implementation on the shoulders of the robot manufacturers, physicians, and the healthcare facilities where robotic surgery is utilized [1]. As such, no single federal mandate currently exists to describe the specific training requirements. Multiple agencies, including the manufacturers themselves, SAGES and ASMBS, have published guidelines they believe will help standardize this new technology and its learning curve.

K. A. Rona
Department of Surgery, Tulane Medical Center, New Orleans, LA, USA

M. N. Marturano · L. P. Chan
Department of Surgery, Tulane University School of Medicine, New Orleans, LA, USA

C. G. DuCoin (✉)
Department of Surgery, University of South Florida, Tampa, FL, USA
e-mail: CDucoin@health.usf.edu

J. Ettinger et al. (eds.), *Gastric Bypass*, https://doi.org/10.1007/978-3-030-28803-7_40

Intuitive Company Credentialing

As required by the FDA, Intuitive requires and provides a training curriculum for prospective surgeons [2]. This curriculum is the foundation for all robotic surgeries and does not vary based on subspecialty. Thus following credentialing through Intuitive, fellowship training should proceed the same as laparoscopic bariatric surgery: beginning at bedside and then performing more difficult and complex portions of bariatric surgery gradually. Instructions and the online modules are provided by Intuitive from their website at www.davincisurgerycommunity.com.

Intuitive Surgical's curriculum is composed of the following four components: online modules, skills simulator, bedside cases/precepted cases, and continuing education classes. Initially, fellows are required to complete all online training modules (for both Xi and Si robots) – this will familiarize the surgeon with the console and operation system. Upon completion of the assessments, the surgeon will receive a training certificate. With this training certificate, the surgeon must complete all the skills simulator modules on the robotic training system with a score of 90% or higher. This will instruct the surgeon regarding the manual operation of the robot (clutch, manipulate camera, switch between robot arms, robotic suturing, etc.). After completing the online modules and the skills simulator, the surgeon should be at bedside for at least 10 cases and then on the console for at least 20 cases. With the completion of all these requirements, the surgeon is prepared to use the da Vinci robotic surgery system. For additional training, Intuitive company hosts many advanced robotics courses specific to bariatric surgery in multiple cities across the United States. This would be of benefit to the fellow to gain an understanding of port placement (as it differs from common laparoscopic port placement) and robotic instruments used and learn useful tips/tricks from expert robotic bariatric surgeons [3].

Progression Through Surgical Steps

Like any other surgical procedure, the approach to robotic bariatric surgery training should occur in a stepwise progression with graduated responsibility for the training bariatric surgeon. It is extremely important to stress the importance of self-motivated learning which should occur outside of the operating room. As discussed in the section on laparoscopic bariatric training, a thorough understanding of gastrointestinal anatomy, the pathophysiology and systemic effects of morbid obesity, and the role of surgical management should be obtained prior to pursuing the technical skills required to perform bariatric surgery. Prior to assuming the role of primary surgeon, the training bariatric surgeon should have obtained a certificate of completion of robotic training through Intuitive. Involvement in a specific robotic bariatric course would likely be more beneficial once the training surgeon is reaching the end of his/her fellowship and has a better grasp of both robotic and bariatric surgery.

A learning tool often not utilized sufficiently in surgical training is video review of operative procedures. Even prior to playing the role of operative assistant, the learner should ideally review his/her trainer's technique for common bariatric procedures (sleeve gastrectomy/Roux-en-Y gastric bypass) through intensive and repeated review of the trainer's videos. This would require the trainer to record his/her most common bariatric procedures, but would also prepare the trainee to become an efficient assistant. Once the video review phase is complete, the trainee should observe the trainer in the operating room. This would be to gain an understanding of operative setup, trocar placement, instrument preferences, and ultimately reconfirm the operative steps.

At the point that the trainee has developed familiarity with the steps of the operation he or she should transition to the second phase, which would be the role of the assistant. As the assistant, the trainee can obtain firsthand experience with critical technical aspects such as trocar placement, instrument handling, facilitating the operation for the primary surgeon, and developing an appreciation for the nuances of bariatric surgery. Given the complexity of the Roux-en-Y gastric bypass, experience with the sleeve gastrectomy should precede that of the bypass. Upon achieving proficiency as the first assistant, the trainee can assume the role of the primary surgeon for specific portions of the procedure beginning with the least difficult and transitioning to the most technically complex. The robotic console is unique in that the trainer can easily share the surgeon role and also manipulate the third arm while the trainee is in the surgeon role. In the case of a sleeve gastrectomy, the trainee can begin with mobilization of the greater curvature of the stomach and through subsequent cases advance to mobilization of the cardia and finally performance of the sleeve gastrectomy. There should be emphasis on technique, efficiency, and avoidance of common mistakes. With respect to a gastric bypass, the less complex steps such as splitting the omentum and measuring the roux limb should be perfected before allowing the trainee to perform the more difficult aspects of the procedure including the retrogastric dissection, creating the jejunojejunal anastomosis, and creating the gastrojejunal anastomosis. Once the trainee has proved that he or she can perform all the required steps in a safe and efficient manner, then there should be transition to performing the entire operation with the trainer acting as an assistant and providing constructive feedback. Ideally, if the surgical procedures are recorded, the trainee can review their own performance and identify areas of possible improvement. This would optimize the learning potential for the training surgeon.

Vetting of Credentials

The process of credentialing and granting privileges to bariatric surgeons should be stringent but not significantly limiting as the need for bariatric surgeons increases with the rising obesity epidemic in the nation. The surgeon should demonstrate technical proficiency in the surgical management of bariatric patients, in addition to possessing the knowledge to perform adequate preoperative workup and manage postoperative complications [4].

Although the credentialing process may vary from institution to institution, and is ultimately decided by administrative officials or a credentialing committee, there are guidelines set forth by the major bariatric surgical societies that provide a basic groundwork [4–6]. In 2013, a Joint Task Force composed of leadership from national surgical societies including the ASMBS, American College of Surgeons (ACS), and SAGES established uniform guidelines to aid in the credentialing process of bariatric surgeons [7]. By consolidating the unique credentialing guidelines of the three surgical societies, this facilitated the credentialing process for institutions.

An important factor in the credentialing of bariatric surgeons involves the ability to track and monitor patient data. The Metabolic and Bariatric Surgery Accreditation and Quality Improvement Program (MBSAQIP), introduced in 2012, was a quality improvement program that encouraged close data collection and outcome surveillance in patients undergoing bariatric surgery [8]. It is strongly recommended that bariatric surgeons practice in an institution that utilizes the MBSAQIP or a national data registry to closely monitor outcomes as this has been shown to significantly improve patient outcomes and decrease mortality after bariatric surgery [7].

The following recommendations have been set forth by the Joint Task Force [7]:

1. Evidence of completion of an accredited general surgery residency program
2. Certification or eligibility of certification by the American Board of Surgery
3. Good standing and current medical license
4. Completion of an accredited bariatric surgery fellowship or supporting documentation of surgical and didactic training in bariatric surgery meeting ASMBS guidelines
5. Clinical experience working in a bariatric program that integrates ancillary staff including dietary, counseling, support groups, and psychological assessments for morbidly obese patients
6. Utilization of clinical pathways in bariatric surgery
7. Privileges to perform gastrointestinal surgery and advanced laparoscopy
8. Participation and adherence to MBSAQIP or an equivalent national quality improvement program

With respect to bariatric surgery training, the ASMBS currently requires a minimum of 100 cases, 51 of which need to be as the primary surgeon. The surgeon needs exposure to both restrictive (at least 10 sleeves) and malabsorptive procedures (at least 50 bariatric procedures that require anastamoses) [6]. Eighty percent of the cases must be done laparoscopic or robotic. In addition, the surgeon must demonstrate training in perioperative care of the bariatric patient evidenced through hands-on experience in preoperative workup, postoperative management of complications, and long-term outpatient care. Early and recurrent review of surgeon outcomes is of utmost importance in the credentialing of a new bariatric surgeon [7]. After the first 6 months, outcome data should be reviewed by the institution to confirm patient safety. Any deviation beyond expected outcomes and complication rates should be identified and addressed appropriately. This process should be repeated after the first 50 cases and in regular intervals to maintain a high standard of care.

References

1. Lanfranco AR, Castellanos AE, Desai JP, Meyers WC. Robotic surgery: a current perspective. Ann Surg. 2004;239(1):14–21.
2. Center for Devices and Radiological Health. Computer-Assisted Surgical Systems. US Food and Drug Administration Home Page. https://www.fda.gov/MedicalDevices/ProductsandMedicalProcedures/SurgeryandLifeSupport/ComputerAssistedSurgicalSystems/default.htm. Accessed 18 Oct 2018.
3. da Vinci Surgery Customer Portal Instructions for SimNow Link. Training. http://www.davincisurgery-community.com/. Accessed 18 Oct 2018.
4. Clements R, Saber A, Teixeira J, et al. Guidelines for institutions granting bariatric privileges utilizing laparoscopic techniques. Society of American Gastrointestinal and Endoscopic Surgeons Guidelines Committee. Surg Endosc. 2011;25:671–6.
5. American College of Surgeons Bariatric Surgery Center Network Program Manual, V4.03–01–11.
6. American Society for Metabolic and Bariatric Surgery. Guidelines for granting privileges in bariatric surgery. October 2005.
7. Joint Task Force Recommendations for Credentialing of Bariatric Surgeons. ASMBS. Available at: https://asmbs.org/resources/joint-task-force-recommendations-for-credentialing-of-bariatric-surgeons. Published June, 2013. Accessed 12 Oct 2018.
8. Metabolic and Bariatric Surgery Accreditation and Quality Improvement Program. American College of Surgeons. Available at: https://www.facs.org/quality-programs/mbsaqip. Accessed 12 Oct 2018.

Mechanisms of Control of Type 2 Diabetes with Gastric Bypass

41

Manuel F. Landecho, Carlota Tuero, Víctor Valentí, Rafael Moncada, and Gema Frühbeck

Mechanisms of Control of Type 2 Diabetes with Gastric Bypass

Noncommunicable diseases (NCDs) are currently a leading cause of morbidity and mortality worldwide and are mainly related to obesity and unhealthy habits. Obesity and type 2 diabetes (T2D), its most deleterious travel partner, represent the twenty-first-century pandemia and have proven to be frequently refractory to conventional treatment. The classic therapies, including diet, exercise, behavior modification, and pharmacotherapy, rarely obtain a sustained weight loss and euglycemia.

Evidence accumulated since the early 1980s [1] has proven that surgery is the most effective strategy to improve obesity and T2D. Initially this observation was taken with caution, due to the high rate of intervention-related complications of the old-fashioned surgical procedures. At the beginning, surgery was reserved for morbidly obese patients, but the improvement of the techniques, associated with the cumulative evidence of the specific benefits on glucose metabolism,

M. F. Landecho
General Health Check-Up Unit, Internal Medicine Department, Clinica Universidad de Navarra, Pamplona, Spain

C. Tuero
Department of General Surgery, Clínica Universidad de Navarra, Pamplona, Spain

V. Valentí
Department of General Surgery, Clínica Universidad de Navarra, Pamplona, Spain

CIBER Fisiopatología de la Obesidad y Nutrición (CIBEROBN), Instituto de Salud Carlos III, Pamplona, Spain

Obesity & Adipobiology Group, Instituto de Investigaciones Sanitarias de Navarra (IdiSNA), Clínica Universidad de Navarra, Pamplona, Spain

R. Moncada
CIBER Fisiopatología de la Obesidad y Nutrición (CIBEROBN), Instituto de Salud Carlos III, Pamplona, Spain

Obesity & Adipobiology Group, Instituto de Investigaciones Sanitarias de Navarra (IdiSNA), Clínica Universidad de Navarra, Pamplona, Spain

Department of Anesthesiology, Clínica Universidad de Navarra, Pamplona, Spain

G. Frühbeck (✉)
Metabolic Research Laboratory, University of Navarra, Pamplona, Spain

CIBER Fisiopatología de la Obesidad y Nutrición (CIBEROBN), Instituto de Salud Carlos III, Pamplona, Spain

Obesity & Adipobiology Group, Instituto de Investigaciones Sanitarias de Navarra (IdiSNA), Clínica Universidad de Navarra, Pamplona, Spain

Department of Endocrinology and Nutrition, Clínica Universidad de Navarra, Pamplona, Spain
e-mail: gfruhbeck@unav.es

J. Ettinger et al. (eds.), *Gastric Bypass*, https://doi.org/10.1007/978-3-030-28803-7_41

has placed it in the T2D management algorithm [2]. Although almost all forms of weight loss ameliorate T2D, several studies have demonstrated that glucose control improves more after Roux-en-Y gastric bypass (RYGB) than with equivalent weight loss by other means. Furthermore, among the currently indicated interventions, RYGB achieves higher rates of diabetes remission than restrictive procedures. Although others like the biliopancreatic diversion are more effective in T2D remission, RYGB is preferred due to the better risk-benefit ratio. After surgery, about 80% of diabetic patients experience full remission of this disease, defined as normal blood glucose and hemoglobin A1c (HbA1c) values. Although not reaching full remission in all, the vast majority of patients enjoyed improvements in their glycemic control and reduced medication dependence. Relapse risk seems to be more closely related to the severity of the preoperative pancreatic disease than to any other predictor, including BMI or weight regain [3]. Of note, this evidence has defined the remission of T2D as a main goal after surgery. Due to its relevance, it is critical to try to predict whether a patient is likely or not to succeed under this point of view. A preoperative tool that describes the probability of diabetes remission after RYGB, namely, the DiaRem score [3], has been described. The DiaRem score stratifies the risk based on a weighted system of punctuation (range 0–22) that stratifies subjects into five groups based on scoring for age, glycated hemoglobin, and the medication used: a score of 0–2 has the highest likelihood of T2M remission, followed by the subsequent groups [3–22] with a decreasing probability of remission of T2D (Table 41.1).

Table 41.1 DiaRem score

Prediction factor	Score
Age (years)	
If age <40	*0 points*
If age 40–49	*1 point*
If age 50–59	*2 points*
If age >60	*3 points*
HbA1c (%)	
If HbA1c <6.5	*0 points*
If HbA1c 6.5–6.9	*2 points*
If HbA1c 7.0–8.9	*4 points*
If HbA1c >9.0	*6 points*
Other diabetes medications	
If not using sulfonylureas or not using insulin-sensitizing agents	0 points
If on sulfonylureas and insulin-sensitizing agents	3 points
Treatment with insulin	
If not using insulin	*0 points*
If using insulin	*10 points*
DiaRem score (sum of individual components) →	

Modified from Still et al. [3]

Additionally, T2D tends to improve rapidly and soon after surgery, even before major reductions in body weight occur, suggesting a weight-independent antidiabetic effect of RYGB.

The effectiveness of RYGB in the management of T2D and the rapidly increasing demand for bariatric operations worldwide have converted the description of the physiological mechanisms underlying these procedures in an important research priority. There are multiple mechanisms at different levels that explain the antidiabetic effect of RYGB that go beyond the loss of excess adiposity, and the combination of all is supposed to be responsible for the improvement of T2D. This combined multi-site effect justifies the better results of the RYGB compared to other strategies (Fig. 41.1).

The RYGB effect on T2D is mediated via the combination of gut-related mechanisms (changes in gut hormones, intestinal glucose metabolism, and nutrient sensing) associated with excess of weight loss, reversion of islet cell dysfunction, and the subsequent effects on glucose secretion and insulin sensitivity, as well as adipokine profile modification, modification of bile acid metabolism, and gut microbiota. All these mechanisms will be reviewed here.

RYGB effects could be classified, based on the temporal pattern, in acute effects that are mainly independent of weight and adiposity and chronic effects that depend on weight and adiposity as well as the functional reserve of the subject before surgery.

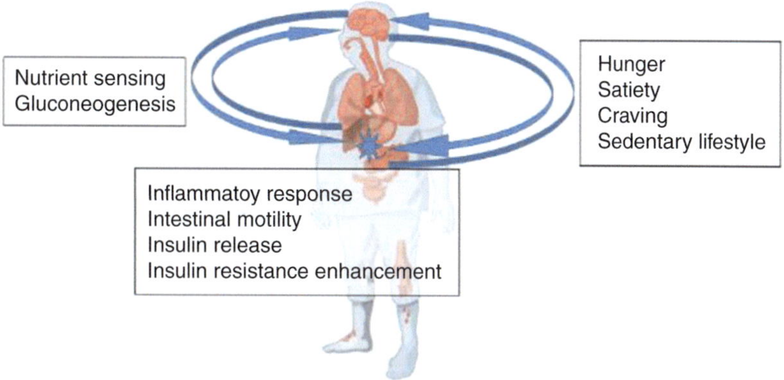

Fig. 41.1 Combined multi-site etiology of obesity and different levels in which RYGB has been shown to exert its effect

Acute Effects of RYGB

Caloric Restriction

The beneficial effect of caloric restriction on glycemia is well established, and RYGB induce significant reductions in caloric intake beginning already in the early postoperative period. The relevance of acute caloric restriction in the immediate improvement of glycemic parameters before weight loss has been stressed with the evidence that subjects under a caloric-restricted diet comparable to the indicated after RYGB display similar changes in meal-stimulated glucose and insulin sensitivity after 4 days [4]. The comparable improvement in glucose tolerance and insulin sensitivity was observed after caloric restriction, and data suggest that decreased caloric intake represents a relevant factor in the rapid improvement in glycemia after RYGB.

Gut

Endocrine Actions of the Gut

Gut Hormones: GLP 1, PYY, and GIP

In this context two of classic hypothesis explaining the possible effects of RYGB in the amelioration of T2D have been proposed. On the one hand, the lower intestinal hypothesis (hindgut hypothesis) which postulates that RYGB creates intestinal shortcuts to expedite delivery of ingested nutrients to the lower bowel that accentuate the secretion of glucagon-like peptide-1 (GLP-1), thereby improving glucose metabolism. In addition to regulating appetite and body weight, elevated levels of peptide YY (PYY) after RYGB could contribute independently to the improved glucose homeostasis. On the other hand, the upper intestinal hypothesis (foregut hypothesis) postulates that exclusion of a short segment of the proximal small intestine from contact with ingested nutrients exerts direct antidiabetic effects, possibly due to downregulation of unidentified anti-incretin factors [5].

Both hypotheses underline the observation that glucose homeostasis is dependent upon a complex interplay of multiple hormones. Some of them exert anorexigenic and/or insulin-sensitizing effects and are enhanced after RYGB. Among them, glucagon-like peptide-1 (GLP-1) and PYY have gained major attention in order to explain RYGB's beneficial effects.

GLP-1 is produced and secreted in L cells of the small intestine in response to nutrients. It exerts a main effect by stimulating glucose-dependent insulin release from the pancreatic islets, accompanied by an inhibition of the inappropriate postprandial glucagon release. This effect is not induced after an intravenous carbohydrate load and explains the greater stimulatory effect on insulin of enteral glucose, compared to intravenous glucose, encompassing the so-called incretin effect. Consistently, blockade of the GLP-1 action results in a significant rise of postprandial glycemia in healthy volunteers. Additionally, GLP-1 stimulates pancreatic beta-cell proliferation and differentiation (Fig. 41.2).

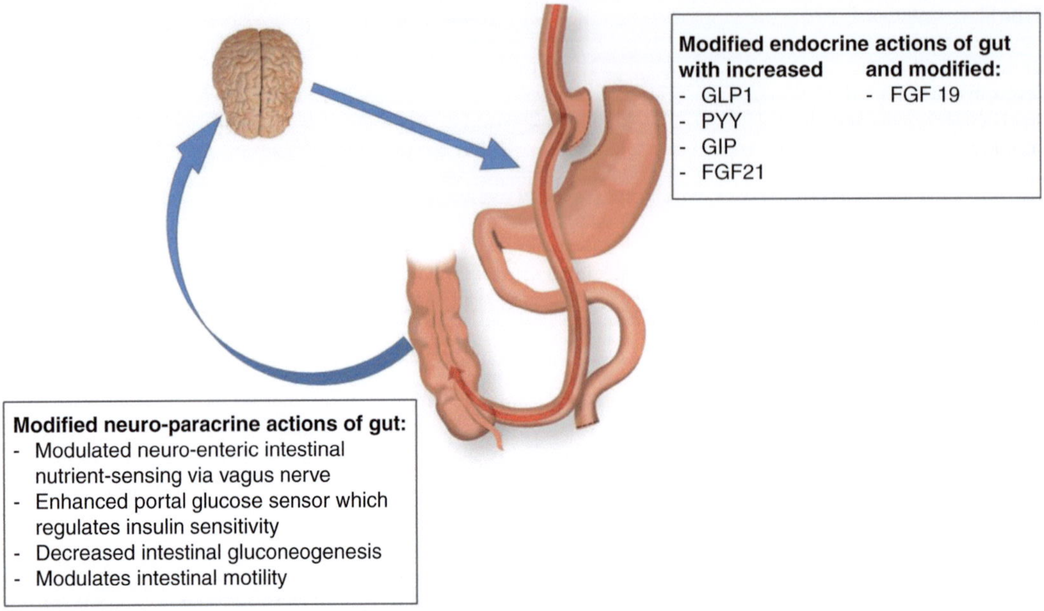

Fig. 41.2 Schematic representation of the neuro-paracrine and endocrine actions that RYGB exerts

In patients with T2D, there is an impaired regulation of GLP-1 that is reversed after RYGB. Furthermore, an enhanced postsurgical GLP-1 secretion has been observed. This enhancement appears few days after surgery and has been proven to last at least for 10 years in subjects with sustained T2D remission. Consistently, it has been shown in an animal model that GLP-1 blockade reverses the improved glucose tolerance resulting from bariatric surgery, and the association between the early improvements of glucose tolerance after RYGBP with a larger GLP-1 response to nutrient intake has been proven [6]. Despite this, GLP-1 is not likely to be the only responsible factor of the T2D improvement observed postsurgically, since it has been described that obese subjects who consumed a post-bariatric liquid diet for 4 days replicated this beneficial effect [7].

PYY is produced by the L cells of the gastrointestinal tract and by the H cells in the ileum and colon. Under normal conditions, PYY release is stimulated by the presence of ingested fat in the intestinal lumen, mainly short-chain and polyunsaturated fatty acids [8]. PYY is an anorexigenic neuroendocrine peptide that exerts its function acting on the brain, gut, and pancreas at least [9]. PYY not only restores normal glucose regulation of insulin but also of glucagon secretion that is also relevant in the pathogenesis of T2D [10] (Fig. 41.2).

Elevated levels of serum PYY following bariatric surgery has been documented, with an increase that is maintained in the long term [11]. The chronic exposure to elevated levels of PYY may be important in the restoration of β-cell functional identity via the NPY receptor 1 [12]. RYGB surgery induces a significant improvement in pancreatic islet structure and function in diabetic GK rats within 10–14 days of the intervention [13]. The rise in PYY levels appear to be a main mediator in the long-term improvement of glucose metabolism, since PYY does not affect glucose metabolism when applied acutely [14].

The increase in circulating PYY concentrations is also believed to be a relevant factor for the "ileal brake," which refers to the inhibition of some gastrointestinal processes, mainly gastric emptying and intestinal motility, thus delaying the delivery of additional food to the intestine. This also decreases circulating fatty acids and consequently increases postprandial insulin sensitivity. PYY also signals to the hypothalamus to reduce food intake and is able to inhibit vagally stimulated gastric acid secretion and pancreatic exocrine secretion and act as a potent vasoconstrictor in many vascular beds. Circulating PYY levels are drastically reduced in obesity and T2D. On the other hand, it has been described that conditions that impair food absorption might increase blood levels of PYY. Consistently RYGB has been shown to increase circulating levels of PYY shortly after surgery, with a rise that is maintained on the long term [15–17]. L cells of the gastrointestinal tract, and by the H cells in the ileum and colon, are also responsible of paracrine functions and the neuro-enteric axis (see neuro-paracrine actions of the gut).

Glucose-dependent insulinotropic polypeptide (GIP) is another endocrine insulinotropic factor, released by the K-type endocrine cells, located in the proximal gut. GIP exhibits also metabolic roles, namely, control of glucose-dependent insulin and postprandial glucagon levels and fatty acid metabolism. Some data had shown decreased levels of GIP in patients after RYGB and a reduction in β-cell stimulation/insulin release. Thus, it can be suggested that this mechanism can contribute to the early resolution of T2D [18, 19].

Fibroblast Growth Factors

Fibroblast growth factor (FGF) is a cytokine superfamily with a wide range of biological functions including regulating cell growth, differentiation, development, and metabolism. Human FGFs contain 22 members which can be divided into 7 subfamilies based on phylogeny and sequence, namely, FGF subfamilies 1, 4, 7, 8, 9, 11, and 19. Among them, the FGF19 subfamily that includes FGF19, FGF21, and FGF23 works in an endocrine manner rather than an autocrine manner as other subfamily members of FGFs. FGF23 regulates phosphate/vitamin D metabolism in a bone-kidney cross talk [20] (Fig. 41.2).

FGF19 is an ileum-derived enterokine in which circulating plasma levels are inversely related to visceral adiposity [21]. FGF19 functions include decreased gluconeogenesis, increased glycogen and protein synthesis, increased metabolic rate, decreased adiposity, regulation of gallbladder filling, and regulation of bile acid (BA) homeostasis via feedback inhibition of the hepatic BA synthesis rate [22]. Intracerebroventricular administration of FGF19 has shown to increase energy expenditure and to reduce 24-h food intake and body weight, as well as acutely improve glucose tolerance. This underlines the importance of FGF19 in the regulation of the neuro-enteric axis in rodents [23]. On the other hand, in humans, it has been also reported that FGF19 and bile acid levels increase after RYGB but not after intensive medical management in subjects who achieved similar improvement in glycemic control [22]. This different behavior might be among the reasons of the long-term differences observed in the evolution of patients undergoing RYGB (Fig. 41.2).

FGF21 is produced mainly in the liver and promotes fatty acid oxidation, improves insulin sensitivity, and increases energy expenditure, with the consequent reduction in fat mass, which entails improvement in insulin sensitivity, lowering of blood glucose, and reduction in hepatic/plasma triglycerides. FGF21 exerts its biologic actions by binding to FGF receptor 1 in the presence of co-receptor β-klotho, which is a FGF receptor co-receptor with a high expression in the liver, fat, and the central nervous system. Adipose tissue is a main FGF21 target as shown by the absence of metabolic effects in mice with fat-specific ablation of either β-klotho or FGF receptor 1. Consistently, it has been demonstrated that FGF21 induces a shift from white to beige-brown adipose tissue due to an increased expression of uncoupling protein 1 (UCP1) and other thermogenic genes in fat tissues. The primary function of brown adipose tissue is to produce heat, a feature which is achieved through the function of UCP1. UCP1 uncouples oxidation from phosphorylation short-circuiting the mitochondrial electron transport chain, driving a futile cycle that produces heat. FGF21 is paradoxically increased in obesity, suggesting that obesity is an FGF21-resistant state; albeit in humans, short-term treatment with an FGF21 analogue has proven to lower body weight and improve dyslipidemia and insulin resistance in obese patients with type 2 diabetes, despite no significant effect on blood glucose.

The change in FGF21 concentrations emerged as a significant predictor of the change in insulin resistance (HOMA) after weight loss. It is noteworthy that FGF21 levels behave differently after caloric restriction (with very low-calorie diet as well as with gastric banding) compared to RYGB. Calorie restriction results in decrease of FGF21 levels, while they rise after RYGB [24]. This different behavior, the correction of FGF21 resistance, might suggest an explanation for the different evolution of T2D after RYGB as compared with calorie restriction, suggesting a possible role for FGF21 in the rapid improvement of T2D after RYGB.

Neuro-paracrine Actions of the Gut

It has been demonstrated that nutrient sensing and carbohydrate metabolism in the intestine influence glucose control and insulin sensitivity, complementing the other intestinal effects. These mechanisms are believed to be relevant in the improvement of diabetes due to RYGB.

Intestinal Lipid Sensing

Small intestinal infusion of small amounts of lipids triggers a gut-brain-liver circuit that regulates glucose production. Thus, the intestine acts as an early responder to ingested food, heralding the conversion from a nonfed to a fed state and preventing mobilization of endogenous fuel stores after meals. This pathway involves intestinal sensing of fatty acyl-coenzyme A molecules and generates signals that are transmitted, via the vagus nerve, first to the hindbrain and second to the liver. These signals enhance hepatic insulin sensitivity and reduce hepatic glucose output. Thus, the intestine acts as an early sensor to ingested food, and works in line with other mechanisms that facilitate an adequate insulin secretion and function [25–28] (Fig. 41.2).

RYGB, by directly delivering unconjugated nutrients (including free fatty acids which are converted to fatty acyl-coenzyme A molecules) to the jejunum, could efficiently activate a fat-stimulated insulin-sensitizing pathway. The precise mechanism remains elusive, but a possible explanation could be mediated by L and H cells, in which a cell neuronal action has been described, since these cells also express synaptic boutons, neurofilaments, and even synaptic vesicles that connect directly with the enteric nerves, providing a pathway to connect the neuro-enteric axis. Consequently they provide an anatomic rationale to explain other main mechanisms of T2D control after RYGB that are the intestinal glucose metabolism and the intestinal nutrient sensing [9, 29].

Intestinal Glucose Metabolism and Portal Glucose Sensor

Intestinal glucose metabolism depends, at least, upon two main components: the intestinal Na /glucose cotransporter SGLT1 and portal glucose sensors. SGLT1, expressed in the small intestine, is the main responsible for the dietary glucose uptake under physiological conditions, and its duodenal SGLT1 expression increases near to threefold in T2D compared with controls [30]. SGLT1 overexpression leads to increased glucose uptake, in association with obesity and T2D in murine models [31], and is induced by the exposure of the proximal intestine to increased glucose load [32]. Consistently, duodenal exclusion of the alimentary limb in the context of RYGB is accompanied by changes in intestinal glucose transport capacity, with a main reduction in SGLT1-mediated glucose uptake prior to onset of feeding [32].

Additionally, some studies suggest that the small intestine might produce about one-third of glucose after a 72-hour fast due to induction of the expression of key enzymes for gluconeogenesis in states of energy deficit [33]. This gluconeogenesis delivers glucose to the portal vein and, when sensed by the portal glucose sensor, mainly the GLUT2 receptor [34], is able per se to activate the hypothalamic nuclei involved in the regulation of food intake and to cause a decrease in subsequent food consumption [35]. The location of glucose sensors, in the portal vein, has been demonstrated by the evidence that when the portal vein is denervated, the effect of the neuro-enteric axis disappears [35].

Portal vein glucose sensor activation engages a neurocircuit that increases hepatic insulin sensitivity and decreases hepatic glucose output, analogous to the lipid-sensing circuit described above, while also inhibiting food intake [29]. The importance of this effect in the context of RYGB has been stressed in a rodent model, in which authors confirm that a gastric bypass model in mice is able to promote intestinal gluconeogenesis and stimulate the hepatoportal glucose sensor via a GLUT2-dependent pathway [36]. Consequently, the gastric bypass procedure, through the regulation of the intestinal gluconeogenic function, appears to be a crucial actor not only in the control of food intake but also for the regulation of glucose homeostasis.

Bile Acid Metabolism

Bile acids are synthesized in the liver from oxidation of cholesterol and stored in the gallbladder as the main constituents of bile. Bile acids are amphipathic molecules synthesized from cholesterol in the liver. This amphipathic property (that means they have a hydrophobic and a hydrophilic side) is essential for facilitating the excretion of hydrophobic molecules and allowing the absorption of dietary lipids from the intestinal lumen, which has been classically considered as the main bile acid biological function. However, recent progress in bile acid research suggests that they are important signaling molecules that play a role in glucose homeostasis [37] (Fig. 41.3).

Chenodeoxycholic acid (CDCA) and cholic acid (CA) are the two primary bile acids in humans. More than 95% of the bile acid pool is reabsorbed from the terminal ileum and transported back to the liver. A limited pool of bile acids that is not reabsorbed in the small intestine is deconjugated and dehydroxylated by bacteria of the gut microflora, leading to the formation of the secondary bile acids, deoxycholic acid (DCA) from CA and lithocholic acid (LCA) from CDCA. These bile acids are reabsorbed passively from the colon and return to the liver through the portal circulation to exert feedback control on bile acid synthesis. During the second passage through the liver, a small part of the secondary bile acids is again modified by sulfonation or

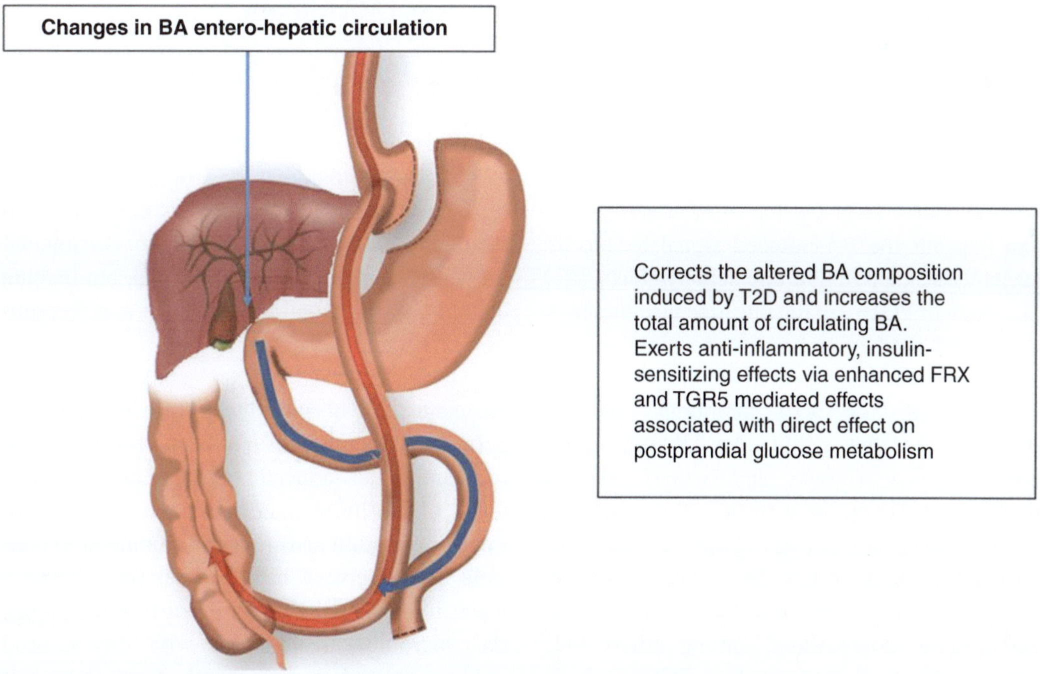

Fig. 41.3 Schematic representation of the RYGB-induced modifications in bile acid circulation

glucuronidation giving rise to tertiary bile acids, which are able to regulate their own synthesis and release.

This enterohepatic circle is altered in patients with T2D in whom, despite an absence of difference in the size of the total bile acid pool, the contribution of specific bile acid species to the pool is altered, with a net effect of CDCA decrease probably due to changes in the gut microbiota. Interestingly, changes in the gut microflora have been associated with the development of metabolic diseases (see below). The relevance of the composition of the bile acid pool is explained by the different metabolic effect of the specific bile acid [38]. CDCA is most effective in activating Farnesoid X receptor (FXR), while LCA, DCA, and CA bind with lower affinity and specificity. LCA is most effective binding the G protein-coupled receptor TGR5.

The nuclear receptor FXR is highly expressed in the liver and intestine, the main sites of bile acid metabolism, but also in the adipose tissue, pancreas, and adrenals [39]. Adipose FXR activation leads to enhanced insulin signaling and insulin-stimulated glucose uptake, acting in an insulin-sensitizing manner [40]. FXR further induces the expression and subsequent secretion of GLP-1 [41] C3 and FGF19. FXR binds to C3 complement genes and induces the rise in C3 that can be observed in the setting of obesity. Circulating C3 might serve as a signal for an immune process that harbors impaired glucose tolerance [42]. On the other hand, FGF19 can transmit the BA-induced signal to specific target tissues and inhibit bile acid synthesis [43]. Secretion of FGF19 in the intestine also increases energy expenditure and reversed weight gain; as a consequence it improves insulin resistance.

TGR5, a bile acid membrane receptor expressed in the gallbladder, ileum, colon, adipose tissue (brown and white), skeletal muscle, and liver, is activated by nanomolar concentrations of LCA and TLCA and micromolar concentrations of CA, DCA, and CDCA. Its activation mediates bile acid functions in energy and glucose homeostasis, among others [44]. Glucose tolerance modulated by TGR5 in high-fat diet-fed mice depends mainly on GLP1 and insulin secretion [45].

Additionally, BA exerts a direct effect on postprandial glucose metabolism. In the context of RYGB, bile diversion affects postprandial glucose metabolism by modulating sodium-glucose intestinal cotransport. The intestinal uptake of ingested glucose is blunted in the bile-deprived alimentary limb (AL) and is restored by the addition of bile or sodium, an observation that stresses the importance of the intestinal sodium-glucose cotransporter [25].

It is noteworthy that total serum bile acid concentrations have been found to be up to twofold higher in the post-RYGB state. The increase in serum bile acids inversely correlates with 2-hour postprandial glucose levels [46] due to the enhancement of all the aforementioned mechanisms. It also correlates positively with adiponectin and peak GLP-1 [46]. All together, these data suggest that modification of bile acid levels and composition may contribute to improved glucose and lipid metabolism in patients who have undergone a RYGB.

Intestinal Microbiota

The gut microbiota has been directly implicated in the etiopathogenesis of a number of pathological states as diverse as obesity, autism, circulatory disease, inflammatory bowel diseases, and type 1 diabetes. The mechanisms through which the microbiota exerts its beneficial or detrimental influences remain largely undefined, but include elaboration of signaling molecules and recognition of bacterial epitopes by both intestinal epithelial and mucosal immune cells [47, 48]. In the context of obesity and insulin resistance, a germ-free mice model has been reported to be resistant to diet-induced obesity, to express lower levels of pro-inflammatory markers, and to have improved insulin sensitivity as compared to controls that receive a high-fat diet [49]. Further, when transplanted to lean germ-free recipients, the microbiota from mice with diet-induced obesity promoted greater fat deposition than

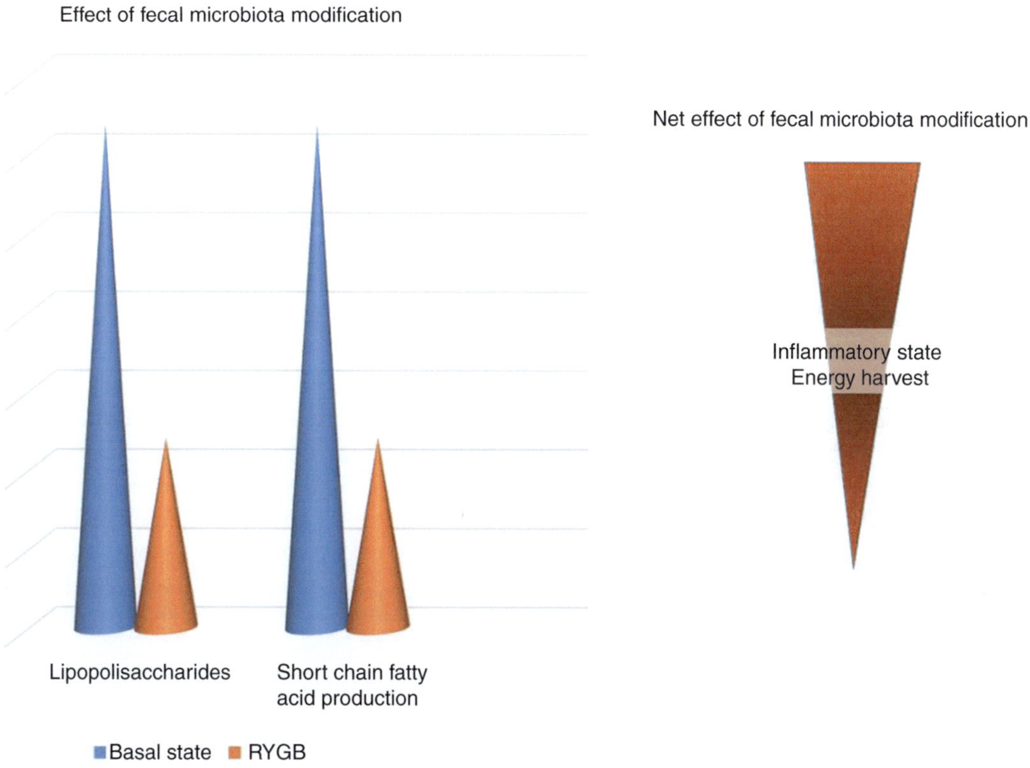

Fig. 41.4 Schematic representation of the RYGB-induced modifications in fecal microbiota

transplants from lean donors [50], suggesting a potential causal involvement of the gut microbiota in weight regulation and the development of obesity (Fig. 41.4).

Several mechanisms have been proposed to explain the influence of gut flora in developing obesity. First, the gut microbiota is essential for processing nondigestible dietary polysaccharides to monosaccharides, which can be absorbed by the host or further fermented to short-chain fatty acids by the microbiota. Short-chain fatty acids serve as substrates for hepatic gluconeogenesis and de novo lipogenesis. Second, the gut microbiota also helps to store calories in adipose tissue since it inhibits the expression of angiopoietin-like 4 in enterocytes. Angiopoietin-like 4 inhibits lipoprotein lipase, the enzyme responsible for the hydrolysis of triglycerides, and enables the uptake of fatty acids in tissues for storage [51].

The development of diet-induced obesity has a well-known travel partner, insulin resistance, and T2D that are also favored by low-grade inflammation [52]. Consistently, diet-induced obesity is accompanied by high levels of lipopolysaccharide (LPS) and other pro-inflammatory markers. LPS is part of the cell membrane of gram-negative bacteria, which are commonly found in the gut microbiota. LPS is able to translocate from the intestine to several tissue sides and, when bound to the toll-like receptor (TLR) 4, trigger a pro-inflammatory response mediated by interleukins 1, 6, and 32 [53] and others, providing a link between diet, microbiota, and insulin resistance. Consistently, inhibition of TLR4 suppressed this inflammatory response and resolved the insulin resistance [54]. In conclusion, chronic higher levels of pro-inflammatory factors such as LPS lead to inhibition of insulin signaling in several tissues, which may lead to insulin resistance and T2D.

A change in the composition of the gut microbiota after RYGB, not dependent on BMI or degree of weight and BF% loss, has been reported. It is also noteworthy that the fecal microbiota modification, which accompanies the metabolic improvement, endures in the long term [55, 56]. The importance of the fecal microbiota in the surgery-related weight loss has been demonstrated after colonizing germ-free rodents with microbiota that had belonged, either to RYGB or obese subjects. After 2 weeks, rodents colonized with RYGB microbiota accumulated 43% less body fat, respectively, than mice colonized with obese microbiota, while mice colonized with RYGB microbiota had the highest average increase in lean mass, with no differences in food intake. In addition, recipients of RYGB microbiota showed a decreased utilization of carbohydrates and increased utilization of lipids as fuel [56]. Among the major changes described, the *Bacteroides/Prevotella* group and *Escherichia coli* species were lower in obese subjects and increased after surgery. The *Bacteroides/Prevotella* group correlated negatively with corpulence (this correlation depended highly on caloric intake); the *Escherichia coli* species inversely correlated with BF%. Lactic acid bacteria (*Lactob acillus/Leuconostoc/Pediococcus* group and *Bifidobacterium* genus) decreased after surgery. *Faecalibacterium prausnitzii* species was lower in subjects with diabetes and associated negatively with inflammatory markers independently of changes in food intake [57]. The explanation for these changes might be due to a decreased short-chain fatty acid production by the gut microbiome after RYGB that entails a reduced energy harvest from the diet [56] and/or the increase in plasmatic secondary bile acid levels of RYGB patients that are regulated by the gut microbiome (see above).

Chronic Effects of RYGB

Islet Cell Dysfunction Improvement

The maintenance of long-term relapse of T2D after RYGB seems to be closely dependent on the preoperative severity of the pancreatic disease and on the pancreatic reserve [3]. T2D progression is accompanied by a decrease in β-cell mass, mainly dependent on apoptosis, while new islet formation and β-cell replication are normal [58]. Several metabolic mechanisms are involved, including mitochondrial dysfunction, oxidative stress, changes in fatty acid metabolism, and increased intracellular Ca^{2+}. Adiponectin, ghrelin, and systemic inflammation have been hypothesized to be the most relevant mediators among the mechanisms that modulate pancreatic beta-cell apoptosis.

Adiponectin is a hormone secreted by adipose tissue that produces beneficial effects on lipid metabolism, enhancing both lipid clearance from plasma and beta-oxidation of fatty acids in muscle [59]. Higher adiponectin levels are associated with better glycemic control, more favorable lipid profile, and reduced inflammation in diabetic women [60]. It has been reported that adiponectin levels rise after RYGB [61] and that adiponectin-induced changes in Akt and ERK signaling lead to protection against apoptosis and stimulate insulin gene expression and secretion in pancreatic beta cells [62].

The second mechanism described that mediates the pancreatic derangement related to diabetes is associated with inflammasome-mediated low-grade, chronic inflammation that may induce pancreatic beta-cell dysfunction and apoptosis. It has been described in an animal model that RYGB also modulates the inflammatory status by suppressing the NLRP3 inflammasome in pancreatic islets and that this effect may contribute to improved glycemic control after bariatric interventions [63].

Ghrelin, which is mainly produced by the stomach, decreases with hyperglycemia and in obesity. It has raised plenty theories about its role in improving glucose tolerance after RYGB due to the variability of ghrelin levels after surgery that depend on the degree of dysfunctionality of the fundus [64–66]. Despite interesting novel theories that suggest a pivotal role of ghrelin in reducing apoptosis of pancreatic islet cells after RYGB surgery [67], no main difference has been observed in the evolution of RYGB depending on ghrelin levels, and thus ghrelin seems not to be the main factors responsible for the metabolic improvement after RYGB.

Adipose Tissue Effects

Obesity is frequently accompanied by lipotoxicity, which entails a pro-inflammatory-prooxidative state that is associated with insulin resistance and pancreatic derangement. This state is mainly due to visceral adiposity, enhanced by a decrease in adipose tissue AMPK activity along with activation of inflammatory genes [68, 69]. AMPK is an energy sensor that restores cellular energy homeostasis. As for the mechanism responsible for the elevated AMPK activity postoperatively, adiponectin, GLP1, and substantial weight loss are candidates [70]. As aforementioned, adiponectin is a hormone secreted by adipose tissue that produces beneficial effects on lipid metabolism [59], glycemic control, and inflammatory profile [60]. After surgery, along with the increased AMPK activity, inflammatory and oxidative stress markers have been reported to diminish significantly [70]. Mitochondrial dysfunction in adipose tissue is among the major adipose tissue-oxidative stress mediators. In adipose tissue, chronic nutrient overload results in mitochondria-driven increased reactive oxygen species leading to carbonylation of proteins that impair mitochondrial function and downregulation of key genes linked to mitochondrial biogenesis. After RYGB, a reduction in adipose protein carbonylation and increased expression of genes linked to mitochondrial biogenesis have been described, starting early after surgery and lasting all along the changes in body composition, suggesting that these mechanisms may collaborate in the postoperative metabolic improvements following RYGB [71].

Conclusions

Obesity is a syndrome that activates a pathophysiological positive feedback circle that induces the development of cardio-metabolic disease that underlies the current pandemia of noncommunicable diseases, which are a main cause of death worldwide [72].

It has been widely demonstrated that nowadays RYGB is among the most efficient treatments for T2D, and evidence has demonstrated that the biliary-microbiota-gut axis is a main organ that regulates food intake as well as insulin secretion and action to improve glucose tolerance. We believe that RYGB exerts a multilinear modulation of all the aforementioned mechanisms that, when combined, act synergistically and achieve the best results in the T2D management currently reported (Fig. 41.5).

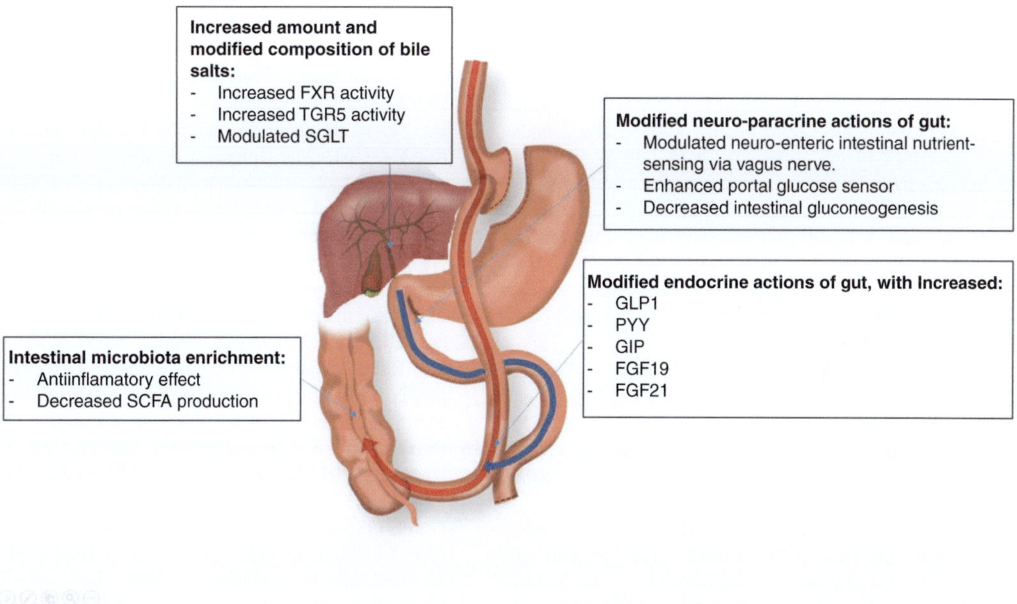

Fig. 41.5 Schematic representation of the RYGB-induced multi-site synergistic effects

RYGB redistributes synchronically and modifies the composition of the products that communicate with the intestinal nutrient-sensing and glucose-control mechanisms. Suddenly bile is delivered at the distal small intestine, which allows a different composition and amount of the circulating bile salts, modifying innate immune response, glucose sensitivity, postprandial glucose metabolism, energy expenditure, and intestinal microbiota. Intestinal microbiota itself is enriched and changes the products derived from their metabolism of the nutrients, leading to less inflammatory and lower-caloric byproducts. The combination of both is sensed in the gut as a less digested content that induces satiety and results in decreased intestinal gluconeogenesis with increased insulin sensitivity, which combined with the less inflammatory and lower-caloric content induces the improvement of diabetes. Additionally, an improved molecular insulin-sensitive phenotype of skeletal muscle and adipose tissue appears to contribute to the improved whole-body insulin action following a substantial weight loss after RYGB [73].

References

1. Pories WJ, Swanson MS, Macdonald KG, Long SB, Morris PGN, Brown BM, et al. Who would have thought it? An operation proves to be the Most effective therapy for adult-onset diabetes mellitus. Ann Surg. 1995;222(3):339–52.
2. Moncada R, Landecho MF, Frühbeck G. Metabolic surgery enters the T2DM treatment algorithm. Trends Endocrinol Metab [Internet]. 2016 [cited 2016 Oct 17];27(10):678–80.
3. Still CD, Wood GC, Benotti P, Petrick AT, Gabrielsen J, Strodel WE, et al. Preoperative prediction of type 2 diabetes remission after Roux-en-Y gastric bypass surgery: a retrospective cohort study. lancet Diabetes Endocrinol [Internet]. 2014 [cited 2016 Nov 3];2(1):38–45.
4. James M. Isbell, Robyn A. Tamboli, Erik N. Hansen, Jabbar Saliba, Julia P. Dunn, Sharon E. Phillips, et al. The importance of caloric restriction in the early improvements in insulin sensitivity after roux-en-Y gastric bypass surgery. Diabetes Care [Internet]. 2010 [cited 2016 Nov 4];33(7):1438–42.
5. Dirksen C, Jørgensen NB, Bojsen-Møller KN, Jacobsen SH, Hansen DL, Worm D, et al. Mechanisms of improved glycaemic control after Roux-en-Y gastric bypass. Diabetologia. 2012;55(7):1890–901.
6. Jiménez A, Casamitjana R, Viaplana-Masclans J, Lacy A, Vidal J. GLP-1 action and glucose tolerance in subjects with remission of type 2 diabetes after gastric bypass surgery. Diabetes Care. 2013;36(7):2062–9.
7. Vetter ML, Wadden TA, Teff KL, Khan ZF, Carvajal R, Ritter S, et al. GLP-1 plays a limited role in improved glycemia shortly after Roux-en-Y gastric bypass: a comparison with intensive lifestyle modification. Diabetes. 2015;64(2):434–46.
8. Adrian TE, Ferri GL, Bacarese-Hamilton AJ, Fuessl HS, Polak JM, Bloom SR. Human distribution and release of a putative new gut hormone, peptide YY. Gastroenterology [Internet]. 1985 [cited 2016 Oct 21];89(5):1070–1077.
9. Bohórquez D V, Shahid RA, Erdmann A, Kreger AM, Wang Y, Calakos N, et al. Neuroepithelial circuit formed by innervation of sensory enteroendocrine cells. J Clin Invest [Internet]. 2015 [cited 2016 Oct 21];125(2):782–786.
10. Unger RH, Cherrington AD. Glucagonocentric restructuring of diabetes: a pathophysiologic and therapeutic makeover. J Clin Invest [Internet]. 2012 [cited 2016 Nov 3];122(1):4–12.
11. Chan JL, Mun EC, Stoyneva V, Mantzoros CS, Goldfine AB. Peptide YY levels are elevated after gastric bypass surgery*. Obesity [Internet]. 2006 [cited 2016 Nov 3];14(2):194–198.
12. Persaud SJ, Bewick GA. Peptide YY: more than just an appetite regulator. Diabetologia. 2014;57(9):1762–9.
13. Ramracheya RD, McCulloch LJ, Clark A, Wiggins D, Johannessen H, Olsen MK, et al. PYY-dependent restoration of impaired insulin and glucagon secretion in type 2 diabetes following Roux-En-Y gastric bypass surgery. Cell Rep [Internet]. 2016;15(5):944–50.
14. Tan TM, Salem V, Troke RC, Alsafi A, Field BCT, De Silva A, et al. Combination of peptide YY3-36 with GLP-1(7-36) amide causes an increase in first-phase insulin secretion after IV glucose. J Clin Endocrinol Metab [Internet]. 2014 [cited 2016 Nov 3];99(11):E2317–E2324.
15. Pancreatic polypeptide, peptide YY, and neuropeptide Y – UpToDate [Internet]. Available from: https://www.uptodate.com/contents/pancreatic-polypeptide-peptide-yy-and-neuropeptide-y?source=search_result&search=pancreaticpolypeptide&selectedTitle=1~19.
16. Nä Slund E, Kral JG. Impact of gastric bypass surgery on gut hormones and glucose homeostasis in type 2 diabetes. Diabetes. 2006;55(Suppl 2):S92–7.
17. Sala PC, Torrinhas RS, Giannella-Neto D, Waitzberg DL. Relationship between gut hormones and glucose homeostasis after bariatric surgery. Diabetol Metab Syndr [Internet]. 2014;6(1):87.
18. Rao RS, Kini S. GIP and bariatric surgery. Obes Surg [Internet]. 2011 [cited 2016 Oct 21];21(2):244–252.
19. Hickey MS, Pories WJ, MacDonald KG, Cory KA, Dohm GL, Swanson MS, et al. A new paradigm for type 2 diabetes mellitus: could it be a disease of the foregut? Ann Surg [Internet]. 1998 [cited 2016 Oct 21];227(5):637–43-4.

20. Cheng P, Zhang F, Yu L, Lin X, He L, Li X, et al. Physiological and pharmacological roles of FGF21 in cardiovascular diseases. J Diabetes Res. 2016;2016:1.
21. Gómez-Ambrosi J, Gallego-Escuredo JM, Catalán V, Rodríguez A, Domingo P, Moncada R, et al. FGF19 and FGF21 serum concentrations in human obesity and type 2 diabetes behave differently after diet- or surgically-induced weight loss. Clin Nutr [Internet]. 2017;36(3):861–8.
22. Sachdev S, Wang Q, Billington C, Connett J, Ahmed L, Inabnet W, et al. FGF 19 and bile acids increase following Roux-en-Y gastric bypass but not after medical Management in Patients with type 2 diabetes. Obes Surg [Internet]. 2016 [cited 2016 Oct 21];26(5):957–965.
23. Ryan KK, Kohli R, Gutierrez-Aguilar R, Gaitonde SG, Woods SC, Seeley RJ. Fibroblast growth factor-19 action in the brain reduces food intake and body weight and improves glucose tolerance in male rats. Endocrinology [Internet]. 2013 [cited 2016 Oct 21];154(1):9–15.
24. Lips MA, de Groot GH, Berends FJ, Wiezer R, van Wagensveld BA, Swank DJ, et al. Calorie restriction and Roux-en-Y gastric bypass have opposing effects on circulating FGF21 in morbidly obese subjects. Clin Endocrinol (Oxf) [Internet]. 2014 [cited 2016 Oct 21];81(6):862–870.
25. Baud G, Daoudi M, Hubert T, Raverdy V, Pigeyre M, Hervieux E, et al. Bile diversion in roux-en-y gastric bypass modulates sodium-dependent glucose intestinal uptake. Cell Metab. 2016;23(3):547–53.
26. Wang PYT, Caspi L, Lam CKL, Chari M, Li X, Light PE, et al. Upper intestinal lipids trigger a gut-brain-liver axis to regulate glucose production. Nature [Internet]. 2008 [cited 2016 Oct 21];452(7190):1012–1016.
27. Rasmussen BA, Breen DM, Lam TKT. Lipid sensing in the gut, brain and liver. Trends Endocrinol Metab. 2012;23(2):49–55.
28. Breen DM, B a R, Kokorovic A, Wang R, Cheung GWC, Lam TKT. Jejunal nutrient sensing is required for duodenal-jejunal bypass surgery to rapidly lower glucose concentrations in uncontrolled diabetes. Nat Med [Internet]. 2012;18(6):950–5.
29. Thaler JP, Cummings DE. Minireview: hormonal and metabolic mechanisms of diabetes remission after gastrointestinal surgery. Endocrinology. 2009;150(6):2518–25.
30. Dyer J, Wood IS, Palejwala A, Ellis A, Shirazi-Beechey SP. Expression of monosaccharide transporters in intestine of diabetic humans. Am J Physiol – Gastrointest Liver Physiol. 2002;282(2):241–8.
31. Osswald C, Baumgarten K, Stümpel F, Gorboulev V, Akimjanova M, Knobeloch K-P, et al. Mice without the regulator gene Rsc1A1 exhibit increased Na+ -D-glucose cotransport in small intestine and develop obesity. Mol Cell Biol. 2005;25(1):78–87.
32. Stearns AT, Balakrishnan A, Tavakkolizadeh A. Impact of Roux-en-Y gastric bypass surgery on rat intestinal glucose transport. Am J Physiol Gastrintest. 2009;297:950–7.
33. Mithieux G, Bady I, Gautier A, Croset M, Rajas F, Zitoun C. Induction of control genes in intestinal gluconeogenesis is sequential during fasting and maximal in diabetes. Am J Physiol Endocrinol Metab [Internet]. 2004 [cited 2016 Oct 21];286(3):E370–E375.
34. Burcelin R, Dolci W, Thorens B. Glucose sensing by the hepatoportal sensor is GLUT2-dependent: in vivo analysis in GLUT2-null mice. Diabetes [Internet]. 2000 [cited 2016 Oct 21];49(10):1643–1648.
35. Mithieux G, Misery P, Magnan C, Pillot B, Gautier-Stein A, Bernard C, et al. Portal sensing of intestinal gluconeogenesis is a mechanistic link in the diminution of food intake induced by diet protein. Cell Metab [Internet]. 2005 [cited 2016 Oct 21];2(5):321–329.
36. Troy S, Soty M, Ribeiro L, Laval L, Migrenne S, Fioramonti X, et al. Intestinal gluconeogenesis is a key factor for early metabolic changes after gastric bypass but not after gastric lap-band in mice. Cell Metab [Internet]. 2008 [cited 2016 Oct 21];8(3):201–211.
37. Nguyen A, Bouscarel B. Bile acids and signal transduction: role in glucose homeostasis. Cell Signal [Internet]. 2008;20(12):2180–97.
38. Prawitt J, Caron S, Staels B. Bile acid metabolism and the pathogenesis of type 2 diabetes. Curr Diab Rep. 2011;11(3):160–6.
39. Lefebvre P, Cariou B, Lien F, Kuipers F, Staels B. Role of bile acids and bile acid receptors in metabolic regulation. Physiol Rev [Internet]. 2009 [cited 2016 Oct 20];89(1):147–191.
40. Cariou B, van Harmelen K, Duran-Sandoval D, van Dijk TH, Grefhorst A, Abdelkarim M, et al. The farnesoid X receptor modulates adiposity and peripheral insulin sensitivity in mice. J Biol Chem [Internet]. 2006 [cited 2016 Oct 20];281(16):11039–11049.
41. Pournaras DJ, Glicksman C, Vincent RP, Kuganolipava S, Alaghband-Zadeh J, Mahon D, et al. The role of bile after Roux-en-Y gastric bypass in promoting weight loss and improving glycaemic control. Endocrinology. 2012;153(8):3613–9.
42. Onat A, Can G, Rezvani R, Cianflone K. Complement C3 and cleavage products in cardiometabolic risk. Clin Chim Acta [Internet]. 2011 [cited 2016 Oct 20];412(13–14):1171–1179.
43. Inagaki T, Choi M, Moschetta A, Peng L, Cummins CL, McDonald JG, et al. Fibroblast growth factor 15 functions as an enterohepatic signal to regulate bile acid homeostasis. Cell Metab [Internet]. 2005 [cited 2016 Oct 20];2(4):217–225.
44. Thomas C, Pellicciari R, Pruzanski M, Auwerx J, Schoonjans K. Targeting bile-acid signalling for metabolic diseases. Nat Rev Drug Discov [Internet]. 2008 [cited 2016 Oct 20];7(8):678–693.
45. Thomas C, Gioiello A, Noriega L, Strehle A, Oury J, Rizzo G, et al. TGR5-mediated bile acid sensing controls glucose homeostasis. Cell Metab [Internet]. 2009 [cited 2016 Oct 20];10(3):167–177.
46. Patti M-E, Houten SM, Bianco AC, Bernier R, Larsen PR, Holst JJ, et al. Serum bile acids are higher in humans with prior gastric bypass: potential contribution to improved glucose and lipid metabolism.

Obesity (Silver Spring) [Internet]. 2009 [cited 2016 Oct 20];17(9):1671–1677.
47. Sekirov I, Russell SL, Caetano L, Antunes M, Finlay BB. Gut microbiota in health and disease. Physiol Rev. 2010;90:859–904.
48. Kinross JM, Darzi AW, Nicholson JK. Gut microbiome-host interactions in health and disease. Genome Med [Internet]. 2011 [cited 2016 Oct 20];3(3):14.
49. Rabot S, Membrez M, Bruneau A, Gérard P, Harach T, Moser M, et al. Germ-free C57BL/6J mice are resistant to high-fat-diet-induced insulin resistance and have altered cholesterol metabolism. FASEB J [Internet]. 2010 [cited 2016 Oct 20];24(12):4948–4959.
50. Turnbaugh PJ, Bäckhed F, Fulton L, Gordon JI. Diet-induced obesity is linked to marked but reversible alterations in the mouse distal gut microbiome. Cell Host Microbe [Internet]. 2008 [cited 2016 Oct 20];3(4):213–223.
51. Scheithauer TPM, Dallinga-Thie GM, de Vos WM, Nieuwdorp M, van Raalte DH. Causality of small and large intestinal microbiota in weight regulation and insulin resistance. Mol Metab [Internet]. 2016;5(9):1–12.
52. Cani PD, Amar J, Iglesias MA, Poggi M, Knauf C, Bastelica D, et al. Metabolic endotoxemia initiates obesity and insulin resistance. Diabetes [Internet]. 2007 [cited 2016 Oct 21];56(7):1761–1772.
53. Catalán V, Gómez-Ambrosi J, Rodríguez A, Ramírez B, Valentí V, Moncada R, et al. Increased IL-32 levels in obesity promote adipose tissue inflammation and extracellular matrix remodeling. Effect of weight loss. Diabetes [Internet]. 2016 [cited 2016 Oct 17].
54. Liang H, Hussey SE, Sanchez-Avila A, Tantiwong P, Musi N, Cani P, et al. Effect of Lipopolysaccharide on Inflammation and Insulin Action in Human Muscle. Wolfe A, editor. PLoS One [Internet]. 2013 [cited 2016 Oct 21];8(5):e63983.
55. Palleja A, Kashani A, Allin KH, Nielsen T, Zhang C, Li Y, et al. Roux-en-Y gastric bypass surgery of morbidly obese patients induces swift and persistent changes of the individual gut microbiota. Genome Med [Internet]. 2016;8(67):1–13.
56. Tremaroli V, Karlsson F, Werling M, Ståhlman M, Kovatcheva-Datchary P, Olbers T, et al. Roux-en-Y gastric bypass and vertical banded Gastroplasty induce Long-term changes on the human gut microbiome contributing to fat mass regulation. Cell Metab. 2015;22(2):228–38.
57. Furet J-P, Kong L-C, Tap J, Poitou C, Basdevant A, Bouillot J-L, et al. Differential adaptation of human gut microbiota to bariatric surgery-induced weight loss: links with metabolic and low-grade inflammation markers. Diabetes [Internet]. 2010 [cited 2016 Oct 21];59(12):3049–3057.
58. Butler AE, Janson J, Bonner-Weir S, Ritzel R, Rizza RA, Butler PC. β-cell deficit and increased β-cell apoptosis in humans with type 2 diabetes. Diabetes. 2003;52(1):102–10.
59. Xu A, Wang Y, Keshaw H, Xu LY, Lam KSL, Cooper GJS. The fat-derived hormone adiponectin alleviates alcoholic and nonalcoholic fatty liver diseases in mice. J Clin Invest [Internet]. 2003 [cited 2016 Nov 4];112(1):91–100.
60. Mantzoros CS, Li T, Manson JE, Meigs JB, Hu FB. Circulating adiponectin levels are associated with better glycemic control, more favorable lipid profile, and reduced inflammation in women with type 2 diabetes. J Clin Endocrinol Metab [Internet]. 2005 [cited 2016 Nov 4];90(8):4542–4548.
61. Chai F, Wang Y, Zhou Y, Liu Y, Geng D, Liu J. Adiponectin downregulates hyperglycemia and reduces pancreatic islet apoptosis after Roux-En-Y gastric bypass surgery. Obes Surg [Internet]. 2011 16 [cited 2016 Nov 4];21(6):768–773.
62. Wijesekara N, Krishnamurthy M, Bhattacharjee A, Suhail A, Sweeney G, Wheeler MB. Adiponectin-induced ERK and Akt phosphorylation protects against pancreatic beta cell apoptosis and increases insulin gene expression and secretion. J Biol Chem [Internet]. 2010 [cited 2016 Nov 4];285(44):33623–33631.
63. Mocanu AO, Mulya A, Huang H, Dan O, Schauer PR, Dinischiotu A, et al. Effect of Roux-en-Y Gastric Bypass on the NLRP3 Inflammasome in Pancreatic Islets from Zucker Diabetic Fatty Rats. Obes Surg [Internet]. 2016 [cited 2016 Nov 4];September(Epub ahead of print).
64. Frühbeck G, Diez-Caballero A, Gil MJ, Montero I, Gómez-Ambrosi J, Salvador J, et al. The decrease in plasma ghrelin concentrations following bariatric surgery depends on the functional integrity of the fundus. Obes Surg [Internet]. 2004 [cited 2016 Nov 6];14(5):606–612.
65. Frühbeck G, Rotellar F, Hernández-Lizoain JL, Gil MJ, Gómez-Ambrosi J, Salvador J, et al. Fasting plasma ghrelin concentrations 6 months after gastric bypass are not determined by weight loss or changes in insulinemia. Obes Surg [Internet]. 2004 [cited 2016 Nov 6];14(9):1208–1215.
66. Frühbeck G, Díez Caballero A, Gil MJ. Fundus functionality and ghrelin concentrations after bariatric surgery. NEJM. 2004;350(3):308–9.
67. Yang J, Feng X, Zhong S, Wang Y, Liu J. Gastric bypass surgery may improve Beta cell apoptosis with ghrelin overexpression in patients with BMI ≥ 32.5 kg/m2. Obes Surg [Internet]. 2014 [cited 2016 Nov 4];24(4):561–571.
68. Gauthier M-S, O'Brien EL, Bigornia S, Mott M, Cacicedo JM, Xu XJ, et al. Decreased AMP-activated protein kinase activity is associated with increased inflammation in visceral adipose tissue and with whole-body insulin resistance in morbidly obese humans. Biochem Biophys Res Commun. 2011;404(1):382.
69. Xu XJ, Gauthier M-S, Hess DT, Apovian CM, Cacicedo JM, Gokce N, et al. Insulin sensitive and resistant obesity in humans: AMPK activity, oxidative stress, and depot-specific changes in gene expression

in adipose tissue. J Lipid Res [Internet]. 2012 [cited 2016 Nov 6];53(4):792–801.

70. Xu XJ, Apovian C, Hess D, Carmine B, Saha A, Ruderman N. Improved insulin sensitivity 3 months after RYGB surgery is associated with increased subcutaneous adipose tissue AMPK activity and decreased oxidative stress. Diabetes. 2015;64(9):3155–9.
71. Jahansouz C, Serrot FJ, Frohnert BI, Foncea RE, Dorman RB, Slusarek B, et al. Roux-en-Y gastric bypass acutely decreases protein carbonylation and increases expression of mitochondrial biogenesis genes in subcutaneous adipose tissue. Obes Surg. 2015;25(12):2376–85.
72. Frühbeck G, Toplak H, Woodward E, Halford JCG, Yumuk V, European Association for the Study of Obesity. Need for a paradigm shift in adult overweight and obesity management – an EASO position statement on a pressing public health, clinical and scientific challenge in Europe. Obes Facts [Internet]. 2014 [cited 2016 Oct 21];7(6):408–416.
73. Albers PH, Bojsen-Møller KN, Dirksen C, Serup AK, Kristensen DE, Frystyk J, et al. Enhanced insulin signaling in human skeletal muscle and adipose tissue following gastric bypass surgery. Am J Physiol – Regul Integr Comp Physiol. 2015;309(5):510–24.

The Gut and Type 2 Diabetes Mellitus

42

Stephen Boyce

Introduction

Obesity and T2DM are among the most devastating health crises worldwide [1, 2]. Diet, exercise, and pharmacotherapy are the cornerstones of T2DM management; nonetheless, long-term success rates with lifestyle modification and pharmacotherapy are disappointing, and long-term glycemic control is often suboptimal. T2DM is a chronic, relentless, progressive disease in which the *delay* of end-organ complications is the major treatment goal. However, bariatric and metabolic surgery offers the promising endpoint of complete disease remission [3]. In fact, numerous randomized clinical trials have demonstrated that bariatric surgery achieves superior glycemic control and reduction of cardiovascular risk factors in obese patients with T2DM when compared with medical and lifestyle changes [4–19] (Fig. 42.1).

Although bariatric surgery was designed to facilitate weight loss, anecdotal reports of rapid postoperative remission of T2DM emerged as early as the 1950s [20]. Similarly, gastrectomy for ulcer disease or cancer has been shown to produce rapid postoperative normalization of hyperglycemia [21, 22]. It has also been observed that operations involving intestinal bypass exert an even greater and more durable improvement on glycemic control than does gastrectomy alone. For example, 84% of obese diabetic patients who undergo RYGB experience complete remission of T2DM and maintain euglycemia without medication for at least 14 years [23–25].

Current research supports the notion that the gastrointestinal tract is an important contributor to normal glucose homeostasis and that bariatric and metabolic surgery is viable for *prevention and treatment* of T2DM [3–19, 26–28] and represents a unique model for studying glucose metabolism. Interestingly, some bariatric surgical procedures employ mechanisms that improve glucose homeostasis prior to significant weight loss [6]. Changes in gut hormones, bile acid metabolism, intestinal glucose metabolism, gut microbiota, and nutrient sensing of the intestines are all mechanisms that have influence on improving postoperative glycemic control [3, 29–38]. This postoperative glycemic control has been shown to be a long-lasting effect, with one observational study concluding that bariatric and metabolic surgery provided sustained improvements in glucose metabolism for up to 20 years [39]. Bariatric and metabolic surgeries have consistently demonstrated superior efficacy in reducing weight and achieving glycemic control when compared to medical therapy and lifestyle interventions alone. These trials

S. Boyce (✉)
Department of Surgery, Turkey Creek Medical Center, Knoxville, TN, USA
e-mail: sboyce@premiersurgical.com

J. Ettinger et al. (eds.), *Gastric Bypass*, https://doi.org/10.1007/978-3-030-28803-7_42

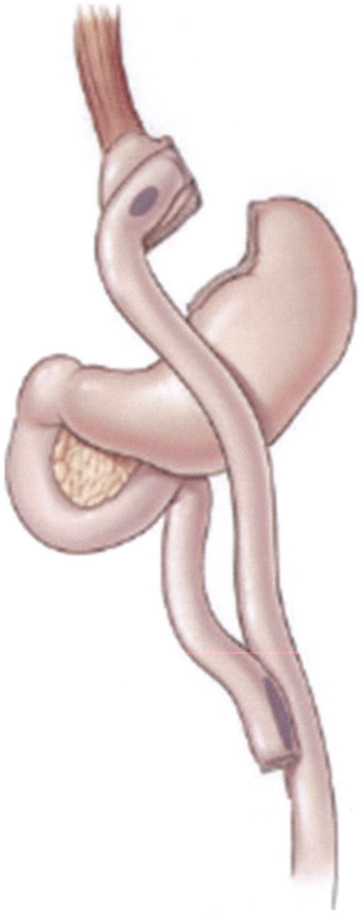

Fig. 42.1 (Used with permission from Rubino et al. [3])

show reduction in the hemoglobin A1c (HbA1c) of 2% for surgery versus 0.5% for conventional therapies ($P < 0.001$) (Fig. 42.2) [4–19, 40].

Though published data reveals that diabetes may recur in up to 30–50% of patients who initially achieve complete remission of T2DM after surgery, the median disease-free period among individuals' status-post RYGB is 8.3 years [39, 41]. Even with T2DM recurrence, the majority of patients who undergo bariatric surgery actually maintain substantial improvement in glycemic control from their preoperative baseline for anywhere from 5 to 15 years [39, 41–45]. In addition to improving glycemic control, bariatric surgery also reduces vascular complications of T2DM, cardiovascular disease (Fig. 42.3), cancer, and death [26, 39, 43, 46–50].

When comparing the efficacy of bariatric surgery to maximum medical therapy in the treatment of T2DM, available randomized clinical trials and nonrandomized studies show surgical efficacy is dependent upon the specific surgical procedure performed. The efficacy of weight loss and T2DM remission following bariatric surgery has been found to be highest with the biliopancreatic diversion (BPD) (Fig. 42.4), followed by the RYGB, sleeve gastrectomy (SG) (Fig. 42.5), and laparoscopic adjustable gastric banding (LAGB) (Fig. 42.6), respectively (Table 42.1) [4–19, 51–55].

Mechanism of T2DM Remission Following Gastrointestinal Surgery

The gut produces greater than 100 known bioactive peptides [3]. Although numerous physiological consequences of bariatric and metabolic operations contribute to the antidiabetic benefits of surgery, the exact mechanisms mediating T2DM remission after the various operations are far from being fully understood [3, 29, 32–38].

Starvation

Before discussing the effects of intestinal bypass on glucose homeostasis, one must consider the antidiabetic mechanisms of starvation. It is hypothesized that remission of T2DM following surgery is achieved as a result of postoperative starvation and rapid weight loss. In this model, T2DM resolves because pancreatic beta cells are no longer challenged with nutrients. By the time the early postoperative dietary restrictions have been lifted, the patient begins to experience the hepatic insulin-sensitizing effects of weight loss resulting from severe energy restriction. Given the known effects of acute starvation and weight loss to improve diabetes, this hypothesis has merit.

In starvation and in the post RYGB patient, there are comparable reductions in insulin levels, basal

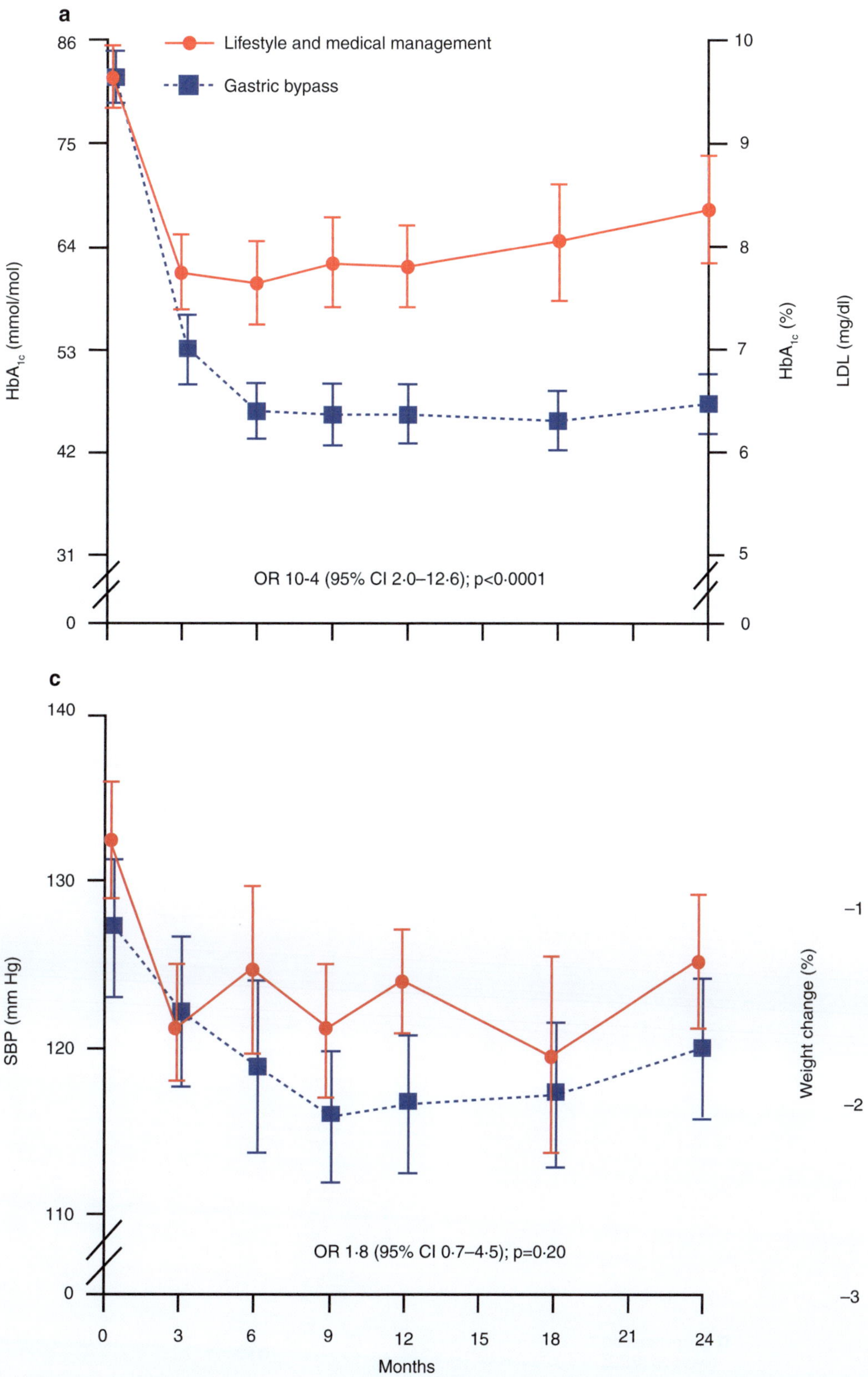

Fig. 42.2 (Used with permission from Ikramuddin et al. [15])

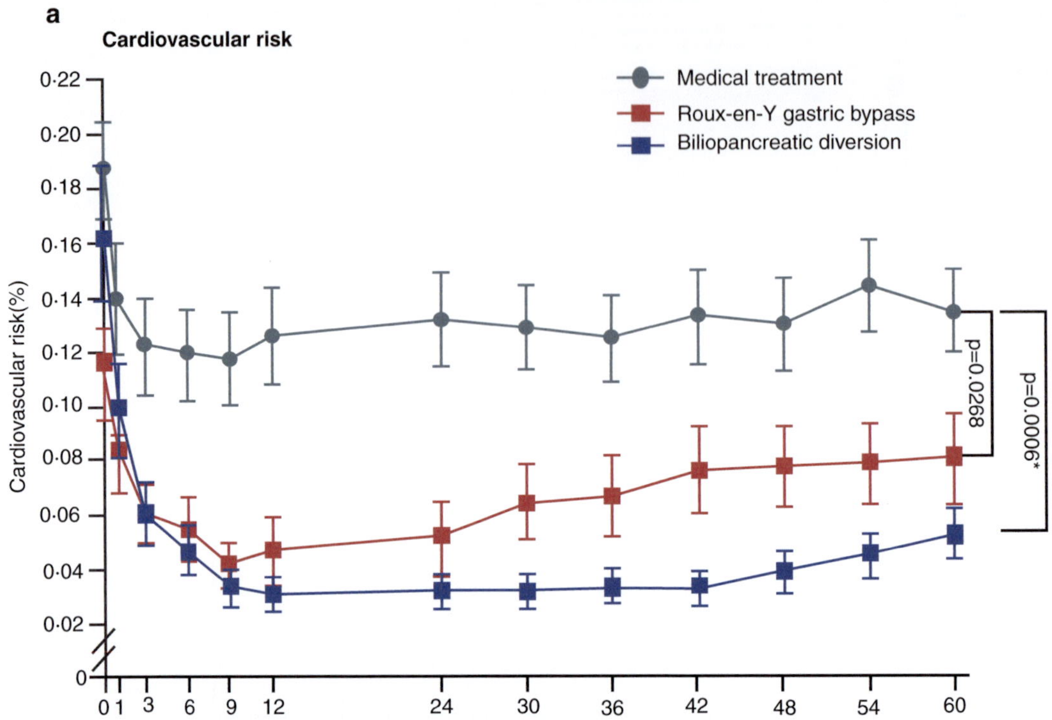

Fig. 42.3 Mean number of cardiovascular drugs (including blood pressure and lipid-lowering drugs). (Reproduced with permission from Mingrone et al. [14])

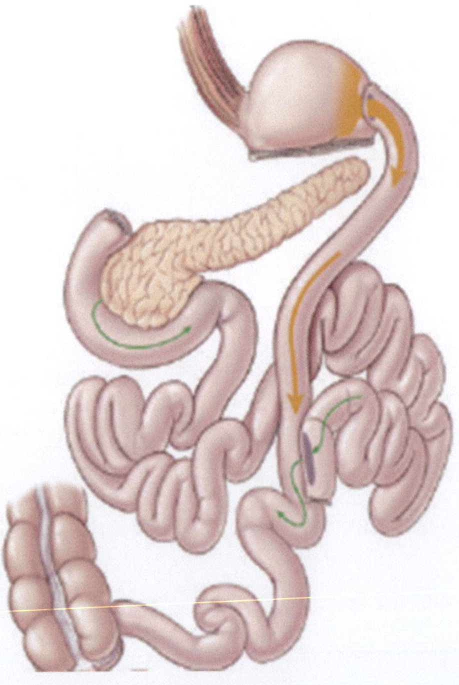

Fig. 42.4 (Used with permission from Rubino et al. [3])

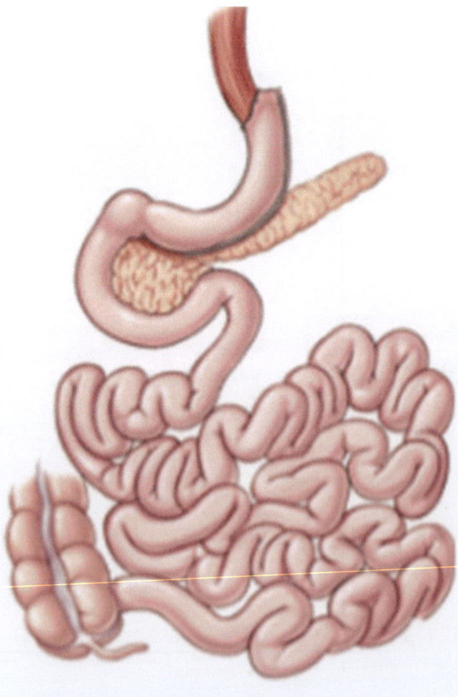

Fig. 42.5 (Used with permission from Rubino et al. [3])

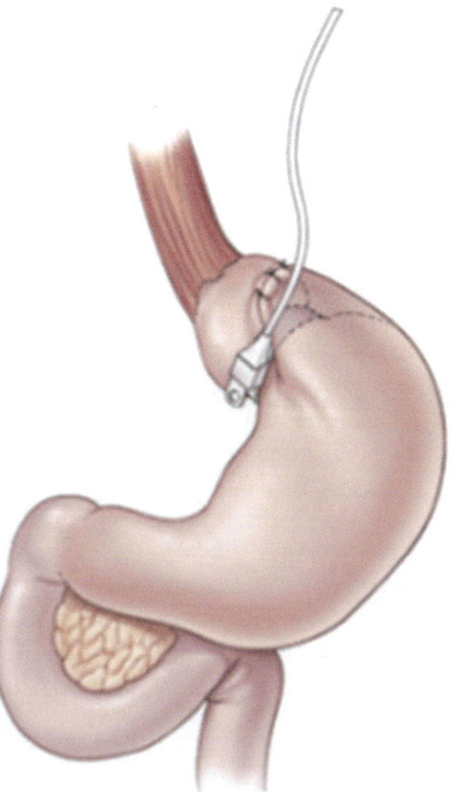

b Adjustable gastric banding (LAGB)

Fig. 42.6 (Used with permission from Rubino et al. [3])

Table 42.1

	LAGB	RYGB	BPD
Resolution of T2DM	48%	84%	98%
Resolution of hypertension	43%	68%	83%
Improvement of hyperlipidemia	59%	97%	99%
% Excess weight loss	47%	62%	70%

Used with permission from Rubino et al. [3]
Abbreviations: *LAGB* laparoscopic adjustable gastric banding, *RYGB* Roux-en-Y gastric bypass, *BPD* biliopancreatic diversion, *T2DM* type 2 diabetes mellitus

rate of hepatic glucose production, and intrahepatic lipid content, and there is increased hepatic insulin sensitivity in obese patients with T2DM after only 1 week [56–58]. Intracellular lipids in the liver and peripherally in the muscle are the most significant known contributors to blood glucose levels and contribute to insulin resistance [59]. Thus, improved hepatic insulin sensitivity induced by postoperative starvation may explain the isolated reduction in the homeostatic model assessment for evaluating pancreatic beta cell function and insulin resistance (HOMA-IR) seen early after gastric bypass.

However, if starvation were the only mechanism at work, one would predict that LAGB patients would achieve similar T2DM remission rates as the RYGB and the BPD. However, T2DM resolves in only 48% of cases after LAGB compared with 84% and a greater than 95% after RYGB and BPD, respectively (Table 42.1) [23]. Additionally, resolution of T2DM after LAGB occurs over many weeks to months, whereas T2DM resolution after the RYGB and BPD occurs almost immediately and, importantly, before significant weight loss has occurred [25]. In a landmark study by Schauer et al., in patients undergoing RYGB with T2DM severe enough to be treated with oral medications and/or insulin, 30% were discharged from their initial surgical hospitalization with normal plasma glucose levels off all diabetes medications after an average hospital stay of the only 2.8 days. Most of the remaining patients discontinued their diabetes treatments within a few weeks. The eventual complete remission rate was 83% [25].

Mounting evidence shows that certain intestinal diversionary operations resolve T2DM through mechanisms beyond weight loss and reduced caloric intake. Data favoring this assertion are derived from the following observations:

- Rapid postoperative T2DM remission before substantial weight loss is common.
- Greater improvements in glucose homeostasis occur after RYGB when compared to equivalent weight loss from purely gastric restrictive operations or nonsurgical interventions.
- Glucose tolerance improvement is found following experimental intestinal procedures that cause little or no weight loss.
- Occasional development of late-onset beta cell hyperactivity is noted after intestinal bypass procedures.

Potential mechanisms underlying the direct antidiabetic effect of RYGB include enhanced nutrient stimulation of the lower intestinal hormones, altered physiology from excluding ingested nutrients from the upper intestines, compromised ghrelin secretion, modulation of intestinal nutrient sensing, and regulation of insulin sensitivity [30, 60–62].

The Stomach

As mentioned above a link between gastrectomy and glycemic control has been recognized for over 60 years [20]. The stomach produces three peptide hormones known to be directly and indirectly involved in glucose homeostasis.

The first, ghrelin, is a 28-amino acid hormone. Ghrelin, the only known circulating orexigenic hormone, is produced (90%) in the stomach and to a lesser extent in the duodenum and pancreatic islet epsilon cells [30, 63–68]. Ghrelin is primarily produced in the gastric fundus, and normally plasma levels increase before a meal and decrease postprandially (Fig. 42.7). Ghrelin is thought to stimulate meal initiation [69–71], and in addition to its orexigenic properties, ghrelin also has the effect of being pro-diabetic through:

- Stimulating insulin counter-regulatory hormones
- Suppressing the insulin-sensitizing hormone adiponectin
- Blocking hepatic insulin signaling
- Inhibiting insulin secretion
- Increasing food intake
- Increasing the use of glucose by adipose tissue
- Increasing cortisol levels

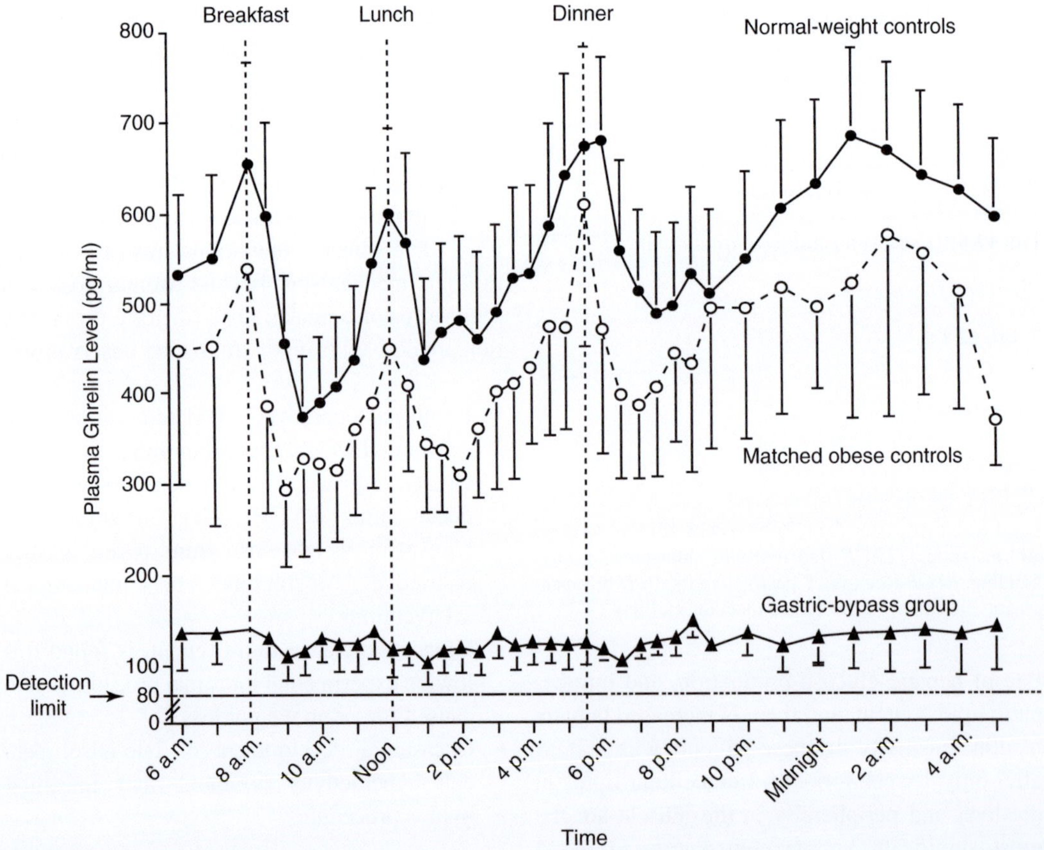

Fig. 42.7 24-hour plasma ghrelin profiles in subjects who underwent gastric bypass and in controls. Reproduced with permission from Cummings et al. [62])

- Increasing epinephrine levels
- Interfering with hepatocyte glucose metabolism [69, 72–76]

Ghrelin plasma levels are generally inversely proportional to the degree of adiposity, yet, immediately after RYGB, plasma levels are relatively constant and may be reduced up to 75% preprandially (Fig. 42.7). RYGB is thought to inhibit production of ghrelin through "override inhibition." Override inhibition is a theory that states that if a hormone secretion is triggered by an episodic stimulus, then its secretion will be paradoxically inhibited when the stimulus occurs continuously. Ghrelin secretion would be stimulated continuously after gastric bypass by an empty stomach; thus, ghrelin levels and its pro-diabetic effect are paradoxically lower postoperatively [69, 70, 77].

Ghrelin acts as an anti-incretin (an incretin is a hormone that stimulates insulin secretion in response to a meal) to limit peripheral glucose use, and the suppression of ghrelin after gastric bypass improves glucose homeostasis [62].

The second hormone produced by the stomach that contributes to glucose homeostasis is gastrin. G-cells in the pyloric antrum, duodenum, and pancreas produce gastrin. Gastrin is stimulated by gastric nutrient exposure, and its effects include satiety, increased gastric secretions, increased pancreatic exocrine secretions, stimulation of glucagon release, and a proliferative effect on pancreatic islet beta cells [78, 79]. Gastrin-deficient mice exhibit mild hypoglycemia and a defective glucagon secretory response to insulin-induced hypoglycemia. This, combined with its proliferative effects on pancreatic beta cells, has the effect of improving T2DM [80]. Grong et al. have recently shown that gastrin levels are significantly reduced after RYGB. This would be expected since RYGB isolates the gastric antrum from nutrient stimulation [81] (Fig. 42.8).

Glucose-dependent insulinotropic polypeptide (GIP) is the third gastric hormone involved in glucose homeostasis. GIP is a 42-amino acid peptide secreted by the stomach, and proximal small intestine K-cells in response to a nutrient exposure and levels are elevated after RYGB. As with most intestinal hormones, GIP's half-life is very short (only about 5 minutes) [82]. GIP potentiates glucose-stimulated insulin secretion through transmembrane GIP receptors (GIPR) located in the pancreas, stomach, small intestine, and adipose tissue [83]. GIP is a classic incretin hormone and acts to increase beta cell insulin release, increase muscle cell uptake of glucose, increase liver uptake of glucose, decrease pancreatic alpha cell glucagon secretion, decrease hepatic gluconeogenesis, and increase beta cell

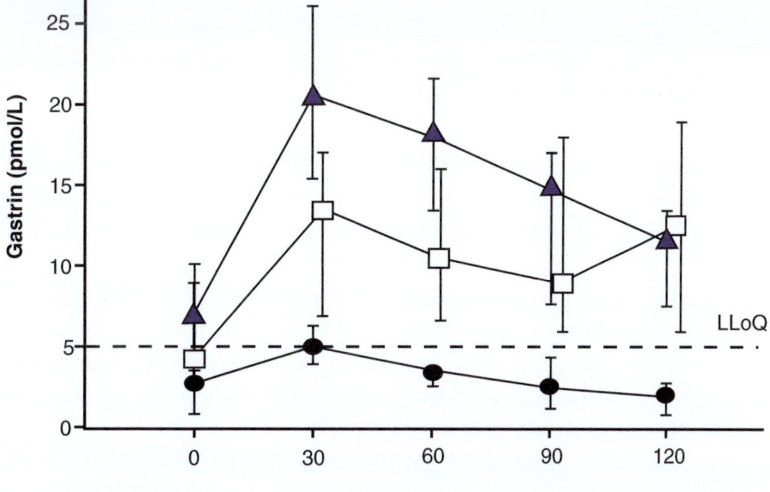

Fig. 42.8 Gastrin levels during mixed-meal tolerance test for control group and Roux-en-Y gastric bypass. (Reproduced with permission from Grong et al. [66])

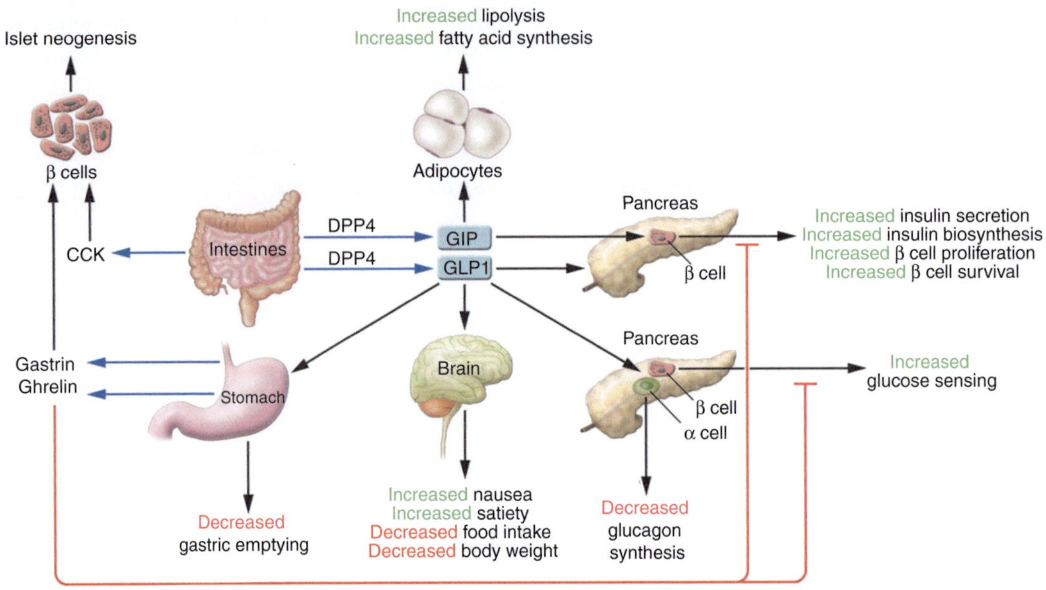

Fig. 42.9 Actions of selected peptides on key tissues important for the control of glucose homeostasis. (From Drucker et al. [84])

mass and pancreatic islets all of which lead to improved glucose homeostasis in the patient suffering from T2DM (Fig. 42.9) [84, 85].

GIP appears to increase beta cell secretion of insulin by increasing the beta cell exocytosis, increasing beta cell insulin synthesis, activating beta cell antiapoptotic pathways, reducing proapoptotic protein BAX, and increasing antiapoptotic protein BCL2 in diabetic rodents [86]. GIP additionally enhances adipocyte energy storage and decreases insulin's effect on adipocytes [87].

The Upper Intestinal Hypothesis

The upper intestinal hypothesis proposes that the exclusion of a short-segment proximal small intestine from contact with ingested nutrients produces direct antidiabetic effects through unidentified factors or processes that influence glucose homeostasis in a manner that is independent of weight loss [30]. The proximal bypass, primarily the duodenum, is short enough that it is unlikely that it would promote rapid delivery of nutrients to the distal small intestine enteroendocrine cells.

Some of the strongest supports for this model come from studies performed with a gastric-sparing variant of the RYGB known as the duodenal-jejunal bypass (DJB) developed by Francesco Rubino. In the DJB the stomach is left intact, and a modest bypass of proximal small intestines is created similar to that in a standard RYGB (Fig. 42.10). When this operation is performed on diabetic Goto-Kakizaki rats, diabetes improves rapidly and durably even though it caused no reduction in food intake, body weight, or nutrient absorption compared with sham-operated controls [29, 60, 88]. Drs. Cohen and Ramos performed DJB on nonobese patients with T2DM. Postoperatively, the patients had lower fasting blood glucose levels, normalization of HbA1c levels (8–9% preoperatively compared to 5–6% postoperatively), and cessation of all diabetic medications with or without weight loss [89, 90].

Additional support for the upper intestinal hypothesis comes from experiments with the endoscopic duodenal-jejunal liner sleeve (ELS), a flexible plastic sleeve implanted in the upper intestine causing food to move from the pylorus to the beginning of the jejunum without coming in contact with intestinal mucosa (Fig. 42.11).

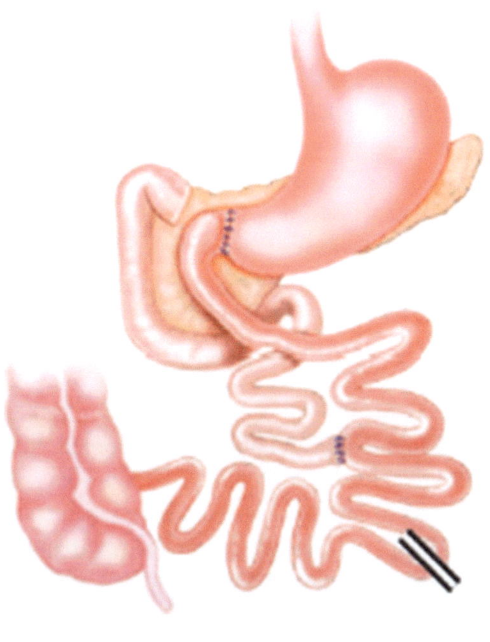

Fig. 42.10 (Used with permission from Rubino et al. [3])

Prospective randomized clinical trials of the ELS produced lower fasting blood glucose levels, improved glucose tolerance, and showed a decrease in the hemoglobin A1c (HbA1c) of 2.9% compared to controls which had a decrease of the HbA1c of only 0.8% with diet and exercise [91–93]. These findings indicate that, if you can keep nutrient exposure from the duodenum and proximal jejunum, it blocks signals that promote T2DM in patients suffering from the disease. Additionally, the antidiabetic effect of the DJB and the ELS is reversed with reconstitution of bowel anatomy or with removal of the endoscopic sleeve [60].

Duodenal sensing of a high-protein or high-fat meal generates neural signals via the afferent vagus nerve to the hindbrain and then down the efferent vagus nerve to the liver, enhancing hepatic insulin sensitivity and decreasing hepatic gluconeogenesis. This normal intestine-brain-liver neural circuit increases hepatic insulin sensitivity and is bypassed by the RYGB and DJB [94]. Bypassing this glucose homeostatic

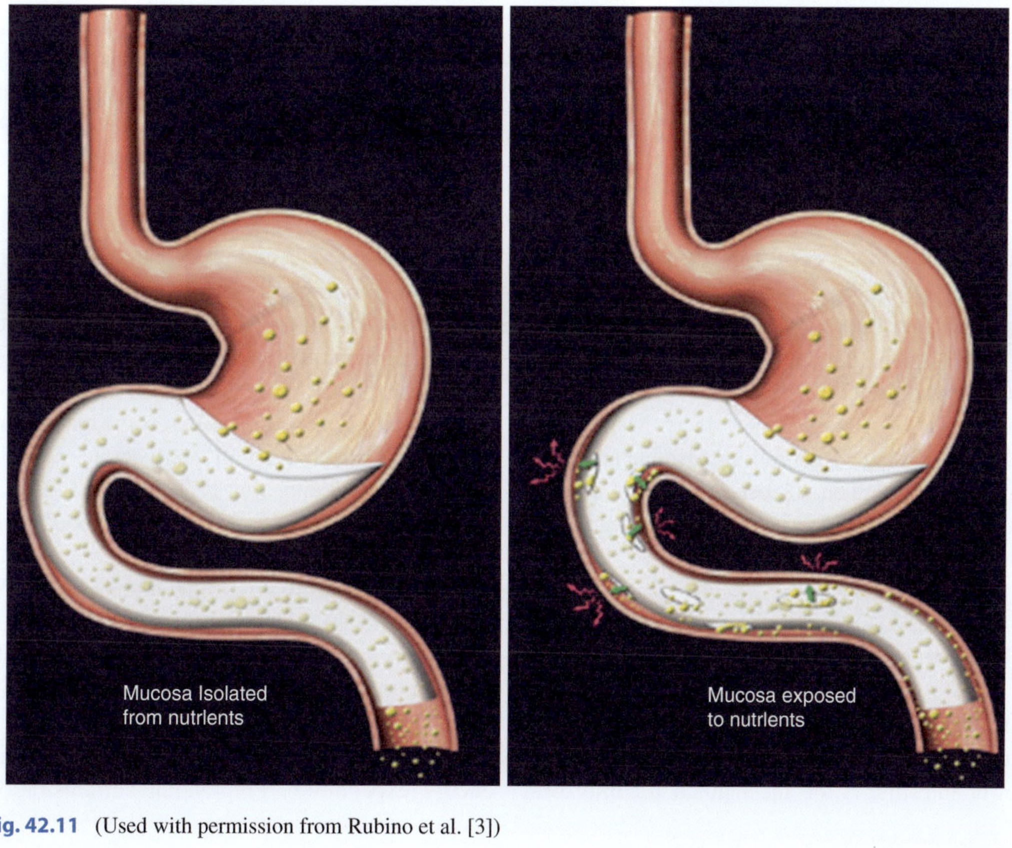

Fig. 42.11 (Used with permission from Rubino et al. [3])

mechanism and still achieving improved glucose homeostasis are paradoxical in the diabetic patient who undergoes DJB, RYGB, or BPD.

The above notwithstanding, proximal small intestinal bypass also delivers nutrients directly to the small bowel, and doing so has also been shown to activate neural and metabolic feedback circuits that counteract energy excess and glucose imbalance via a gut-brain-liver neuroendocrine axis [95–102]. In fact intra-jejunal lipid infusion lowers food intake in humans [103, 104]. The underlying mechanisms of jejunal lipid sensing are unclear, but a gut-brain contribution appears to be in effect [105, 106].

Interestingly, small intestinal bypass after RYGB also induces intestinal gluconeogenesis in the Roux limb. Saeidi et al. evaluated the Roux limb contribution to glucose homeostasis after RYGB in diet-induced obese rats [38]. The Roux limb underwent adaptive changes including upregulation of glucose transporter 1 expression, increased basolateral glucose uptake, increased aerobic glycolysis, decreased gluconeogenesis, increased cholesterol production, and increased glucose utilization and uptake. The aforementioned produces increased glucose levels in the portal vein which then activate portal vein glucose sensors which in turn engage a neural circuit that increases hepatic insulin sensitivity, decreases hepatic gluconeogenesis, and decreases food intake [107]. Post RYGB the intestines became a major tissue for glucose disposal and improved glycemic control. After RYGB the intestine actually had the highest tissue glucose uptake in the body per gram of tissue. The adaptive changes were felt to be secondary to exposure of the Roux limb to undigested nutrients and were an important factor in glucose homeostasis. Many questions remain regarding nutrient-stimulated neural circuits influence on glucose metabolism, as well has how these pathways are affected after RYGB and DJB in the diabetic patient [30].

The Lower Intestinal Hypothesis

The lower intestinal hypothesis proposes that expedited delivery of ingested nutrients to the lower intestine is the mechanism for improved glucose homeostasis after gastric bypass or other intestinal bypass procedures. The concept that rapid delivery of nutrients to the distal intestines could influence the actions of the proximal bowel was first described as the "ileal brake" in 1983 [108]. Rapid delivery of nutrients to the lower intestines decreases gastric emptying, decreases food intake, and decreases small bowel transit of nutrients [108–110]. Consistent with the lower intestinal hypothesis, the bariatric operations most noted for rapid T2DM remission, the RYGB, and the BPD create intestinal shortcuts for food to access the distal intestines. When high concentrations of unabsorbed nutrients are expedited to the distal intestine, the secretion of intestinal hormones such as peptide YY (PYY) and proglucagon-derived peptides (PGDPs) glucagon-like polypeptide 1 (GLP-1), glucagon-like polypeptide 2 (GLP-2), and oxyntomodulin (OXM) are hyperstimulated from enteroendocrine L-cells in the ileal and colonic mucosae [111–115].

GLP-1 is another classic incretin that increases 5–10-fold postprandially with a half-life of less than 2 minutes being cleared by dipeptidyl peptidase 4 (DPP-4 inactivates both GLP-1 and GIP) [115–119]. GLP-1 secretion is elevated after RYGB by nutrient stimulation of enteroendocrine L-cells [111]. GLP-1 improves glucose homeostasis by stimulating glucose-dependent insulin secretion, inhibiting glucagon secretion, enhancing beta cell response to glucose, inducing beta cell neogenesis and proliferation, inhibiting beta cell apoptosis, increasing muscle uptake of glucose, increasing liver uptake of glucose, decreasing hepatic gluconeogenesis, and increasing beta cell mass (Fig. 42.9) [84, 85]. It is the expansion of beta cell mass that some claim may cause hyperinsulinemic hypoglycemia seen in over 30% of patients after RYGB [120–122].

Another PGDP peptide, oxyntomodulin, is a 29-amino acid sequence of glucagon with an 8-amino acid carboxy-terminal extension. OXM is also produced in ileal enteroendocrine L-cells. OXM improves glucose homeostasis after RYGB by stimulating intestinal glucose uptake and insulin secretion, delaying gastric emptying, decreasing food intake, increasing satiety, and increasing energy expenditure. Preprandial administration of oxyntomodulin reduced voluntary energy intake by 17% and increased activity-related energy expenditure by 26% and total energy expenditure by 9.4% in overweight and obese patients [123–126].

GLP-2 is a 33-amino acid PGDP secreted with GLP-1 from enteroendocrine L-cells in a nutrient-dependent manner. GLP-2 appears to have an intestinotrophic effect on the bowel, but there is no evidence that it directly regulates insulin secretion or glucose homeostasis in humans. This intestinotrophic effect may have future utility in patients with short bowel syndrome [127, 128].

GLP-1 and PYY are substantially and durably elevated after RYGB but not after LAGB [129–136]. Exogenous PYY stimulates a neuroendocrine pathway via the vagus nerve and produces the effect of satiety [137, 138]. These effects are mediated presumably through inhibition of gut motility by way of vagal efferent neurons that descend from the hindbrain and via inhibition of neuropeptide Y2 receptors in the hypothalamus, leading to disinhibition of neurons that express the anorectic peptides α-MSH and cocaine- and amphetamine-regulated transcript [131]. Madsbad et al. nicely summarize the effects of PYY and PGDPs after RYGB in Fig. 42.12.

Further support for the lower intestinal hypothesis comes from a novel operation involving ileal interposition or ileal transposition (IT) first described by Koopmans et al. in 1982 [139]. In this operation a segment of the L-cell-rich ileum is transplanted in an isoperistaltic fashion into the upper intestine near the ligament of Treitz (Fig. 42.13). This proximal positioning directly exposes the ileal mucosa to high concentrations of undigested nutrients. IT greatly enhances postprandial levels of GLP-1 and PYY and results in satiety and improved glycemic control without significant weight loss, gastric restriction, or malabsorption [108, 109, 140, 141]. In a study of 60 patients with T2DM and a body mass index of only 24–34, De Paula et al. reported resolution of T2DM in 87% of the patients after IT [108, 142].

Understanding the roles of GLP-1 and DPP-4 has led to therapeutic benefits for the patient suffering from T2DM. Both GLP-1 receptor agonist (Byetta, Bydureon, Tanzeum, Trulicity, and Victoza) and DPP-4 inhibitors (Sitagliptin Saxagliptin) are currently useful adjuncts in the treatment of T2DM.

Bile Acids

Bile acids (BA) are amphipathic molecules synthesized from cholesterol in the liver. They are physiological detergents that play important roles in facilitating hepatobiliary secretion of endobiotic and xenobiotic metabolites. In the intestines, BA help intestinal absorption of dietary fats, fat-soluble vitamins, and other nutrients. Over the past decade, it has become evident that BA function as more than just digestive surfactants but are involved as signaling molecules in a wide range of biological functions, including glucose and lipid metabolism, energy homeostasis, and the modulation of immune response. Among the changes to gut physiology that occur following bariatric surgery is an altered enterohepatic circulation of BA. RYGB is associated with a substantial increase in circulating total BA in humans and in rodent models. It is now clear that BA bind to the nuclear receptor FXR (farnesoid x receptor, NR1H4) and cell surface G-protein-coupled receptors such as TGR5 to function as signaling molecules contributing to the regulation of various metabolic processes including glucose homeostasis [143, 144]. FXR is expressed in the liver, intestine, and adipose tissue and appears to be involved in regulating BA synthesis as well as lipid and glucose metabolism in the liver and intestines. FXR-deficient mice develop insulin resistance with hyperglycemia, impaired glucose tolerance, and severely blunted insulin signaling in both the liver and muscle [144]. TGR5 activation by BA stimulates rapid intracellular cyclic adenosine monophosphate (c-AMP) production and protein kinase A activation. TGR55 appears to be involved in regulating energy metabolism in adipose tissue and in the secretion of GLP-1 from enteroendocrine L-cells [144–147]. A study comparing nondiabetic post RYGB patients with morbidly obese and overweight controls found a more than twofold elevation of fasting BA in the post RYGB group [144]. The FXR pathway appears to be related to sustained weight

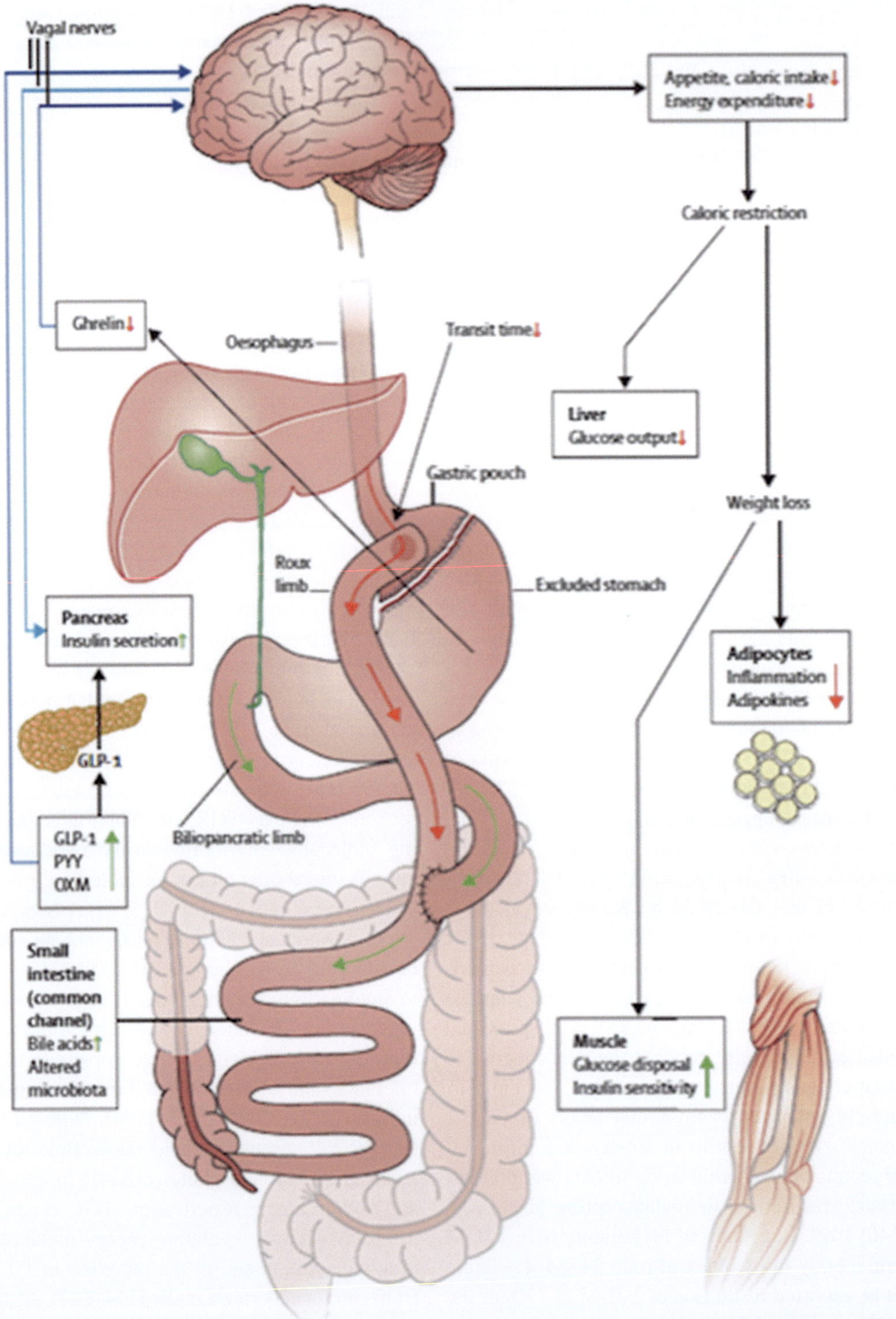

Fig. 42.12 Early effects of RYGB are induction of postprandial increases in GLP-1, PYY, and OXM because of the fast entry of food into the small intestine, while ghrelin secretion is reduced. Together, these changes are probably the main causes of reduced appetite and food intake. The exaggerated GLP-1 response also accounts for the increase in insulin secretion seen in patients with T2DM after RYGB. Reduced postoperative caloric intake increases hepatic insulin sensitivity within a few days after surgery. Later effects include improvements in skeletal muscle insulin sensitivity. (Reproduced with permission from Madsbad et al. [31])

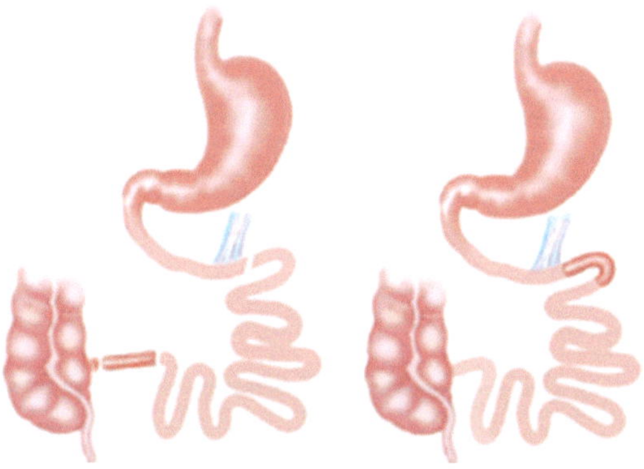

d Ileal interposition (IT)

Fig. 42.13 (Used with permission from Rubino et al. [3])

loss, suppression of rebound hyperphagia, and improved glucose control, but the precise mechanisms require further elucidation [36].

Microbiota

Gut microbial communities are altered in obese individuals compared to their nonobese counterparts. Human microbiota respond to changes in caloric intake and macronutrient content of the diet. Recent evidence implicates dramatic changes in gut microbial communities both in humans and mice, as potential contributors to the benefits of bariatric and metabolic surgery. Patients' microbiota after RYGB demonstrate an increase in *Proteobacteria* in comparison to nonoperated severely obese cohorts [33]. Transplantation of the gut microbiota from obese mice into gnotobiotic mice is associated with weight gain, whereas transplantation of gut microbiota from RYGB patients into gnotobiotic mice is associated with weight loss, reduced fat deposition, and a reduced respiratory quotient indicating a decreased use of carbohydrates as fuel compared to transplantation with sham microbiota [33, 36]. A decrease in adiposity and body weight without a change in food intake suggests that the RYGB-associated microbiota may either reduce the ability to harvest energy from the diet or produce signals regulating energy expenditure and/or lipid metabolism [36]. It is clear from studies that RYGB improves glucose metabolism in animals and in people. However, the degree to which the RYGB-altered microbiota mediates those improvements remains uncertain [37].

Conclusion

RYGB causes complete remission of T2DM in a large majority of cases. This remarkable phenomenon results from effects beyond those related to starvation and weight loss. The evidence supports weight loss-independent antidiabetic actions of RYGB. After RYGB there is a very rapid resolution of T2DM before significant weight loss occurs. There is also greater improvement of glucose homeostasis than after equivalent weight loss from other means, and there is the development of improved pancreatic beta cell function. Several mechanisms likely mediate the direct antidiabetic impact of RYGB, including enhanced nutrient stimulation of L-cell peptides (GLP-1, OXM) from the lower intestine, alterations in nutrient sensing, and the gut-brain-liver axis related to exclusion of the upper intestine from contact with ingested nutrients, compromised ghrelin secretion, altered BA metabolism, altered gut microbiota, and other effects that have yet to be discovered. It is increasingly clear that the gut plays a major role in glucose homeostasis, regulating both insulin secretion and sensitivity in the liver and peripherally, and RYGB probably influences several gastrointestinal pathways in complementary ways to improve glucose control (Fig. 42.12). Sorting out these mechanisms, as well as identifying potential additional pathways, is a compelling research objective that will provide for improved surgical design and novel targets for the treatment of diabetes.

References

1. Koopman PG. Obesity as a medical problem. Nature. 2000;404(6778):635–43.
2. Zimmet P. The burden of type 2 diabetes: are we doing enough? Diabetes Metab. 2003;29(4 Pt 2):6S9–18.

3. Rubino F, Schauer PR, Kaplan LM, Cummings DE. Metabolic surgery to treat type 2 diabetes: clinical outcomes and mechanisms of action. Annu Rev Med. 2010;61:393–411.
4. Dixon JB, O'Brien PE, Playfair J, et al. Adjustable gastric banding and conventional therapy for type 2 diabetes: a randomized controlled trial. JAMA. 2008;299:316–23.
5. Mingrone G, Panunzi S, De Gaetano A, et al. Bariatric surgery versus conventional medical therapy for type 2 diabetes. N Engl J Med. 2012;355:1577–85.
6. Schauer PR, Kashyap SR, Wolski K, et al. Bariatric surgery versus intensive medical therapy in obese patients with diabetes. N Engl J Med. 2012;366:1567–76.
7. Ikramuddin S, Komer J, Lee WJ, et al. Roux-en-Y gastric bypass vs intensive medical management for the control of type 2 diabetes, hypertension and hyperlipidemia: the diabetes surgery study randomized clinical trial. JAMA. 2013;309:2240–9.
8. Courcoulas AP, Goodpaster BH, Eagleton JK, et al. Surgical vs medical treatments for type 2 diabetes mellitus: a randomized clinical trial. JAMA Surg. 2014;149:707–15.
9. Halperin F, Ding SA, Simonson DC, et al. Roux-en-Y gastric bypass or lifestyle with intensive medical management in patients with type 2 diabetes: feasibility and 1-year results of a randomized clinical trial. JAMA Surg. 2014;149:716–26.
10. Liang Z, Wu Q, Chen B, Yu P, Zhao H, Quyang X. Effect of laparoscopic Roux-en-Y gastric bypass surgery on type 2 diabetes mellitus with hypertension: a randomized controlled trial. Diabetes Res Clin Pract. 2013;101:50–6.
11. Wentworth JM, Playfair J, Laurie C, et al. Multidisciplinary diabetes care with and without bariatric surgery in overweight people: a randomized controlled trial. Lancet Diabetes Endocrinol. 2014;2:545–52.
12. Parikh M, Chung M, Sheth S, et al. Randomized pilot trial of bariatric surgery versus intensive medical weight management on diabetes remission in type 2 diabetic patients who do NOT meet NIH criteria for surgery and the role of soluble RAGE as a novel biomarker of success. Ann Surg. 2014;260:617–22.
13. Schauer PR, Bhatt DL, Kirwan JP, et al. STAMPEDE investigators. Bariatric surgery versus intensive medical therapy for diabetes 3-year outcomes. N Engl J Med. 2014;370:2002–13.
14. Mingrone G, Panunzi S, De Gaetano A, et al. Bariatric –metabolic surgery versus conventional medical treatment in obese patients with type 2 diabetes: 5 year follow-up of an open-label, single-centre, randomized controlled trial. Lancet. 2015;386:964–73.
15. Ikramuddin S, Billington CJ, Lee WJ, et al. Roux-en-Y gastric bypass for diabetes (the Diabetes Surgery Study); 2-year outcomes of a 5-year, randomized, controlled trial. Lancet Diabetes Endocrinol. 2015;3:413–22.
16. Ding SA, Simonson DC, Wewalka M, et al. Adjustable gastric band surgery or medical management in patients with type 2 diabetes: a randomized clinical trial. J Clin Endocrinol Metab. 2015;100:2545–56.
17. Cummings DE, Arterburn DE, Westbrook EO, et al. Gastric bypass surgery vs intensive lifestyle and medical intervention for type 2 diabetes: the CROSSROADS randomized controlled trial. Diabetologia. 2016;59:945–53.
18. Courcoulas AP, Belle SH, Neiberg RH, et al. Three-year outcomes of bariatric surgery vs lifestyle intervention for type 2 diabetes mellitus treatment: a randomized clinical trial. JAMA Surg. 2015;150:931–40.
19. Gloy VL, Briel M, Bhatt DL, et al. Bariatric surgery versus non-surgical treatment for obesity: a systematic review and meta-analysis of randomized controlled trials. BMJ. 2013;347:f5934.
20. Friedman NM, Sancetta AJ, Magovern GJ. The amelioration of diabetes mellitus following subtotal gastrectomy. Surg Gynecol Obstet. 1955;100:201–4.
21. Bittner R, Bittner B, Beger HG. Homeostasis of glucose and gastric resection. The influence of the food passage through the duodenum. Z Gastroenterol. 1981;19:698–707.
22. Forgacs S, Halmos T. Improvement of glucose tolerance in diabetics following gastrectomy. Z Gastroenterol. 1973;11:293–6.
23. Buchwald H, Avidor Y, Braunwald E, et al. Bariatric surgery: a systematic review and meta-analysis. JAMA. 2004;292:1724–37.
24. Pories WJ, Swanson MS, MacDonald DG, et al. Who would have thought it? An operation proves to be the most effective therapy for adult-onset diabetes mellitus. Ann Surg. 1995;222:339–50.
25. Schauer PR, Burguera B, Ikramuddin S, et al. Effect of laparoscopic Roux-en-Y gastric bypass on type 2 diabetes mellitus. Ann Surg. 2003;238:467–84.
26. Sjostrom L, Lindroos AK, Peltonen M, Swedish Obese Subjects Study Scientific Group, et al. Lifestyle, diabetes, and cardiovascular risk factors 10 years after bariatric surgery. N Engl J Med. 2004;351:2683–93.
27. Carlisson LM, Peltonen M, Ahlin S, et al. Bariatric surgery and prevention of type 2 diabetes in Swedish obese subjects. N Engl J Med. 2012;367:695–704.
28. Sjoholm K, Pajunen P, Jaconson P, et al. Incidence and remission of type 2 diabetes in relation to degree of obesity at baseline and 2 year weight change: the Swedish obese subjects (SOS) study. Diabetologia. 2015;58:1448–53.
29. Rubino F, Marescaux J. Effect of duodenal- jejunal exclusion in a non-obese animal model of type 2 diabetes: a new perspective for an old disease. Ann Surg. 2004;239:1–11.
30. Thaler JP, Cummings DE. Mini review: hormonal and metabolic mechanisms of diabetes remission after gastrointestinal surgery. Endocrinology. 2009;150:2518–25.

31. Madsbad S, Dirksen C, Holst JJ. Mechanisms of changes in glucose metabolism and body- weight after bariatric surgery. Lancet Diabetes Endocrinol. 2014;2:152–64.
32. Salehi M, Woods SC, D'Alessio DA. Gastric bypass alters both glucose-dependent and glucose-independent regulation of islet hormone secretion. Obesity (Silver Spring). 2015;23:2046–52.
33. Tremaroli V, Karlsson F, Werling M, et al. Roux-en-Y gastric bypass and vertical banded gastroplasty induce long-term changes on the human gut microbiome contributing to fat mass regulation. Cell Metab. 2015;22:228–38.
34. Dirksen C, Jørgensen NB, Bojsen-Møller KN, et al. Mechanisms of improved glycaemic control after Roux-en-Y gastric bypass. Diabetologia. 2012;55:1890–901.
35. Breen DM, Rasmussen BA, Kokorovic A, Wang R, Cheung GW, Lam TK. Jejunal nutrient sensing is required for duodenal-jejunal bypass surgery to rapidly lower glucose concentrations in uncontrolled diabetes. Nat Med. 2012;18:950–5.
36. Ryan KK, Tremaroli V, Clemmensen C, et al. FXR is a molecular target for the effects of ver- tical sleeve gastrectomy. Nature. 2014;509:183–8.
37. Liou AP, Paziuk M, Luevano JM Jr, Machineni S, Turnbaugh PJ, Kaplan LM. Conserved shifts in the gut microbiota due to gastric bypass reduce host weight and adiposity. Sci Transl Med. 2013;5:178ra41.
38. Saeidi N, Meoli L, Nestoridi E, et al. Reprogramming of intestinal glucose metabolism and glycemic control in rats after gastric bypass. Science. 2013;341:406–10.
39. Sjostrom L, Peltonen M, Jacobson P, et al. Association of bariatric surgery with long-term remission of type 2 diabetes and with microvascular and macrovascular complications. JAMA. 2014;311:2297–304.
40. Rubino S, Nathan DM, Eckel RH, Schauer PR, et al. Metabolic surgery in the treatment algorithm for type 2 diabetes: a joint statement by international diabetes organizations. Diabetes Care. 2016;39:861–77.
41. Arterburn DE, Bogart A, Sherwood NE, et al. A multisite study of long-term remission and relapse of type 2 diabetes mellitus following gastric bypass. Obes Surg. 2013;23:93–102.
42. Cohen RV, Pinheiro JC, Schiavon CA, Salles JE, Wajchenberg BL, Cummings DE. Effects of gastric bypass surgery in patients with type 2 diabetes and only mild obesity. Diabetes Care. 2012;35:1420–8.
43. Adams TD, Davidson LE, Litwin SE, et al. Health benefits of gastric bypass surgery after 6 years. JAMA. 2012;308:1122–31.
44. Brethauer SA, Aminian A, Romero-Talamás H, et al. Can diabetes be surgically cured? Long- term metabolic effects of bariatric surgery in obese patients with type 2 diabetes mellitus. Ann Surg. 2013;258:628–36.
45. Hsu CC, Almulaifi A, Chen JC, et al. Effect of bariatric surgery vs medical treatment on type 2 diabetes in patients with body mass index lower than 35: five-year outcomes. JAMA Surg. 2015;150:1117–24.
46. Sjostrom L, Gummesson A, Sjöström CD, Swedish Obese Subjects Study, et al. Effects of bariatric surgery on cancer incidence in obese patients in Sweden (Swedish Obese Subjects Study): a prospective, controlled intervention trial. Lancet Oncol. 2009;10:653–62.
47. Sjostrom L, Peltonen M, Jacobson P, et al. Bariatric surgery and long-term cardiovascular events. JAMA. 2012;307:56–65.
48. Sjostrom L, Narbro K, Sjostrom CD, Swedish Obese Subjects Study, et al. Effects of bariatric surgery on mortality in Swedish obese subjects. N Engl J Med. 2007;357:741–52.
49. Adams TD, Gress RE, Smith SC, et al. Long- term mortality after gastric bypass surgery. N Engl J Med. 2007;357:753–61.
50. Arterburn DE, Olsen MK, Smith VA, et al. Association between bariatric surgery and long-term survival. JAMA. 2015;313:62–70.
51. Flum DR, Belle SH, King WC, Longitudinal Assessment of Bariatric Surgery (LABS) Consortium, et al. Perioperative safety in the longitudinal assessment of bariatric surgery. N Engl J Med. 2009;361:445–54.
52. Birkmeyer NJ, Dimick JB, Share D, Michigan Bariatric Surgery Collaborative, et al. Hospital complication rates with bariatric surgery in Michigan. JAMA. 2010;304:435–42.
53. Altieri MS, Yang J, Telem DA, et al. Lap band outcomes from 19,221 patients across centers and over a decade within the state of New York. Surg Endosc. 2016;30:1725–32. https://doi.org/10.1007/s00464-015-4402-8.
54. Hutter MM, Schirmer BD, Jones DB, et al. First report from the American College of Surgeons Bariatric Surgery Center Network: laparoscopic sleeve gastrectomy has morbidity and effectiveness positioned between the band and the bypass. Ann Surg. 2011;254:410–20; discussion 420–422.
55. Nguyen NT, Slone JA, Nguyen XM, Hartman JS, Hoyt DB. A prospective randomized trial of laparoscopic gastric bypass versus laparoscopic adjustable gastric banding for the treatment of morbid obesity: outcomes, quality of life, and costs. Ann Surg. 2009;250:631–41.
56. Isbell JM, Tamboli RA, Hansen EN, et al. The importance of caloric restriction in the early improvements in insulin sensitivity after Roux-en-Y gastric bypass surgery. Diabetes Care. 2010;33:1438–42.
57. Laferrere B, Teixeira J, McGinty J, et al. Effect of weight loss by gastric bypass surgery versus hypocaloric diet on glucose and incretin levels in patients with type 2 diabetes. J Clin Endocrinol Metab. 2008;93:2479–85.
58. Lim EL, Hollingsworth KG, Aribasale B, Chen MJ, Mathers JC, Taylor R. Reversal of type 2 diabetes is associated with decrease in pancreas and liver fat levels. Diabetologia. 2011;54:2506–14.

59. Cummings DE. Endocrine mechanisms mediating remission of diabetes after gastric bypass surgery. Int J Obes (Lond). 2009;33:533–40.
60. Rubino F, Forgione A, Cummings DE, et al. The mechanism of diabetes control after gastrointestinal bypass surgery reveals a role of the proximal small intestine in the pathophysiology of type 2 diabetes. Ann Surg. 2006;244:741–9.
61. Rubino F, Gagner M, Gentileschi P, et al. The early effect of the Roux-en-Y gastric bypass on hormones involved in body weight regulation and glucose metabolism. Ann Surg. 2004;240:236–42.
62. Cummings DE, Overduin J, Shannon MH, et al. Hormonal mechanisms of weight loss and diabetes resolution after bariatric surgery. Surg Obes Relat Dis. 2005;1:358–68.
63. Kojima M, Hosoda H, Date Y, et al. Ghrelin is a growth hormone– releasing acylated peptide from stomach. Nature. 1999;402:656–60.
64. Tschop M, Smiley DL, Heiman ML. Ghrelin induces adiposity in rodents. Nature. 2000;407:908–13.
65. Nakazato M, Murakami N, Date Y, et al. A role for ghrelin in the central regulation of feeding. Nature. 2001;409:194–8.
66. Wren AM, Small CJ, Ward HL, et al. The novel hypothalamic peptide ghrelin stimulates food intake and growth hormone secretion. Endocrinology. 2000;141:4325–8.
67. Ariyasu H, Takaya K, Tagami T, et al. Stomach is a major source of circulating ghrelin, and feeding state determines plasma ghrelin-like immunoreactivity levels in humans. J Clin Endocrinol Metab. 2001;86:4753–8.
68. Ahren B, Holst JJ, Efendic S. Anti-diabetogenic action of cholecystokinin-8 in type 2 diabetes. J Clin Endocrinol Metab. 2000;85:1043–8.
69. Cummings DE, Shannon MH. Roles for ghrelin in the regulation of appetite and body weight. Arch Surg. 2003;138:389–96.
70. Cummings DE, Purnell JQ, Frayo RS, et al. A preprandial rise in plasma ghrelin levels suggests a role in meal initiation in humans. Diabetes. 2001;50:1714–9.
71. Cummings DE, Frayo RS, Marmonier C, et al. Plasma ghrelin levels and hunger scores in humans initiating meals voluntarily without time-and food-related cues. Am J Physiol Endocrinol Metab. 2004;287:E297–304.
72. Cummings DE, Foster-Schubert KE, Overduin J. Ghrelin and energy balance: focus on current controversies. Curr Drug Targets. 2005;6:153–69.
73. Dezaki K, et al. Endogenous ghrelin in pancreatic islets restricts insulin release by attenuating Ca2+ signaling in beta-cells: implication in the glycemic control in rodents. Diabetes. 2004;53:3142–51.
74. Sun Y, Asnicar M, Saha PK, Chan L, Smith RG. Ablation of ghrelin improves the diabetic but not obese phenotype of ob/ob mice. Cell Metab. 2006;3:379–86.
75. Theander-Carrillo C, et al. Ghrelin action in the brain controls adipocyte metabolism. J Clin Invest. 2006;116:1983–93. https://doi.org/10.1172/JCI25811.
76. Broglio F, Arvat E, Benso A, et al. Ghrelin, a natural GH secretagogue produced by the stomach, induces hyperglycemia and reduces insulin secretion in humans. J Clin Endocrinol Metab. 2001;86:5083–6.
77. Cummings DE, Weigle DS, Frayo RS, et al. Human plasma ghrelin levels after diet-induced weight loss and gastric bypass surgery. N Engl J Med. 2002;346:1623–30.
78. Kuntz E, Pinget M, Damge P. Cholecystokinin octapeptide: a potential growth factor for pancreatic beta cells in diabetic rats. JOP. 2004;5:464–75.
79. Suarez-Pinzon WL, Lakey JR, Brand SJ, Rabinovitch A. Combination therapy with epidermal growth factor and gastrin induces neogenesis of human islet beta-cells from pancreatic duct cells and an increase in functional beta-cell mass. J Clin Endocrinol Metab. 2005;90:3401–9.
80. Boushey RP, et al. Hypoglycemia, defective islet glucagon secretion, but normal islet mass in mice with a disruption of the gastrin gene. Gastroenterology. 2003;125:1164–74.
81. Grong E, Graeslei H, Munkvold B, et al. Gastrin secretion after bariatric surgery-response to a protein-rich mixed meal following Roux-en-Y gastric bypass and sleeve gastrectomy: a pilot study in normoglycemic women. Obes Surg. 2016;26:1448–56.
82. Deacon CF, Nauck MA, Meier J, Hucking K, Holst JJ. Degradation of endogenous and exogenous gastric inhibitory polypeptide in healthy and in type 2 diabetic subjects as revealed using a new assay for the intact peptide. J Clin Endocrinol Metab. 2000;85:3575–81.
83. Mentlein R, Gallwitz B, Schmidt WE. Dipeptidyl-peptidase IV hydrolyses gastric inhibitory polypeptide, glucagon-like peptide- 1(7-36)amide, peptide histidine methionine and is responsible for their degradation in human serum. Eur J Biochem. 1993;214:829–35.
84. Drucker DJ. The role of gut hormones in glucose homeostasis. J Clin Invest. 2007;117(1):24–32.
85. Drucker DJ. Glucagon-like peptides: regulators of cell proliferation, differentiation, and apoptosis. Mol Endocrinol. 2003;17:161–71.
86. Kim SJ, et al. GIP stimulation of pancreatic beta-cell survival is dependent upon phosphatidylinositol 3-kinase (PI3-K)/protein kinase B (PKB) signaling, inactivation of the forkhead transcription factor Foxo1 and downregulation of bax expression. J Biol Chem. 2005;280:22297–307.
87. Gault VA, et al. Chemical ablation of gastric inhibitory polypeptide receptor action by daily (Pro3) GIP administration improves glucose tolerance and ameliorates insulin resistance and abnormalities of islet structure in obesity-related diabetes. Diabetes. 2005;54:2436–46.

88. Rubino F, Zizzari P, Tomasetto C, et al. The role of the small bowel in the regulation of circulating ghrelin levels and food intake in the obese Zucker rat. Endocrinology. 2005;146:1745–51.
89. Cohen RV, Schiavon CA, Pinheiro JS, et al. Duodenal-jejunal bypass for the treatment of type 2 diabetes in patients with body mass index of 22–34 kg/m^2. Surg Obes Relat Dis. 2007;3:195–7.
90. Ramos AC, Neto MPG, de Souza YM, et al. Laparoscopic duodenal-jejunal exclusion in the treatment of type 2 diabetes mellitus in patients with BMI <30 kg/m^2. Obes Surg. 2009;19:307–12.
91. Tarnoff M, Sorli C, Rodriguez L, et al. Interim report of a prospective, randomized sham-controlled trial investigating a completely endoscopic duodenal-jejunal bypass sleeve for the treatment of type 2 diabetes. Diabetes. 2008;57:A32.
92. Tarnoff M, Rodriguez L, Escalona A, et al. Open label, prospective, randomized controlled trial of an endoscopic duodenal-jejunal bypass sleeve versus low calorie diet for preoperative weight loss in bariatric surgery. Surg Endosc. 2009;23:650–6.
93. Sorli C, Rodriguez L, Reyes E, et al. Pilot clinical study of an endoscopic, removable duodenal- jejunal bypass liner for the treatment of type 2 diabetes. Diabetes Technol Ther. 2009;11(11):725–32.
94. Wang PY, Caspi L, Lam CK, Chari M, Li X, Light PE, Gutierrez-Juarez R, Ang M, Schwartz GJ, Lam TK. Upper intestinal lipids trigger a gut-brain-liver axis to regulate glucose production. Nature. 2008;452:1012–6.
95. Badman MK, Flier JS. The gut and energy balance: visceral allies in the obesity wars. Science. 2005;307:1909–14.
96. Cummings DE, Overduin J. Gastrointestinal regulation of food intake. J Clin Invest. 2007; 117:13–23.
97. Murphy KG, Bloom SR. Gut hormones and the regulation of energy homeostasis. Nature. 2006;444:854–9.
98. Coll AP, Farooqi IS, O'Rahilly S. The hormonal control of food intake. Cell. 2007;129:251–62.
99. Lam TK. Neuronal regulation of homeostasis by nutrient sensing. Nat Med. 2010;16:392–5.
100. Greenberg D, Smith GP, Gibbs J. Intraduodenal infusions of fats elicit satiety in sham-feeding rats. Am J Physiol. 1990;259:R110–8.
101. Matzinger D, Degen L, Drewe J, et al. The role of long chain fatty acids in regulating food intake and cholecystokinin release in humans. Gut. 2000;46:688–93.
102. Cheung GW, Kokorovic A, Lam CK, Chari M, Lam TK. Intestinal cholecystokinin controls glucose production through a neuronal network. Cell Metab. 2009;10:99–109.
103. Drewe J, Gadient A, Rovati LC, Beglinger C. Role of circulating cholecystokinin in control of fat-induced inhibition of food intake in humans. Gastroenterology. 1992;102:1654–9.
104. Ogawa N, Yamaguchi H, Shimbara T, et al. The vagal afferent pathway does not play a major role in the induction of satiety by intestinal fatty acid in rats. Neurosci Lett. 2008;433:38–42.
105. Lal S, Kirkup AJ, Brunsden AM, Thompson DG, Grundy D. Vagal afferent responses to fatty acids of different chain length in the rat. Am J Physiol Gastrointest Liver Physiol. 2001;281:G907–15.
106. Randich A, Chandler PC, Mebane HC, et al. Jejunal administration of linoleic acid increases activity of neurons in the paraventricular nucleus of the hypothalamus. Am J Physiol Regul Integr Comp Physiol. 2004;286:R166–73.
107. Troy S, Soty M, Ribeiro L, Laval L, Migrenne S, Fioramonti X, Pillot B, Fauveau V, Aubert R, Viollet B, Foretz M, Leclerc J, Duchampt A, Zitoun C, Thorens B, Magnan C, Mithieux G, Andreelli F. Intestinal gluconeogenesis is a key factor for early metabolic changes after gastric bypass but not after gastric lap-band in mice. Cell Metab. 2008;8:201–11.
108. De Paula AL, Macedo AL, Prudente AS, et al. Laparoscopic sleeve gastrectomy with ileal interposition ("neuroendocrine brake")-pilot study of a new operation. Surg Obes Relat Dis. 2006;2:464–7.
109. Strader AD, Vahl TP, Jandacek RJ, et al. Weight loss through ileal transposition is accompanied by increased ileal hormone secretion and synthesis in rats. Am J Physiol Endocrinol Metab. 2005;288:E447–53.
110. Drucker DJ. Enhancing incretin action for the treatment of type 2 diabetes. Diabetes Care. 2003;26:2929–40.
111. Cummings DE, Overduin J, Foster-Schubert KE, et al. Role of the bypassed proximal intestine in the anti-diabetic effects of bariatric surgery. Surg Obes Relat Dis. 2007;3(2):109–15.
112. Reimer RA, McBurney MI. Dietary fiber modulates intestinal proglucagon messenger ribo- nucleic acid and postprandial secretion of glucagon-like peptide-1 and insulin in rats. Endocrinology. 1996;137:3948–56.
113. Tappenden KA, Thomson AB, Wild GE, McBurney MI. Short-chain fatty acids increase proglucagon and ornithine decarboxylase messenger RNAs after intestinal resection in rats. JPEN J Parenter Enteral Nutr. 1996;20:357–62.
114. Tappenden KA, McBurney MI. Systemic short-chain fatty acids rapidly alter gastro- intestinal structure, function, and expression of early response genes. Dig Dis Sci. 1998;43:1526–36.
115. Brubaker PL, Anini Y. Direct and indirect mechanisms regulating secretion of glucagon- like peptide-1 and glucagon-like peptide-2. Can J Physiol Pharmacol. 2003;81:1005–12.
116. Orskov C, Rabenhoj L, Wettergren A, Kofod H, Holst JJ. Tissue and plasma concentrations of amidated and glycine-extended glucagon- like peptide I in humans. Diabetes. 1994;43:535–9.

117. Vilsboll T, Krarup T, Deacon CF, Madsbad S, Holst JJ. Reduced postprandial concentrations of intact biologically active glucagon-like peptide 1 in type 2 diabetic patients. Diabetes. 2001;50:609–13.
118. Hansen L, Deacon CF, Orskov C, Holst JJ. Glucagon-like peptide-1-(7-36)amide is transformed to glucagon-like peptide-1-(9- 36)amide by dipeptidyl peptidase IV in the capillaries supplying the L cells of the porcine intestine. Endocrinology. 1999;140:5356–63.
119. Deacon CF, Nauck MA, Toft-Nielsen M, et al. Both subcutaneously and intravenously administered glucagon-like peptide 1 are rapidly degraded from the NH2-terminus in type II diabetic patients and in healthy subjects. Diabetes. 1995;44:1126–31.
120. Service GJ, Thompson GB, Service FJ, Andrews JC, Collazo-Clavell ML, Lloyd RV. Hyperinsulinemic hypoglycemia with nesidioblastosis after gastric- bypass surgery. N Engl J Med. 2005;353:249–54.
121. Patti ME, McMahon G, Mun EC, Bitton A, Holst JJ, Goldsmith J, Hanto DW, Callery M, Arky R, Nose V, Bonner-Weir S, Goldfine AB. Severe hypoglycaemia post-gastric bypass requiring partial pancreatectomy: evidence for inappropriate insulin secretion and pancreatic islet hyperplasia. Diabetologia. 2005;48:2236–40.
122. Foster-Schubert KE. Hypoglycemia complicating bariatric surgery: incidence and mechanisms. Curr Opin Endocrinol Diabetes Obes. 2011;18(2):129–33.
123. Collie NL, Zhu Z, Jordan S, Reeve JR. Oxyntomodulin stimulates intestinal glucose uptake in rats. Gastroenterology. 1997;112:1961–70.
124. Jarrousse C, Bataille D, Jeanrenaud B. A pure enteroglucagon, oxyntomodulin (glucagon 37), stimulates insulin release in perfused rat pancreas. Endocrinology. 1984;115:102–5.
125. Wynne K, Park AJ, Small CJ, et al. Oxyntomodulin increases energy expenditure in addition to decreasing energy intake in overweight and obese humans: a randomised controlled trial. Int J Obes (Lond). 2006;30(12):1729–36.
126. Wynne K, Park AJ, Small CJ, et al. Subcutaneous oxyntomodulin reduces body weight in overweight and obese subjects: a double-blind, randomized, controlled trial. Diabetes. 2005;54:2390–5.
127. Cheeseman CI, Tsang R. The effect of gastric inhibitory polypeptide and glucagon like peptides on intestinal hexose transport. Am J Physiol Gastrointest Liver Physiol. 1996;271:G477–82.
128. Jeppesen PB, Hartmann B, Thulesen J, et al. Glucagon-like peptide 2 improves nutrient absorption and nutritional status in short-bowel patients with no colon. Gastroenterology. 2001;120:806–15.
129. le Roux CW, Aylwin SJ, Batterham RL, Borg CM, Coyle F, Prasad V, Shurey S, Ghatei MA, Patel AG, Bloom SR. Gut hormone profiles following bariatric surgery favor an anorectic state, facilitate weight loss, and improve metabolic parameters. Ann Surg. 2006;243:108–14.
130. Korner J, Bessler M, Inabnet W, Taveras C, Holst JJ. Exaggerated glucagon-like peptide-1 and blunted glucose-dependent insulinotropic peptide secretion are associated with Roux-en-Y gastric bypass but not adjustable gastric banding. Surg Obes Relat Dis. 2007;3:597–601.
131. Korner J, Bessler M, Cirilo LJ, Conwell IM, Daud A, Restuccia NL, Wardlaw SL. Effects of Roux-en-Y gastric bypass surgery on fasting and postprandial concentrations of plasma ghrelin, peptide YY, and insulin. J Clin Endocrinol Metab. 2005;90:359–65.
132. Laferrère B, Heshka S, Wang K, Khan Y, McGinty J, Teixeira J, Hart AB, Olivan B. Incretin levels and effect are markedly enhanced 1 month after Roux-en-Y gastric bypass surgery in obese patients with type 2 diabetes. Diabetes Care. 2007;30:1709–16.
133. Morínigo R, Moizé V, Musri M, Lacy AM, Navarro S, Marín JL, Delgado S, Casamitjana R, Vidal J. Glucagon-like peptide-1, peptide YY, hunger, and satiety after gastric bypass surgery in morbidly obese subjects. J Clin Endocrinol Metab. 2006;91:1735–40.
134. Rodieux F, Giusti V, D'Alessio DA, Suter M, Tappy L. Effects of gastric bypass and gastric banding on glucose kinetics and gut hormone release. Obesity (Silver Spring). 2008;16:298–305.
135. Borg CM, le Roux CW, Ghatei MA, Bloom SR, Patel AG, Aylwin SJ. Progressive rise in gut hormone levels after Roux-en-Y gastric bypass suggests gut adaptation and explains altered satiety. Br J Surg. 2006;93:210–5.
136. Vincent RP, le Roux CW. Changes in gut hormones after bariatric surgery. Clin Endocrinol (Oxf). 2008;69:173–9.
137. Batterham RL, Cowley MA, Small CJ, et al. Gut hormone PYY(3-36) physiologically inhibits food intake. Nature. 2002;418:650–4.
138. Batterham RL, Cohen MA, Ellis SM, et al. Inhibition of food intake in obese subjects by peptide YY3-36. N Engl J Med. 2003;349:941–8.
139. Koopmans HS, Sclafani A, Fichtner C, Aravich PF. The effects of ileal transposition on food intake and body weight loss in VMH-obese rats. Am J Clin Nutr. 1982;35:284–93.
140. Patriti A, Facchiano E, Annetti C, Aisa MC, Galli F, Fanelli C, Donini A. Early improvement of glucose tolerance after ileal transposition in a non-obese type 2 diabetes rat model. Obes Surg. 2005;15:1258–64.
141. Patriti A, Aisa MC, Annetti C, Sidoni A, Galli F, Ferri I, Gullà N, Donini A. How the hindgut can cure type 2 diabetes. Ileal transposition improves glucose metabolism and -cell function in Gotokakizaki rats through an enhanced Proglucagon gene expression and L-cell number. Surgery. 2007;142:74–85.
142. DePaula AL, Macedo AL, Rassi N, et al. Laparoscopic treatment of type 2 diabetes mellitus for patients with a body mass index less than 35. Surg Endosc. 2008;22:706–16.
143. Patti ME, Houten SM, Bianco AC, et al. Serum bile acids are higher in humans with prior gastric bypass:

potential contribution to improved glucose and lipid metabolism. Obesity. 2009;17:1671–7.
144. Ding L, Yang L, Wang Z, et al. Bile acid nuclear receptor FXR and digestive system diseases. Acta Pharm Sin B. 2015;5(2):135–44.
145. Makishima M, Okamoto AY, Repa JJ, et al. Identification of a nuclear receptor for bile acids. Science. 1999;284:1362–5.
146. Parks DJ, Blanchard SG, Bledsoe RK, et al. Bile acids: natural ligands for an orphan nuclear receptor. Science. 1999;284:1365–8.
147. Wang H, Chen J, Holister K, et al. Endogenous bile acids are ligands for the nuclear receptor FXR/BAR. Mol Cell. 1999;3:543–53.

Shifts in the Intestinal Microbiota After Gastric Bypass

43

Meera Nair, Carel W. le Roux, and Neil G. Docherty

Context and Objectives

Current estimates by the World Health Organisation suggest that more than 600 million individuals or approximately 8% of the global population have a body mass index (BMI) $\geq$30 kg/m^2 and are hence classifiable as obese [1]. Recent designation of obesity as a disease by influential bodies such as the American Medical Association means that by extrapolation obesity can objectively be quantified as constituting one of the most pressing health challenges of our time.

The development of molecular microbiology has led to a growing recognition that the essential functions of the human body arise as a synthesis of interactions between a collaborative consortium of host eukaryotic cells, microbial eukaryotic and prokaryotic cells and commensal virions (microbiome) [2]. Recognising alterations in these symbiotic relationships as an essential element of disease pathogenesis represents a paradigmatic shift and a challenge to modern medicine as it considers new approaches to the diagnosis and management of disease. Obesity and diabetes are in the vanguard of these new directions in medicine being as they are inextricably linked to one of the major sites of microbial colonisation in the body, namely, the gastrointestinal tract (GT) [3–5].

Diet, exercise and host genetics cannot fully explain the pathogenesis of obesity and diabetes. The present chapter firstly summarises current theory on the major means by which alterations in the gut microbiome may be causally linked to the development of these diseases. Subsequently the objectives, methodological approaches and key findings from the major studies in the literature examining changes in the gut microbiota after gastric bypass surgery are described. The chapter concludes by bringing together some of the potential mechanisms by which changes in the gut microbiota after gastric bypass might play an active causative

M. Nair · C. W. le Roux · N. G. Docherty (✉)
Diabetes Complications Research Centre, Conway Institute, School of Medicine, University College Dublin, Dublin, Ireland
e-mail: neil.docherty@ucd.ie

J. Ettinger et al. (eds.), *Gastric Bypass*, https://doi.org/10.1007/978-3-030-28803-7_43

role in the bariatric and metabolic effects of gastric bypass and outlines some perspective on future focus.

Structure and Function of the Gut Microbiota

The gastrointestinal tract (GIT) constitutes the major reservoir of microorganisms in the human body. The density of microbial (bacterial) colonisation increases aborally from 10^3 organisms/gram of contents in the duodenum to 10^{11} organisms/gram of contents in the large intestine [6]. The marked increase in density arising with increased distance along the tract can be attributed to the provision of a more stable niche in terms of (1) segment motility/transit, (2) chemical environment with increasing pH developing distally as the influence of gastric acids and bile acids dissipates (3) a less marked innate mucosal immune response evidenced by reduced release of bactericidal factors and (4) provision of a more developed mucous gel layer substrate for bacterial growth. Growth characteristics of colonising species become progressively more anaerobic in character with increasingly distal location.

The number of bacterial species supported by the human intestine has been estimated to be in the region on 1000. Within any given individual, the total number of colonising bacterial species is estimated to be around 150–160 being constituted by a core membership drawn from five main phyla, namely, *Firmicutes*, *Bacteroidetes* (together accounting for 90%), *Proteobacteria* and *Verrucobacteria* [7]. Functional clustering of microbiota results in the identification of three overarching enterotypes in humans stable over race, age, sex and location [6]. Interindividual differences in the fine structure of composition can be explained to some degree by diverse factors including age, diet and mode of delivery at birth (vaginal versus Caesarian section) [8, 9]. The last point emphasises the crucial importance of the first species colonising the sterile neonatal gut in setting the basic core structure of the microbiota. This then stabilises and becomes rather resistant to major changes from the age of 2 to 3 years onwards.

The key contributions to symbiosis provided for by the gut microbiota are classically considered to be the provision of short-chain fatty acids for colonocyte health, fermentation products suitable for energy synthesis as the result of digestion of fibre and the provision of vitamins such as vitamin K. More recent advances have demonstrated that the gut microbiota play a critical role in the overall digestion, absorption and utilisation/storage of ingested nutrient through maintenance of gut barrier function [10] and modulation of dietary energy harvest and modification of post-absorptive metabolism [11]. Linkages to higher control of ingestive behaviour through changes in gut hormone profiles and hypothalamic satiety signalling are also increasingly being revealed [11].

Thus the general recognition that the gut microbiota might play a role in the coordination of multiple aspects of metabolism and ingestive behaviour has led to a large body of research effort focussed on describing associations between microbiota composition and the development and progression of obesity and diabetes.

Theories on the Role of the Gut Microbiota in Obesity and Diabetes

The gut presents the largest internal surface area in the body in continuity with the external world [12]. A critical tension thus exists between maintaining the separation and protection of the internal milieu and the assimilation of nutrient from and extrusion of waste to the exterior. This relies on highly selective permeability achieved through the inherent structural integrity of the intestinal epithelium coupled to epithelial and lamina propria lymphocyte-derived secretion of a mucus gel layer, associated bactericidal factors and secretory IgA immunoglobulin, all of which require a degree of collaboration between host and "friendly" microbe [13].

A fundamental line of evidence linking the microbiota to adiposity was elucidated in 2004 when Backhed and colleagues demonstrated that conventionalisation of germ-free mice with transfer of caecal microbiota from specific pathogen-free mice resulted in increased body weight through augmented energy uptake and storage in fat [14]. This implied that weight gain following excessive caloric intake must rely on the microbiota and/or that shifts in microbiota composition that increase energy harvest could be involved in extracting higher levels of energy from diets of normal caloric content. Turnbaugh and colleagues demonstrated that increases in *Firmicutes/Bacteroidetes* ratios in obese mice were associated with adiposity and transmission of the obese phenotype to lean mice through cross-colonisation [15].

Diets enriched in saturated fats have been proposed to play a major permissive role in allowing the intestinal microbiota to negatively influence host metabolism and adiposity [16, 17]. Lipopolysaccharide (LPS) is the major pathogen-associated molecular pattern (PAMP) derived from gram-negative bacteria. LPS stimulates innate immune reactivity through activation of the CD14/Toll-like receptor-4 complex. Increased dietary fat intake results in elevation of circulating LPS through increases in intestinal epithelial micellar uptake of LPS, its packaging within chylomicrons and distribution to the adipose depots [18, 19]. Enhanced paracellular flux of LPS and bacterial translocation via increases in intercellular permeability secondary to reduced tight-junction patency have also been described in obesity [17]. Resulting metabolic endotoxaemia as it is termed is implicated as a driver of peripheral insulin resistance through the establishment of adipose insulin resistance and subsequent skeletal muscle insulin resistance occurring secondary to ectopic fat storage.

Another means by which the intestinal microbiota has been implicated in obesity and diabetes is through modulation of energy harvest and storage from the diet. Gut microbiota catalyse the enzymatic generation of absorbable saccharides from fibre and the generation of short-chain fatty acids through subsequent fermentation reactions. Aside from their ascribed roles in colonocyte health, the major short-chain fatty acids butyrate, acetate and propionate can be used as substrates for gluconeogenesis and hepatic lipogenesis providing for anabolic effects [11].

Simultaneously the intestinal microbiota exerts a tonic inhibition on the expression and release of the anti-anabolic factor angiopoietin-like 4 (Angptl4) from the intestinal epithelium. Angptl antagonises the actions of lipoprotein lipase in adipose tissue, and restriction of its bioactivity promotes the discharge and uptake into adipose tissue of lipid cargo from circulating lipoprotein complexes [14]. High levels of SCFA production can also limit fat catabolism through inhibition of the AMP-activated protein kinase (AMPK) which when activated drives fatty acids into mitochondrial respiration for utilisation rather than storage through anabolic pathways [14].

Convergent studies in animal models of diet-induced obesity and profiling of faecal microbiota in humans with obesity reveal that the obese gut microbiome has reduced diversity and a relative increase in *Firmicutes* phylum versus a relative loss of the *Bacteroidetes* phylum [20]. Loss of candidate individual species such as *F. prausnitzii* and *A. muciniphila* which are associated with preservation of anti-inflammatory tone and gut barrier integrity has been identified in several studies of the obese and diabetic faecal microbiome [21].

Key Studies Examining Changes in the Gut Microbiota after Gastric Bypass

Since 2009, seven principle original research communications can be identified that have contributed to understanding of the impact of gastric bypass on the composition and activity of the gut microbiota. These encompass studies in rodents and man both cross-sectional and longitudinal in design. All characterise compositional changes, and some make compositional change-function inferences based on microbiota transplantation experiments and functional metagenomic annotation. The study design, methodological approaches and major findings of these studies are summarised below.

Studies Describing Compositional Alterations

Zhang and colleagues [22] used 454 pyrosequencing methods to define and cross-sectionally compare the human gut microbiota in three categories of individual: normal weight (NW, $n = 3$), morbidly obese (OB, $n = 3$) and post-gastric bypass (GB $n = 3$). The study aimed to identify specific microbial lineages that may play a vital role in obesity development and to determine whether presence or abundance of these microorganisms changed after gastric bypass. A total of 184,094 16S rRNA gene sequence tags derived from 16S rRNA PCR amplicons were subjected to sequencing.

UniFrac distance matrix analysis showed separation of the NW and OB groups with two out of three samples from the GB group forming a discrete cluster. The gut microbiota was shown to contain sequences from six phyla. Most sequences belonged to *Firmicutes* and *Bacteroidetes*, with the rest drawn from *Proteobacteria*, *Actinobacteria*, *Fusobacteria* and *Verrucomicrobia*. Sequences from the families *Prevotellaceae* (phylum = *Bacteroidetes*) and *Erysipelotrichaceae* (phylum = *Firmicutes*) were mostly harboured in patients from the OB group. *Fusobacteria* and the family *Enterobacteriaceae* (within *Proteobacteria*) were found only in the RYGB group. GB markedly altered the stool microbial community structure towards an increase in *Gammaproteobacteria* with proportional decreases in *Firmicutes*.

Higher numbers of Archaea were observed in the OB group, a finding which segregated with the almost exclusive presence in this group of the order *Methanobacteriales* from the archaeal phylum *Euryarchaeota*. The mechanism connecting obesity to methanogens may be in part due to the transfer of H_2 from H_2-producing bacteria to a H_2 using methanogens. Methanogen metabolism may boost host energy extraction from indigestible polysaccharides by removing fermentation intermediates to allow for greater production and absorption of SCFAs across the intestinal epithelium. Syntrophic partnerships between H_2-producing bacteria such as *Prevotellaceae* which are increased in obesity may signal that specific bacteria-archaea interdependent relationships could be of functionally importance in the development of the obese phenotype.

Furet and colleagues [23] conducted a longitudinal study involving 30 female patients with morbid obesity undergoing gastric bypass surgery and 13 lean control volunteers. The faecal microbiota was profiled at low coverage using specific genus- and species-level quantitative PCR techniques at the time of surgery and 3 and 6 months thereafter. *Bacteroides* was lower in obese subjects than in control subjects at baseline and increased by the third month. *Escherichia coli* species were increased by the third post-operative month M3. Lactic acid bacteria including *Lactobacillus*/*Leuconostoc*/*Pediococcus* group and the *Bifidobacterium* genus were decreased by 3 months after surgery. Copy number of the anti-inflammatory *Faecalibacterium prausnitzii* species associated negatively with inflammatory markers at baseline and post-surgery time points.

The authors of the above detailed study subsequently conducted a deeper study of longitudinal changes in the gut microbiota profile in the obese cohort undergoing surgery using pyrosequencing [24]. A correlation analyses with changes in the white adipose tissue transcriptome at 3 months after surgery was also conducted. Principal component analysis showed bacterial profiles at baseline differed from those at 3- and 6-month post-surgery. Gastric bypass was associated with an increase in gut microbiota richness with 58 genera undetectable before surgery and detected after surgery in all patients. A total of 37% of these new sequences were assigned as *Proteobacteria* in origin. Gut bacterial genera belonging to *Firmicutes*, e.g. *Lactobacillus*, *Dorea* and *Blautia* and *Bifidobacterium* (phylum = *Actinobacteria*) decreased after gastric bypass, while *Escherichia* (*Proteobacteria*), *Bacteroides* and *Alistipes* (phylum = *Bacteroides*) increased after RYGB. The authors demonstrated significant correlation between beneficial alterations in the white adipose tissue transcriptome and dominant bacterial genera changes after surgery suggesting that the gut microbiota is a modulator of adipose tissue health.

Studies Assessing Functional Changes and Assigning Functional Annotation

The human studies described thus far point principally to consistent and characteristic changes in the gut microbiome occurring after gastric bypass with notable shifts observable at the phylum level. However empirical data showing a cause-effect relationship between microbiome shifts and decreased adiposity and improved metabolic control are best generated in experimental animal models that permit more agility in testing causality through microbiota transplant studies, etc.

Using a murine model of gastric bypass, Liou and colleagues [25] set out to examine whether changes in the gut microbiota after gastric bypass are conserved among humans, rats and mice and whether reconfiguration of the GI tract is more dominant in these changes than changes in caloric intake. Lastly the authors sought to identify whether the gastric bypass-modified microbiota when transplanted into unoperated mice conferred transferability of the weight loss effect.

The authors used the high-fat diet model of diet-induced obesity in the susceptible C57BL/6J strain to develop mice weighing 40–50 g (33–66% body weight excess) at 22–26 weeks of age. Three experimental groups were derived to test the hypothesis that procedure-dependent transplantable alterations in the gut microbiome akin to those seen in humans and rats would be induced following gastric bypass. The first group received a sham operation (SHAM), and a second group underwent sham operation and were subsequently weight matched through food restriction (WMS) to a 3rd group of mice that underwent gastric bypass (GB). Sequencing analysis of the faecal microbiome was carried out longitudinally, while caecal contents from donor animals representing each group were obtained at harvest, characterised and administered by oral gavage to germ-free mice to observe impact on adiposity.

A decrease in body weight of 30% was observed by 3 weeks post-GB. Food intake did not differ between GB and SHAM groups, but increased faecal calorie loss occurred in the GB group signalling energy wasting. The WMS required a 25% reduction in ad libitum food intake to achieve a body weight trajectory similar to GB group.

UniFrac analysis revealed that distal stomach and ileal, caecal and colonic microbiota were strongly affected by GB. GB markedly altered the faecal microbiota from 1 week after surgery and reconfiguration stabilised by 5 weeks after surgery. No alterations were noted between the faecal microbiome of SHAM and WMS animals indicating procedure-specific effects of GB that are independent of body weight change. Weight loss per se (GB or WMS) was accompanied by some similar proportional changes in the abundance of taxonomic groups within the *Firmicutes* phylum with both groups harbouring higher *Clostridiales* and lower levels of *Lactobacillales* and *Erysipelotrichales.* Unique changes after GB included increases in *Enterobacteriales* and higher *Verrucomicrobiales*. Three phylum level increases predominated in *Bacteroidetes*, *Verrucomicrobia* and *Proteobacteria*, with resolution at the genus level of *Alistipes*, *Akkermansia* and *Escherichia*.

Lean, germ-free mice inoculated with caecal contents from GB operated animals had reduced body weight, decreased fat deposition and improvements in insulin sensitivity versus animals inoculated with SHAM- or WMS-derived microbiota.

Tremaroli and colleagues [26] extended the above studies by performing shotgun sequencing of the human faecal metagenome to functionally analyse the gut microbiota of weight-stable women 9 years after gastric bypass and interrogate whether changes in the microbiota after gastric bypass were stable at long-term follow-up. The authors also assessed whether stably altered microbiota from humans could likewise transfer a reduction in adiposity in an animal model.

Significant differences in microbiota composition were observed in the gastric bypass samples versus a BMI-, sex- and age-matched comparator control group with genera differing significantly between groups. Increased presence of *Gammaproteobacteria* was notable after gastric bypass, while within the *Firmicutes* phylum (*Clostridium difficile*, *Clostridium hiranonis* and *Gemella sanguinis*), lower levels were recorded for the gastric bypass group. Facultative anaerobes within *Proteobacteria* (*Escherichia*, *Klebsiella* and *Pseudomonas*) were increased in relative abundance in the gastric bypass group.

From a functional genomic annotation perspective, alignment of reads to the MetaHIT human gut microbial gene catalogue revealed that 928 KEGG orthologs (Kos) were enriched and 60 depleted in gastric bypass samples with reporter pathways for phosphotransferase systems, fluorobenzoate degradation, nitrogen metabolism and fatty acid metabolism enriched in gastric bypass. Two component systems that enable bacteria to sense and respond to changes in the surrounding environment (nitrogen availability, phosphoglycerate transport, SCFA metabolism, response for antimicrobial peptides, outer membrane stress) were enriched in gastric bypass samples.

Metabolomic comparisons revealed a decrease in SCFA/branched chain fatty acid ratio after gastric bypass suggesting a shift from carbohydrate to amino acid fermentation after surgery with reductions in SCFA in faeces indicative of reduced energy harvest for the host. Genetic signatures for microbial enzymes involved in the generation of secondary bile acids were increased and correlated with shifts in the ratio of secondary to primary bile acid profiles.

Transplantation of faecal microbiota from humans after gastric bypass into mice resulted in a 43% reduction in body fat at 2-week post-inoculation coincident with a lower respiratory quotient [ratio between CO_2 produced and O_2 consumed], suggesting that decreased utilisation of carbohydrates and increased utilisation of lipids as fuel occurring in recipients of RYGB microbiota may participate in reductions in adiposity after surgery.

Graessler and colleagues [27] conducted pre-post surgery (3 months) metagenomic annotation of the faecal microbiota in six male diabetic recipients of gastric bypass and correlated changes with improvements in metabolic and inflammatory profiles. Consistent with other studies, expansion of *Proteobacteria* and increases in the *Bacteroidetes*/*Firmicutes* ratio were evident. As in the study of Tremaroli [26] and colleagues and a more recent longitudinal study by Palleja and colleagues [28], a striking increase in annotation of sequences to phosphotransferase systems was detected, while significant correlations between individual species and reductions in C-reactive protein and lipid and glucose homeostasis were found. Inflammatory improvements were however not independently associated with the microbiota when adjusted for BMI change.

Perspectives and Future Challenges

Review of the key publications in the field focussing on the effect of gastric bypass on the gut microbiome reveals that some common features are conserved across heterogenous study designs and species.

Phylogenetic comparison is the first lens through which comparisons can be made. Perhaps the most striking change in this regard is the consistent increase in the representation of the *Proteobacteria* phylum. One explanation for their increased prevalence may come from the preponderance of facultative anaerobes in this phylum which could drive proportional increases in abundance as a consequence of elevations in colonic oxygen tension secondary to reduced intestinal length. Small intestinal microbiota from the *Proteobacteria* such as *Enterobacteriaceae* may more readily colonise the large intestine due to more rapid transit of ingested materials to the colon. *Bacteroidetes* are also less acid-tolerant than *Firmicutes*, and elevated luminal pH after gastric bypass may provide a narrowing of the growth capacity differential between the phyla, thus explaining the consistent increase in *Bacteroidetes*/*Firmicutes* ratios.

Diversity assessed by species-level coverage is also increased by gastric bypass, but the profiles obtained suggest that gastric bypass increases diversity by the inclusion of new species within microbiome that are exclusive to the reconfigured gut rather than increased diversity being indicative of regression of the microbiome to that of nonobese individuals with intact gastrointestinal anatomy.

Phylogenetic changes do not in and of themselves provide particular insight into causality. However studies examining the microbiota through the lens of metagenomics and back-translation in rodents have been useful in this regard. Faecal transplantation experiments coupled to metagenomic annotation have been highly informative in assigning relevant functionality to the shifted microbiome after gastric bypass. Whether mechanistic improvements can ultimately be assigned to individual bacteria at the genus level or small groups of bacteria remains to be determined. However it appears clear that after gastric bypass the adapted microbiota shifts its preference in terms of metabolic substrate and does so in a fashion that favours reduced energy transfer to the host. Alterations in bile acid profile and enteroendocrine cell activity secondary to shifts in microbiota composition may also be important. Systematic description of the minimally effective microbiome would have enormous potential from a therapeutic perspective if the altered microbiota from gastric bypass could be stably adopted in intact recipients.

A direct and weight-independent causative role of changes in the microbiome in improvements in metabolic control and inflammation remains to be convincingly demonstrated in the same way that effects on adiposity have been.

Overall shifts in the microbiota after gastric bypass seem likely to be involved in the therapeutic effect and offer an exciting prospect in relation to the development of non-surgical "bariatric mimetic" approaches to the control of obesity and diabetes.

References

1. Organisation WH. Global health obervatory data-overweight and obesity. 2014. Available from: http://www.who.int/gho/ncd/risk_factors/overweight_text/en/.
2. Human Microbiome Project Consortium. Structure, function and diversity of the healthy human microbiome. Nature. 2012;486(7402):207–14.
3. Cani PD, Osto M, Geurts L, Everard A. Involvement of gut microbiota in the development of low-grade inflammation and type 2 diabetes associated with obesity. Gut Microbes. 2012;3(4):279–88.
4. Cox LM, Blaser MJ. Pathways in microbe-induced obesity. Cell Metab. 2013;17(6):883–94.
5. Scheithauer TP, Dallinga-Thie GM, de Vos WM, Nieuwdorp M, van Raalte DH. Causality of small and large intestinal microbiota in weight regulation and insulin resistance. Mol Metab. 2016;5(9):759–70.
6. Arumugam M, Raes J, Pelletier E, Le Paslier D, Yamada T, Mende DR, et al. Enterotypes of the human gut microbiome. Nature. 2011;473(7346):174–80.
7. Eckburg PB, Bik EM, Bernstein CN, Purdom E, Dethlefsen L, Sargent M, et al. Diversity of the human intestinal microbial flora. Science (New York, NY). 2005;308(5728):1635–8.
8. Adlerberth I, Wold AE. Establishment of the gut microbiota in Western infants. Acta Paediatr (Oslo, Norway: 1992). 2009;98(2):229–38.
9. Harmsen HJ, de Goffau MC. The human gut microbiota. Adv Exp Med Biol. 2016;902:95–108.
10. Zhang K, Hornef MW, Dupont A. The intestinal epithelium as guardian of gut barrier integrity. Cell Microbiol. 2015;17(11):1561–9.
11. Tremaroli V, Backhed F. Functional interactions between the gut microbiota and host metabolism. Nature. 2012;489(7415):242–9.
12. Helander HF, Fandriks L. Surface area of the digestive tract – revisited. Scand J Gastroenterol. 2014;49(6):681–9.
13. Caricilli AM, Castoldi A, Camara NO. Intestinal barrier: a gentlemen's agreement between microbiota and immunity. World J Gastrointest Pathophysiol. 2014;5(1):18–32.
14. Backhed F, Ding H, Wang T, Hooper LV, Koh GY, Nagy A, et al. The gut microbiota as an environmental factor that regulates fat storage. Proc Natl Acad Sci U S A. 2004;101(44):15718–23.
15. Turnbaugh PJ, Ley RE, Mahowald MA, Magrini V, Mardis ER, Gordon JI. An obesity-associated gut microbiome with increased capacity for energy harvest. Nature. 2006;444(7122):1027–31.
16. Cani PD, Amar J, Iglesias MA, Poggi M, Knauf C, Bastelica D, et al. Metabolic endotoxemia initiates obesity and insulin resistance. Diabetes. 2007;56(7):1761–72.
17. Cani PD, Bibiloni R, Knauf C, Waget A, Neyrinck AM, Delzenne NM, et al. Changes in gut microbiota control metabolic endotoxemia-induced inflammation in high-fat diet-induced obesity and diabetes in mice. Diabetes. 2008;57(6):1470–81.
18. Hersoug LG, Moller P, Loft S. Gut microbiota-derived lipopolysaccharide uptake and trafficking to adipose tissue: implications for inflammation and obesity. Obes Rev. 2016;17(4):297–312.
19. Vors C, Pineau G, Drai J, Meugnier E, Pesenti S, Laville M, et al. Postprandial endotoxemia linked with chylomicrons and lipopolysaccharides handling

in obese versus lean men: a lipid dose-effect trial. J Clin Endocrinol Metab. 2015;100(9):3427–35.
20. Ley RE, Turnbaugh PJ, Klein S, Gordon JI. Microbial ecology: human gut microbes associated with obesity. Nature. 2006;444(7122):1022–3.
21. Remely M, Aumueller E, Jahn D, Hippe B, Brath H, Haslberger AG. Microbiota and epigenetic regulation of inflammatory mediators in type 2 diabetes and obesity. Benefic Microbes. 2014;5(1):33–43.
22. Zhang H, DiBaise JK, Zuccolo A, Kudrna D, Braidotti M, Yu Y, et al. Human gut microbiota in obesity and after gastric bypass. Proc Natl Acad Sci U S A. 2009;106(7):2365–70.
23. Furet JP, Kong LC, Tap J, Poitou C, Basdevant A, Bouillot JL, et al. Differential adaptation of human gut microbiota to bariatric surgery-induced weight loss: links with metabolic and low-grade inflammation markers. Diabetes. 2010;59(12):3049–57.
24. Kong LC, Tap J, Aron-Wisnewsky J, Pelloux V, Basdevant A, Bouillot JL, et al. Gut microbiota after gastric bypass in human obesity: increased richness and associations of bacterial genera with adipose tissue genes. Am J Clin Nutr. 2013;98(1):16–24.
25. Liou AP, Paziuk M, Luevano JM Jr, Machineni S, Turnbaugh PJ, Kaplan LM. Conserved shifts in the gut microbiota due to gastric bypass reduce host weight and adiposity. Sci Transl Med. 2013;5(178):178ra41.
26. Tremaroli V, Karlsson F, Werling M, Stahlman M, Kovatcheva-Datchary P, Olbers T, et al. Roux-en-Y gastric bypass and vertical banded gastroplasty induce long-term changes on the human gut microbiome contributing to fat mass regulation. Cell Metab. 2015;22(2):228–38.
27. Graessler J, Qin Y, Zhong H, Zhang J, Licinio J, Wong ML, et al. Metagenomic sequencing of the human gut microbiome before and after bariatric surgery in obese patients with type 2 diabetes: correlation with inflammatory and metabolic parameters. Pharmacogenomics J. 2013;13(6):514–22.
28. Palleja A, Kashani A, Allin KH, Nielsen T, Zhang C, Li Y, et al. Roux-en-Y gastric bypass surgery of morbidly obese patients induces swift and persistent changes of the individual gut microbiota. Genome Med. 2016;8(1):67.

44 Infection: Diagnosis and Treatment

Álvaro Antônio Bandeira Ferraz and Luciana Teixeira de Siqueira

Postoperative Infection in Bariatric Surgery

At present, surgical complications and postoperative mortality in bariatric surgery have a mean incidence of 5.2% and 0.05%, respectively, at specialized centers [5].

The most common complications include anastomosis dehiscence, bleeding, infection of site of surgery, and pulmonary embolism. The most important infectious complications are infection of the site of surgery and dehiscence of the suture lines or stapling, leading to intra-abdominal infection by fistulas or peritonitis [6].

Intra-abdominal Infection

Management of intra-abdominal infection patients should be aggressive, precise, and timely. Identification of this complication is solely clinical in 72% of cases, with complementary image exams necessary in 25% [7]. In severely obese patients, clinical exteriorization is non-specific, and imaging exams do little to aid diagnosis. An infectious intra-abdominal complication should thus be suspected when the patient presents with tachypnea, tachycardia, and later fever; chills; shoulder pain, especially on the left; and pleural effusion.

Adequate control of the focus of infection is the main factor in reducing postoperative mortality.

The principles for management of abdominal sepsis thus include [8, 9]:

1. When to indicate reoperation
2. What to do

When to Indicate Reoperation

It is important to identify the characteristics specific to obese patients, such as unfavorable postoperative evolution with minimal signs and symptoms, physical examination of limited use for evaluation, and low resistance to progressively serious diseases [10]. Biotype and clinical limitations may pose technical obstacles for radiological studies requested after surgery to investigate complications [11].

Diagnosis of intra-abdominal infection is thus based on clinical symptoms, with or without the aid of radiology [12]. Patients whose condition

Á. A. B. Ferraz (✉)
Federal University of Pernambuco, Department of Surgery, Recife, Brazil

L. T. de Siqueira
Federal University of Pernambuco, Recife, Brazil

General Surgery Residence Program at the Federal University of Pernambuco Clinical Hospital, Recife, Brazil

J. Ettinger et al. (eds.), *Gastric Bypass*, https://doi.org/10.1007/978-3-030-28803-7_44

does not evolve favorably after the first day after surgery and experience increased abdominal pain, persistent tachycardia, fever, tachypnea, oliguria, or any combination of these symptoms require prompt investigation [12–14], and tachycardia above 120 beats per minute appears to be a good indicator of an infectious complication [12].

The imaging methods that can be used to detect leakage include upper gastrointestinal seriography and computerized tomography. Another test that may be useful, especially when radiology is of limited effectiveness, is oral administration of methylene blue to evaluate the outflow of coloring through intra-abdominal drainage [14].

The radiological findings usually encountered when investigating this complication are collections of liquid adjacent to the gastric pouch, diffuse abdominal fluid, free intraperitoneal air, and oral contrast in drainage. These findings can determine surgical conduct, depending on the clinical condition of the patient.

Conservative treatment may be effective in hemodynamically stable patients with contained discharge and may include 4–6 weeks of intravenous administration of broad spectrum antibiotics, monitoring of drained secretions, and nasoenteric or full parenteral nutrition, and, if the abscess identified is accessible, percutaneous drainage may be carried out [14]. However, image-guided percutaneous drains usually have a diameter of less than 24 French, which may result in ineffective drainage. Endoscopic treatment may be combined with the introduction of self-expandable esophageal stents, which remain in place for a maximum of 3–4 weeks as one more component of the array of therapeutic tools used to control infection, whether its etiology lies in a gastric fistula, normally in the angle of His and generally associated with gastric stenosis, in the gastric pouch or anastomosis. In these cases outpatient sessions of endoscopic pneumatic balloon dilations and argon scalpel septotomies may also be used to facilitate gastric emptying, guiding salivary secretion into the gastric pouch and helping to close the fistula.

Surgical treatment is indicated in hemodynamically unstable patients, with leakage complicated by peritonitis, especially if there is no intra-abdominal drainage, whether or not an imaging exam has been employed, since the fundamental aims of re-intervention are to confirm and repair the leak, if indicated, remove gastrointestinal content from the abdominal cavity, and bring about broad and effective abdominal drainage.

What to Do

Hemodynamic, Immunological, and Metabolic Support

In addition to the hydroelectrolytic and metabolic care that the abdominal sepsis patient should receive, the aims of management of this type of patient should be outlined [15]:

Hemodynamic Support

Maximize O_2 support for tissues:

- Hydroelectrolytic replacement
- Inotropic agents
- Vasoactive agents
- Mechanical ventilation

Metabolic Support

The aim is, essentially, to reverse the state of catabolism. Nutritional support should be aggressive, preferably through enteral nutrition, which has the clear advantage of modulating the inflammatory response and reducing the tumor necrosis factor response (TNF) [16]. Enteral nutrition generally improves the capacity of the organism by reducing bacterial translocation by diminishing the catabolic response, lowering levels of plasma cortisol, and preventing atrophy of the intestinal mucosa [17]. If gut functioning is inadequate but the patient is hemodynamically stable, parenteral nutrition should be initiated.

Nutritional therapy, in addition to preventing and treating dietary deficiencies, has been used to obtain similar responses to pharmacological agents, in order to improve the immune response of patients to certain types of aggression. A large variety of nutrients bring about immunostimulant alterations, including the fatty acids omega 3, glutamine, and arginine.

Balanced enteral nutrition plays an important role, both in recovery and maintenance of nutritional status and in modulation of the inflammatory response. Studies show that a balanced diet supplemented with arginine, nucleotides, and fish oil reduces the length of time patients stay in ICU and the incidence of infectious complications [18].

Enteral nutrition in gastric fistula patients requires special care when passing through the endoscope and placing the tube, once the site of the fistula has been identified during reoperation. The tube should ideally be positioned after the duodenal portion in cases of sleeve gastrectomy and in a more distal part of the jejunum in cases of Roux-en-Y gastric bypass, for reason of reflux of food content from the tube and gut, causing contamination and perpetuation of the fistula orifice. Parenteral nutrition should be provided in cases of reflux of enteral diet through the tube and consequent outflow through the abdominal drain. It is not advisable to initiate oral diet in patients without an esophageal stent, even though methylene blue oral ingestion tests are negative for outflow. The best test for this is seriography of the upper gastrointestinal tract.

Immunological Support

Immunological support aims to prevent nosocomial infections, eradicate existing infections, and minimize the effects of the metabolic response to infection. Immunomodulation is the treatment intervention that aims to modify the compromised immune response [19, 20]. Precise identification of immunocompromised patients, who have an exaggerated inflammatory response, is one route for diagnosis of patients prone to present an inadequate organic response to anesthesiological and surgical intervention. Surgery may be immunomodulatory in so far as it controls the focus of infection and also immunosuppressive if it reduces the reserves and resistance of the immune response of the host [21]. Attempts have been made to modulate the immune response of the surgery patient, but few have been able to interfere in this response. This is probably because the timing of each of the numerous variables involved in sepsis and systemic inflammatory response syndrome (SIRS) is still not fully understood. According to the current state of knowledge, it is understood that current medical intervention regarding the healing of tissue is inadequate, causing selection of multiresistant bacteria through inappropriate use of antibiotics, irresponsible use of invasive devices, and surgical techniques that are inadequate for controlling foci of infection [22]. However, the reduction in mortality among surgery patients has not been insignificant in the past decade with greater application of this knowledge, although there is clearly a long way to go.

Antimicrobial Treatment

Owing to their body composition, obese patients absorb, metabolize, and excrete drugs differently [23]. Recent studies have investigated the relation between body size, physiological functions, and pharmacokinetic variables in this population. Some physiological alterations peculiar to the morbidly obese have potential consequences for the kinetics of drugs. These include:

- Increased body mass
- Increased cardiac deficit and total blood volume
- Increased renal clearance
- Increased deposition of fat in the liver
- Alterations in plasma levels of proteins

Antibiotic treatment of intra-abdominal infection is usually initiated empirically and should cover a polymicrobial flora composed essentially of Gram-negative and anaerobic microorganisms. Gram staining is highly recommended, and a culture will indicate the correct sensitivity of bacterial pathogens.

After removal of the focus of infection, antibiotic treatment should be maintained until the patient presents with the following [24]:

- Normal leukogram for more than 48 hours
- No fever peaks for more than 48 hours
- No anorexia
- Level of consciousness re-established

Inadequate use of antibiotics, especially in this type of patient, may lead to infection by multiresistant pathogens and massive release of endotoxins, which, depending on the action of the antibiotics, are related to increased mortality and should be taken into consideration when selecting the treatment regimen [25, 26].

Vancomycin and the aminoglycosides are some of the few antibiotics whose pharmacokinetics has been extensively studied in the obese population. Although there are as yet no definitive data, some initial recommendations may be suggested. Doses of vancomycin should be calculated according to total body weight (TBW). Doses of aminoglycosides should be based on the volume of distribution, using an FCDP of approximately 0.4. The interval between doses should be determined on a case-by-case basis by measuring serum concentrations of these drugs [27].

Allard et al. [28] studied the volume of distribution and clearance of ciprofloxacin in obese patients and found that the maximum plasma concentration of ciprofloxacin is lower in obese individuals than in the nonobese after intravenous infusion of 400 mg, although concentrations still lie within the recommended range. These authors conclude that the dose of ciprofloxacin should be based on ideal body weight (IBW) plus FCDP of 0.45.

Tables 44.1 and 44.2 provide some suggestions for optimal doses in obese patients [29, 30].

Table 44.1 Dose of antibiotic by patient weight

Antibiotic	Calculation of dose based on weight
Beta lactams	IBW + 0.30 (TBW – IBW)
Cefazolin	Double dose (2 g/6–6 hours)
Cefoxitin	Empirical – IBW
Ceftriaxone	IBW + 0.40 (TBW – IBW)
Cefepime	Empirical (2 g/12–12 hours)
Ceftazidime	Empirical – IBW
Ampicillin	Empirical – IBW
Imipenem	Empirical – IBW
Metronidazole	TBW
Gentamicin	IBW + 0.43 (TBW – IBW)
Amikacin	IBW + 0.38 (TBW – IBW)
Vancomycin	TBW
Ciprofloxacin	IBW + 0.45 (TBW – IBW)
Macrolides	IBW
Amphotericin B	TBW
Aciclovir	IBW

Ferraz et al. [29]
IBW ideal body weight, *TBW* total body weight

Table 44.2 Recommended dose for antibiotics, according to body mass index

Antimicrobial	Half-life if normal renal function (h)	Recommended infusion time (min)	Standard intravenous dose	Recommended intravenous dose per BMI group	Redosing interval (h)
Cefazolin	1.2–2.5	3–5[a] 15–60[b]	1 g	BMI ≥30 to ≤50 kg/m^2: 2 gBMI >50 kg/m^2: 3 g	2–5
Cefoxitin	0.5–1.1	3–5[a] 15–60[b]	1 g	BMI ≥30 to ≤50 kg/m^2: 2 gBMI >50 kg/m^2: 3 g	2–3
Ceftriaxone	5–11	3–5[a] 15–60[b]	1 g	BMI ≥30 to ≤50 kg/m^2: 2 gBMI >50 kg/m^2: 3 g	10
Metronidazole	6–14	30–60	500 mg	1 g	6–8
Clindamycin	2–5.1	10–60 (not to exceed 30 mg/min)	600 mg	BMI ≥30 to ≤50 kg/m^2: 900 mg BMI >50 kg/m^2: 1200 mg	6–8
Ciprofloxacin	3–7	60	400 mg	400 mg	4–10
Levofloxacin	5.7–9.6	60 90	500 mg–	– 750 mg	– 24
Aztreonam	1.5–2	3–5[a]	1 g	BMI ≥30 to ≤50 kg/m^2: 2 g BMI ≥50 kg/m^2: 3 g	3–5
Vancomycin	4–6	1 h/g	1 g	25 mg/kg (TBW)[#] Maximum initial dose: 2.5 g Maximum redose: 1.5 g	8–12

[a, b]From Chopra et al. [30]
BMI body mass index

Control of Focus of Infection and Underlying Disease

On diagnosis of the discharge, surgical repair is initially the ideal strategy for controlling the focus of infection, but the local suture may pose a challenge, owing to the intensive acute inflammatory process in the tissue creating a greater risk of worsening the lesion if there is local manipulation with a new suture. In such cases, removal of the gastrointestinal contents and placement of drainage tubes may be the safest option. Depending on the abilities of the surgical team, the surgery may be laparoscopic or open. Maintenance of nutrition requires being able to heal the tissue at the site of the leakage.

On the other hand, bariatric surgery related intra-abdominal infection presents essentially in one of two ways: in the form of secondary peritonitis or intra-abdominal abscess.

In the case of secondary peritonitis, surgical treatment is recommended for the purpose of:

1. Elimination of the focus of contamination
2. Removal of secondary sources of contamination
3. Drainage of established abscesses
4. Deep cleaning of cavity
5. Primary fascial closure

In cases of secondary peritonitis, re-laparotomies every 48 hours are indicated until the cavity presents no macroscopic signs of infection. Thereafter re-laparotomies are performed when necessary, if the clinical and laboratory profile deteriorates [31].

Peritoneostomy is indicated only in exceptional circumstances, as it may be harmful to the patient and its benefits need to be clearly established. It is indicated if primary closure of the abdominal cavity is impossible, in cases of fecal etiology and diffuse peritonitis, with patient in an unstable condition with secondary foci of necrosis and tissue ischemia.

Treatment of intra-abdominal abscess invariably involves drainage, which can be performed percutaneously or through open surgery. Analysis of the correlation between type of drainage and APACHE II score has found no difference between types of drainage in patients with low risk of mortality. However, in patients with high APACHE II scores, better outcomes have been achieved when the abscess is treated using open surgery [32]. The outcome is excellent for percutaneous drainage when the following conditions pertain [33]:

1. Well-established unilocular collection of fluid
2. Well-established drainage route
3. Adequate material and equipment

Surgical drainage is indicated in cases of:

1. Failure of percutaneous drainage
2. Multiple abscesses
3. Abscesses associated with abdominal pathology and fistulas

The most important thing, however, is that drainage is effective, especially in cases of diagnosis of fistula leakage, usually at the level of the angle of His, to prevent the development of chronic fistulas that require complex treatment, such as gastrobronchial and gastrocutaneous ones. It is known that factors affecting the persistence of this condition include the presence of inadequately drained subphrenic abscess and stenosis distal to the fistula orifice (at the level of the angular incisure in sleeve gastrectomy or the gastrojejunal anastomosis in Roux-en-Y gastric bypass). Intra-abdominal drainage is accompanied by early endoscopic treatment of fistulas by placement of esophageal stent, preferably at the time of reoperation, which reduces the length of stay in hospital and enables more rapid return to an oral diet, reducing catabolism and improving the organic response to the infection. It is important to avoid insertion of the nasoenteric tube along with the stent, because of the risk of distal migration, as this may cause intestinal obstruction and emergency laparotomies or partial covering of the fistula orifice, which may perpetuate the contamination through secretion of saliva. Periodical radiological examinations should therefore be carried out to check for possible dislocation of the stent and even partially covered metal ones. If the fistula has become chronic or evolved into a gastrobronchial or gastrocutaneous fistula, the prognosis changes, and, in most cases, patients are found to be malnourished, with multiresistant infections. Such cases require various sessions of endoscopic treatment, including dilation and stenostomy. Thoracic surgery or reoperation of the abdomen to carry out gastrostomy of the excluded stomach or esophagostomy in severe cases, or even conversion of sleeve gastrectomy into RYGB to reduce gastric reflux of bilioenteric secretion and hence contamination of the fistula, may be needed in cases refractory to endoscopic treatment. It is thus imperative that the patient be accompanied by a multidisciplinary team including a nutritionist, a physiotherapist, a psychologist, an endoscopist, and chest and abdomen surgeons [34–37].

The use of antibiotics for treatment of intra-abdominal abscess is still a matter of controversy. Stable patients with a single clearly limited, purulent collection, precisely diagnosed by radiological imaging, may undergo extra-serous or puncture drainage with or without the aid of ultrasound or computerized tomography, with a single dose of antibiotics, 30–60 minutes prior to the procedure. The antibiotic should cover anaerobic and aerobic Gram-negative bacteria.

With the exception of these cases, antibiotics are indicated for most intra-abdominal abscess patients.

Final Considerations

In the light of the above discussion, reoperation should thus be indicated for infectious complications after bariatric surgery, principally on the basis of the clinical profile. Intervention should be as early as possible and involve concomitant endoscopic treatment and effective drainage, with the support of intensive care and a multidisciplinary team, in order to better control the focus of infection and reduce damage and consequent heightened organic response, which may culminate in multiple organ failure, in view of the specific physiopathological profile of obese patients (chronic inflammation with the immunological repercussion of low resistance to progressively more severe diseases).

References

1. World Health Organization (WHO) Obesity. Retrieved from http://www.who.int/mediacentre/factsheets.fs311/en/. 15 Aug 2015.
2. Chong AJ, Dellinger EP. Infectious complications of surgery in morbidly obese patients. http://www.biomedcentral.com/1523-3820/5/387. Accessed 27 Dec 2005.
3. Chang SH, Stoll CR, Song J, Varela JE, Eagon CJ, Colditz GA. The effectiveness and risks of bariatric surgery: an updated systematic review and meta-analysis, 2003–2012. JAMA Surg. 2014;149:275.
4. Ferraz AAB, Ferraz EM. Antibioticoprofilaxia em cirurgia. In: Colégio Brasileiro de Cirurgiões. Programa de atualização. Ano I. 2002;1(2):4–18.
5. Birkmeyer JD, Finks JF, O'Reilly A, et al. Surgical skill and complications rates after bariatric surgery. N Engl J Med. 2013;369(15):1434–42.
6. Lyons T, Neff KJ, Benn J, Chuah LL, le Roux CW, Gilchrist M. Body mass index and diabetes status do not affect postoperative infection rates after bariatric surgery. Surg Obes Relat Dis. 2014;10(2):291–7.
7. Conor TJ, Garcha IS, Ramshaw BJ, Mitchell CW, Wilson JP, Mason EM, Duncan TD, Dozier FA, Lucas GW. Diagnostic laparoscopy for suspected appendicitis. Am Surg. 1995;61(2):187–9.
8. Christou NV, Barie PS, Dellinger EP, Waymack JP, Stone HH. Surgical Infection Society intra-abdominal infection study. Prospective evaluation of management techniques and outcome. Arch Surg. 1993;128(2):193–8.
9. Ferraz AAB, Ferraz EM. Abordagem cirúrgica da sepse abdominal. In: Petroianu A, editor. Terapêutica cirúrgica. Rio de Janeiro: Guanabara Koogan; 2001. p. 640–5.
10. Karmali S, Stoklossa CJ, Sharma A, Stadnyk J, Christiansen S, Cottreau D, et al. Bariatric surgery. Can Fam Physician. 2010;56:873–9.
11. Labrunie EM, Marchiori E, Tubiana JM. Fístulas de anastomose superior pós-gastroplastia redutora pela técnica de Higa para tratamento da obesidade mórbida: aspectos por imagem. Radiol Bras. 2008;41:75–9.
12. Kravetz AJ, Reddy S, Murtaza G, et al. A comparative study of handsewn versus stapled gastrojejunal anastomosis in laparoscopic Roux-en-Y gastric bypass. Surg Endosc. 2011;25:1287–92.
13. Raman R, Raman B, Raman P, et al. Abnormal findings on routine upper GI series following laparoscopic Roux-en-Y gastric bypass. Obes Surg. 2007;17(3):311–6.
14. Rogula T, Yenumula PR, Schauer PR. A complication of Roux- en-Y gastric bypass: intestinal obstruction. Surg Endosc. 2007;21(11):1914–8. Epub 2007 Sep 22.
15. Wittmann DH. Tratamento cirúrgico das peritonites. In: Ferraz EM, editor. Infecção em cirurgia. Rio de Janeiro: MEDSI; 1997. p. 387–420.

16. Marshall JC, Nathens AB. Multiple organ dysfunction syndrome. In: Wilmore DW, Cheung LY, Harken AH, Holcroft JW, Meakins JL, Soper NT, editors. ACS surgery: principles & practice. New York: WEBMD Corporation; 2001. p. 1473–94.
17. Fong, Y; Lowry, S. Cytokines and the cellular response to injury and infection. In. Meakins JL (ed) Surgical infections. Scientific American Inc. New York, 65–86; 1994.
18. Faist E, Storck M, Hueltner L, et al. Functional analysis of monocyte (MO) activity via synthesis patterns of interleukin 1, 6, 8 (IL-1, IL-6, IL-8) and neopterin (NPT) in surgical intensive care patients. Surgery. 1992;9:562–72.
19. Alexander W. Can nutrition influence translocation? The effect of nutrition on translocation and host defense. J Intensive Care Med. 1994;20(1):134.
20. Horn JK. Origem da Sepse. In: Ferraz EM, editor. Infecção em Cirurgia. Rio de Janeiro: MEDSI; 1997.
21. Faist E, Bawe AE. Imunoconseqüências do Trauma, do Choque e da Sepse: mecanismos e abordagens contra-reguladoras. In: Ferraz EM, editor. Infecção em Cirurgia. Rio de Janeiro: MEDSI; 1997.
22. Meakins JL. Surgical infections in critical care medicine. New York: Churchill Livingstone; 1985.
23. Condon RE. Infecções Cirúrgicas nos hospedeiros comprometidos. In: Ferraz EM, editor. Infecção em Cirurgia. Rio de Janeiro: MEDSI; 1997.
24. Ferraz EM, Bacelar TS, Aguiar JLA, et al. Wound infection rates in clean surgery: a potentially misleading risk classification. Infect Control Hosp Epidemiol. 1992;13(8):457–62.
25. Cossu ML, Caccia S, Coppola M, et al. Orally administered ranitidine plasma concentrations before and after bibliopancreatic diversion in morbidly obese patients. Obes Surg. 1999;9(1):36–9.
26. Mock CN, Jurkovich GJ, Dries DJ, Maier RV. Clinical significance of antibiotic endotoxin-releasing properties in trauma patients. Arch Surg. 1995;130(11):1234–40.
27. Bearden DT, Rodvold KA. Dosage adjustments for antibacterials in obese patients. Clin Pharmacokinet. 2000;38(5):415–26.
28. Allard S, Kinzing M, Boivin G, Sorgel F, Lebel M. Intravenous ciprofloxacin disposition in obesity. Clin Pharmacol Ther. 1993;54:368–73.
29. Ferraz AAB, et al. Profilaxia antimicrobiana na cirurgia bariátrica. Rev Col Bras Cir. 2007;34(2):73–7.
30. Chopra T, Zhao JJ, Alangaden G, Wood MH, Kaye KS. Preventing surgical site infections after bariatric surgery: value of perioperative antibiotic regimens. Expert Rev Pharmacoecon Outcomes Res. 2010;10(3):317–28.
31. Adeodato LCL, Pagnosin G, Ferraz EM. Relaparotomias programadas. In: Ferraz EM, editor. Infecção em cirurgia. Rio de Janeiro: MEDSI; 1997. p. 441–68.
32. Levison MA, Zeigler D. Correlation of APACHE II score, drainage technique and outcome in postoperative intra-abdominal abscess. Surg Gynecol Obstet. 1991;172:89–94.
33. Ferraz EM, Ferraz AAB. Abscesso intra-abdominais. In: Coelho JCU, editor. Aparelho Digestivo: Clínica e Cirurgia. Rio de Janeiro: ATHENEU; 2005. p. 1929–39.
34. Ramos AC, Ramos MG, Campos JM, Galvão Neto Mdos P, Bastos EL. Laparoscopic total gastrectomy as an alternative treatment to postsleeve chronic fistula. Surg Obes Relat Dis. 2015;11(3):552–6.
35. Nedelcu AM, Skalli M, Deneve E, Fabre JM, Nocca D. Surgical management of chronic fistula after sleeve gastrectomy. Surg Obes Relat Dis. 2013;9(6):879–84.
36. Campos JM, Pereira EF, Evangelista LF, Siqueira L, Neto MG, Dib V, Falcão M, Arantes V, Awruch D, Albuquerque W, Ettinger J, Ramos A, Ferraz Á. Gastrobronchial fistula after sleeve gastrectomy and gastric bypass: endoscopic management and prevention. Obes Surg. 2011;21(10):1520–9.
37. Simon F, Siciliano I, Gillet A, Castel B, Coffin B, Msika S. Gastric leak after laparoscopic sleeve gastrectomy: early covered self-expandable stent reduces healing time. Obes Surg. 2013;23(5):687–92.

Gastric Bypass in Patients with Metabolic Syndrome

45

Mariano Palermo, Maria del Pilar Quevedo, Edgardo Serra, and Marianela Aguirre Ackermann

Metabolic surgery was defined by Varco and Buchwald as "the operative manipulation of a normal organ or organ system to achieve a biological result for a potential health gain" (Buchwald [1]).

Introduction

Type 2 diabetes (T2DM) is one of the largest health emergencies of the twenty-first century. During the past decades, we have been witnesses of the world-increasing pandemic of obesity and diabetes. Currently, some 415 million people worldwide are estimated to have diabetes, and if these trends continue, by 2040 some 642 million people, or 1 adult in 10, will have diabetes [2]. The World Health Organization (WHO) estimates that globally, high blood glucose is the third highest risk factor for premature mortality, after high blood pressure and tobacco use; therefore, in order to prevent cardiovascular complications aiming to reduce mortality, a broader management focusing in glucose control, lipids, and blood pressure is necessary [3]. Conventional management for T2DM includes lifestyle interventions and medication [4], but despite the increasing number and variety of antidiabetic drugs that have emerged during the last two decades to achieve optimal glycemic control, T2DM control remains suboptimal [5, 6]. Numerous aspects must be considered when setting glycemic targets. The ADA proposes optimal targets, but each target must be individualized to the needs of each patient and his or her disease factors. Current treatment goals proposed by the American Diabetes Association (ADA) are glycated hemoglobin (A1c) <7%, low-density lipoprotein cholesterol levels <100 mg/dl, and blood pressure <130–80 mm Hg [4].

Hyperglycemia defines diabetes, and glycemic control is fundamental to diabetes management. Several trials have provided evidence that appropriate glycemic control could lead to a significant reduction in the risk of long-term diabetic complications. The *UK Prospective Diabetes Study* (UKPDS) demonstrated over 10 years of follow-up that tight glycemic control in the intensive treatment arm was associated with significantly decreased rates of micro- and macrovascular complications when compared with conventional management (HbA1c 7% vs. HbA1c 7.9%, respectively) and correlated with a 10% reduction in the risk of any diabetes-related death and 6% for all causes of mortality. Long-term follow-up of the UKPDS cohort showed enduring effects of early glycemic control on most microvascular complications [7]. Three landmark trials (Action to Control Cardiovascular

M. Palermo (✉) · M. del Pilar Quevedo
M. A. Ackermann
Division of Bariatric Surgery Centro CIEN – DIAGNOMED, Institution to the University of Buenos Aires, Buenos Aires, Argentina

E. Serra
Division of Bariatric Surgery Centro CIEN – DIAGNOMED, Affiliated Institution to the University of Buenos Aires and DAICIM Foundation, Buenos Aires, Argentina

J. Ettinger et al. (eds.), *Gastric Bypass*, https://doi.org/10.1007/978-3-030-28803-7_45

Risk in Diabetes [ACCORD], Action in Diabetes and Vascular Disease: Preterax and Diamicron MR Controlled Evaluation [ADVANCE], and Veterans Affairs Diabetes Trial [VADT]) showed that lower A1C levels were associated with reduced onset or progression of microvascular complications [8–10]. In diabetic patients, *cardiovascular disease (CVD) is a more common cause of death than microvascular complications, and there is strong evidence that more intensive control of glycemic may reduce long-term CVD rates. The UKPDS* reported a 16% risk reduction of CVD events (combined fatal or nonfatal myocardial infarction (MI) and sudden death) in the intensive glycemic control arm, but it was not statistically significant ($p = 0.0052$). However, after long-term follow-up, those originally assigned to the intensive group had significant long-term reduction in MI and in all-cause mortality (13% vs. 27%). *Therefore, achieving glycemic control of A1c target <7% has been shown to reduce microvascular complications of diabetes.*

Bariatric surgery was initially developed as a tool for weight reduction in severely obese patients. The prospective controlled Swedish Obese Subjects (SOS) study compared obese subjects who underwent bariatric surgery versus contemporaneously matched conventionally treated patients. It demonstrated that the surgery group arm not only had more drastic and sustainable average changes in body weight but also showed remarkable effects on risk factor values, such as waist circumference; glucose and insulin levels; uric acid, triglyceride, and HDL cholesterol levels; as well as blood pressure, when compared with conventionally treated patients [11]. The SOS also found reduced number of cardiovascular events and overall mortality reduction in the surgery group compared with the conventional arm (HR 0.76, CI95%) [12, 13], but one of the most interesting findings in this study was that there was no significant relationship between cardiovascular mortality and body mass index (BMI) [14]. More than two decades later, gastrointestinal surgery provides a unique opportunity to improve our understanding of glucose homeostasis, diabetes, and B-cell growth.

Gastrointestinal operations have demonstrated, especially those that involve food rerouting through the gastrointestinal tract that are safe and provide better outcomes for weight loss and improvement in glucose metabolism in obese patients with type 2 diabetes (T2DM) in comparison to conventional strategies. Bariatric/metabolic procedures have even shown to cause remission of the disease [15, 16] as well as demonstrated extraordinary benefits on lipids and blood pressure control, suggesting good long-term effects on cardiovascular risk profile and mortality [6, 12, 17, 18]. Better glucose control was observed in patients following Roux-en-Y gastric bypass (RYGB) when compared with patients that lost the same amount of weight after lifestyle intervention [19, 20]. Early improvement of metabolic control in the postoperative population was observed days or weeks after the surgical procedure, long before considerable weight loss, preluding a direct antidiabetic effect [6]. This remarkable effect has been described not only in morbidly obese patients but also with class I obesity patients, making it a promising tool to treat T2DM.

The mechanisms by which these operations control diabetes have become the subject of intense research, fueled by the experimental evidence that gastrointestinal bypass surgery can induce very rapid antidiabetes, independent of weight loss [21].

The pathophysiology of T2DM is complex, but it's characterized by a combination of insulin resistance and progressive defective insulin secretion with ends in hyperglycemia and its deletereal effects. The metabolic abnormalities of T2DM are ameliorated by an increase in insulin availability or a decrease in insulin resistance. Improving hyperglycemia decreases glucose toxicity and thus insulin secretion function. Furthermore, insulin resistance in overweight and obese subjects overcomes as a consequence of adiposopathy. The dysfunction of adipose tissue seems to be the beginning of the deposition of excess quantities of lipid, lipid metabolites, and adipokines into non-adipose tissue cells. This ectopic fat deposit in muscle and liver interferes with insulin physiological actions and results in insulin resistance (Savage et al. [22]); therefore, decreasing hepatic fat infiltration and reducing visceral fat may be the best predictor of improvement in insulin resistance. One of the most relevant points in this pathophysiological context is that BMI does not reflect adipose tissue distribution; therefore, it becomes a poor index of metabolically significant obesity (Pories et al. [23]). In this way, BMI should not be considered as a stringent eligibility criteria for metabolic procedures as well as to determine the potential benefits for resolution or improvement because it does not represent a measure of metabolically significant abnormalities associated with obesity.

In this background, it's reasonable to expect that treatments that attack both defects would be more effective and could achieve diabetes remission.

Mechanisms

Metabolic surgery is a highly effective treatment of T2DM, inducing improvement and/or remission in obese patients [15, 16, 19].

GI surgical procedures that involve food rerouting can improve both insulin sensitivity and production [24, 25], especially RYGB, which restores first-phase insulin response [25] and results in hypersecretion of C-peptide and insulin after a meal, suggesting enhancement of B-cell function and increase of B-cell mass. There exist numerous mechanisms proposed to explain how RYGB exerts its effects on B-cell islets. The incretin effect, a hormonal response of B cells to exacerbate insulin secretion after an oral load of glucose, is mediated by GLP-1, an intestinal hormone released by L cell in the ileum. This response appears to be enhanced after surgery; in fact, RYGB causes a three- to fourfold increase in postprandial levels of GLP-1 [26] resulting in further stimulation to insulin release from the pancreas as well as an antiapoptotic effect on the B cell. On the other side, the anti-incretin theory postulates that in addition to the well-known uncertain effect (GLP-1, glucose-dependent insulinotropic polypeptide (GIP)), nutrient passage through the small bowel could also activate "anti-incretins" or feedback mechanisms to balance the actions of GLP-1 and GIP such as to enhance insulin secretion, insulin action, and B-cell function and growth. In the absence of one or more of these feedback mechanisms, these effects would expose to exacerbated insulin hypersecretion and B-cell function and growth, with the concomitant risk of postprandial hyperinsulinemic hypoglycemia and uncontrolled B-cell proliferation. Reduction of nutrient passage and stimuli on the gut by surgical procedures that exclude parts of the foregut and the arrival of them to the handgun could restore appropriate incretin/anti-incretin balance explaining improvement of T2DM [27, 28]. Besides, some operations engage mechanisms that improve glucose homeostasis independent of weight loss, such as changes in gut hormones, bile acid metabolism, microbiota, intestinal glucose metabolism, and nutrient sensing [21, 29–38].

Eligibility Criteria for Metabolic Surgery

Bariatric and metabolic surgery might be misunderstood as synonymous, but they are not since bariatric operation primary indication is to achieve weight loss in morbidly obese patients and the metabolic benefits (improvement in T2DM, hypertension, dyslipidemia) and reduction of overall mortality might be considered beneficial side effects. In 1978, Varco and Buchwald defined metabolic surgery as "the operative manipulation of a normal organ or organ system to achieve a biological result for a potential health gain" [1]. This definition involves the notion of an anatomical and functional procedure on a normal gastrointestinal tract aimed at reducing or reverting an altered function that causes a metabolic disease. Therefore, metabolic surgery can be considered only if the goal of the functional change is to correct or counteract a metabolic alteration [39].

Gastrointestinal surgery for the specific intention to treat T2DM was first recommended at the 2007 Diabetes Surgery Summit (DSS) [40] and implicated a shift in the primary focus of surgery from mere weight management to treatment or improvement of metabolic illness that may have significant and practical ramification [41]. After the DSS recommendations for considering gastrointestinal surgery to intentionally treat T2DM, the concept of "metabolic surgery" has emerged to more broadly indicate a surgical approach to control metabolic illness, not just excess weight. In 2011 the International Federation of Diabetes (IDF) concluded that surgery could be considered in the treatment of poorly controlled T2DM among white individuals with BMI of ≧30 Kg/m² and in Asian individuals (especially susceptible to T2DM) with a BMI as low as 27.5 kg/m² [42 IDF].

Currently, eligibility criteria for metabolic surgery do not include metrics of metabolic disease severity, predictor of success of treatment, or an evaluation of risks and benefits of surgery as contrasted to those alternative diabetes treatment options [43]. The preoperative evaluation for metabolic surgery should include clinical considerations such as inadequate response of glycemia to optimal medical therapy or the presence of other cardiovascular risk factors, as well as the need to identify and monitor diabetes-related parameters and complications instead of focusing on BMI or body weight criteria solely [1, 44]. In fact, the SOS study demonstrated that baseline BMI does not predict the benefits of surgery related to T2DM development, cancer, cardiovascular events, or death [44, 45] but surgical benefits were notably predicted by high baseline insulin and/or glucose levels, presumably reflecting insulin resistance. In this background, BMI cutoff at 35 kg/m² is not an accurate parameter to predict the potential of surgery to induce glycemic and metabolic control, so it should not be considered a *stand-alone* criterion for surgical selection.

Given its role in metabolic regulation, the gastrointestinal (GI) tract constitutes a clinically and biologically meaningful target for the management of T2DM. The DSS position statement recognized for the first time the legitimacy of GI surgery to specifically treat T2DM in carefully selected patients. The DSS delegates agreed that patients with *inadequately controlled diabetes* and BMI ≥35 kg/m² should be considered for GI surgery; and in patients with BMI <35 kg/m², there was good consensus regarding the legitimacy of GI surgery as a non-primary therapeutic alternative to treat mildly to moderately obese patients (BMI 30–35 kg/m²) with T2DM inadequately controlled by lifestyle and medications [40].

In 2016, the 2nd Diabetes Surgery Summit (DDS-2) was published on the basis of a substantial body of evidence that demonstrated that gastrointestinal surgery achieved superior glycemic control and reduction of cardiovascular risk factors in obese patients with T2DM compared with various medical/lifestyle interventions; so, based on these evidence, several international professional organizations have recently suggested expanding the indications for bariatric/metabolic surgery to include patients with inadequately controlled T2DM and BMI as low as 30 kg/m² and down to 27,7 kg/m² for Asians [43].

The DSS-2 recommendations for metabolic surgery include:

- Metabolic surgery should be a *recommended* option to treat T2DM in appropriate surgical candidates with class III obesity (BMI ≥ 40 kg/m²), regardless of the level of glycemic control or complexity of glucose-lowering regimens, as well as in patients with class II obesity (BMI 35–39.9 kg/m²) with inadequately controlled hyperglycemia despite lifestyle and optimal medical therapy
- Metabolic surgery should be also *considered* to be an option to treat T2DM in patients with class I obesity (BMI 30–35 kg/m²) and inadequately controlled hyperglycemia despite optimal medical treatment by either oral or injectable medications (including insulin).
- All BMI threshold should be considered depending on the ancestry of the patient. For example, for patients of Asian descent, the BMI values above should be reduced by 2.5 kg/m².

So, on the basis of these evidence that demonstrated that metabolic surgery achieves excellent glycemic control and reduces cardiovascular risk factors, selecting a population with greater metabolic illness and hence with greater potential to benefit from treatment might further enhance the cost-effectiveness of the surgery, implicating a shift in the paradigm of the eligibility criteria for surgery, focusing more on the treatment of the diseases and complications related to obesity rather than simply on body weight.

Results of Metabolic Surgery and Prognostic Factors

The GI tract is an important contributor to normal glucose homeostasis [1] and increasing evidence has demonstrated that gastrointestinal operations can dramatically ameliorate or prevent T2DM. Beyond inducing weight loss-related metabolic improvements, some operations engage mechanisms that improve glucose homeostasis independent of weight loss. Moreover, when comparing medical therapy (conventional and/or intensive) for T2DM versus surgical GI procedures, surgery resulted in significantly better glucose control than did medical therapy alone; so it's not surprising that bariatric-metabolic surgery is being used throughout the world to treat diabetes [39].

Based on data from growing evidence that demonstrate that metabolic surgery achieves excellent glycemic control and reduces cardiovascular risks factors, improvement of metabolic diseases and cardiovascular disease risk reduction are more rational measures of outcomes becoming mandatory to change goals of bariatric-metabolic surgery and to redefine the success and failure of surgical treatment.

Defining the idea of *T2DM remission* following surgery has been controversial [43, 44].

Currently, based on 2009 consensus criteria, T2DM remission is defined as being off diabetes medication with normal fasting blood glucose (6.6 mmol/L) or HbA1c level of less than 6% [1]. These criteria rely on more stringent cutoff points and implicate that rates of remission are likely to be lower [44]. The American Diabetes Association (ADA) also defined criteria for total and partial remission of T2DM. Specifically *partial remission* was defined as HbA1c <6.5%, fasting blood glucose <7.0 mmol/L, and the absence of antidiabetic drugs for at least 12 months after the surgery; and *complete remission* was defined as HbA1c <6%, fasting blood glucose concentrations <5.6 mmol/L, and without hypoglycemic pharmacological therapies for at least 12 months. Prolonged remission was defined as complete remission of at least 5 years' duration. These criteria may emphasize surgery as a superior tool for achieving glycemic control rather than as a tool for achieving T2DM remission.

Various factors have been proposed as predictor of remission T2DM after RYGB [44]. Durable remission has been seen in early stage of T2DM [1], loss of a large percentage of excess bodyweight, young age, and low BMI (25–35 kg/m^2). Duration of diabetes, usage of insulin, and duration of insulin usage have all been reported to negatively predict the likelihood of diabetes remission after surgery [44, 45].

The DiaRem scoring system is a method that uses four preoperative clinical variables (use of insulin before surgery, age, HbA1c, and diabetes drugs before surgery) to predict the probability of remission of T2DM after RYGB surgery. It predicts remission irrespective of early or late occurrence and includes patients in partial remission who might be progressing to complete remission [43].

However, the major benefit of surgery would probably not be to improve glycemic control per se but rather to reduce microvascular and macrovascular complications associated with T2DM [44], so in the selection of T2DM patients for metabolic surgery, a balance between the diabetes-related risk of micro- and macrovascular complications and the potential benefits of surgery rather than BMI solely should be considered [1]. BMI-associated risk varies with sex and ethnicity and is not a reliable prognostic factor for mortality and morbidity in patients with fully established diabetes; therefore, IDF recommends the use of diabetes-specific parameters as a measure of efficacy of treatment when surgery is performed with the intent to treat diabetes [43]. The IDF recommendations include mandatory assessment of glycated hemoglobin levels, C-peptide, fasting glycemic, insulin levels, lipid profile, and regular monitoring of arterial blood pressure among others.

Finally, metabolic surgery should be considered as a broad surgical specialty where the gastrointestinal operations are used with the primary intent to treat diabetes and metabolic disease. This definition is not based on the assumption of whether the site of surgery is normal or pathological, yet it is consistent with the evidence that gastrointestinal procedures engage mechanisms of action beyond the mechanical restriction of energy intake and altered nutrient absorption. According to such definition, standard Roux-en-Y gastric bypass should be thought as a "metabolic" rather than "bariatric" surgery [44].

Surgical Technique

In the last 10 years, multiple publications demonstrated improvement of blood glucose levels and concomitant reduction of morbidity and mortality related to CV events after BS/MS [29–32]. RYGB technique was the first technique that proved its effectiveness in remission of T2DM in morbidly obese patients. Laparoscopic RYGB is the most accepted and effective procedure; it is also the safest and has the best long-term T2DM remission rates compared with other restrictive techniques. These characteristics postulate laparoscopic RYGB as the gold standard [33, 34].

RYGB Technique Description

The patient is positioned in a split-leg position and carefully strapped to the operating room table, with the surgeon between the patient's legs. The laparoscopy tower is placed on the right of the patient's head [30, 35–38]. The surgery is performed under general anesthesia with endotracheal intubation. Abdominal insufflation up to 15 mmHg was obtained with the insertion of a Veress needle at the patient's umbilicus [30, 46, 47]. Trocars were placed as follows: 10 mm just to the left of the midline; 12 mm in the right upper quadrant on the midclavicular line; 12 mm in the left upper quadrant on the midclavicular line at the same level as the optical trocar; 5 mm used for liver retraction just distal and to the left of the xiphoid; and, finally, 5 mm on the left anterior axillary line 5 mm distal to the costal margin (Fig. 45.1a, b).

Gastric pouch of approximate volume 30–50 ml is calibrated with 34–36 Fr boogies. It must be isolated completely from the gastric fundus.

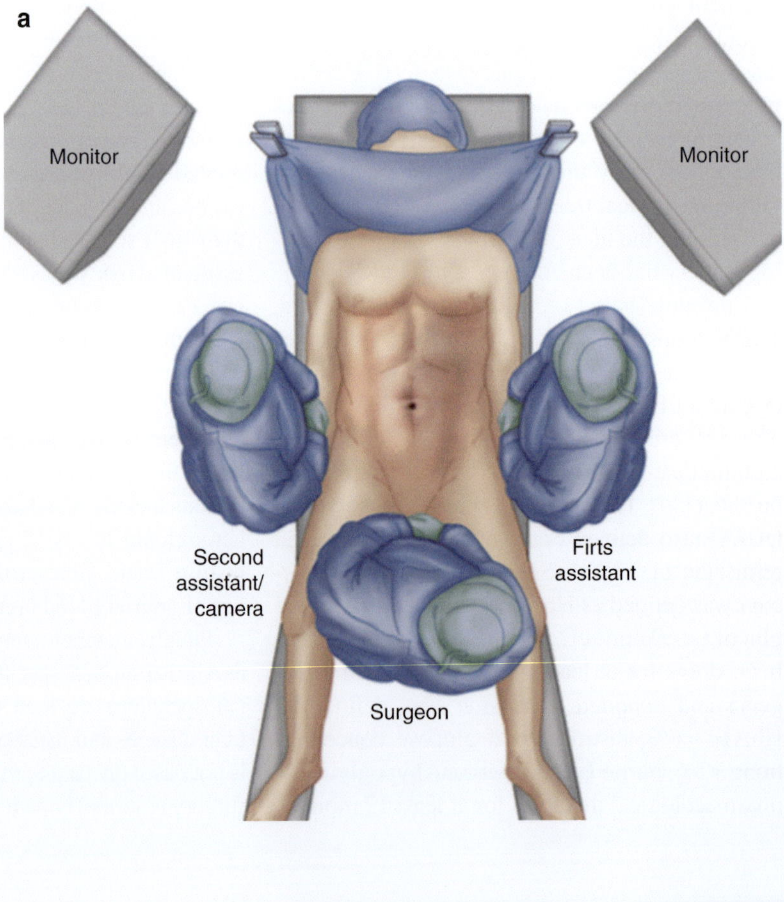

Fig. 45.1 (**a**, **b**) Patient and trocar position

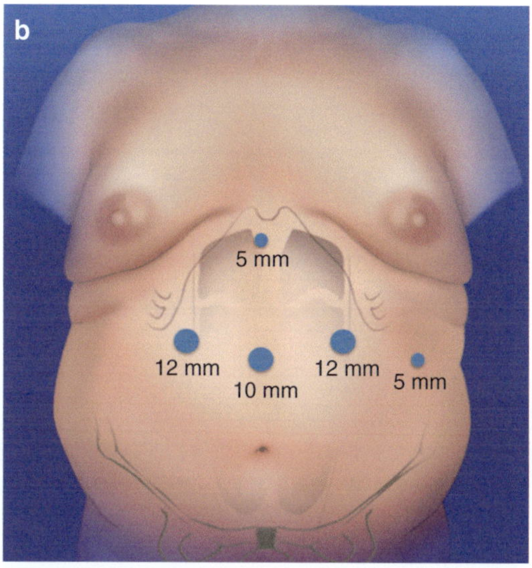

Fig. 45. 1 (continued)

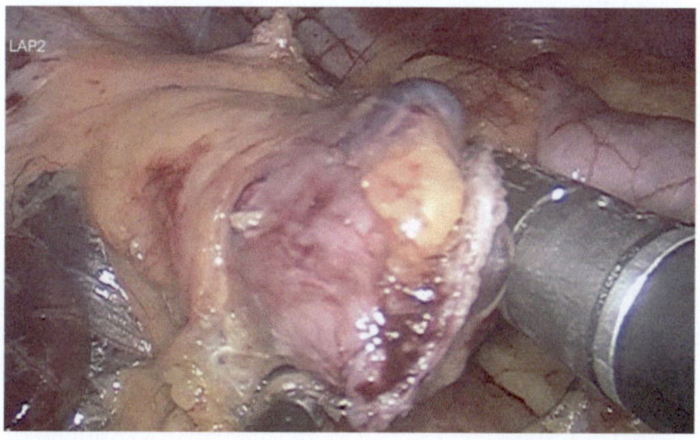

Fig. 45.2 The gastric pouch is manufactured using blue loads

The approximated size should be about 4 × 7 cm. The stomach is transected horizontally at the level described above firing a blue load linear stapler introduced through the right upper quadrant 12 mm trocar. The stapler is introduced in the left upper quadrant 12 mm trocar and aiming the left lateral horizontal section toward the esophagogastric angle. Two stapler firings disconnected the small upper stomach from the remaining portion of the stomach. The vertical resection is performed as close as possible to the lesser curve by using a 34 Fr boogie (Fig. 45.2) [30, 45, 48].

For gastrojejunostomy recommended is a hybrid technique (manual-mechanic), although it can be performed fully hand sewn. It should

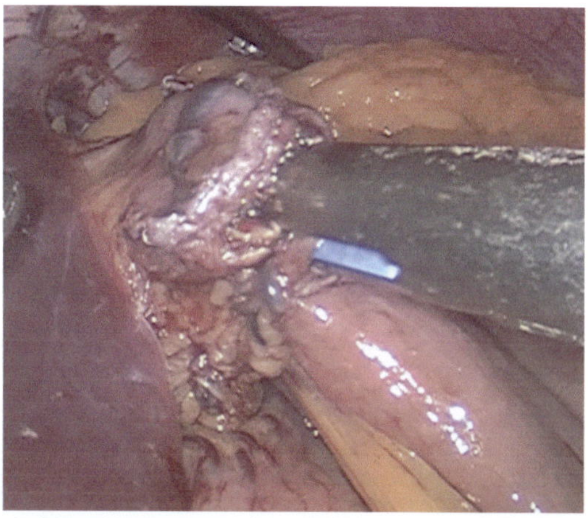

Fig. 45.3 A 2.5 cm gastrojejunal anastomosis by using blue loads is performed

be always calibrated with a 34–36 Fr boogie. The omentum is divided and the duodenojejunal angle is identified. From that site, the bowel was lifted toward the hiatus, and a loop was identified that could reach this level with acceptable traction. A side-to-side jejunojejunostomy is performed by using a white cartridge. For this step, a blue load linear stapler is inserted only half way into the pouch hole in order to create an anastomosis that is about 2 cm in length before firing. This anastomosis is located on the posterior part of the gastric pouch and with 2 cm in diameter (Fig. 45.3). A running suture using Vicryl® 3.0 is used to close the stapler openings (Fig. 45.4) [30, 45].

A biliary limb of 100 cm of length from duodenojejunal flexure, a 150 cm alimentary limb from gastrojejunostomy, and a jejunojejunostomy with hybrid mechanic-manual techniques are recommended (Fig. 45.5). The antecolic/antegastric loop ascent is also suggested to decrease the risk of vowel obstruction. The closure of mesenteric gaps, Petersen's, and intermesenteric spaces is advisable to decrease the risk of internal hernia (Fig. 45.6). Blue test is done before performing the last small bowel division in order to test both anastomoses at the same time. After the blue test is done, the last stapler is fired in the jejunum (Fig. 45.7). Finally, the abdominal cavity is drained with a JP drain for about 7 days [30, 45].

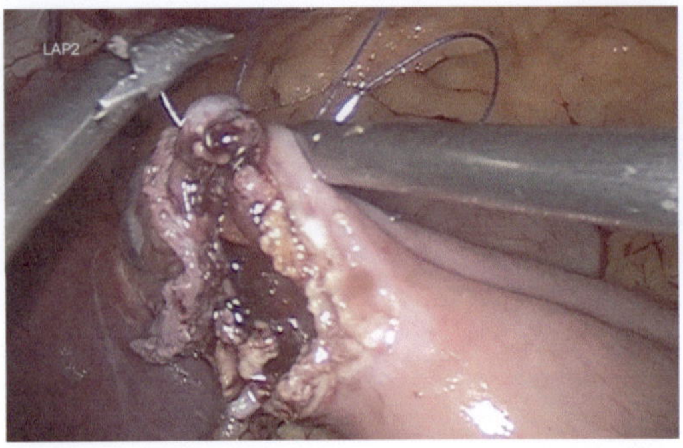

Fig. 45.4 Running suture using Vicryl 3.0 for the closure of the anastomotic defect

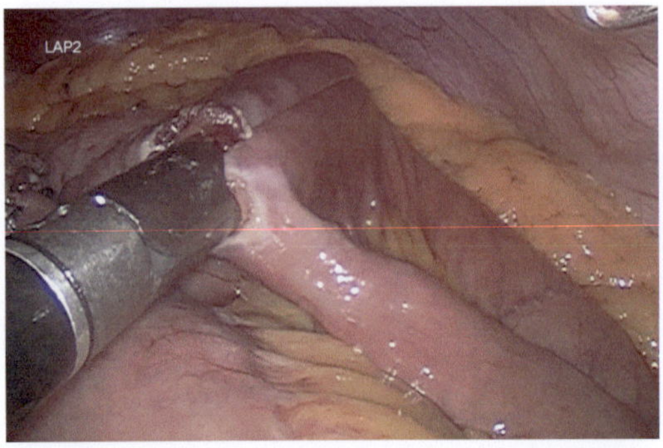

Fig. 45.5 A side to side jejuno-jejunostomy is performed with a white load

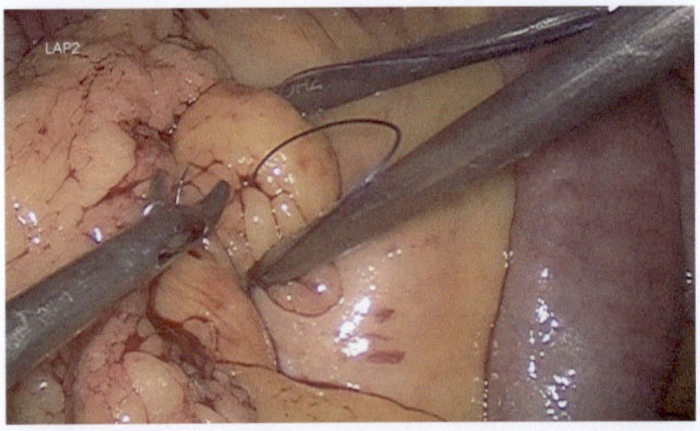

Fig. 45.6 The closure of the Petersen defect is routinely performed

References

1. Buchwald H. Metabolic surgery. In: Lucchese M, Scopinaro N, editors. Bariatric and metabolic mini-invasive surgery. New York: Springer; 1978.
2. IDF Atlas 7th. Edition 2015. www.diabetesatlas.org.

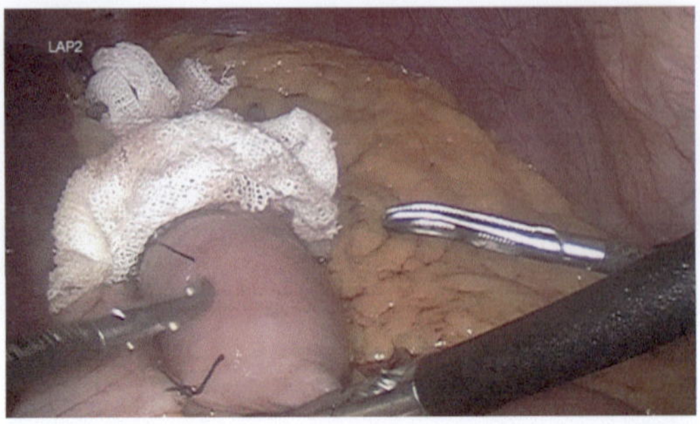

Fig. 45.7 Blue test before the last cut of the jejunum in order to demonstrate leaks

3. Gaede P, Lund-Andersen H, Parving H-H, Pedersen O. Effect of a multifactorial intervention on mortality in type 2 diabetes. N Engl J Med. 2008;358: 580–91.
4. American Diabetes Association. Standards of medical care in diabetes. Diabetes Care. 2016;39: 88–99(Suppl.1).
5. Stark Casagrande S, Fradkin JE, Sayad SH, Rust KF, Cowie CC. The prevalence of meeting A1c, blood pressure, and LDL goals among people with diabetes, 1998–2010. Diabetes Care. 2013;36:2271–9.
6. Cohen R, Caravatto PP, Petry T. Surgery for diabetes. Curr Surg Rep. 2013;1:160.
7. UK Prospective Diabetes Study (UKPDS) Group. Intensive blood glucose control with sulfonylureas or insulin compared with conventional treatment and risk for complications in patients with type 2 diabetes (UKPDS 33). Lancet. 1998;352:837–53.
8. Ismail-Beigi F, Craven T, Banerji MA, ACCORD Trial Group, et al. Effect of intensive treatment of hyperglycaemia on microvascular outcomes in type 2 diabetes: an analysis of the ACCORD randomised trial. Lancet. 2010;376:419–30.
9. Patel A, Mac Mahon S, Chalmers J, ADVANCE Collaborative Group, et al. Intensive blood glucose control and vascular outcomes in patients with type 2 diabetes. N Engl J Med. 2008;358:2560–72.
10. Duckworth W, Abraira C, Moritz T, VADT Investigators, et al. Glucose control and vascular complications in veterans with type 2 diabetes. N Engl J Med. 2008;359:1577–89.
11. Sjöström L, et al. Lifestyle, diabetes and cardiovascular risk factors 10 years after bariatric surgery. N Engl J Med. 2004;351(26):2683–93.
12. Sjostrom L, Peltonen M, Jacobson P, et al. Bariatric surgery and long term cardiovascular events. JAMA. 2012;307:56–65.
13. Sjostrom L, et al. Effects of bariatric surgery on mortality in Swedish obese subjects. N Engl J Med. 2007;357(8):741–52.
14. Cohen R, Caravatto PP, Petry T. Metabolic surgery for type 2 diabetes in patients with BMI of <35 kg/m^2: a surgeon's perspective. Obes Surg. 2013;23:809–18.

Comprehensive review of metabolic surgery in BMI below 35 kg/m^2.
15. Mingrone G, Panunzi S, De Gaetano A, et al. Bariatric surgery versus conventional medical therapy in obese patients with diabetes. N Engl J Med. 2012;366:1577–85.
16. Schauer PR, Kashyap SR, Wolski K, et al. Bariatric surgery versus intensive medical therapy in obese patients with diabetes. N Engl J Med. 2012;366:1567–76.
17. Cohen R, Caravatto PP, Petry T, Cummings D. Role of metabolic surgery in less obese or non-obese subjects with type 2 diabetes: influence over cardiovascular events. Curr Atheroscler Rep. 2013;15:355.
18. Cummings DE, Flum DR. Gastrointestinal surgery as a treatment for diabetes. JAMA. 2008;299:341–3.
19. Ikkramudin S, Korner J, Lee WJ, et al. Roux-en-Y gastric bypass vs intensive medical management for the control of type 2 diabetes, hypertension and hyperlipidemia: the Diabetes Surgery Study randomized clinical trial. JAMA. 2013;309:2240–9.
20. Laferrere B, Texeira J, McGinty J, et al. Effect of weight loss by gastric bypass surgery versus hypocaloric diet on glucose and uncertain levels in patients with type 2 diabetes. J Clin Endocrinol Metab. 2008;93:2479–85.
21. Rubino F, Marescaux J. Effect of duodenal-jejunal exclusion in a non-obese animal model type 2 diabetes: a new perspective for an old disease. Ann Surg. 2004;239:1–11.
22. Savage DB, Petersen KF, Schulman GI. Disordered lipid metabolism and pathogenesis of insulin resistance. Phys Rev. 2007;87:507–20.
23. Pories WJ, Dohm LG, Mansfield CJ. Beyond the BMI: the search for better guidelines for bariatric surgery. Obesity. 2010;18:865–71.
24. Bojsen-Moller KN, Dirksen C, Jorgensen NB, et al. Early enhancements of hepatic and later of peripheral insulin sensitivity combined with increased postprandial insulin secretion contribute to improved glycemic control after Roux-en-Y gastric bypass. Diabetes. 2014;63:1725–37.
25. Salinari S, Bertuzzi A, Guidone C, Previti E, Rubino F, Mingrone G. Insulin sensitivity and secretion changes after gastric by pass in normotolerant and diabetic obese subjects. Ann Surg. 2013;257:462–8.
26. Dirksen C, Bojsten- Moller KN, Jorgensen NB, et al. Exaggerated release and preserved insulinotropic action of glucagon-like-peptide 1underlie insulin hypersecretion in glucose-tolerant individual after Roux-en Y gastric bypass. Diabetologia. 2013;56:2679–87.
27. Lindqvist A, Spegel P, Ekelund M, et al. Gastric by pass improves B-cell function and increases B-cell mass in a porcine model. Diabetes. 2014;63:1665–71.
28. Rubino F, Amiel SA. Is the gut the "sweet spot" for the treatment of diabetes ? Diabetes. 2014;63:2225–8.
29. Jacob BP, Gagner M. New developments in gastric bypass procedures and physiological mechanisms. Surg Technol Int. 2003;11:119–26.
30. Palermo M, Gimenez M, Gagner M. Laparoscopic gastrointestinal surgery. Novel techniques, extending the limits. Caracas: AMOLCA; 2015.
31. Himpens JM. The gastrojejunostomy in laparoscopic Roux-en-Y gastric bypass. Semin Laparosc Surg. 2004;11(3):171–7.
32. Cadière GB, Himpens J, Dapri G. Laparoscopic stomach bypass surgery. Chirurg. 2005;76(7):668–77.
33. Palermo M, Dapri G. Single port laparoscopic surgery. Medellin, Colombia: AMOLCA; 2015.
34. Collins BJ, Miyashita T, Schweitzer M, Magnuson T, Harmon JW. Gastric bypass: why Roux-en-Y? A review of experimental data. Arch Surg. 2007;142(10):1000–3; discussion 1004.
35. Madan AK, Harper JL, Tichansky DS. Techniques of laparoscopic gastric bypass: on-line survey of American Society for Bariatric Surgery practicing surgeons. Surg Obes Relat Dis. 2008;4(2):166–72; discussion172–3.
36. Franco JV, Ruiz PA, Palermo M, Gagner M. A review of studies comparing three laparoscopic procedures in bariatric surgery: sleeve gastrectomy, Roux-en-Y gastric bypass and adjustable gastric banding. Obes Surg. 2011;21(9):1458–68.
37. Acquafresca P, Palermo M, Duza G, Blanco L, Serra E. Gastric Bypass versus Sleeve gastrectomy: comparison between type 2 Diabetes weight loss and complications. Review of randomized control trails. Acta Gastroenterol Latinoam. 2015;45:284–7.
38. Acquafresca PA, Palermo M, Rogula T, Duza GE, Serra E. Early complications after gastric by-pass: a literature review. Arq Bras Cir Dig. 2015;28(1):74–80.
39. De Luca M, Angrisani L, Himpens J, et al. Indications for surgery for obesity and weight- related diseases: position statements from the International Federation for the Surgery of Obesity an Metabolic Disorders (IFSO). Obes Surg. 2016;26:1659–96.
40. Rubino R, Kaplan LM, Schauer PR, Cummings DE. The diabetes surgery summit consensus conference: recommendations for the evaluation and use of gastrointestinal surgery to treat type 2 diabetes mellitus. Ann Surg. 2010;251:399–405.
41. Rubino F, et al. Bariatric, metabolic and diabetes surgery: what's in a name? Ann Surg. 2012;34:1–6.
42. Rubino F, Cummings DE, et al. Metabolic surgery in the treatment algorithm for type 2 diabetes. A joint statement by international diabetes organizations. Diabetes Care. 2016;39:861.
43. Carlsson LM, et al. Bariatric surgery and prevention of type 2 diabetes in Swedish obese subjects. N Engl J Med. 2012;367:695–704.
44. Rubino F, Nathan DM, Eckel RH, Schauer PR, Alberti KG, Alberti MM, Zimmet PZ, Del Prato S, Ji L, Sadikot SM, Amiel SA, Kaplan LM, Herman WH, Taroncher-Oldenburg G, Cummings DE. Metabolic surgery in the treatment algorithm for type 2 diabetes: a joint statement by international diabetes organizations. Diabetes Care. 2016;39:861–77.

45. Ramos AC, Silva ACS, Ramos MG, Cansaco EGC, dos Passos Galvao Neto M, de Almeida Menexes M, Galvao TD. Eduardo Lemos de Souza Bastos. ABCD Arq Bras Cir Dig. 2014;27(Suppl. 1):2–8.
46. Fletcher R, Deal R, Kubasiak J, Torquati A, Omotosho P. Predictors of Increased Length of Hospital Stay Following Laparoscopic Sleeve Gastrectomy from the National Surgical Quality Improvement Program. J Gastrointest Surg. 2018;22(2):274–8. https://doi.org/10.1007/s11605-017-3642-4. Epub 2017 Dec 5.
47. Bussetto L, Dixon J, De Luca M, Shikora S, Pories W, Angrisani L. Bariatric surgery in class I obesity: a position statement from the International Federation For De Surgery Of Obesity And Metabolic Disorders. Obes Surg. 2014;24:487–519.
48. Henry B, Estok R, Fahrbach K, Banel D, Jensen MD, Pories W, Bantle J, Sledge I. Weight and type 2 diabetes after bariatric surgery: systematic review and meta-analysis. Am J Med. 2008;122:248–256.e5. https://doi.org/10.1016/j.amjmed.2008.09.041.

46 Gastric Bypass for Type 2 Diabetes Mellitus on BMI >35

Jad Khoraki, Matthew G. Browning,
Bernardo M. Pessoa, and Guilherme M. Campos

Introduction

The estimated number of people with diabetes worldwide increased from 108 million (4.7%) in 1980 to 422 million (8.5%) in 2014; and this worldwide epidemic has been driven by the increase in type 2 diabetes (T2D) that represents 95% of all cases of diabetes [1, 2]. Similarly, in the USA, the prevalence of diabetes has substantially risen from 3.6% in 1983 to 8.7% in 2015, again mostly due to the increase in cases of T2D [3]. Not surprisingly, prevalence of obesity shows similar trends of a steady increase and the proportion of individuals with obesity, defined as a body mass index (BMI) of 30 kg/m^2 or more, and those with class 3 obesity (BMI $\geq$ 40 kg/m^2) have reached 37.7% and 7.7% of adults in 2014, respectively [4]. BMI is a strong and modifiable risk factor for T2D [5, 6]. Relative to normal weight, severe obesity (BMI $\geq$ 35 kg/m^2) increases the lifetime risk of diabetes from 19.8% to 70.3% in males and from 17.1% to 74.4% in females [6].

Importantly, in individuals with severe obesity, bariatric surgery has been shown to be superior to conventional medical therapy alone in producing remission of T2D, reducing T2D-related end-organ complications and long-term premature mortality [7–10].

Roux-en-Y gastric bypass (RYGB) is currently 1 of the 2 most common bariatric procedures done worldwide, with an estimated 40,584 primary cases done in the USA in 2017 [11].

In this chapter, we present:

- A brief overview of the pathophysiology of T2D in patients with severe obesity
- Outcomes of the disease following RYGB surgery, including rates and predictors of T2D remission and relapse, and effects on T2D-related complications and long-term premature mortality
- A summary of the current evidence comparing RYGB with conventional medical therapy and with other bariatric procedures as provided by the randomized controlled trials
- A briefing on the proposed mechanisms by which RYGB promotes remission of T2D

Pathophysiology of Type 2 Diabetes in Severe Obesity

T2D pathogenesis is multifactorial and includes excess accumulation of adipose tissue, absolute or relative deficiency in pancreatic β-cell insulin

J. Khoraki · M. G. Browning · B. M. Pessoa
G. M. Campos (✉)
Division of Bariatric and Gastrointestinal Surgery, Department of Surgery, Virginia Commonwealth University, Richmond, VA, USA
e-mail: guilherme.campos@vcuhealth.org

J. Ettinger et al. (eds.), *Gastric Bypass*, https://doi.org/10.1007/978-3-030-28803-7_46

production, and insulin resistance. All these factors combined lead to the primary clinical manifestation of T2D, hyperglycemia. Chronic hyperglycemia over time results in multiple tissue and organ damage. Importantly, while many patients with T2D may not be classified as obese by traditional BMI criteria [6], the central part of the pathogenesis of the disease in all patients with T2D involves excess adiposity that is usually distributed in the abdominal region, the liver, and/or the skeletal muscle [12–15].

In individuals with severe obesity, the role of excess adipose tissue accumulation in the pathophysiology of T2D is not in dispute, as adipose tissue is increased in deferent degrees in all and can often account for 50% or more of the total body mass in these individuals.

However, the reasons for why only some individuals with severe obesity develop T2D rest on the fact that the disease develops based on when and where excess adipose tissue accumulation occurs and how each individual responds to that excess adipose tissue accumulation, that is, when and what type of obesity triggers insulin resistance. In addition, after developing insulin resistance, the pancreas initially responds by secreting more insulin producing a temporary hyperinsulinemic state that over time ends up in an absolute or relative failure of the pancreatic β-cell to maintain normoglycemia.

The timeline for an individual to develop this pancreatic dysfunction depends on the severity of insulin resistance and the ability of the pancreas to maintain hyperinsulinemia and, thus, normoglycemia. Each individual's ability to maintain hyperinsulinemia is also dependent on the varied individual initial adult β-cell mass and the rate that these cells are slowly destroyed in the setting of insulin resistance and hyperinsulinemia [16].

One of the mechanisms by which excess fat accumulation leads to insulin resistance is that it creates low-grade inflammation in the adipocyte that then can damage the adipocyte architecture. The adipocyte (and any other cell with excess fat accumulation) becomes resistant to insulin-mediated glucose uptake and suppression of lipolysis as a defense mechanism for its own survival. In other words, its cell membrane resists glucose uptake attempting to prevent further intracellular fat synthesis and additional damage, leading to further impairment in triglyceride synthesis and storage, a characteristic component of T2D [12]. All these then result in an elevation in the bloodstream concentrations of glucose and free-fatty acids (FFAs) that individual patients will differentially attempt to traffic to other tissues, including skeletal muscle and the liver. Compared to patients with severe obesity without T2D, glycogen content is significantly reduced in skeletal muscle but not in the liver of T2D patients [13, 17]. It follows that, in the setting of peripheral tissue insulin resistance, the liver maintains glucose homeostasis through increases in glycogen synthesis and/or tricarboxylic acid cycle activity. However, as the capacity for hepatic glycogen storage becomes saturated, partitioning of glucose is shifted toward mitochondrial oxidation to provide substrates for de novo lipogenesis (DNL), the process where surplus glucose is used to synthesize FFAs.

The liver is the most lipogenic non-adipose organ, and chronic hyperinsulinemia and/or hyperglycemia in T2D stimulates DNL (lipid synthesis) through upregulation of two transcription factors responsible for DNL (sterol response element-binding protein-1c or SREBP-1c and carbohydrate response element-binding protein-β or ChREBP-β). Studies where intraoperative liver biopsies were performed in patients with T2D undergoing bariatric surgery have shown that SREBP-1c and the DNL gene program is markedly upregulated in the liver but downregulated alongside lower glucose transporter expression in peripheral adipose tissue [12, 18, 19]. Along with the influx of FFAs released from insulin-resistant adipose tissue, DNL-produced FFAs may then be esterified into triglycerides for storage. This is in agreement with the established associations among high adiposity, insulin resistance, and nonalcoholic fatty liver disease (NAFLD), a spectrum of conditions defined clinically by triglyceride accumulation in >5% of hepatocytes on liver histology.

An inability of worsening hyperinsulinemia to compensate for insulin resistance and/or β-cell exhaustion eventually results in hyperglycemia that hallmarks T2D pathophysiology. The latter mechanisms also highlight a possible causative role of hepatic fat accumulation in β-cell failure, as insulin secretion and peripheral appearance but not insulin resistance or glucose concentrations were significantly higher in T2D patients with NAFLD relative to those with T2D and normal liver fat content [20].

Importantly, RYGB is known to favorably impact most if not all of the above pathways to normalize adipose tissue and liver metabolism and restore glucose homeostasis. We discuss these facts at the end of this chapter.

Outcomes of Gastric Bypass in Patients with Severe Obesity and Type 2 Diabetes

We conducted an electronic search in PubMed for all bariatric surgery studies published in English that contained data on weight loss and T2D-related outcomes for patients with BMI ≥35 kg/m^2 treated with RYGB. Search terms were "type 2 diabetes," "gastric bypass," "obese," "bariatric surgery," "metabolic," "comorbidities," "remission," "relapse," "glycemic," "outcomes," "microvascular," "macrovascular," and "mortality."

We included observational and randomized studies that reported outcomes of open and/or laparoscopic RYGB only and those comparing RYGB with conventional medical therapy (Medical) or other nonsurgical control groups and studies that reported RYGB outcomes in comparison with three other bariatric procedures [sleeve gastrectomy (SG), biliopancreatic diversion (BPD) with or without duodenal switch (BPD/DS), and laparoscopic adjustable gastric banding (LAGB)]. Some studies with a large sample size and/or long-term followup that collectively reported outcomes of RYGB and other bariatric studies were included in this literature review but not in the sections comparing RYGB with medical therapy and other bariatric procedures. RYGB was the bariatric surgery performed for the majority of patients in those studies. If two or more studies reported results of the same series or clinical trial, only the one with the longer follow-up was included.

We excluded studies that combined RYGB with other RYGB-like procedures such as mini-gastric bypass or studies reporting outcomes only for patients with a BMI less than 35 kg/m^2. Data was collected by two independent researchers and vetted by the senior author.

Rates of Remission and Relapse of T2D After Gastric Bypass

Two criteria are commonly used to define T2D remission [21, 22]. The first is a 2009 consensus statement in which a complete remission is considered if glycated hemoglobin (HbA1c) <6% and fasting plasma glucose (FPG) <100 mg/dl [<5.6 mmol/l] and a partial remission if HbA1c <6.5% and FPG 100–125 mg/dl (5.6–6.9 mmol/l), in both cases in the absence of drug therapy or ongoing procedures, for a duration of at least 1 year. The other comes from the American Diabetes Association (ADA) that states that remission occurs if HbA1c <5.7% and improvement if HbA1c 5.7–6.5%, in both cases without hypoglycemic treatment and a duration of at least 1 year, and no remission if these criteria were not met. However, many publications have used modifications of these definitions, and one must always revisit remission and relapse definitions in each reporting.

Initial remission of T2D after RYGB has been reported, using varied definitions, in about 80% of the patients and has been observed to occur soon thereafter surgery or months to years after surgery [23–26]. It is important, however, to note that relapse of T2D has been observed to occur in 12–54% of those with initial remission [8, 24, 27–33]. When compared to medical therapy alone though, RYGB have been shown to yield better glycemic control, greater rates of remission of T2D, lower rates of relapse, reduction of T2D complications and other cardiovascular risk factors, and reduction in premature T2D-related deaths [8, 30, 34–38].

Table 46.1 summarizes T2D remission and relapse rates in 16 studies from multiple countries that reported T2D outcomes at a minimum of 5 years after RYGB. Durable remission rates between 22% and 100% have been reported in these studies (Table 46.1).

Table 46.1 Long-term remission and relapse of type 2 diabetes (T2D) after gastric bypass (RYGB) in studies with 5 years or more of follow-up

Author (year)	Follow-up duration	Study design	Groups	Country	RYGB N_{BL}/N^a (%T2D)	T2D[a] N_{FU}	Race (%)	Definition of remission	Remission, *n* (%)	Relapse, *n* (%)	Findings
Xiaosong (2019)[b] [33]	5 years	Retrospective cohort	RYGB	China	24/24 (100)	24	NR	HbA1c <6% and FPG[c] <5.6 for 1 year without medication	NR	13/24 (54.2)	Rates of relapse after initial remission increased from 4% at 1 year to 54% at 5 years. Preoperative HbA1c and C-peptide levels predict relapse
Nguyen (2017) [117]	10 years	RCT	RYGB, LAGB	USA	NR/111 (NR)	48	NR	Improvement: reduction in dosage or the number of diabetic medicationsRemission: patient no longer required the use of diabetes medication	NR (86.4%)	NR	RYGB was associated with better long-term weight loss, lower rate of late reoperations, and improved remission of diabetes compared to LAGB
Peterli (2018) [95]	5 years	RCT	RYGB, SG	Switzerland	28/104 (27)	28	NR	HbA1c <6% and FPG[c] <5.6 at least 1 year with no active pharmacologic therapy	19 (67.9)	NR	There were no significant differences in excess BMI loss or T2D remission between SG and RYGB at 5 years
Salminen (2018) [96]	5 years	RCT	RYGB, SG	Finland	41/95 (43)	40	NR	HbA1c <6% and FPG[c] <5.6 and at least 1 year with no pharmacologic therapy	10/40 (25)	NR	RYGB was associated wtih a statistically similar rate of T2D remission and a greater % excess weight loss at 5 years compared to SG (the difference did not meet the criteria for clinical significance)
Schauer (2017)[d] [8]	5 years	RCT	RYGB, SG, medical therapy	USA	50/50 (100)	49	White (74)	HbA1c ≤6% without medication	11 (22.4)	10/20 (50)	RYGB was superior to medical therapy and similar to SG

Jammu (2016) [142]	7 years	Prospective cohort	RYGB, SG, mini-gastric bypass	India	33 (23.1)	NR	NR	NR	NR (75.8)	NR	Mini-gastric bypass was superior to RYGB and LSG
Mingrone (2015) [30]	5 years	RCT	RYGB, BPD, medical therapy	Italy	19/19 (100)	19	NR	HbA1c ≤ 6.5% and FPG[c] ≤5.6 for 1 year without medication	7 (37)	8/15 (53)	RYGB and BPD were superior to medical therapy and BPD was superior to RYGB
Bhasker (2015) [143]	5 years	Prospective cohort	RYGB	India	106/106 (100)	90	Indian	HbA1c <6.0%, FPG[c] <5.6 without medication for a continuous minimum period of 6 months	NR	0 (0%)	Weight regain did not lead to T2D relapse
Leyba (2014) [108]	5 years	Prospective cohort	RYGB, SG	Venezuela	3/75 (0.04)	3	NR	HbA1c <6% without medication	2 (66.7)	NA	There was no difference between RYGB and SG
Arterburn (2013) [28]	5 years	Retrospective cohort	RYGB	USA	4,434/4,434 (100)	3006	NR	HbA1c <6.0%, FPG[c] <5.6 occurring ≥180 days without medications	2,050 (68.2)	NR (35.1)	RYGB results in durable remission but not in all patients. One-third experience relapse
Brethauer (2013) [29]	5 years or more	Retrospective cohort	RYGB, SG, LAGB	USA	162/162 (100)	162	NR	HbA1c <6%, FPG[c] <5.6 for 1 year without medication	50 (31)	20/115 (17)	RYGB is superior to SG and LAGB
Adams (2012) [144]	6 years	Prospective cohort	RYGB, 2 control groups	USA	93/418 (22.2)	87	White (95)	Normal FPG[c] and HbA1c without medication	54 (62.1)	NR	RYGB had high rates of remission compared to nonsurgical control groups
Zhang 2014 [26]	5 years	RCT	RYGB, SG	China	8/32 (25)	8	NR	Resolution: discontinuation of T2D medications Improvement: reduction of T2D medications	7 (87.5)	NR	RYGB was superior to LSG in weight loss, but the difference in resolution or improvement of comorbidities did not reach the statistical significance

(continued)

Table 46.1 (continued)

Author (year)	Follow-up duration	Study design	Groups	Country	RYGB N_{BL}/N^a (%T2D)	T2D[a] N_{FU}	Race (%)	Definition of remission	Remission, *n* (%)	Relapse, *n* (%)	Findings
DiGiorgi 2010 [31]	5 years	Retrospective cohort	RYGB	USA	42 (100)	NR	NR	HbA1c ≤ 6% without medication	27 (64)	7/27 (26)	There were significant rates of T2D recurrence or worsening after initial resolution
Chikunguwo (2009) [24]	5 years or more	Retrospective cohort	RYGB	USA	177/177 (100)	177	NR	No longer requiring any diabetic medication or dietary management	157 (88.7)	68/157 (43.3)	High early remission rate of 89% was followed by 43% relapse rate
Alexandrides (2007) [145]	5 years	Retrospective cohort	RYGB, BPD	Greece	26/26 (100)	9	NR	5.6≤FPG[c] ≤6.9 on two occasions or 2-hour glucose≤11.1 after a 75 g oral glucose tolerance test	6 (66.7)	NR	BPD was more effective than RYGB in diabetes and impaired fasting glucose resolution

LAGB laparoscopic adjustable gastric banding, *SG* sleeve gastrectomy, *BPD* biliopancreatic diversion, *RCT* randomized control trial, *NR* not reported

[a]*N*, total number of patients who underwent RYGB; N_{BL}, all patients with T2D at baseline; N_{FU}, patients with baseline T2D at last follow-up

[b]Xiaosong et al. [33] included only 24 patients with complete remission 6 months after surgery in their study. The authors did not report data on their entire cohort (n = 91). Relapse at 5 years of follow-up occurred in 12 (50%) in addition to another patient with relapse at year 6 [13 patients with overall observed relapse (54.2%)]

[c]FPG (fasting plasma glucose) is expressed in mmol/L

[d]Schauer et al. [8] included patients with BMI 27–43 in their study. 14 patients had BMI <35 in the RYGB group

Again and importantly, different definitions of remission are adopted by authors of these studies and can partly explain the large variations in remission and relapse rates found in the literature [39].

The mechanisms by which RYGB produces these remarkable effects involve weight loss-dependent and weight loss-independent factors as explained later in this chapter.

In the following sections, we review predictors of remission and relapse of T2D after RYGB and compare the outcomes of RYGB versus medical therapy and other bariatric procedures in randomized controlled trials (RCTs).

Predictors of Remission and Relapse of Type 2 Diabetes Following Gastric Bypass

It is of great relevance to identify patient-level characteristics that could independently predict remission (and relapse) after surgery. It helps physicians better counsel patients with T2D who are being evaluated for gastric bypass surgery especially when the principal consideration is the treatment of their T2D. It also provides the necessary evidence to guide policymakers (including insurance companies) in the efforts to include metabolic surgery and expand its indication for the treatment algorithm and guidelines of T2D [40, 41]. These predictors can also help researchers understand the mechanisms of glycemic control after RYGB (discussed later in this chapter). We found 26 articles reporting on remission and relapse of T2D after RYGB (Tables 46.2 and 46.3). Table 46.2 summarizes preoperative and postoperative factors that have been reported as predictors of T2D remission and relapse following RYGB.

Although most of these predictors of remission and relapse were statistically independent, as demonstrated by multivariate analyses conducted in many studies (Table 46.3), they seem to be physiologically interconnected. Greater rates of remission are achieved in younger patients (likely associated with shorter duration of the disease), who may have greater residual β-cell function (lack of insulin requirement and better glycemic control preoperatively). C-peptide measurement provides a practical tool to assess insulin secretion and reflect islet cell mass. Thus, higher baseline C-peptide levels indicate relatively adequate pancreatic β-cell function. Similarly, glucagon-like peptide (GLP-1), an incretin produced in the L-cells of the distal ileum and colon, is a modula-

Table 46.2 Predictors of type 2 diabetes (T2D) remission and relapse after gastric bypass

Time of prediction	Predictors of remission	Predictors of relapse
Preoperative	Younger age [32, 47, 49, 58, 61, 143, 145]	Older age [24, 28, 56]
	Shorter T2D duration [8, 29, 32, 45–47, 56, 59, 65, 143, 145, 146]	Longer T2D duration [28]
	Better glycemic control (lower HbA1c and/or fasting blood glucose) [28, 32, 45, 48, 49, 56, 61, 65, 146]	Poor glycemic control (higher HbA1c and/or fasting blood glucose) [28] [33]
	Lack of insulin requirement [24, 28, 31, 48, 55, 56, 61, 65, 143, 147] or lower insulin dose in patients with insulin-dependent T2D [57, 145]	Insulin requirement [24, 28, 32, 56]
	Higher BMI [46–49]	Lower BMI [31]
	Male gender [24, 28] Female gender [146]	Female gender [24]
	Higher C-peptide level [46, 47, 49, 143]	Lower C-peptide level [33]
	Smaller waist circumference [25, 147]	
	Longer alimentary limb (long-limb RYGB) [24]	
	Higher baseline triglyceride level [30]	
Postoperative	Weight loss [8, 24, 28, 29, 46, 49, 55–58]	Weight regain [24, 29, 31, 56]
	Higher GLP-1 secretion at 1 month after surgery [43]	

HbA1c glycated hemoglobin, *GLP-1* glucagon-like peptide-1, *BMI* body mass index

Table 46.3 Predictors of type 2 diabetes (T2D) remission and relapse after gastric bypass

Author (year)	Study design	n/N^a(%T2D)	Predictors of remission	Predictors of relapse
Xiaosong (2019) [33]	Retrospective cohort	24/24 (100)	NR	Higher preoperative HbA1c and lower C-peptide (2 h and 3 h)
Huang (2018) [45]	Meta-analysis	1,160/1,160 (100)	Shorter duration of T2D and lower preoperative HbA1c	NR
de Oliveira (2018) [32]	Retrospective cohort	254/254 (100)	Younger age, better glycemic control, and shorter duration of diabetes prior to surgery.	Preoperative use of insulin or any antidiabetic agent other than metformin
Schauer (2017)[b] [8]	RCT	50/50 (100)	Duration of diabetes <8 years	Not associated with weight regain
Aminian (2017)[b] [65]	Retrospective cohort	659/659 (100)	Fewer diabetes medications, absence of insulin use, shorter duration of T2D, and glycemic control (HbA1C <7%)	NR
Casajoana (2017) [43]	RCT	15/15 (100)	Preoperative insulin use and higher GLP-1 secretion at 1 month after surgery. Weight loss not predictive	NR
Park (2016) [49]	Retrospective cohort	134/403 (33)	Younger age at operation, lower HbA1c and higher C-peptide levels, and % total body weight loss after surgery	NR
Panunzi (2015) [25]	Meta-analysis	2,415/4,944 (49)	Smaller baseline waist circumference	NR
Mingrone (2015) [30]	RCT	19/19 (100)	Higher baseline triglycerides. Weight loss not predictive	Not associated with weight regain
Khanna (2015) [59]	Prospective cohort	27/27 (100)	Shorter duration of diabetes (<5 years). Weight loss not predictive	NR
Bhasker (2015) [143]	Prospective cohort	106/106 (100)	Fasting C-peptide levels ≥3 ng/mL, duration of T2D ≤5 years, BMI ≥40 kg/m², not on insulin preoperatively and age <60 years	NR
Still (2014) [61]	Retrospective cohort	NR//2,365 (NR)	Younger age, lower HbA1c, absence of use of insulin and insulin-sensitizing agent (not metformin) with sulfonylureas	NR
Dixon (2013) [46]	Prospective cohort	103/103 (100)	Diabetes duration <4 years, BMI >35 kg/m², fasting C-peptide concentration >2.9 ng/m and %WL	NR
Arterburn (2013) [28]	Retrospective cohort	4,434/4,434 (100)	Male gender, preoperative HbA1c <6.5%, not requiring insulin or oral hypoglycemic agents and shorter DM duration	Older age, preoperative HbA1c ≥6.5%, insulin requirement, and longer T2D duration
Brethauer (2013) [29]	Retrospective cohort	162/162 (100)	Duration of DM <5 y and % excess weight loss	Weight regain
Lee (2013)[b] [47]	Prospective cohort	2,523/5,467 (46)	Younger age, higher BMI and C-peptide level, and shorter duration of T2D	NR
Jimenez (2012) [56]	Prospective cohort	98/98 (100)	Shorter duration of diabetes, lower baseline HbA1c, lack of insulin treatment and greater weight loss	Insulin use, older age, and weight regain

Table 46.3 (continued)

Author (year)	Study design	*n*/*N*[a](%T2D)	Predictors of remission	Predictors of relapse
Hayes (2011) [48]	Retrospective cohort	130/130 (100)	Lower HbA1c, lower fasting plasma glucose, no hypertension, higher BMI and no requirement for insulin	NR
Hall (2010) [146]	Retrospective cohort	110/110 (100)	Shorter duration (<10 years) and better control (HbA1c <8%) of diabetes prior to surgery	NR
DiGiorgi (2010) [31]	Retrospective cohort	42/42 (100)	Not being on insulin or oral hypoglycemic agents	Lower preoperative BMI, lower weight loss and weight regain
Chikunguwo (2010) [24]	Retrospective cohort	177/177 (100)	Excess weight loss, long-limb RYGB. Durability: male gender and absence insulin requirement before surgery	Older age, female gender, preoperative insulin requirement, lower weight loss, and weight regain
Kadera (2009) [57]	Retrospective cohort	318/1,546 (21)	Preoperative insulin dose and % excess weight loss	NR
Alexandrides (2007) [145]	Retrospective cohort	137/137 (100)	Younger age, shorter duration of diabetes (<5 years), and lower insulin dose for insulin-dependent T2D	NR
Torquati (2005) [147]	Retrospective cohort	117/117 (100)	Smaller preoperative waist circumference and absence of insulin treatment	NR
Schauer (2003) [55]	Retrospective cohort	240/1,160 (21)	Shorter duration (<5 years), diet controlled, and greater weight loss	NR
Sugerman (2003) [58]	Retrospective cohort	154/1,025 (15)	Younger age and greater % excess weight loss	NR

HbA1c glycated hemoglobin, *GLP-1* glucagon-like peptide-1, *NR* not reported
[a]*N*, patients at the last year of the follow-up duration; *n*, patients with T2D at follow-up
[b]Studies that included a subset of patients with body mass index (BMI) <35 kg/m^2

tor of β-cell function and may prevent further loss of pancreatic beta cell mass. It plays a key role in the increased insulin and decreased glucose response to a meal, and changes in GLP-1 have been linked to greater weight loss and metabolic improvements after bariatric surgery [42]. Therefore, the finding that restoration of endogenous GLP-1 soon after RYGB provides a prognostic value is not surprising [43].

Additionally, patients with T2D remission after RYGB likely have favorable fat distribution pattern with less central adiposity (smaller waist circumference) compared to those who don't achieve remission or have T2D relapse. A meta-analysis by Panunzi et al. studied predictors of remission of T2D in severely obese individuals after bariatric surgery found waist circumference to be the only predictor of HbA1c reduction after surgery [25]. The finding is in agreement with a study by Blaha and colleagues demonstrating a similar negative correlation between waist circumference and glycemic control following an intensive intervention aimed at controlling diabetes in 164 adult patients with a history of poor glycemic control [44]. Another meta-analysis of predictors of glycemic control after RYGB vs sleeve gastrectomy found that the duration of T2D and preoperative HbA1C were correlated with glycemic control after RYGB [45].

Higher preoperative BMI has been shown to predict T2D remission by some studies [46–49]; however, it's likely influenced by other factors included in the multivariate analysis models of some of those studies such as weight loss [49] and by inclusion of patients with BMI <35 kg/m^2 by others [46, 47]. BMI per se is a poor predictor of T2D or its remission after bariatric surgery [50, 51]. In fact, fat distribution (central obesity and intrahepatic fat deposition) rather than BMI is a more accurate representative of the adverse metabolic consequences of obesity [15, 52], and the T2D-related complications are highly associated with an elevated HbA1c and not the BMI [53, 54].

Weight loss [24, 28, 29, 46, 49, 55–58] and regain [24, 29, 31] after RYGB have been found to play a major role in T2D remission and relapse, respectively.

Other studies, however, did not find an association between weight outcomes and T2D remission [30, 43, 59] and relapse [8, 30] suggesting that in some patients the presence of weight-independent mechanisms that contribute to the glycemic control may have a larger role than weight change itself.

Scoring Systems for Predicting T2D Remission (and Relapse) After Gastric Bypass

In attempts to possibly adopt a personalized approach to better counsel individual patients who are being considered for surgery as to their specific chances of achieving glycemic control, several scoring systems have been proposed to predict the likelihood of T2D remission after surgery.

Lee et al. used the results of a large prospective study to develop the Diabetes Surgery Score which utilizes four baseline patient characteristics [age, BMI, C-peptide level, and duration of T2D (ABCD score)] to predict remission with RYGB and sleeve gastrectomy. An ABCD score > 6 predicts failure to achieve remission at 1 year [47, 60].

The DiaRem score is another scoring system that utilizes the results of independent predictors of remission of a large cohort of patients who underwent RYGB [61]. It combines preoperative age, insulin use, HbA1c level, and type of antidiabetic medication with the highest weight given to insulin use. It gives a score between 0 and 22 with the lower scores having higher probability of remission at 1 year. In a cohort of 136 patients with complete follow-up data on the four components of the score, Aminian et al. provided external validation up to 2 years after surgery [62]. However, two later studies showed limitations of the DiaRem score [63, 64] including its lack of accuracy for predicting long-term durable outcomes as remission was only achieved in 50% of patients with the lowest score of 0–2 after 8 years of follow-up [63].

Recently, an individualized metabolic surgery (IMS) score was later developed and externally validated by Aminian and colleagues in a large cohort of 900 patients with T2D who underwent RYGB and sleeve gastrectomy with more than 5 years of follow-up. It has the benefit of selecting the appropriate surgical procedure in addition to predicting success of treatment [65–67].

Lastly, in an effort to apply a scoring system to predict long-term remission and relapse after surgery, Debédat et al. proposed the 5y-Ad-DiaRem with an ability to predict 5-year remission and identify patients at risk for relapse utilizing 1-year follow-up data (glycemia, number of antidiabetic treatments, remission status, 1-year weight loss) in addition to baseline information [68].

These scoring systems, although not widely adopted yet, provide useful tools for bariatric surgeons and a promising step toward personalized patient care for improving outcomes of metabolic surgery.

Effects of Gastric Bypass on T2D-Related Complications and Long-Term Premature Mortality

In patients with T2D, morbidity is related to both macrovascular (atherosclerosis) and microvascular (nephropathy, neuropathy, and retinopathy) complications [69]. It has been estimated that 12% of all mortalities in the USA could be attributable to T2D, making it, in essence, the third leading cause of death despite it being listed as the underlying cause of death in only 2.8% of death certificates [70]. Cardiovascular disease, including coronary artery disease, stroke, and heart failure, remains the leading cause of mortality in patients with T2D [71]. In addition, increasing evidence has shown that T2D is not unimpeachable of premature deaths from other causes including several types of cancer and infectious diseases [72]. Furthermore, severe obesity further exacerbates these risks owing to the detrimental role of increased adiposity in insulin resistance and glycemic impairment [73–76].

Improved glycemic control after RYGB and other bariatric-metabolic procedures (including complete and durable remission of T2D in a subset of patients) leads to decreased risk of macrovascular and microvascular complications [10, 30, 71, 74, 77–81].

Recently, Fisher et al. retrospectively analyzed two cohorts of patients with BMI ≥35 and T2D who underwent bariatric surgery ($n = 5{,}301$, RYGB 76%) and control patients ($n = 14{,}934$) matched by baseline age, sex, BMI, HbA1c, insulin use, and diabetes duration. They found a lower composite incidence of macrovascular events and coronary artery disease at 5 years following bariatric surgery (2.1% and 1.6%, respectively) compared to controls (4.3% and 2.8%, respectively) [10].

A prospective matched case-control study of patients with BMI >34 kg/m^2 and T2D (Swedish Obese Subjects Study) reported short-term and long-term outcomes following bariatric surgery [$n = 343$ (55 RYGB)] and compared them to contemporaneous obese control ($n = 260$) who received conventional medical management [79, 82]. Sjöström et al. found that bariatric surgery produced higher rates of T2D remission and fewer micro- and macrovascular complications than medical therapy median follow-up of 18 years.

Similarly, Johnson et al., using a large cohort from administrative data of obese patients with T2D who underwent bariatric surgery ($n = 2{,}580$) compared to nonsurgical control group matched by insurance status ($n = 13{,}371$). At 5 years, bariatric surgery was associated with a 60% to 70% reduction in any first major macrovascular complication (myocardial infarction, stroke, or death) or microvascular complication (new blindness, laser eye or retinal surgery, non-traumatic amputation, or requiring long-term dialysis) [83].

The effects on cardiovascular risk following RYGB alone were studied in a smaller prospective cohort of 92 patients with predicted baseline 10-year cardiovascular risk of 6.7%. This was decreased to 5.4% at 1 year after surgery, representing absolute risk reduction of 1.3% [77]. Long-term outcomes of diabetes-related complications are studied in a few RCT which reported reduction in cardiovascular events [30], nephropathy [30], neuropathy [30], and retinopathy [8, 30] 5 years after bariatric surgery. Due to the small sample size of the RCTs, prevalence of these complications were not powered enough to draw any definitive conclusion.

On the other hand, data showing long-term survival benefits after RYGB (or other bariatric procedures) is limited to observational studies [9, 83–86] as it may be infeasible to conduct RCTs given the large sample size and long duration of follow-up required in addition to ethical consideration of assigning patients to nonsurgical arms with expected inferior outcomes [87]. Results from three meta-analyses [74, 84, 86] comparing mortality between bariatric surgery and nonsurgical treatment found a 41–50% mortality reduction in patients after bariatric surgery [84, 86] and even a larger reduction of 79% in patients with T2D who underwent bariatric surgery [74].

All of these observational studies with one exception [9] analyzed their results combining all types of bariatric surgery and did not report procedure-specific outcomes. In a retrospective review of a large cohort of consecutive patients who underwent RYGB at a single practice in Utah ($n = 7{,}925$), Adams et al. compared long-term all-cause and disease-specific mortality compared to a control group matched for age, sex, and self-reported BMI of driver license applicants in the same state. At a mean of

7.1 years of follow-up, they found that all-cause mortality decreased by 40%, in the RYGB group compared with controls. Interestingly and relevant to the focus of this chapter, mortality associated with diabetes decreased by 92%, whereas mortality associated with coronary artery disease and cancer decreased by 56% and 60%, respectively [9].

Notwithstanding the evidence provided by the Adams, one should be cautious to not generalize these findings to all bariatric patients' populations as patients with higher risk may not have similar favorable outcomes [88].

Comparisons Between Outcomes of Gastric Bypass and Other Medical and Surgical Interventions in Randomized Controlled Trials

Gastric Bypass vs Medical Management

Results from seven RCT's (Table 46.4) have shown superior outcomes of RYGB compared to well-structured and supervised programs of optimal/intensive medical management and lifestyle modifications for the treatment of T2D. Remission rates from 15% to 90% were achieved 1–5 years following RYGB compared to only 0–9% following medical management alone. This variation in remission rates can be explained, in part, by the different definitions of T2D remission in these trials in addition to differences in the inclusion criteria and patient populations. Of the seven RCT's, six included a subset of patients with BMI <35 kg/m^2 (29–60% of patients) without reporting T2D remission outcomes for those separately [8, 35, 38, 116, 148, 149]. As expected, patients had a substantially higher percentage of weight loss with RYGB compared to medical management (22–28% vs 5–8% at 1–5 years of follow-up). These studies did not control for weight loss, rather studied outcomes at certain time-points following the two interventions.

Therefore, one cannot answer the question of whether the superior outcomes associated with RYGB are solely related to weight loss. Interestingly, however, Liang et al. compared patients who underwent RYGB ($n = 31$) with two medical management groups, one of which involved adding glucagon-like peptide-1 (GLP-1) receptor agonist (exenatide) to the treatment regimen. Exenatide is known to have a weight loss effect in obese diabetic patients [38], and as expected in this group ($n = 34$), BMI decreased from a mean of 30.3 to 26.8 kg/m^2 which was a significantly higher reduction than that observed in the second medical management group ($n = 36$) without exenatide and barely any BMI change from baseline. This better weight loss in the exenatide group yielded a greater improvement in insulin resistance (measured by HOMA-IR); however, it failed to translate into remission of T2D as none of the patient in either of the two medical management groups had remission of T2D at 1 year of follow-up compared to 90% of those in the RYGB group [38]. In-depth physiologic mechanistic studies comparing medical vs surgical interventions controlling for weight loss are needed to better understand the reasons behind superior outcomes observed with RYGB when compared to medical management alone.

Gastric Bypass vs Sleeve Gastrectomy

Sleeve gastrectomy (SG) is the most common bariatric surgery performed in the USA [11] and worldwide [89]. Conflicting results exist on whether SG provides comparable weight loss and glycemic control outcomes compared to RYGB.

We identified ten RCT's that studied outcomes of RYGB in comparison with SG in patients with severe obesity (Table 46.5), six of which reported short-term outcomes of 1–3 years of follow-up [43, 90–94] and a few reported relatively long-term outcomes 5 years after surgery [8, 26, 95, 96].

Contrary to a large body of observational studies, including very large comparative studies [97, 98], some of which included matched cohorts [98], showing superior weight loss [97, 98] and T2D resolution with RYGB [98], most RCT's showed little or no difference (at least statisti-

Table 46.4 Summary of randomized controlled trials comparing gastric bypass (RYGB) to intensive medical and lifestyle management (Medical) for type 2 diabetes (T2D)

Author (year)	Follow-up duration	Country	RYGB n/N^a (%T2D)	Medical n/N^a (%T2D)	BMI[b] Inclusion	BMI[b] <35 n (%)	Definition of remission or glycemic control	Remission or glycemic control n (%)	Weight loss outcomes	Findings
Schauer (2017) [8]	5 years	USA	49/49 (100)	38/38 (100)	27–43	RYGB 14 (29), Medical 17 (45)	Partial: HbA1c ≤6% without medical treatment Complete: HbA1c ≤6% without medical treatment	Partial remission: RYGB 15 (31), Medical 0 (0); Complete remission: RYGB 11 (22), Medical 0 (0)	Mean (SD) % weight loss: RYGB 23.2 (9.6), Medical 5.3 (10.8)	RYGB plus intensive medical therapy was more effective than intensive medical therapy alone in decreasing, or resolving, hyperglycemia
Mingrone (2015) [30]	5 years	Italy	19/19 (100)	15/15 (100)	≥35	0 (0)	Partial: 5.6 ≤FPG[b] ≤6.9 and HbA1c <6.5% for 1 year, without medications Complete: FPG[b]<5.6 and HbA1c <6% for 1 year, without medication	Partial remission: RYGB 7 (37), Medical 0 (0) Complete remission RYGB 0 (0), Medical 0 (0)	Mean (SD) % weight loss: RYGB 28.4 (7.4), Medical 6.9 (8.4)	RYGB is more effective than medical treatment for the long-term control of obese patients with T2D
Simonson (2018) [148]	3 years	USA	19/19 (100)	19/19 (100)	30–42	RYGB 6 (32), Medical 9 (47)	Glycemic control: HbA1c <6.5% and FPG1[b] <7, regardless of medication	HbA1c <6.5% without medications: RYGB 7 (37), Medical 0 (0); HbA1c <6.5% regardless of medications: RYGB 8 (42), Medical 0 (0)	Median (interquartile range) BMI[b] unit loss: RYGB 8.7 (7.1–10.3), Medical 1.8 (0–3.5)	RYGB provided superior weight loss and metabolic outcomes compared to lifestyle and medical management
Courcoulas (2015) [116]	3 years	USA	20/20 (100)	20/20 (100)	30–40	26 (43) in all study groups combined	Partial: HbA1c <6.5% and FPG[b] ≤6.9 without medication Complete: HbA1c <5.7% and FPG[b] ≤5.6 without medication	Partial or complete: RYGB 8 (40), Medical 0 (0) Complete: RYGB 3 (15), Medical 0 (0)	Mean (SE) % weight loss: RYGB 25 (2), Medical 5.7 (2.4)	RYGB is superior to lifestyle intervention alone for the remission of T2D

(continued)

Table 46.4 (continued)

Author (year)	Follow-up duration	Country	RYGB *n*/*N*[a] (%T2D)	Medical *n*/*N*[a] (%T2D)	BMI[b] Inclusion	BMI[b] <35 *n* (%)	Definition of remission or glycemic control	Remission or glycemic control *n* (%)	Weight loss outcomes	Findings
Ikramuddin (2015) [35]	2 year	USA and Taiwan	56/56[c] (100)	59/59 (100)	30≥BMI[b] >40	RYGB 36 (60), Medical 35 (58)	Partial: HbA1c ≤6.5% for 1 year without medications Complete: HbA1c ≤6% for 1 year, without medication	HbA1c <6%: RYGB 25 (44), Medical 5 (9)	Mean (SD) % weight loss: RYGB 26.1 (8.7), Medical 7.9 (7.8)	Adding RYGB to lifestyle and medical management was associated with higher rates of T2D remission
Cummings (2016) [149]	1 year	USA	15/15 (100)	17/17 (100)	30–45	RYGB 5 (33), Medical 6 (35)	HbA1c <6, without medication	RYGB 9 (60), Medical 1 (5.9)	Mean (SD) % weight loss: RYGB 25.8 (14.5), Medical 6.4 (5.8)	RYGB yielded greater T2D remission in mild to moderately obese patients compared to a rigorous intensive lifestyle and medical intervention
Liang (2013) [38]	1 year	China	31/31 (100)	65/65 (100)	>28	NR	NR	RYGB 28 (90), Medical 0 (0)	Mean BMI[b] (baseline to 1 year): RYGB 30.5 to 24.5, Medical 30.9 to 30.4, Medical+exenatide 30.3 to 26.8	RYGB is effective for treatment of obese hypertensive people with T2D and demonstrate cardiovascular benefit compared with conventional medical treatment

HbA1c glycated hemoglobin, *SD* standard deviation, *SE* standard error, *NR* not reported
[a]*N*, patients at the last year of the follow-up duration; *n*, patients with T2D at follow-up
[b]BMI (body mass index) is expressed in kg/m^2 and FPG (fasting plasma glucose) is expressed in mmol/L
[c]2-year data was available for 56/61 in the RYGB group and 54/59 in the Medical group

Table 46.5 Summary of randomized controlled trials comparing gastric bypass (RYGB) to sleeve gastrectomy (SG) for type 2 diabetes (T2D)

Author (year)	Follow-up duration	Country	RYGB n/N[a] (%T2D)	SG n/N[a] (%T2D)	BMI[b] inclusion	BMI[b] <35 N[a] (%)	Definition of remission or glycemic control	Remission or glycemic control n (%)	Weight loss outcome	Findings
Peterli (2018) [95]	5 years	Switzerland	28/104 (27)	26/101 (26)	>35[c]	0 (0)	HbA1c <6% and FPG[b] <5.6 for 1 year, without medication	RYGB19/28 (67.9), SG 16/26 (61.5)	Mean % excess BMI loss: RYGB 68.3, SG 61.1	No significant differences in excess BMI loss or T2D remission between SG and RYGB at 5 years
Salminen (2018) [96]	5 years	Finland	41/95 (43)	41/98 (42)	>35[c]	0 (0)	Partial: HbA1c <6.5% and 5.6 ≤ FPG[b] ≤6.9 for 1 year, and no medical/surgical treatment Complete: HbA1c <6% and FPG[a] <5.6 for 1 year, without medication	Partial or complete remission:RYGB 18/40 (45), SG 15/41 (36.6) Complete remission: RYGB 10/40 (25), SG 5/41 (12.2)	Mean % excess weight loss: RYGB 57, SG 49 Mean difference % excess weight loss, between groups: All patients[c] 8.2, patients with T2D 11.7	RYGB was associated a statistically similar rate of T2D remission and a greater % excess weight loss at 5 years compared to SG, but the difference did not meet the criteria for clinical significance[d]
Schauer (2017) [8]	5 years	USA	49/49 (100)	47/47 (100)	27–43	RYGB 14 (29.1) SG 18 (38.3)	Partial: HbA1c ≤6% without medical treatment Complete: HbA1c ≤6% without medication	Partial remission: RYGB 15 (30.6), SG 11 (23.4) Complete remission: RYGB 11 (22.4), SG 7 (14.9)	Mean (SD) % weight loss: RYGB 23.2 (9.6), SG 18.6 (7.5)	A trend for greater % of remission of T2D and weight after RYGB than SG at 5 years but without statistical significance
Zhang (2014) [26]	5 years	China	9/30 (30)	8/30 (27)	50 > BMI > 32	NR	Resolution: discontinuation of T2D medications, Improvement: reduction of T2D medications	Resolution or improvement: RYGB 7 (87.5), SG 8 (88.9)	% excess weight loss: RYGB 76.2, SG 63.2	RYGB and SG are equally effective in improvement or resolution of T2D and RYGB possesses the superiority in terms of weight loss

(continued)

Table 46.5 (continued)

Author (year)	Follow-up duration	Country	RYGB *n*/*N*[a] (%T2D)	SG *n*/*N*[a] (%T2D)	BMI[b] inclusion	BMI[b] <35 *N*[a] (%)	Definition of remission or glycemic control	Remission or glycemic control *n* (%)	Weight loss outcome	Findings
Kehagias (2011) [90]	3 years	Greece	10/30 (16)	5/30 (16)	≤50	0 (0)	FPG[b] <6.9 or 2H-PG[b] <11.1 (OGTT), without medical treatment	RYGB 4 (80), SG 4 (80)	Mean % excess weight loss: RYGB 62.1, SG 68.5	RYGB and SG are equally effective in weight reduction and amelioration of comorbidities at 3 years
Tang[e] (2016) [91]	2 years	China	38/38 (100)	34/34 (100)	≥28[e, f]	NR	Partial: HbA1c <6.5% and FPG[b] ≤6.9 for 1 year, without medical/surgical treatment Complete: HbA1c <6% and FPG[b] <5.6 for 1 year, without medication	Partial remission[e]: RYGB 22 (57.9), SG 26 (76.5) Complete remission[e]: RYGB 14/38 (36.8), SG 17/34 (50)	Mean (SD) % excess weight loss[e]: RYGB 53.7 (30.1), SG 69.4 (39.9)	Similar weight loss with a trend for more T2D remission after RYGB compared to SG, but no statistical significance[e]. SG was more cost-effective
Murphy (2017) [92]	1 year	New Zealand	7/7 (100)	7/7 (100)	35–65	0 (0)	HbA1c <6.5%, without medication	RYGB 5/7 (71), SG 5/7 (71)	Mean BMI[b] baseline to 1 year: RYGB: 38.4 to 28 SG: 36.9 to 29.3	Similar rates of T2D remission and weight reduction 1 year after RYGB vs SG with differences in gut microbiota taxonomy
Keidar (2013) [93]	1 year	Israel	19/19 (100)	18/18 (100)	>35	0 (0)	HbA1c <6%	RYGB = SG[g]	Mean (SD) % weight loss: RYGB 25.9 (5.4), SG 28.4 (5.9)	RYGB and SG had similar T2D remission rates, HbA1c and weight changes at 1 year
Kalinowski (2017) [94]	1 year	Poland	14/36 (39)	12/36 (33)	60 > BMI ≥ 35	0 (0)	FPG[b] <5.6 and HbA1c <6%, without medication	RYGB 5/14 (35.7), SG 6/12 (50)	Mean (SD) % weight loss: RYGB 30.4 (8.3), SG 29.2 (7.1)	RYGB and SG induce comparable weight loss and improvement in glucose metabolism at 1 year

Casajoana (2017) [43]	1 year	Spain	15/15 (100)	14/14 (100)	35–43	0 (0)	HbA1c <6% and FPG[b] <5.6 for 1 year, without medication	RYGB 12/15 (80), SG 8/14 (53.3)	Mean (SD) % weight loss: RYGB 35.3 (8.2), SG 27.2 (5.5)	RYGB achieved superior rates of weight loss and T2D remission at 1 year compared to SG

HbA1c glycated hemoglobin, *SD* standard deviation, *SE* standard error, *NR* not reported

[a]*N*, patients at the last year of the follow-up duration; *n*, patients with T2D at follow-up

[b]BMI (body mass index) data is in kg/m^2. Results of FPG (fasting plasma glucose) and 2-H-PG (2-hour plasma glucose) are in mmol/L; OGTT, oral glucose tolerance test

[c]Patients with 40 > BMI ≥ 35 kg/m^2 were eligible if they had at least one obesity-associated comorbidity. Studies of patients with only BMI <35 kg/m^2 were not included in this table

[d]The difference in %weight loss was not clinically significant, as the pre-specified minimal clinically important difference of 9 is within the confidence interval

[e]Tang et al. reported higher % partial and complete remission (without statistical significance) after SG compared to RYGB. However, in the Discussion, the authors comment on a finding of a trend for higher % remission after RYGB. They refer to their small sample size and explain this finding by the higher baseline BMI in the SG group with higher % excess weight loss, a finding consistent between the Results and Discussion sections of this study

[f]Tang et al. explained the rationale of the inclusion criterion of BMI ≥28 kg/m[b] by referring to the different definition of obesity in China (BMI ≥ 28 kg/m[b]) compared to the USA

[g]Keidar et al. did not report % remission (NR, not reported). Rather, they stated that there was no difference in remission rate between the groups. They reported mean (SD) HbA1c (RYGB 6.2 ± 0.5%, SG 6 ± 1%) at 1 year, which was similar between the two groups

cally) between the two procedures in their ability to reduce weight and improve T2D [8, 90–96]. Only two RCT's, one from Spain [43] and another China [26], found clear statistically significant differences in T2D remission rates and/or weight loss. At 1-year follow-up, Casajoana et al. found superior outcomes with RYGB with higher T2D remission rate (RYGB 12/15 80%, 8/14 53.3%, $p < 0.001$) and % total body weight loss (RYGB 35.3, SG 27.2, $p < 0.001$) compared to SG [43]. In another RCT, Zhang et al. found higher % excess weight loss following RYGB than SG (76.2 vs 63.2, $p = 0.02$) at 5 years; however, remission rates of T2D were similar between groups (RYGB 7/8, 87.5%, vs SG 8/9, 88.9%) [26].

Three recent RCTs, one from the USA [8] and two from Europe [95, 96], reported 5-year outcomes. They observed that RYGB and SG had equivalent effects on weight loss and glycemic control. Interestingly, these authors and others reported weight loss [92, 94–96] and T2D remission rates [8, 95, 96] that were higher in the RYGB group compared to SG but lacking statistical significance. This could be partly attributed to the small sample size in these studies, inclusion and exclusion criteria, patient population, and associated diseases, compared to large cohort studies that found statistical significance even with smaller differences in percent of weight loss and remission rates between procedures [97, 98].

Although considered the gold standard for clinical research, bariatric surgery RCT's have several limitations that, in many cases, preclude their ability to produce generalizable evidence. Patients in these trials may have clinical and demographic characteristics that differ from those in the routine practice of surgeons. Some of the factors to consider when interpreting the results of the RCTs comparing RYGB to SG are:

1. Lack of diversity and inclusion of racial minorities.
2. Different patient populations have different outcomes, LAGB in the USA vs Europe and Australia as an example [99, 100].
3. Variation (and potential selectivity) in reported measures of weight loss and their interpretation [96].
4. Differences between patients consenting to research and non-consenting [98].
5. Power-effect/sample size especially for SG [101, 102].
6. Inclusion of patients with BMI <35 kg/m^2, who aren't otherwise eligible for standard of care bariatric surgery [8, 91]
7. Dropout, lost to follow-up, and crossover effects in relatively small sample sizes [102] and the use of intention-to-treat vs per-protocol analysis [8, 95, 96, 103, 104].
8. The trial effect [105, 106].
9. Lack of long-term outcomes (more than 5 years) after SG [102, 107].

In a meta-analysis of midterm and long-term comparative studies of RYGB and SG (with at least 3 years of follow-up), Shoar et al. found that despite the insignificant difference between the two bariatric techniques in midterm weight loss, RYGB produced better weight loss in the long-term but similar rates of T2D remission [107]. This meta-analysis, however, included both randomized and observational studies, only two of which reported long-term T2D remission rates (one observational study from Venezuela [108] with very small sample size and the RCT from China by Zhang et al. [26]).

Another meta-analysis analyzing predictors of T2D remission after bariatric surgery found that among the four main subgroups of surgical treatments (RYGB, LAGB, SG, and BPD with 567, 2,377, 601, and 622 total patients, respectively), SG had the lowest remission rate (60%) which was similar to gastric banding (62%) but lower than remission rates associated with RYGB (71%) and biliopancreatic diversion (89%) [25].

Gastric Bypass vs Biliopancreatic Diversion (Duodenal Switch)

Biliopancreatic diversion (BPD) with or without duodenal switch (BPD/DS) comprises less than 1% of all bariatric surgeries performed in the USA [11]. It produces profound weight loss and metabolic effects due to its malabsorptive nature. It's associated with higher perioperative complications and risk of severe nutritional deficiencies compared with RYGB [109–111].

Nevertheless, BPD is associated with better weight loss and comorbidity outcomes, especially among the super-obese (BMI > 50 kg/m^2) [109]. Results from a RCT [30] comparing patients with T2D after RYGB (n = 19) vs BPD (n = 19) confirmed the findings of previous large retrospective cohort studies [109] and showed that patients treated with BPD had significantly better weight loss and higher rate of initial remission at 2 years (95% vs 75%) with a lower risk of relapse at 5 years (37% vs 53%) which resulted in a durable remission rate of 63% compared to 37% after RYGB [30]. On the other hand, another RCT by Risstad et al. comparing the outcomes of RYGB vs BPD/DS in super-obese patients (BMI = 50–60 kg/m^2) found similar rates of diabetes remission at 5 years (RYGB 80%, BPD/DS 100%) and argued that RYGB provided excellent glycemic control and metabolic outcomes, with fewer complications and nutritional deficiencies and a better quality of life than BPD/DS. However, this trial was limited by a small number of patients with T2D in each group (RYGB 5/31, BPD/DS 6/29) [112].

Hedberg et al. studied patients with a mean BMI of 55 (all > 48) kg/m^2 who were randomized to undergo either RYGB (n = 23) or BPD/DS (n = 24) with only one patient in the RYGB group (4%) and seven in the BPD/DS (29%) suffering from T2D. And although the authors did not report diabetes remission outcomes in this small subset of patients, they did find lower glucose and HbA1c levels at 3 years after BPD/DS compared with RYGB [113], a finding also observed in the RCT by Mingrone et al. that included patients with lower preoperative BMI (mean BMI = 45 kg/m^2), all of which had T2D [30]. Findings of the three RCT's are summarized in Table 46.6.

Based on these results, it is recommended that BPD/DS should be utilized only in a select patient population due to the increased risk of perioperative and nutritional complications. Some centers currently offer this procedure for super-obese patients as a second part of a two-step approach following sleeve gastrectomy in those with good compliance to postoperative regimens but suboptimal weight loss and glycemic control [30, 114, 115].

Gastric Bypass vs Laparoscopic Adjustable Gastric Banding

Laparoscopic adjustable gastric banding (LAGB) is a restrictive bariatric procedure that has been associated to poor long-term weight loss outcomes and high reoperation and failure rates in the USA [99]. However, many surgeons continue to offer it for the treatment of severe obesity with an estimated 6,316 new LAGBs implanted in 2017 [11]. Only two RCT's have studied the outcomes of RYGB in comparison to LAGB (Table 46.7). They show inferior short-term [116] and long-term [117] weight loss and T2D remission outcomes after LAGB compared to RYGB. Courcoulas et al. compared 41 patients with T2D who were randomized to undergo either RYGB (n = 20) or LAGB (n = 21) and found that complete remission at 3 years was achieved in only 5% after LAGB (29% partial remission) compared to 15% after RYGB (40% partial remission) [116].

A recent study with 10 years of follow-up showed that improvement or remission of T2D occurred in 50% following LAGB compared to 86% following RYGB based on the reduction of the dose or number of diabetic medications [117]. In these two RTC's, % weight loss was superior after RYGB (25–33%) compared to LAGB (15–21%) [116, 117]. LAGB is not an effective procedure for the glycemic control in patients with severe obesity and T2D, and its utilization should be discouraged.

Table 46.6 Summary of randomized controlled trials comparing gastric bypass (RYGB) to biliopancreatic diversion with [112, 113] or without [30] duodenal switch (BPD/DS) for type 2 diabetes (T2D)

Author (year)	Follow-up duration	Country	RYGB n/N^a (%T2D)	BPD n/N^a (%T2D)	BMI[b] inclusion	BMI[b] <35 n (%)	Definition of remission/glycemic control	Remission or glycemic control n (%)	Weight loss outcome	Findings
Mingrone (2015) [30]	5 years	Italy	19/19 (100)	19/19 (100)	≥35	0 (0)	Partial: 5.6≤ FPG[b] ≤6.9 and HbA1c <6.5% for 1 year, without medication Complete: FPG[b] <5.6 and HbA1c <6% for 1 year, without medication	Partial remission: RYGB 7 (37), BPD 12 (63) Complete remission: 0 (0) HbA1c ≤6·5% without treatment: RYGB 8 (42), BPD 13 (68)	Mean (SD) % weight loss: RYGB 28·4 (7·4), BPD 31·1 (9·3)	BPD resulted in a significantly higher rate of diabetes remission and a lower risk of disease recurrence than RYGB, but RYGB induced optimum glycemic and metabolic control, with fewer nutritional side effects and a better quality of life than BPD
Risstad (2015) [112]	5 years	Sweden and Norway	5/31 (16)	6/29 (21)	50–60	0 (0)	FPG[b] <5.6 for 1 year, without medication	RYGB 4 (80), BPD/DS 6 (100)	Mean (range) % BMI units loss: RYGB 13.6 (11–16.1), BPD/DS 22.1 (19.5–24.7)	BPD/DS resulted in greater weight loss and improvements in blood lipids and glucose than RYGB across 5 years in super-obese patients but was associated with more long-term surgical and nutritional complications

Hedberg (2012) [113]	3 years	Sweden	1/23 (4)	7/24 (29)	>48	0 (0)	NR[c]	NR[c]	Mean (SD) % excess BMI loss: RYGB 80 (15), BPD/DS 51 (23)	BPD/DS produces superior weight loss and improved glucose control compared with RYGB in the long term, without substantial nutritional risks or intolerable side effect

HbA1c glycated hemoglobin, *SD* standard deviation, *NR* not reported

[a]*N*, patients at the last year of the follow-up duration; *n*, patients with T2D at follow-up

[b]BMI (body mass index) is expressed in kg/m^2 and FPG (fasting plasma glucose) is expressed in mmol/L

[c]Hedberg et al. did not report remission rates, possibly due to their small sample size of patients with diabetes but they reported HbA1c and fasting glucose levels

Table 46.7 Summary of randomized controlled trials comparing gastric bypass (RYGB) to laparoscopic adjustable gastric banding (LAGB) for type 2 diabetes (T2D)

Author (year)	Follow-up duration	Country	RYGB *n*/*N*[a](% T2D)	LAGB *n*/*N*[a](% T2D)	BMI[b] inclusion	BMI[b] <35 *n* (%)	Definition of remission or glycemic control	Remission or glycemic control *n* (%)	Weight loss outcome	Findings
Nguyen (2018) [117]	10 years	USA	NR/48 (NR)	NR/52 (NR)	35–60	0 (0)	Improvement: reduction in dosage or the number of diabetic medications Remission: patient no longer required the use of diabetes medication	Remission or improvement RYGB 86.4%, LAGB 50%	Mean ± SD % weight loss: RYGB 32.7 ± 13.6, LAGB 21.2 ± 11.9	RYGB was associated with better long-term weight loss, lower rate of late reoperation, and improved remission of diabetes compared to LAGB
Courcoulas (2015) [116]	3 years	USA	20/20 (100)	21/21 (100)	30–40	26 (43) in all study groups combined	Partial: absence of antidiabetics with HbA1c <6.5% and FPG[b] ≤6.9 Complete: absence of antidiabetics with HbA1c <5.7% and FPG[b] ≤5.6	Partial or complete: RYGB 8 (40), LAGB 6 (29) Complete: RYGB 3 (15), LAGB 1 (5)	Mean ± SE % weight loss: RYGB 25 ± 2, LAGB 15 ± 2	RYGB is superior to LAGB for the remission of T2D

HbA1c glycated hemoglobin, *SD* standard deviation, *SE* standard error, *NR* not reported
[a]*N*, patients at the last year of the follow-up duration; *n*, patients with T2D at follow-up
[b]BMI (body mass index) is expressed in kg/m^2 and FPG (fasting plasma glucose) is expressed in mmol/L
RYGB, Roux-en-Y gastric bypass; SD, standard deviation; SE, standard error; ADA, American Diabetes Association

Mechanisms of Glycemic Control Following Gastric Bypass

Table 46.8 summarizes the signaling changes of weight loss-dependent and weight loss-independent mechanisms involved in glycemic control after RYGB.

Weight-Dependent Mechanisms of Glycemic Control After Gastric Bypass

Given the central role of excess adiposity in the pathogenesis of insulin resistance, nonalcoholic fatty liver disease (NAFLD), and hyperglycemia, reducing body weight through fat mass loss is a primary goal in co-managing severe obesity and T2D. Even modest weight loss (5–10% of the initial body mass) with diet, physical activity, and/or pharmacologic therapies can significantly improve glycemic control and insulin sensitivity. However, the absolute amount of weight reduction needed to meet these minimal thresholds makes attainment of such goals difficult in patients with severe obesity, and clinical improvements wane as weight is generally regained over time. On the other hand, RYGB is one of the most efficacious current treatment options for T2D in individuals with severe obesity and results in at least partial long-term T2D remission in most patients. When compared to even the most intensive combinations of lifestyle and medical T2D treatment strategies, RYGB remains superior with regard to both weight loss and T2D-related outcomes.

Importantly, RYGB can begin to reverse these pathophysiologic changes within the first postoperative week, likely due to caloric restriction and short-term changes in liver fat, glucose, and lipid storage, while subsequent substantial and durable reductions in fat mass continue to drive long-term remission of T2D in approximately 50% of patients. Indeed, greater postoperative weight loss coincides with up to fivefold higher rates of T2D remission following RYGB compared to

Table 46.8 Signaling changes involved in glycemic control after gastric bypass (RYGB)

Signaling Molecule	Source	Function	Change after RYGB
Insulin	Pancreatic β-cells	↑ Glucose uptake and storage ↑ Adipose tissue triglyceride storage ↓ Adipose tissue lipolysis	↑ Insulin secretion ↑ Hepatic insulin clearance ↓ Insulin resistance
Glucagon	Pancreatic α-cells	↑ Endogenous glucose production ↑ Fatty acid oxidation in the liver, brown and white adipose tissue, and skeletal muscle	↑ In systemic and portal blood
Bile acids	Liver	↑ Fatty acid oxidation in the liver, brown and white adipose tissue, and skeletal muscle ↑ Intestinal GLP-1 and FGF-19 secretion	↑ In systemic blood ↓ Hepatic reuptake
GLP-1 GIP PYY FGF-19	Intestine	Insulin-sensitizing; support of appetite control↑ Hepatic and whole-body glucose and lipid metabolism regulation of BA's homeostasis	↑ In systemic, portal, and (perhaps) cerebral circulation
Adiponectin Leptin	Adipose tissue	Insulin sensitizer Satiety factor	↑ In systemic circulation

GLP-1 glucagon-like peptide-1, *GIP* glucose-dependent inhibitory polypeptide, *PYY* peptide tyrosine-tyrosine, *FGF-19* fibroblast growth factor 19, *BA's* bile acids nonsurgical treatment options or LAGB [118–120], while suboptimal weight loss and weight regain are independent predictors of persistent T2D and T2D relapse in RYGB patients. Nevertheless, differences in body weight change alone cannot fully explain why some patients achieve sustained durable T2D remission after RYGB while others do not [120, 121].

Here, it is of interest to consider that weight loss parameters alone cannot provide information regarding pre- to postoperative improvements in body composition and do not account for baseline pancreatic β-cell function that is left over. Excess body weight in severe obesity is attributed to adipose tissue expansion with increased fat mass and, to a lesser extent, accretion of non-adipose fat-free mass (primarily skeletal muscle). Similarly, weight loss following RYGB is comprised mostly of fat mass, with decreased skeletal muscle mass accounting for 15–20% of the total weight change 1 year after surgery [122]. Declines in skeletal muscle mass seem confined to the first 12 months following RYGB, while subsequent changes up to 5 years are minimal and reflect sarcopenic effects of aging as opposed to proteolytic effects of RYGB per se [122]. Since skeletal muscle is a far more important site for glucose disposal than adipose tissue, underlying changes in muscle mass after RYGB could further influence glycemic control beyond reductions in body weight or BMI. However, this seems inconsistent with reports that patients with severe obesity and either normal glucose tolerance or T2D demonstrate similar skeletal muscle glucose uptake and insulin signaling (as evidenced by gene expression of the insulin receptor β and GLUT4 glucose transporter expression) [123, 124]. Furthermore, it is unlikely that the low variability in skeletal muscle mass between the first and fifth postoperative years can explain why a significant proportion of patients will experience new-onset T2D remission and/or relapse of T2D in parallel with divergent weight loss trajectories over this same time period [28, 32].

Rather, the association between successful weight loss and T2D outcomes following RYGB reflects the powerful insulin-sensitizing and antidiabetic effect of decreased adiposity. Indeed, reductions in total adiposity correlate strongly with improved whole-body insulin sensitivity 1 year after RYGB in a cohort of 30 patients with severe obesity and T2D [125], and improvement in peripheral glucose uptake after RYGB was observed only after substantial weight loss has occurred and correlated with the magnitude of weight lost in subjects with severe obesity and insulin resistance [126]. It should be noted that T2D has also been linked to a disproportionate increase in visceral adipose tissue and impaired visceral depot insulin-stimulated glucose uptake in patients with severe obesity [127, 128], while a lower ratio of more metabolically harmful visceral relative to subcutaneous adipose tissue is a positive predictor of T2D remission after RYGB [129].

However, evidence from a recent meta-analysis that relative reductions in visceral adiposity are more pronounced than in subcutaneous depots following both surgical and nonsurgical weight loss [130] exclude a role for preferential targeting of visceral fat in superior T2D remission rates with RYGB relative to conventional treatment options. It follows that, in addition to the strong association between postoperative weight loss and glycemic outcomes, additional factors other than changes in body weight and adiposity also contribute to the pathogenesis of T2D in severe obesity and its reversal after RYGB.

Weight-Independent Mechanisms of Glycemic Control After Gastric Bypass

The shared pathophysiology of severe obesity and T2D is characterized by multiple disruptions to an adipose tissue-liver-gut-brain axis, the latter of which is made intact following successful weight loss with RYGB [131]. Findings from studies in both rodent surgical models and in human patients have shown that RYGB induces a cascade of alterations in neuroendocrine and gut hormone signaling that are not conserved with nonsurgical dieting [132, 133]. The latter effects of surgery are presumed to further support restoration of insulin sensitivity and glycemic control, independently of weight loss.

Reversal of T2D may begin in the early postoperative period. In a study of nine patients with severe obesity (five with T2D), RYGB significantly reduced both homeostasis model of insulin resistance (HOMA-IR) and fasting insulin concentrations within just 1 week after surgery [134]. However changes in HOMA-IR are indeed expected in any subject with minimal changes in body weight and to insulin-sensitizing effects of severe caloric restriction. Matched caloric restriction through nonsurgical dieting also reduces HOMA-IR and fasting insulin concentrations, and suppresses hepatic glucose production similarly to RYGB [126] but cannot recapitulate the post-surgery increases in postprandial secretion of GLP-1 and glucose-dependent inhibitory polypeptide (GIP), both of which promote β-cell insulin secretion [126, 134]. Indeed, administration of the competitive GLP-1 antagonist exendin-(9-39) to RYGB patients 4 weeks after surgery effectively eliminated the stimulatory effect of increased GLP-1 concentrations on glucose-induced β-cell insulin secretion [135]. It is of interest to point out that postprandial GLP-1 but not GIP concentrations continue to increase throughout the first 6 months after RYGB [126].

Along with the rerouting of gastrointestinal macronutrient flow, RYGB promotes antidiabetic gut hormone signaling changes by modulating metabolism and enterohepatic transport of bile acids (BA's). Here, it is of interest to point out that RYGB-induced alterations in the size and/or composition of the circulating BA pool are not conserved with nonsurgical weight loss or LAGB [136, 137]. In addition to supporting digestion and absorption of lipophilic nutrients, BA's stimulate enterocyte release of GLP-1, as well as peptide tyrosine-tyrosine (PYY), by activating the G protein-coupled BA receptor (GPBAR1) on enteroendocrine L-cells [138, 139]. In contrast to GPBAR1, mRNA, and protein expression of the other major BA targets, the nuclear farnesoid x receptor (FXR) is downregulated in ileal enterocytes after RYGB [138]. This is consistent with reports that experimental inhibition of intestinal FXR reversed insulin resistance and glucose intolerance in mice. On the other hand, the limited available evidence in humans suggests that FXR and another member of the nuclear receptor superfamily, lower hepatic FXR, expression at the time of surgery correlates positively with postoperative T2D remission [140]. Although the exact mechanisms linking altered BA metabolism and signaling through GPBAR1 and/or FXR to T2D remission are incompletely understood, results from an RYGB minipig model suggest that hepatic reuptake of BA's returning from the portal vein is inhibited in favor of elevated systemic BA concentrations after RYGB [141].

References

1. Mathers CD, Loncar D. Projections of global mortality and burden of disease from 2002 to 2030. PLoS Med. 2006;3(11):e442.
2. World Health Organization. Diabetes; 2017. Available from: http://www.who.int/news-room/fact-sheets/detail/diabetes.
3. Centers for Disease Control and Prevention, United States diabetes surveillance system. Diagnosed diabetes, total, adults with diabetes, age-adjusted percentage, natural breaks, all states; 2018. Available from: https://gis.cdc.gov/grasp/diabetes/DiabetesAtlas.html.
4. Flegal KM, Kruszon-Moran D, Carroll MD, Fryar CD, Ogden CL. Trends in obesity among adults in the United States, 2005 to 2014. JAMA. 2016;315(21):2284–91.
5. Ganz ML, Wintfeld N, Li Q, Alas V, Langer J, Hammer M. The association of body mass index with the risk of type 2 diabetes: a case-control study nested in an electronic health records system in the United States. Diabetol Metab Syndr. 2014;6(1):50.
6. Gregg EW, Cheng YJ, Narayan KM, Thompson TJ, Williamson DF. The relative contributions of different levels of overweight and obesity to the increased prevalence of diabetes in the United States: 1976–2004. Prev Med. 2007;45(5):348–52.
7. Ribaric G, Buchwald JN, McGlennon TW. Diabetes and weight in comparative studies of bariatric surgery vs conventional medical therapy: a systematic review and meta-analysis. Obes Surg. 2014;24(3):437–55.
8. Schauer PR, Bhatt DL, Kirwan JP, Wolski K, Aminian A, Brethauer SA, et al. Bariatric surgery versus intensive medical therapy for diabetes – 5-year outcomes. N Engl J Med. 2017;376(7):641–51.

9. Adams TD, Gress RE, Smith SC, Halverson RC, Simper SC, Rosamond WD, et al. Long-term mortality after gastric bypass surgery. N Engl J Med. 2007;357(8):753–61.
10. Fisher DP, Johnson E, Haneuse S, Arterburn D, Coleman KJ, O'Connor PJ, et al. Association between bariatric surgery and macrovascular disease outcomes in patients with type 2 diabetes and severe obesity. JAMA. 2018;320(15):1570–82.
11. American Society for Metabolic and Bariatric Surgery. Estimate of bariatric surgery numbers, 2011–2017; 2018. Available from: https://asmbs.org/resources/estimate-of-bariatric-surgery-numbers.
12. Pereira MJ, Skrtic S, Katsogiannos P, Abrahamsson N, Sidibeh CO, Dahgam S, et al. Impaired adipose tissue lipid storage, but not altered lipolysis, contributes to elevated levels of NEFA in type 2 diabetes. Degree of hyperglycemia and adiposity are important factors. Metab Clin Exp. 2016;65(12):1768–80.
13. Macauley M, Smith FE, Thelwall PE, Hollingsworth KG, Taylor R. Diurnal variation in skeletal muscle and liver glycogen in humans with normal health and Type 2 diabetes. Clin Sci (London, England: 1979). 2015;128(10):707–13.
14. Lorenzo C, Hanley AJ, Wagenknecht LE, Rewers MJ, Stefanovski D, Goodarzi MO, et al. Relationship of insulin sensitivity, insulin secretion, and adiposity with insulin clearance in a multiethnic population: the insulin Resistance Atherosclerosis study. Diabetes Care. 2013;36(1):101–3.
15. Khoraki J, Wiens CN, McMillan AB, Artz NS, Haufe W, Campo CA, et al. Intrahepatic fat, not obesity, is a main driver of the metabolic syndrome in obese patients and is significantly reduced by weight loss surgery. J Am Coll Surg. 2016;223(4):e1.
16. Costes S, Langen R, Gurlo T, Matveyenko AV, Butler PC. beta-cell failure in type 2 diabetes: a case of asking too much of too few? Diabetes. 2013;62(2):327–35.
17. Gerhard GS, Styer AM, Wood GC, Roesch SL, Petrick AT, Gabrielsen J, et al. A role for fibroblast growth factor 19 and bile acids in diabetes remission after Roux-en-Y gastric bypass. Diabetes Care. 2013;36(7):1859–64.
18. Eissing L, Scherer T, Todter K, Knippschild U, Greve JW, Buurman WA, et al. De novo lipogenesis in human fat and liver is linked to ChREBP-beta and metabolic health. Nat Commun. 2013;4:1528.
19. Auguet T, Guiu-Jurado E, Berlanga A, Terra X, Martinez S, Porras JA, et al. Downregulation of lipogenesis and fatty acid oxidation in the subcutaneous adipose tissue of morbidly obese women. Obesity (Silver Spring, MD). 2014;22(9):2032–8.
20. Chai SY, Pan XY, Song KX, Huang YY, Li F, Cheng XY, et al. Differential patterns of insulin secretion and sensitivity in patients with type 2 diabetes mellitus and nonalcoholic fatty liver disease versus patients with type 2 diabetes mellitus alone. Lipids Health Dis. 2014;13:7.
21. Buse JB, Caprio S, Cefalu WT, Ceriello A, Del Prato S, Inzucchi SE, et al. How do we define cure of diabetes? Diabetes Care. 2009;32(11):2133–5.
22. American Diabetes Association. Executive summary: standards of medical care in diabetes--2012. Diabetes Care. 2012;35(Suppl 1):S4–s10.
23. Buchwald H, Estok R, Fahrbach K, Banel D, Jensen MD, Pories WJ, et al. Weight and type 2 diabetes after bariatric surgery: systematic review and meta-analysis. Am J Med. 2009;122(3):248–56.e5.
24. Chikunguwo SM, Wolfe LG, Dodson P, Meador JG, Baugh N, Clore JN, et al. Analysis of factors associated with durable remission of diabetes after Roux-en-Y gastric bypass. Surg Obes Relat Dis. 2010;6(3):254–9.
25. Panunzi S, De Gaetano A, Carnicelli A, Mingrone G. Predictors of remission of diabetes mellitus in severely obese individuals undergoing bariatric surgery: do BMI or procedure choice matter? A meta-analysis. Ann Surg. 2015;261(3):459–67.
26. Zhang Y, Zhao H, Cao Z, Sun X, Zhang C, Cai W, et al. A randomized clinical trial of laparoscopic Roux-en-Y gastric bypass and sleeve gastrectomy for the treatment of morbid obesity in China: a 5-year outcome. Obes Surg. 2014;24(10):1617–24.
27. Yu J, Zhou X, Li L, Li S, Tan J, Li Y, et al. The long-term effects of bariatric surgery for type 2 diabetes: systematic review and meta-analysis of randomized and non-randomized evidence. Obes Surg. 2015;25(1):143–58.
28. Arterburn DE, Bogart A, Sherwood NE, Sidney S, Coleman KJ, Haneuse S, et al. A multisite study of long-term remission and relapse of type 2 diabetes mellitus following gastric bypass. Obes Surg. 2013;23(1):93–102.
29. Brethauer SA, Aminian A, Romero-Talamas H, Batayyah E, Mackey J, Kennedy L, et al. Can diabetes be surgically cured? Long-term metabolic effects of bariatric surgery in obese patients with type 2 diabetes mellitus. Ann Surg. 2013;258(4):628–36; discussion 36–7.
30. Mingrone G, Panunzi S, De Gaetano A, Guidone C, Iaconelli A, Nanni G, et al. Bariatric-metabolic surgery versus conventional medical treatment in obese patients with type 2 diabetes: 5 year follow-up of an open-label, single-centre, randomised controlled trial. Lancet. 2015;386(9997):964–73.
31. DiGiorgi M, Rosen DJ, Choi JJ, Milone L, Schrope B, Olivero-Rivera L, et al. Re-emergence of diabetes after gastric bypass in patients with mid- to long-term follow-up. Surg Obes Relat Dis. 2010;6(3):249–53.
32. de Oliveira VLP, Martins GP, Mottin CC, Rizzolli J, Friedman R. Predictors of long-term remission and relapse of type 2 diabetes mellitus following gastric bypass in severely obese patients. Obes Surg. 2018;28(1):195–203.
33. Xiaosong W, Chongyu S, Xuqi S, Peiwu Y, Yongliang Z. Risk factors for relapse of hyperglycemia after laparoscopic Roux-en-Y gastric bypass in T2DM

obese patients: a 5-year follow-up of 24 cases. Obes Surg. 2019;29:1164.
34. Yan Y, Sha Y, Yao G, Wang S, Kong F, Liu H, et al. Roux-en-Y gastric bypass versus medical treatment for type 2 diabetes mellitus in obese patients: a systematic review and meta-analysis of randomized controlled trials. Medicine (Baltimore). 2016;95(17):e3462.
35. Ikramuddin S, Billington CJ, Lee WJ, Bantle JP, Thomas AJ, Connett JE, et al. Roux-en-Y gastric bypass for diabetes (the Diabetes Surgery Study): 2-year outcomes of a 5-year, randomised, controlled trial. Lancet Diabetes Endocrinol. 2015;3(6):413–22.
36. Smith MD, Adeniji A, Wahed AS, Patterson E, Chapman W, Courcoulas AP, et al. Technical factors associated with anastomotic leak after Roux-en-Y gastric bypass. Surg Obes Relat Dis. 2015;11(2):313–20.
37. Halperin F, Ding SA, Simonson DC, Panosian J, Goebel-Fabbri A, Wewalka M, et al. Roux-en-Y gastric bypass surgery or lifestyle with intensive medical management in patients with type 2 diabetes: feasibility and 1-year results of a randomized clinical trial. JAMA Surg. 2014;149(7):716–26.
38. Liang Z, Wu Q, Chen B, Yu P, Zhao H, Ouyang X. Effect of laparoscopic Roux-en-Y gastric bypass surgery on type 2 diabetes mellitus with hypertension: a randomized controlled trial. Diabetes Res Clin Pract. 2013;101(1):50–6.
39. Pournaras DJ, Aasheim ET, Sovik TT, Andrews R, Mahon D, Welbourn R, et al. Effect of the definition of type II diabetes remission in the evaluation of bariatric surgery for metabolic disorders. Br J Surg. 2012;99(1):100–3.
40. Rubino F, Nathan DM, Eckel RH, Schauer PR, Alberti KG, Zimmet PZ, et al. Metabolic surgery in the treatment algorithm for type 2 diabetes: a joint statement by international diabetes organizations. Diabetes Care. 2016;39(6):861–77.
41. Dixon JB, Fitzgerald DA, Kow L, Bailey D, Baur LA. Adolescent bariatric surgery: ANZ guidance and recommendations. ANZ J Surg. 2011;81(12):854–5.
42. Hutch CR, Sandoval D. The role of GLP-1 in the metabolic success of bariatric surgery. Endocrinology. 2017;158(12):4139–51.
43. Casajoana A, Pujol J, Garcia A, Elvira J, Virgili N, de Oca FJ, et al. Predictive value of gut peptides in T2D remission: randomized controlled trial comparing metabolic gastric bypass, sleeve gastrectomy and greater curvature plication. Obes Surg. 2017;27(9):2235–45.
44. Blaha MJ, Gebretsadik T, Shintani A, Elasy TA. Waist circumference, not the metabolic syndrome, predicts glucose deterioration in type 2 diabetes. Obesity (Silver Spring, MD). 2008;16(4):869–74.
45. Huang X, Liu T, Zhong M, Cheng Y, Hu S, Liu S. Predictors of glycemic control after sleeve gastrectomy versus Roux-en-Y gastric bypass: a meta-analysis, meta-regression, and systematic review. Surg Obes Relat Dis. 2018;14(12):1822–31.
46. Dixon JB, Chuang LM, Chong K, Chen SC, Lambert GW, Straznicky NE, et al. Predicting the glycemic response to gastric bypass surgery in patients with type 2 diabetes. Diabetes Care. 2013;36(1):20–6.
47. Lee WJ, Hur KY, Lakadawala M, Kasama K, Wong SK, Chen SC, et al. Predicting success of metabolic surgery: age, body mass index, C-peptide, and duration score. Surg Obes Relat Dis. 2013;9(3):379–84.
48. Hayes MT, Hunt LA, Foo J, Tychinskaya Y, Stubbs RS. A model for predicting the resolution of type 2 diabetes in severely obese subjects following Roux-en Y gastric bypass surgery. Obes Surg. 2011;21(7):910–6.
49. Park JY, Kim YJ. Prediction of diabetes remission in morbidly obese patients after Roux-en-Y gastric bypass. Obes Surg. 2016;26(4):749–56.
50. Mingrone G, Panunzi S, De Gaetano A, Guidone C, Iaconelli A, Leccesi L, et al. Bariatric surgery versus conventional medical therapy for type 2 diabetes. N Engl J Med. 2012;366(17):1577–85.
51. Carlsson LM, Peltonen M, Ahlin S, Anveden A, Bouchard C, Carlsson B, et al. Bariatric surgery and prevention of type 2 diabetes in Swedish obese subjects. N Engl J Med. 2012;367(8):695–704.
52. Livingston EH. Inadequacy of BMI as an indicator for bariatric surgery. JAMA. 2012;307(1):88–9.
53. Yokoyama H, Okudaira M, Otani T, Watanabe C, Takaike H, Miuira J, et al. High incidence of diabetic nephropathy in early-onset Japanese NIDDM patients. Risk analysis. Diabetes Care. 1998;21(7):1080–5.
54. The relationship of glycemic exposure (HbA1c) to the risk of development and progression of retinopathy in the diabetes control and complications trial. Diabetes. 1995;44(8):968–83.
55. Schauer PR, Burguera B, Ikramuddin S, Cottam D, Gourash W, Hamad G, et al. Effect of laparoscopic Roux-en Y gastric bypass on type 2 diabetes mellitus. Ann Surg. 2003;238(4):467–84; discussion 84–5.
56. Jimenez A, Casamitjana R, Flores L, Delgado S, Lacy A, Vidal J. GLP-1 and the long-term outcome of type 2 diabetes mellitus after Roux-en-Y gastric bypass surgery in morbidly obese subjects. Ann Surg. 2013;257(5):894–9.
57. Kadera BE, Lum K, Grant J, Pryor AD, Portenier DD, DeMaria EJ. Remission of type 2 diabetes after Roux-en-Y gastric bypass is associated with greater weight loss. Surg Obes Relat Dis. 2009;5(3):305–9.
58. Sugerman HJ, Wolfe LG, Sica DA, Clore JN. Diabetes and hypertension in severe obesity and effects of gastric bypass-induced weight loss. Ann Surg. 2003;237(6):751–6; discussion 7–8.
59. Khanna V, Malin SK, Bena J, Abood B, Pothier CE, Bhatt DL, et al. Adults with long-duration type 2 diabetes have blunted glycemic and beta-cell function improvements after bariatric surgery. Obesity (Silver Spring, MD). 2015;23(3):523–6.
60. Lee WJ, Almulaifi A, Tsou JJ, Ser KH, Lee YC, Chen SC. Laparoscopic sleeve gastrectomy for type

2 diabetes mellitus: predicting the success by ABCD score. Surg Obes Relat Dis. 2015;11(5):991–6.
61. Still CD, Wood GC, Benotti P, Petrick AT, Gabrielsen J, Strodel WE, et al. Preoperative prediction of type 2 diabetes remission after Roux-en-Y gastric bypass surgery: a retrospective cohort study. Lancet Diabetes Endocrinol. 2014;2(1):38–45.
62. Aminian A, Brethauer SA, Kashyap SR, Kirwan JP, Schauer PR. DiaRem score: external validation. Lancet Diabetes Endocrinol. 2014;2(1):12–3.
63. Wood GC, Mirshahi T, Still CD, Hirsch AG. Association of DiaRem score with cure of type 2 diabetes following bariatric surgery. JAMA Surg. 2016;151(8):779–81.
64. Tharakan G, Scott R, Szepietowski O, Miras AD, Blakemore AI, Purkayastha S, et al. Limitations of the DiaRem score in predicting remission of diabetes following Roux-En-Y gastric bypass (RYGB) in an ethnically diverse population from a single institution in the UK. Obes Surg. 2017;27(3):782–6.
65. Aminian A, Brethauer SA, Andalib A, Nowacki AS, Jimenez A, Corcelles R, et al. Individualized metabolic surgery score: procedure selection based on diabetes severity. Ann Surg. 2017;266(4):650–7.
66. Aminian A, Andalib A. Individualized metabolic surgery (IMS) score. Surg Obes Relat Dis. 2018;14(12):1921–2.
67. Cleveland Clinic Lerner Research Institute. Individualized metabolic surgery score; 2018. Available from: http://riskcalc.org/Metabolic_Surgery_Score/.
68. Debedat J, Sokolovska N, Coupaye M, Panunzi S, Chakaroun R, Genser L, et al. Long-term relapse of type 2 diabetes after Roux-en-Y gastric bypass: prediction and clinical relevance. Diabetes Care. 2018;41(10):2086–95.
69. Gregg EW, Sattar N, Ali MK. The changing face of diabetes complications. Lancet Diabetes Endocrinol. 2016;4(6):537–47.
70. Stokes A, Preston SH. Deaths attributable to diabetes in the United States: comparison of data sources and estimation approaches. PLoS One. 2017;12(1):e0170219.
71. Low Wang CC, Hess CN, Hiatt WR, Goldfine AB. Clinical update: cardiovascular disease in diabetes mellitus: atherosclerotic cardiovascular disease and heart failure in type 2 diabetes mellitus – mechanisms, management, and clinical considerations. Circulation. 2016;133(24):2459–502.
72. Rao Kondapally Seshasai S, Kaptoge S, Thompson A, Di Angelantonio E, Gao P, Sarwar N, et al. Diabetes mellitus, fasting glucose, and risk of cause-specific death. N Engl J Med. 2011;364(9):829–41.
73. Gallagher EJ, LeRoith D. Obesity and diabetes: the increased risk of cancer and cancer-related mortality. Physiol Rev. 2015;95(3):727–48.
74. Sheng B, Truong K, Spitler H, Zhang L, Tong X, Chen L. The long-term effects of bariatric surgery on type 2 diabetes remission, microvascular and macrovascular complications, and mortality: a systematic review and meta-analysis. Obes Surg. 2017;27(10):2724–32.
75. Lu Y, Hajifathalian K, Ezzati M, Woodward M, Rimm EB, Danaei G. Metabolic mediators of the effects of body-mass index, overweight, and obesity on coronary heart disease and stroke: a pooled analysis of 97 prospective cohorts with 1.8 million participants. Lancet. 2014;383(9921):970–83.
76. Chang AR, Grams ME, Ballew SH, Bilo H, Correa A, Evans M, et al. Adiposity and risk of decline in glomerular filtration rate: meta-analysis of individual participant data in a global consortium. BMJ (Clinical research ed). 2019;364:k5301.
77. Arterburn D, Schauer DP, Wise RE, Gersin KS, Fischer DR, Selwyn CA Jr, et al. Change in predicted 10-year cardiovascular risk following laparoscopic Roux-en-Y gastric bypass surgery. Obes Surg. 2009;19(2):184–9.
78. Adams TD, Arterburn DE, Nathan DM, Eckel RH. Clinical outcomes of metabolic surgery: microvascular and macrovascular complications. Diabetes Care. 2016;39(6):912–23.
79. Sjostrom L, Peltonen M, Jacobson P, Ahlin S, Andersson-Assarsson J, Anveden A, et al. Association of bariatric surgery with long-term remission of type 2 diabetes and with microvascular and macrovascular complications. JAMA. 2014;311(22):2297–304.
80. Miras AD, Chuah LL, Khalil N, Nicotra A, Vusirikala A, Baqai N, et al. Type 2 diabetes mellitus and microvascular complications 1 year after Roux-en-Y gastric bypass: a case-control study. Diabetologia. 2015;58(7):1443–7.
81. Gorman DM, le Roux CW, Docherty NG. The effect of bariatric surgery on diabetic retinopathy: good, bad, or both? Diabetes Metab J. 2016;40(5):354–64.
82. Sjostrom L, Lindroos AK, Peltonen M, Torgerson J, Bouchard C, Carlsson B, et al. Lifestyle, diabetes, and cardiovascular risk factors 10 years after bariatric surgery. N Engl J Med. 2004;351(26):2683–93.
83. Johnson BL, Blackhurst DW, Latham BB, Cull DL, Bour ES, Oliver TL, et al. Bariatric surgery is associated with a reduction in major macrovascular and microvascular complications in moderately to severely obese patients with type 2 diabetes mellitus. J Am Coll Surg. 2013;216(4):545–56; discussion 56–8.
84. Kwok CS, Pradhan A, Khan MA, Anderson SG, Keavney BD, Myint PK, et al. Bariatric surgery and its impact on cardiovascular disease and mortality: a systematic review and meta-analysis. Int J Cardiol. 2014;173(1):20–8.
85. Arterburn DE, Olsen MK, Smith VA, Livingston EH, Van Scoyoc L, Yancy WS Jr, et al. Association between bariatric surgery and long-term survival. JAMA. 2015;313(1):62–70.
86. Cardoso L, Rodrigues D, Gomes L, Carrilho F. Short- and long-term mortality after bariatric

surgery: a systematic review and meta-analysis. Diabetes Obes Metab. 2017;19(9):1223–32.
87. Kim J, Eisenberg D, Azagury D, Rogers A, Campos GM. American Society for Metabolic and Bariatric Surgery position statement on long-term survival benefit after metabolic and bariatric surgery. Surg Obes Relat Dis. 2016;12(3):453–9.
88. Maciejewski ML, Livingston EH, Smith VA, Kavee AL, Kahwati LC, Henderson WG, et al. Survival among high-risk patients after bariatric surgery. JAMA. 2011;305(23):2419–26.
89. Angrisani L, Santonicola A, Iovino P, Vitiello A, Zundel N, Buchwald H, et al. Bariatric surgery and endoluminal procedures: IFSO worldwide survey 2014. Obes Surg. 2017;27(9):2279–89.
90. Kehagias I, Karamanakos SN, Argentou M, Kalfarentzos F. Randomized clinical trial of laparoscopic Roux-en-Y gastric bypass versus laparoscopic sleeve gastrectomy for the management of patients with BMI <50 kg/m^2. Obes Surg. 2011;21(11):1650–6.
91. Tang Q, Sun Z, Zhang N, Xu G, Song P, Xu L, et al. Cost-effectiveness of bariatric surgery for type 2 diabetes mellitus: a randomized controlled trial in China. Medicine (Baltimore). 2016;95(20):e3522.
92. Murphy R, Tsai P, Jullig M, Liu A, Plank L, Booth M. Differential changes in gut microbiota after gastric bypass and sleeve gastrectomy bariatric surgery vary according to diabetes remission. Obes Surg. 2017;27(4):917–25.
93. Keidar A, Hershkop KJ, Marko L, Schweiger C, Hecht L, Bartov N, et al. Roux-en-Y gastric bypass vs sleeve gastrectomy for obese patients with type 2 diabetes: a randomised trial. Diabetologia. 2013;56(9):1914–8.
94. Kalinowski P, Paluszkiewicz R, Wroblewski T, Remiszewski P, Grodzicki M, Bartoszewicz Z, et al. Ghrelin, leptin, and glycemic control after sleeve gastrectomy versus Roux-en-Y gastric bypass-results of a randomized clinical trial. Surg Obes Relat Dis. 2017;13(2):181–8.
95. Peterli R, Wolnerhanssen BK, Peters T, Vetter D, Kroll D, Borbely Y, et al. Effect of laparoscopic sleeve gastrectomy vs laparoscopic Roux-en-Y gastric bypass on weight loss in patients with morbid obesity: the SM-BOSS randomized clinical trial. JAMA. 2018;319(3):255–65.
96. Salminen P, Helmio M, Ovaska J, Juuti A, Leivonen M, Peromaa-Haavisto P, et al. Effect of laparoscopic sleeve gastrectomy vs laparoscopic Roux-en-Y gastric bypass on weight loss at 5 years among patients with morbid obesity: the SLEEVEPASS randomized clinical trial. JAMA. 2018;319(3):241–54.
97. Arterburn D, Wellman R, Emiliano A, Smith SR, Odegaard AO, Murali S, et al. Comparative effectiveness and safety of bariatric procedures for weight loss: a PCORnet cohort study. Ann Intern Med. 2018;169(11):741–50.
98. Sudan R, Jain-Spangler K. Tailoring bariatric surgery: sleeve gastrectomy, Roux-en-Y gastric bypass and biliopancreatic diversion with duodenal switch. J Laparoendosc Adv Surg Tech A. 2018;28(8):956–61.
99. Khoraki J, Moraes MG, Neto APF, Funk LM, Greenberg JA, Campos GM. Long-term outcomes of laparoscopic adjustable gastric banding. Am J Surg. 2018;215(1):97–103.
100. Mazzini GS, Khoraki J, Brownning MG, et al. Virginia is not Switzerland: challenging the external validity of the European randomized controlled trials comparing laparoscopic gastric bypass and sleeve gastrectomy. J Am Coll Surg. 2018;227(4):e76–7.
101. Kodama S, Fujihara K, Horikawa C, Harada M, Ishiguro H, Kaneko M, et al. Network meta-analysis of the relative efficacy of bariatric surgeries for diabetes remission. Obes Rev. 2018;19(12):1621–9.
102. Puzziferri N, Roshek TB 3rd, Mayo HG, Gallagher R, Belle SH, Livingston EH. Long-term follow-up after bariatric surgery: a systematic review. JAMA. 2014;312(9):934–42.
103. Mostazir M, Taylor RS, Henley W, Watkins E. An overview of statistical methods for handling nonadherence to intervention protocol in randomised control trials (RCTs): a methodological review. J Clin Epidemiol. 2019;108:121–31.
104. Sedgwick P. Intention to treat analysis versus per protocol analysis of trial data. BMJ (Clinical research ed). 2015;350:h681.
105. Vist GE, Bryant D, Somerville L, Birminghem T, Oxman AD. Outcomes of patients who participate in randomized controlled trials compared to similar patients receiving similar interventions who do not participate. Cochrane Database Syst Rev. 2008;(3):Mr000009.
106. Clarke M, Loudon K. Effects on patients of their healthcare practitioner's or institution's participation in clinical trials: a systematic review. Trials. 2011;12:16.
107. Shoar S, Saber AA. Long-term and midterm outcomes of laparoscopic sleeve gastrectomy versus Roux-en-Y gastric bypass: a systematic review and meta-analysis of comparative studies. Surg Obes Relat Dis. 2017;13(2):170–80.
108. Leyba JL, Llopis SN, Aulestia SN. Laparoscopic Roux-en-Y gastric bypass versus laparoscopic sleeve gastrectomy for the treatment of morbid obesity. A prospective study with 5 years of follow-up. Obes Surg. 2014;24(12):2094–8.
109. Nelson DW, Blair KS, Martin MJ. Analysis of obesity-related outcomes and bariatric failure rates with the duodenal switch vs gastric bypass for morbid obesity. Arch Surg (Chicago, IL: 1960). 2012;147(9):847–54.
110. Sovik TT, Aasheim ET, Taha O, Engstrom M, Fagerland MW, Bjorkman S, et al. Weight loss, cardiovascular risk factors, and quality of life after gastric bypass and duodenal switch: a randomized trial. Ann Intern Med. 2011;155(5):281–91.
111. Aasheim ET, Bjorkman S, Sovik TT, Engstrom M, Hanvold SE, Mala T, et al. Vitamin status

after bariatric surgery: a randomized study of gastric bypass and duodenal switch. Am J Clin Nutr. 2009;90(1):15–22.
112. Risstad H, Sovik TT, Engstrom M, Aasheim ET, Fagerland MW, Olsen MF, et al. Five-year outcomes after laparoscopic gastric bypass and laparoscopic duodenal switch in patients with body mass index of 50 to 60: a randomized clinical trial. JAMA Surg. 2015;150(4):352–61.
113. Hedberg J, Sundbom M. Superior weight loss and lower HbA1c 3 years after duodenal switch compared with Roux-en-Y gastric bypass--a randomized controlled trial. Surg Obes Relat Dis. 2012;8(3):338–43.
114. Dapri G, Cadiere GB, Himpens J. Superobese and super-superobese patients: 2-step laparoscopic duodenal switch. Surg Obes Relat Dis. 2011;7(6):703–8.
115. Iannelli A, Schneck AS, Topart P, Carles M, Hebuterne X, Gugenheim J. Laparoscopic sleeve gastrectomy followed by duodenal switch in selected patients versus single-stage duodenal switch for superobesity: case-control study. Surg Obes Relat Dis. 2013;9(4):531–8.
116. Courcoulas AP, Belle SH, Neiberg RH, Pierson SK, Eagleton JK, Kalarchian MA, et al. Three-year outcomes of bariatric surgery vs lifestyle intervention for type 2 diabetes mellitus treatment: a randomized clinical trial. JAMA Surg. 2015;150(10):931–40.
117. Nguyen NT, Kim E, Vu S, Phelan M. Ten-year outcomes of a prospective randomized trial of laparoscopic gastric bypass versus laparoscopic gastric banding. Ann Surg. 2018;268(1):106–13.
118. Adams TD, Davidson LE, Litwin SE, Kim J, Kolotkin RL, Nanjee MN, et al. Weight and metabolic outcomes 12 years after gastric bypass. N Engl J Med. 2017;377(12):1143–55.
119. Ikramuddin S, Korner J, Lee WJ, Thomas AJ, Connett JE, Bantle JP, et al. Lifestyle intervention and medical management with vs without Roux-en-Y gastric bypass and control of hemoglobin A1c, LDL cholesterol, and systolic blood pressure at 5 years in the diabetes surgery study. JAMA. 2018;319(3):266–78.
120. Purnell JQ, Selzer F, Wahed AS, Pender J, Pories W, Pomp A, et al. Type 2 diabetes remission rates after laparoscopic gastric bypass and gastric banding: results of the longitudinal assessment of bariatric surgery study. Diabetes Care. 2016;39(7):1101–7.
121. Sala P, Torrinhas RS, Fonseca DC, Heymsfield S, Giannella-Neto D, Waitzberg DL. Type 2 diabetes remission after Roux-en-Y gastric bypass: evidence for increased expression of jejunal genes encoding regenerating pancreatic islet-derived proteins as a potential mechanism. Obes Surg. 2017;27(4):1123–7.
122. Davidson LE, Yu W, Goodpaster BH, DeLany JP, Widen E, Lemos T, et al. Fat-free mass and skeletal muscle mass five years after bariatric surgery. Obesity (Silver Spring, MD). 2018;26(7):1130–6.
123. Ferrannini E, Iozzo P, Virtanen KA, Honka MJ, Bucci M, Nuutila P. Adipose tissue and skeletal muscle insulin-mediated glucose uptake in insulin resistance: role of blood flow and diabetes. Am J Clin Nutr. 2018;108(4):749–58.
124. Albers PH, Bojsen-Moller KN, Dirksen C, Serup AK, Kristensen DE, Frystyk J, et al. Enhanced insulin signaling in human skeletal muscle and adipose tissue following gastric bypass surgery. Am J Physiol Regul Integr Comp Physiol. 2015;309(5):R510–24.
125. Mor A, Tabone L, Omotosho P, Torquati A. Improved insulin sensitivity after gastric bypass correlates with decreased total body fat, but not with changes in free fatty acids. Surg Endosc. 2014;28(5):1489–93.
126. Campos GM, Rabl C, Peeva S, Ciovica R, Rao M, Schwarz JM, et al. Improvement in peripheral glucose uptake after gastric bypass surgery is observed only after substantial weight loss has occurred and correlates with the magnitude of weight lost. J Gastrointest Surg. 2010;14(1):15–23.
127. Dadson P, Landini L, Helmio M, Hannukainen JC, Immonen H, Honka MJ, et al. Effect of bariatric surgery on adipose tissue glucose metabolism in different depots in patients with or without type 2 diabetes. Diabetes Care. 2016;39(2):292–9.
128. Immonen H, Hannukainen JC, Iozzo P, Soinio M, Salminen P, Saunavaara V, et al. Effect of bariatric surgery on liver glucose metabolism in morbidly obese diabetic and non-diabetic patients. J Hepatol. 2014;60(2):377–83.
129. Kim MK, Lee HC, Kwon HS, Baek KH, Kim EK, Lee KW, et al. Visceral obesity is a negative predictor of remission of diabetes 1 year after bariatric surgery. Obesity (Silver Spring, MD). 2011;19(9):1835–9.
130. Merlotti C, Ceriani V, Morabito A, Pontiroli AE. Subcutaneous fat loss is greater than visceral fat loss with diet and exercise, weight-loss promoting drugs and bariatric surgery: a critical review and meta-analysis. Int J Obes (2005). 2017;41(5):672–82.
131. Sinclair P, Brennan DJ, le Roux CW. Gut adaptation after metabolic surgery and its influences on the brain, liver and cancer. Nat Rev Gastroenterol Hepatol. 2018;15(10):606–24.
132. Albaugh VL, Flynn CR, Cai S, Xiao Y, Tamboli RA, Abumrad NN. Early increases in bile acids post Roux-en-Y gastric bypass are driven by insulin-sensitizing, secondary bile acids. J Clin Endocrinol Metab. 2015;100(9):E1225–33.
133. Magkos F, Bradley D, Eagon JC, Patterson BW, Klein S. Effect of Roux-en-Y gastric bypass and laparoscopic adjustable gastric banding on gastrointestinal metabolism of ingested glucose. Am J Clin Nutr. 2016;103(1):61–5.
134. Isbell JM, Tamboli RA, Hansen EN, Saliba J, Dunn JP, Phillips SE, et al. The importance of caloric restriction in the early improvements in insulin sensitivity after Roux-en-Y gastric bypass surgery. Diabetes Care. 2010;33(7):1438–42.

135. Shah M, Laurenti MC, Man CD, Ma J, Cobelli C, Rizza RA, et al. Contribution of endogenous glucagon-like Peptide-1 to changes in glucose metabolism and islet function in people with type 2 diabetes four weeks after roux-en-Y gastric bypass (RYGB). Metab Clin Exp. 2019;93:10–7.
136. Kohli R, Bradley D, Setchell KD, Eagon JC, Abumrad N, Klein S. Weight loss induced by Roux-en-Y gastric bypass but not laparoscopic adjustable gastric banding increases circulating bile acids. J Clin Endocrinol Metab. 2013;98(4):E708–12.
137. Jahansouz C, Xu H, Hertzel AV, Serrot FJ, Kvalheim N, Cole A, et al. Bile acids increase independently from hypocaloric restriction after bariatric surgery. Ann Surg. 2016;264:1022–8.
138. Zhai H, Li Z, Peng M, Huang Z, Qin T, Chen L, et al. Takeda G protein-coupled receptor 5-mechanistic target of rapamycin complex 1 signaling contributes to the increment of glucagon-like peptide-1 production after Roux-en-Y gastric bypass. EBioMedicine. 2018;32:201–14.
139. Ullmer C, Alvarez Sanchez R, Sprecher U, Raab S, Mattei P, Dehmlow H, et al. Systemic bile acid sensing by G protein-coupled bile acid receptor 1 (GPBAR1) promotes PYY and GLP-1 release. Br J Pharmacol. 2013;169(3):671–84.
140. Roesch SL, Styer AM, Wood GC, Kosak Z, Seiler J, Benotti P, et al. Perturbations of fibroblast growth factors 19 and 21 in type 2 diabetes. PLoS One. 2015;10(2):e0116928.
141. Chavez-Talavera O, Baud G, Spinelli V, Daoudi M, Kouach M, Goossens JF, et al. Roux-en-Y gastric bypass increases systemic but not portal bile acid concentrations by decreasing hepatic bile acid uptake in minipigs. Int J Obes (2005). 2017;41(4):664–8.
142. Jammu GS, Sharma R. A 7-year clinical audit of 1107 cases comparing sleeve gastrectomy, Roux-En-Y gastric bypass, and mini-gastric bypass, to determine an effective and safe bariatric and metabolic procedure. Obes Surg. 2016;26(5):926–32.
143. Bhasker AG, Remedios C, Batra P, Sood A, Shaikh S, Lakdawala M. Predictors of remission of T2DM and metabolic effects after laparoscopic Roux-en-y gastric bypass in obese Indian diabetics-a 5-year study. Obes Surg. 2015;25(7):1191–7.
144. Adams TD, Davidson LE, Litwin SE, Kolotkin RL, LaMonte MJ, Pendleton RC, et al. Health benefits of gastric bypass surgery after 6 years. JAMA. 2012;308(11):1122–31.
145. Alexandrides TK, Skroubis G, Kalfarentzos F. Resolution of diabetes mellitus and metabolic syndrome following Roux-en-Y gastric bypass and a variant of biliopancreatic diversion in patients with morbid obesity. Obes Surg. 2007;17(2):176–84.
146. Hall TC, Pellen MG, Sedman PC, Jain PK. Preoperative factors predicting remission of type 2 diabetes mellitus after Roux-en-Y gastric bypass surgery for obesity. Obes Surg. 2010;20(9):1245–50.
147. Torquati A, Lutfi R, Abumrad N, Richards WO. Is Roux-en-Y gastric bypass surgery the most effective treatment for type 2 diabetes mellitus in morbidly obese patients? J Gastrointest Surg. 2005;9(8):1112–6; discussion 7–8.
148. Simonson DC, Halperin F, Foster K, Vernon A, Goldfine AB. Clinical and patient-centered outcomes in obese patients with type 2 diabetes 3 years after randomization to Roux-en-Y gastric bypass surgery versus intensive lifestyle management: the SLIMM-T2D study. Diabetes Care. 2018;41(4):670–9.
149. Cummings DE, Arterburn DE, Westbrook EO, Kuzma JN, Stewart SD, Chan CP, et al. Gastric bypass surgery vs intensive lifestyle and medical intervention for type 2 diabetes: the CROSSROADS randomised controlled trial. Diabetologia. 2016;59(5):945–53.

47 Gastric Bypass for Type 2 Diabetes Mellitus on BMI < 35

Admar Concon-Filho, Andre Fernandes Teixeira, Eduardo Grecco, Luiz Gustavo de Quadros, Manoel Galvão Neto, and Thiago Ferreira de Souza

Obesity and Diabetes

Morbid obesity has been defined by the National Institutes of Health (NIH) as a body mass index (BMI, the weight in kilograms divided by the square of the height in meters) of 40 kg/m^2 or more or 35 kg/m^2 or more in the presence of obesity comorbidities. Buchwald study clearly demonstrated that bariatric surgery can cause resolution of the clinical manifestations of type 2 diabetes, as well as improvement, and that this resolution is verified by serum insulin levels. This study also showed that the resolution or improvement in type 2 diabetes is related to the weight loss achieved by morbidly obese diabetic patients. There are, however, data that do not allow the assumption of an absolute cause-and-effect relationship between body weight and type 2 diabetes.

The simplest contradictory evidence is that 10% of type 2 diabetic patients are thin and that approximately three quarters of the morbidly obese are not diabetic [1].

The prevalence of obesity-induced type 2 diabetes mellitus is increasing worldwide [1].

T2DM was defined based on the American Diabetes Association (ADA) criteria: [1] fasting glucose ≥126 mg/dL or [2] glucose ≥200 at 120 minutes after 75 g oral glucose load or [3] HbA1c ≥ 6.5%. Diabetes remission was defined as no longer meeting the ADA criteria for T2DM, without the use of diabetes medications [2].

The primary risk factor for type 2 diabetes is obesity, and 90% of all patients with type 2 diabetes are overweight or obese [1].

Type 2 diabetes mellitus (DM) and obesity are chronic diseases that often coexist. Combined, they account for tremendous morbidity and mortality.

A. Concon-Filho (✉)
Faculty of Medicine of ABC – FMABC, Santo André, Brazil

Concon Clinic, Valinhos, Brazil

Galileo Hospital and Maternity, Valinhos, Brazil

A. F. Teixeira
Bariatric and Laparoscopy Center, Orlando Health, Orlando, FL, USA

E. Grecco
ABC Medical School (FMABC), São Paulo, Brazil

L. G. de Quadros
Department of Bariatric endoscopy, Kaiser day hosptial, São José do Rio Preto, Brazil

M. Galvão Neto
Faculty of Medicine of ABC – FMABC, Santo André, Brazil

Florida International University – FIU, Miami, FL, USA

EndoVitta Institute, São Paulo, Brazil

T. F. de Souza
ABC Medical School (FMABC), São Paulo, Brazil

Faculty of Medicine of ABC – FMABC, Santo André, Brazil

EndoVitta Institute, São Paulo, Brazil

University of São Paulo – USP, São Paulo, Brazil

J. Ettinger et al. (eds.), *Gastric Bypass*, https://doi.org/10.1007/978-3-030-28803-7_47

Approximately 85% of all patients with type 2 DM have a body mass index (BMI) categorizing them as overweight (BMI 25.0–29.9 kg/m^2) or obese (BMI > 30.0 kg/m^2). Obesity is strongly associated with diabetes and is a major cause of insulin resistance that leads to the cascade of hyperglycemia, glucotoxicity, and beta-cell failure, which ultimately leads to the development of microvascular (neuropathy, nephropathy, retinopathy) and macrovascular (myocardial infarction, stroke) complications. Treatment guidelines emphasize that both diabetes and obesity should be treated to optimize long-term outcomes [3].

The National Health and Nutrition Examination Survey III (1988–1994) data showed that the risk for chemical diabetes is approximately 50% at a BMI of 30 kg/m^2 or more and more than 90% at a BMI of 40 kg/m^2 or more.

Virtually all morbidly obese adults have a measurably impaired glucose tolerance; 36% of individuals with impaired glucose tolerance will progress to type 2 diabetes within 10 years [1].

Bariatric/Metabolic Surgery

A study using data from the National Health and Nutrition Examination Survey (N = 4926) to evaluate success rates of lifestyle management plus drug therapy found that just 53% of patients with type 2 DM maintained a hemoglobin A1c (HbA1c) below 7%. For patients with obesity and type 2 DM in whom lifestyle management and medications do not achieve desired treatment goals, bariatric surgery has emerged as the most effective treatment for attaining significant and durable weight loss. Research has shown that these effects are not only secondary to weight loss but also depend on neuroendocrine mechanisms secondary to changes in GI physiology [3].

Metabolic surgery is the only diabetes treatment proven to result in long-term remission in 23–60% of patients depending upon preoperative duration of diabetes and disease severity. The most common procedures are sleeve gastrectomy (SG, 49%), Roux-en-Y gastric bypass (RYGB, 43%), laparoscopic adjustable gastric banding (LAGB, 6%), and biliopancreatic diversion with duodenal switch (BPD-DS, 2%) [3].

Meta-analysis of weight loss overall was 38.5 kg or 55.9% excess body weight loss. Overall, 78.1% of diabetic patients had complete resolution, and diabetes was improved or resolved in 86.6% of patients [1].

Insulin levels declined significantly postoperatively, as did hemoglobin A1c and fasting glucose values. Weight and diabetes parameters showed little difference at less than 2 years and at 2 years or more. The clinical and laboratory manifestations of type 2 diabetes are resolved or improved in the greater majority of patients after bariatric surgery; these responses are more pronounced in procedures associated with a greater percentage of excess body weight loss and is maintained for 2 years or more [1].

Some bariatric procedures improve glycemic control in people with diabetes beyond that expected for weight loss, and understanding this additional effect could provide insights into the pathogenesis of type 2 diabetes and assist in the development of new procedures, devices, and drugs both for obese and nonobese patients [4].

Bariatric/Metabolic Surgery Effects

Bariatric surgery has been shown to have profound glucoregulatory effects. These include rapid improvement in hyperglycemia and reduction in exogenous insulin requirements that occur early after surgery and before the patient has any significant weight loss. Although the exact molecular mechanisms underlying the effects of metabolic surgery on diabetes are not fully understood, many factors appear to play a role, including changes in bile acid metabolism, GI tract nutrient sensing, glucose utilization, insulin resistance, and intestinal microbiomes. These changes, acting through peripheral or central pathways, or perhaps both, lead to reduced hepatic glucose production, increased tissue glucose uptake, improved insulin sensitivity, and enhanced beta-cell function [3].

The term metabolic surgery describes bariatric surgical procedures used primarily to treat type 2 diabetes and related metabolic conditions [3].

Metabolic surgery is more effective than lifestyle or medical management in achieving glycemic control, sustained weight loss, and reducing diabetes comorbidities. Perioperative adverse events are similar to other gastrointestinal surgeries. New guidelines for type 2 diabetes expand use of metabolic surgery to patients with a lower body mass index [3].

Randomized clinical trials have shown that metabolic surgery is statistically superior to medical treatment in achieving targeted glycemic levels along with improvements in weight loss, remission of metabolic syndrome, reduction in medications, and improvements in lipid levels [3].

Metabolic Surgical Procedures

Weight loss and diabetes resolution were greatest for patients undergoing biliopancreatic diversion/duodenal switch, followed by gastric bypass, and least for banding procedures [1].

Dixon et al., on randomized trial, demonstrate that weight loss associated with adjustable gastric banding results in diabetes remission in the majority of obese participants recently diagnosed as having diabetes and was associated with greater improvements in features of the metabolic syndrome and use of related medications [5].

Ding compared laparoscopic adjustable gastric band (LAGB) to an intensive medical diabetes and weight management (IMWM) program for T2D. This was designed as a prospective, randomized clinical trial. LAGB and a multidisciplinary IMWM program have similar 1-year benefits on diabetes control, cardiometabolic risk, and patient satisfaction, which should be considered in the context of other factors, such as personal preference, when selecting treatment options with obese T2D patients [6].

Mingrone randomly assigned 60 patients (BMI 35 or more) to receive either medical treatment (n = 20) or surgery by gastric bypass (n = 20) or biliopancreatic diversion (n = 20); 53 (88%) patients completed 5 years' follow-up. Overall, 19 (50%) of the 38 surgical patients (7 [37%] of 19 in the gastric bypass group and 12 [63%] of 19 in the biliopancreatic diversion group) maintained diabetes remission at 5 years, compared with none of the 15 medically treated patients [7].

Patients with BMI < 35

There are few studies comparing surgery to medical weight management (MWM) for patients with T2DM and BMI < 35. Up to 78% of patients with type 2 diabetes mellitus (T2DM) may experience diabetes remission within 2 years after bariatric surgery. Currently, only patients with T2DM and body mass index (BMI) above 35 kg/m^2 are eligible for bariatric surgery. This is based on the 1991 National Institutes of Health (NIH) Guidelines and has been endorsed by the Center for Medicare and Medicaid Services. Patients with T2DM and BMI < 35 are primarily offered intensive medical weight management (MWM), including pharmacotherapy and nonsurgical weight loss strategies. Millions of patients with T2DM have BMI < 35—yet metabolic surgery is not an option for them. There is emerging evidence supporting the use of bariatric surgery to treat diabetes in less obese (BMI < 35) patients. However, there are very few randomized trials. The Agency for Healthcare Research and Quality (AHRQ) recently identified this area as a research priority for comparative effectiveness research. The NIH is unlikely to change the bariatric surgery guidelines for patients with T2DM without additional evidence to support such a change [2].

A meta-analysis of 19 mostly observational studies (N = 4070 patients) reported an overall type 2 DM remission rate of 78% after bariatric surgery with 1–3 years of follow-up. Resolution or remission was typically defined as becoming "nondiabetic" with normal HbA1c without medications. RCTs showed that the surgical procedures, especially RYGB and SG, were equally effective in patients with BMI 30–35 kg/m^2. This is particularly important given that most patients with type 2 DM have a BMI less than 35 kg/m^2. The effect of surgery in these patients with mild obesity is also durable out to at least 5 years [3].

The assessed outcomes 5 years after 150 patients who had type 2 diabetes and a body mass index of 27–43 were randomly assigned to receive intensive medical therapy alone or intensive medical therapy plus Roux-en-Y gastric bypass or sleeve gastrectomy [8].

At 5 years, changes from the baseline observed in the gastric bypass and sleeve gastrectomy groups were superior to the changes seen in the medical-therapy group with respect to body weight (−23%, −19%, and −5% in the gastric bypass, sleeve gastrectomy, and medical-therapy groups, respectively) [8].

Five-year outcome data showed that, among patients with type 2 diabetes and a BMI of 27–43, bariatric surgery plus intensive medical therapy was more effective than intensive medical therapy alone in decreasing, or in some cases resolving, hyperglycemia [8].

The CROSSROADS randomized controlled trial compared RYGB vs an intensive lifestyle and medical intervention (ILMI) for type 2 diabetes, including among patients with a BMI <35 kg/m^2. The primary outcome was diabetes remission at 1 year (HbA1c <6.0% [<42.1 mmol/mol], off all diabetes medicines). Compared with the most rigorous ILMI yet tested against surgery in a randomized trial, RYGB yielded greater type 2 diabetes remission in mild-to-moderate obese patients recruited from a well-informed, population-based sample [9].

Abbatini confirmed the efficacy of laparoscopic sleeve gastrectomy (LSG) in the treatment of nonmorbidly obese T2DM patients (BMI 30–35 Kg/m^2), with a remission rate of 88.8% without undesirable excessive weight loss [10].

The metabolic effects of laparoscopic sleeve gastrectomy (LSG) and laparoscopic Roux-en-Y gastric bypass (LRYGB) in type 2 diabetes (T2D) patients who do not meet the National Institutes of Health indications have not been well studied. No significant differences in mean percentage of excess weight loss and BMI were observed between the two groups at 2 years. At 3-year follow-up, the LRYGB group had significantly higher percentage of excess weight loss and lower BMI. The total (complete and partial) remission rate achieved with both bariatric procedures was 75.9% at 1 year and 56.4% at 3 years. Both LSG and LRYGB are safe and effective bariatric procedures for T2D in this Chinese population with diabetes and BMI < 35 kg/m^2 [11].

LRYGB resulted in significant clinical and biochemical improvements in nonobese Asian patients, with HOMA-%B indicating *β-cell* function as the main predictor of T2 DM remission. Appropriate patient selection with better β-cell function and evidence from long-term follow-up may justify this therapeutic approach [12].

Patients with type 2 diabetes (T2D) and body mass index (BMI)<35 may benefit from metabolic surgery. The soluble form of the receptor for advanced glycation end products (sRAGE) may identify patients at greater chance for T2D remission. Metabolic surgery was effective in promoting remission of T2D in 63% of patients with BMI 30–35; higher baseline sRAGE predicted T2D remission with surgery [13].

STAMPEDE

In the Surgical Treatment and Medications Potentially Eradicate Diabetes Efficiently (STAMPEDE) trial, both gastric bypass and sleeve gastrectomy were superior to intensive medical therapy alone in achieving excellent glycemic control (i.e., glycated hemoglobin A ≤6.0%), reducing cardiovascular risk, improving quality of life, and decreasing medication use [8].

The reductions in glycated hemoglobin levels and BMI in the surgical groups were similar among patients with a BMI of less than 35 and those with a BMI of 35 or more [8].

The current 5-year follow-up of patients in STAMPEDE trial showed that the beneficial effects of bariatric surgery on glycemic control were durable, even among patients with mild obesity (BMI of 27–34), which led to a sustained reduction in the use of diabetes and cardiovascular medications [8].

Second Diabetes Surgery Summit: DSS-II

Surgery was very effective short term in patients with T2DM and BMI 30–35. Baseline sRAGE may predict patients most likely to benefit from surgery [2].

In 2015, the 2nd Diabetes Surgery Summit (DSS-II) Consensus Conference published guidelines that were endorsed by more than 50 diabetes and medical organizations. The consensus conference delegates concluded that there is sufficient evidence demonstrating that metabolic surgery achieves excellent glycemic control and reduces cardiovascular risk factors. According to the DSS-II guidelines, metabolic surgery should be recommended to treat type 2 DM in patients with class III obesity (BMI ≥ 40 kg/m^2) regardless of glycemic control and in those with class II obesity (BMI 35.0–39.9 kg/m^2) when hyperglycemia is inadequately controlled by lifestyle and optimal medical therapy. Surgery should also be considered for patients with type 2 DM and BMI 30.0–34.9 kg/m^2 if hyperglycemia is inadequately controlled despite optimal treatment with either oral or injectable medications. These BMI thresholds should be reduced by 2.5 kg/m^2 for Asian patients. The 2017 standards of care for diabetes from the American Diabetes Association include those key indications in the recommendations for metabolic surgery [3].

Recent evidence from multiple RCTs has provided level 1[a] evidence supporting metabolic surgery as an effective treatment for type 2 DM. These studies have shown the superiority of surgery vs medical therapy in achieving excellent and durable glycemic control as well as benefits in the long term. Based on the published evidence, metabolic surgery is now endorsed as a standard treatment option, which provides patients and practitioners with a powerful tool to help combat the life-impairing effects of type 2 DM [3].

Metabolic surgery is now recommended as standard treatment option for type 2 diabetes in patients with body mass index levels as low as 30 kg/m^2 [3].

The safety of metabolic and bariatric surgery has significantly improved with the advent of laparoscopic surgery, resulting in complication profiles similar to those of cholecystectomy and appendectomy [3].

Conclusion

Conventional treatments for patients with type 2 diabetes are often inadequate. Ikramuddin et al. report 2-year outcomes of a 5-year randomized trial (the Diabetes Surgery Study). At the baseline, eligible participants had to have HbA1c of at least 8·0% (64 mmol/mol), BMI between 30·0 and 39·9 kg/m^2, and type 2 diabetes for at least 6 months and be aged 30–67 years. The addition of gastric bypass to lifestyle and medical management in patients with type 2 diabetes improved diabetes control, but adverse events and nutritional deficiencies were more frequent [14].

The overall 30 days or less mortality for all bariatric surgery procedures was 0.28%, placing these procedures in the lowest category of operative mortality of operations performed in the United States [1].

No RCT was sufficiently powered to detect differences in macrovascular or microvascular complications or death. A study from the American College of Surgeons (> 65,000 patients) showed that laparoscopic RYGB had perioperative morbidity and mortality rates of 3.4% and 0.3%, respectively, similar to those for laparoscopic cholecystectomy (3.7% and 0.7%) and appendectomy (4.5% and 0.5%) [3].

Changes in body weight, lipid levels, and quality of life after surgery were superior to the changes observed after medical therapy alone. The potential benefits of bariatric surgery on clinical end points, such as myocardial infarction, stroke, renal failure, blindness, and death, as suggested in nonrandomized trials, can be adequately assessed only through larger, multicenter trials [8].

References

1. Buchwald H, Estok R, Fahrbach K, Banel D, Jensen MD, Pories WJ, Bantle JP, Sledge I. Weight and type 2 diabetes after bariatric surgery:systematic review and meta-analysis. Am J Med. 2009;122(3)
2. Parikh M, Chung M, Sheth S, McMacken M, Zahra T, Saunders JK, Ude-Welcome A, Ogedegbe G, Schmidt AM, Pachter L. Randomized pilot trial of bariatric surgery vs. intensive medical weight management on diabetes remission in type 2 diabetic patients who do NOT meet NIH criteria for surgery and the role of soluble RAGE as a novel biomarker of success. Ann Surg. 2014;260(4):617–24.
3. Schauer PR, Hanipah ZN, Rubino F. Metabolic surgery for treating type 2 diabetes mellitus: now supported by the world's leading diabetes organizations. Cleve Clin J Med. 2017;84

4. Dixon JB, Le Roux C, Rubino F, Zimmet P. Bariatric surgery for type 2 diabetes. Lancet. 2012;379(9833):2213.
5. Dixon JB, O'Brien PE, Playfair J, Chapman L, Schachter LM, Skinner S, Proietto J, Bailey M, Anderson M. Adjustable gastric banding and conventional therapy for type 2 diabetes : a randomized controlled trial. JAMA. 2008;299(3)., (Reprinted).
6. Ding SA, Simonson DC, Wewalka M, Halperin F, Foster K, Goebel-Fabbri A, Hamdy O, Clancy K, Lautz D, Vernon A, Goldfine AB. Adjustable gastric band surgery or medical management in patients with type 2 diabetes: a randomized clinical trial. J Clin Endocrinol Metab. 2015;100(7):2546–56.
7. Mingrone G, Panunzi S, Gaetano AD, Guidone C, Iaconelli A, Nanni G, Castagneto M, Bornstein S, Rubino F. Bariatric–metabolic surgery versus conventional medical treatment in obese patients with type 2 diabetes: 5 year follow-up of an open-label, single-centre, randomised controlled trial. Lancet. 2015;386(9997):932.
8. Schauer PR, Bhatt DL, Kirwan JP, Wolski K, Aminian A, Brethauer SA, Navaneethan SD, Singh RP, Pothier CE, Nissen SE, Kashyap SR. Bariatric surgery versus intensive medical therapy for diabetes — 5-year outcomes. N Engl J Med. 2017;376; 7 nejm.org February 16.
9. Cummings DE, Arterburn DE, Westbrook EO, Kuzma JN, Stewart SD, Chan CP, Bock SN, Landers JT, Kratz M, Foster-Schubert KE, Flum DR. Gastric bypass surgery vs intensive lifestyle and medical intervention for type 2 diabetes: the CROSSROADS randomised controlled trial. Diabetologia. 2016;59:945–53.
10. Abbatini F, Capoccia D, Casella G, Coccia F, Leonetti F, Basso N. Type 2 diabetes in obese patients with body mass index of 30–35 kg/m^2: sleeve gastrectomy versus medical treatment. SOARD. 2012;8(1):20–4.
11. Du X, Zhou HX, Zhang SQ, Tian HM, Zhou ZG, Zhong CZ. A comparative study of the metabolic effects of LSG and LRYGB in Chinese diabetes patients with BMI<35 kg/m2. SOARD. 2017;13(2):189–97.
12. Malapan K, Goel R, Tai CM, Kao YH, Chang PC, Huang CK. Laparoscopic Roux-en-Y gastric bypass for nonobese type II diabetes mellitus in Asian patients. SORD. 2014;10(5):840–1.
13. Horwitz D, Saunders JK, Ude-Welcome A, Schmidt AM, Dunn V, Pachter L, Parikh M. Three-year follow-up comparing metabolic surgery versus medical weight management in patients with type 2 diabetes and BMI 30–35. The role of sRAGE biomarker as predictor of satisfactory outcomes. SORD. 2016;12(7):1342.
14. Ikramuddin S, Billington CJ, Lee WJ, Bantle JP, Thomas AJ, Connett JE, Leslie DB, InabnetIII WB, Jeffery RW, Chong K, Chuang LM, Sarr MG, Jensen MD, Vella A, Ahmed L, Belani K, Schone JL, Olofson AE, Korner J. Roux-en-Y gastric bypass for diabetes (the Diabetes Surgery Study): 2-year outcomes of a 5-year, randomised, controlled trial. Lancet Diabetes Endocrinol. 2015;3(6):394–5.

48 Postoperative Care

Amador García Ruiz de Gordejuela and
Jordi Pujol Gebelli

Postoperative Management After Metabolic Surgery

The patient operated for metabolic surgery is quite different from the typical bariatric one. Patients are usually thinner, but they usually have diabetes, hypertension, and dyslipidemia. Their diabetes is usually not compensated, and they have some complications related to hyperglycemia. Their main complication is not their overweight but its complex associated diseases [1].

Technically surgery might be more complex because intraabdominal fat is usually thicker, hemostasis is more difficult, and anesthetic care is also more complicated [2]. Despite this, the initial protocols for the postoperative time may be the same for a bariatric patient. We may apply some parts of the enhanced recovery protocols, but considering that the management of the associated diseases is another issue that might retard the discharge.

The key points recommended after bariatric surgery are [3, 4]:

- Analgesia → Avoid opioid and primary use of multimodal analgesia with a combination of paracetamol and NSAIDs [3–5].
- Lung expansion protocols → Preoperative training for pulmonary physiotherapy is encouraged. Patients are required to follow this therapy as soon as they can after the effect of anesthesia ends. Patients with preoperative CPAP or BiPAP therapies are required to use them after surgery the same way they use them at home [6].
- Postoperative diet → Patients after RYGB should begin oral tolerance some hours after surgery if nausea and vomiting are well controlled. Six hours after surgery, free fluids can be indicated. The patient has to be instructed about small but repetitive ingestions (20–30 mL every 15–20 minutes) [5].
- Early ambulation → When there is an adequate pain relief, patients may begin ambulator 4–6 hours after surgery. This gesture will prevent deep venous thrombosis and will improve oral tolerance and respiratory function [3–5].
- Avoid any kind of tubes → Orogastric tubes or urinary catheters should be avoided at any time before and after surgery. They have not demonstrated any kind of improvement and are usually painful and badly tolerated, slowing down patient recovery [5].
- Fluid management → Restrictive fluid management is highly recommended, as in coloproctology. These strategies have demonstrated improved pulmonary function during and after surgery and allow quicker recovery [5, 7].
- Thromboprophylaxis → Deep venous thrombosis and pulmonary embolism are the main medical complications after bariatric surgery.

A. García Ruiz de Gordejuela (✉) · J. Pujol Gebelli
Bariatric Surgery Unit, General Surgery Department, Bellvitge University Hospital, Barcelona, Spain

J. Ettinger et al. (eds.), *Gastric Bypass*, https://doi.org/10.1007/978-3-030-28803-7_48

They are not very common, but they are preventable with adequate measures. Phamarcological prophylaxis with low molecular weight or unfractionated heparins should be initiated 6–8 hours after surgery. Mechanical pumps for lower extremities should also be used from the surgery up to the beginning of ambulation. Early ambulation is also a key point for this prophylaxis [8].

Postoperative ICU Admission

Patients after bariatric and metabolic surgery usually do not need to go to ICU. They only need monitorization for the first 24 hours. Even if they are high-risk patients, the ICU is only reserved for those with uncontrolled comorbidities, especially those with respiratory issues prior to surgery [9].

Some centers reserve ICU for patients with high-risk respiratory comorbidities as hypoventilation, high-risk obstructive sleep apnea, or others that are uncontrolled or poorly controlled [10, 11]. In those cases, some respiratory interventions should be done after surgery, and special monitoring may be required. Also patients with very high BMI or with difficult intubation due to oro-cervical anatomy may be good candidates.

Patients with cardiac comorbidities as low-left ventricle output, dilated myocardiopathy, or severe ischemic damage can be also candidates for ICU. In those cases, cardiac monitoring and some therapies may be needed [9, 11].

Finally, in patients with intraoperative unexpected complications for the surgeon or the anesthetist, it could be important to keep the patient under intensive care at least for some hours [12].

Complementary Examinations After Surgery

Patients after bariatric and metabolic surgery do not usually require extensive examinations. The only recommended complementary examination is a blood test on the first 24 hours. This blood test is important to evaluate hemorrhage. It is also useful to check ions and metabolites in order to adjust fluids and other medications with the introduction of the free fluid diet.

Some authors recommend to check C-reactive protein (CRP) as it may predict complications, especially leaks. There is a known correlation between CRP levels and morbidity, but the real correlation in the first postoperative hours is yet to be determined. Other authors examine the use of procalcitonin and other acute-phase reactants [13–15].

Patient Comorbidity Management After Surgery

Patients with metabolic syndrome usually arrive to surgery with at least one of these comorbidities: type 2 diabetes, hypertension, dyslipidemia, and obstructive sleep apnea, among others. Here we are going to try to resume the recommendations for the management of each one after surgery.

Type 2 Diabetes

Glucose homeostasis improves with weight loss, but in patients after Roux-en-Y gastric bypass, long time ago Rubino demonstrated that it will improve even before weight loss begins. Patients candidate for metabolic surgery usually have a poor control of the glycemia with high glycated hemoglobin. They usually have more than one medication, and some of them are under insulin [16, 17].

During surgery and in the early postoperative time, sliding scale of short-term insulin is required. Intensive glucose monitoring is highly recommended; in cases of poor control, intravenous insulin perfusion might be required. Once oral tolerance is achieved, we may move to oral hypoglycemic agents. Metformin is one of the safest medications for the bariatric population. Sulfonylureas and mitiglinides should be discontinued. In cases with poor glycemic control, one dose of night long-acting insulin or sliding scale of short-acting insulin can be recommended but with strictly glycemic monitoring [16].

New drugs like GLP-1 analogs and DPP-IV inhibitors may also be used after surgery, but they are quite expensive medications and may be reserved for difficult cases.

Hypertension

Hypertension is not only related to obesity, and its improvement is not as fast as the glucose homeostasis after surgery. Preoperative diet and the effect of the surgery and other medications may modify blood pressure during the early postoperative period, but this does not mean that all the medications should be discontinued [16].

Patients are recommended to reduce their usual dosing of medications, especially with dose with better control before surgery. Daily monitoring and early checkup with a cardiologist are highly recommended after surgery.

Dyslipidemia

Hypertriglyceridemia and hypercholesterolemia improve after bariatric and metabolic surgery-related weight loss. There is no consensus about resuming or not preoperative medications. Some of these patients usually had had previous cardiovascular events, so these medications are also useful to reduce cardiovascular risk [18].

These medications should not be ruled out initially. Later on, depending on the weight loss results and the evolution of the blood test, this premise can be reconsidered.

Obstructive Sleep Apnea

This condition is quite common among the bariatric population. Patients usually have CPAP or BiPAP therapies. It is strongly recommended to continue the therapy as soon as it is necessary. Patients are encouraged to take their air pumps to the hospital and use them the same way they use them at home [6]. Some surgeons and anesthetists are afraid about the risk of the air pressure swallowed at the pouch of the anastomosis. Until now there is no paper that demonstrates the increased risk of leak related to the use of these devices. Despite this, the pulmonary function improves significantly, and the risk of atelectasia and respiratory failure is reduced.

Other Considerations

After bariatric and metabolic surgery, patients are encouraged to have an active way of life, to go walking, to do some exercise, and to improve their physical condition. These activities should be initiated as soon as they can. After surgery and after discharge, patients are recommended to walk daily for at least 20–30 minutes. It is also important to join in physical activity with moderate to high intensity [19].

Other medications that should be used at the postoperative time are proton pump inhibitors. They are recommended for at least the first postoperative month; some centers recommend it for 3 months, especially if a sleeve gastrectomy has been performed. Nausea and vomiting prophylaxis for the first postoperative days is mandatory. Metoclopramide and ondansetron are the most commonly used drugs [16].

Metabolic deficiency prophylaxis should be initiated as soon as possible. After RYGB the most common deficiencies are iron, calcium, and vitamin D. B family vitamins are also important, especially in patients with increased nausea and vomiting. Some patients will need parenteral B12 supplementation but usually some months later. Multivitamin prescriptions plus calcium and vitamin D supplementation are the most common recommendations after RYGB. Other deficiencies will be checked during the follow-up routinary blood tests [20, 21].

Patient Discharge

The discharge of the patient can be prepared for the first to the third postoperative day depending on the recovery after the surgery. Usually the most limiting factor will be the control of the comorbidities, especially the glycemic control.

Oral tolerance is usually achieved at the first postoperative day.

Prior to sending the patient home, it is mandatory to check that there are no complications. One easy sign to check is tachycardia. It is a classical lesson that no patient with non-explained tachycardia should be discharged. Patients should also be informed about how to take the pulse and to look for a consultation in case of tachycardia.

Patients should go home with a complete information about the procedure that has been performed, the diet recommended, and the possible complications. Health and sanitary education from the surgeon and the allied health professionals will improve the results and will avoid unnecessary consultations [22].

References

1. Rubino F, Nathan DM, Eckel RH, Schauer PR, Alberti KGMM, Zimmet PZ, et al. Metabolic surgery in the treatment algorithm for type 2 diabetes: a joint statement by international diabetes organizations. Surg Obes Relat Dis. 2016;12:1144–62. https://doi.org/10.1016/j.soard.2016.05.018.
2. Santoro S. From bariatric to pure metabolic surgery: new concepts on the rise. Ann Surg. 2014;0:1–2. https://doi.org/10.1097/SLA.0000000000000590.
3. Singh PM, Panwar R, Borle A, Goudra B, Trikha A, van Wagensveld BA, et al. Efficiency and safety effects of applying ERAS protocols to bariatric surgery: a systematic review with meta-analysis and trial sequential analysis of evidence. Obes Surg. 2016:1–13. https://doi.org/10.1007/s11695-016-2442-3.
4. Alvarez A, Goudra BG, Singh PM. Enhanced recovery after bariatric surgery. Curr Opin Anaesthesiol. 2016; https://doi.org/10.1097/ACO.0000000000000404.
5. Hoffmann H, Kettelhack C. Fast-track surgery – conditions and challenges in postsurgical treatment: a review of elements of translational research in enhanced recovery after surgery. Eur Surg Res. 2012;49:24–34. https://doi.org/10.1159/000339859.
6. Martí-Valeri C, Sabaté A, Masdevall C, Dalmau A. Improvement of associated respiratory problems in morbidly obese patients after open Roux-en-Y gastric bypass. Obes Surg. 2007;17:1102–10. https://doi.org/10.1007/s11695-007-9186-z.
7. Gustafsson UO, Scott MJ, Schwenk W, Demartines N, Roulin D, Francis N, et al. Guidelines for perioperative care in elective colonic surgery: enhanced recovery after surgery (ERAS®) society recommendations. World J Surg. 2013;37:259–84. https://doi.org/10.1007/s00268-012-1772-0.
8. Gould MK, Garcia DA, Wren SM, Karanicolas PJ, Arcelus JI, Heit JA, et al. Prevention of VTE in nonorthopedic surgical patients. Antithrombotic therapy and prevention of thrombosis, 9th ed: American College of Chest Physicians evidence-based clinical practice guidelines. Chest. 2012;141:227–77. https://doi.org/10.1378/chest.11-2297.
9. Pompilio CE, Pelosi P, Castro MG. The bariatric patient in the intensive care unit: pitfalls and management. Curr Atheroscler Rep. 2016;18:55. https://doi.org/10.1007/s11883-016-0606-1.
10. Goucham AB, Coblijn UK, Hart-Sweet HB, de Vries N, Lagarde SM, van Wagensveld BA. Routine postoperative monitoring after bariatric surgery in morbidly obese patients with severe obstructive sleep apnea: ICU admission is not necessary. Obes Surg. 2016;26:737–42. https://doi.org/10.1007/s11695-015-1807-3.
11. van den Broek RJC, Buise MP, van Dielen FM, Bindels AJGH, van Zundert AAJ, Smulders JF. Characteristics and outcome of patients admitted to the ICU following bariatric surgery. Obes Surg. 2009;19:560–4. https://doi.org/10.1007/s11695-008-9699-0.
12. Froylich D, Corcelles R, Davis M, Boules M, Daigle CR, Schauer PR, et al. Factors associated with length of stay in intensive care after bariatric surgery. Surg Obes Relat Dis. 2016;12:1391–6. https://doi.org/10.1016/j.soard.2015.11.031.
13. Hamilton EC, Sims TL, Hamilton TT, Mullican MA, Jones DB, Provost DA. Clinical predictors of leak after laparoscopic Roux-en-Y gastric bypass for morbid obesity. Surg Endosc. 2003;17:679–84. https://doi.org/10.1007/s00464-002-8819-5.
14. Lins DC, Campos JM, de Paula PS, Galvão-Neto M, Pachu E, Cavalcanti N, et al. C-reactive protein in diabetic patients before gastric bypass as a possible marker for postoperative complication. Arq Bras Cir Dig. 2015;28(Suppl 1):11–4. https://doi.org/10.1590/S0102-6720201500S100005.
15. Noble F, Curtis NJ, Underwood TJ. C-reactive protein 2 days after laparoscopic gastric bypass surgery reliably indicates leaks and moderately predicts morbidity. J Gastrointest Surg. 2013;17:844–5. https://doi.org/10.1007/s11605-012-2082-4.
16. Schlienger J-L, Pradignac A, Luca F, Meyer L, Rohr S. Medical management of diabetes after bariatric surgery. Diabetes Metab. 2009;35:558–61. https://doi.org/10.1016/S1262-3636(09)73465-2.
17. Elrazek AEMAA, Elbanna AEM, Bilasy SE. Medical management of patients after bariatric surgery: principles and guidelines. World J Gastrointest Surg. 2014;6:220–8. https://doi.org/10.4240/wjgs.v6.i11.220.
18. Gellad WF, Good CB, Lowe JC, Donohue JM. Variation in prescription use and spending for lipid-lowering and diabetes medications in the veterans affairs healthcare system. Am J Manag Care. 2010;16:741–50.
19. Mechanick JI, Youdim A, Jones DB, Timothy Garvey W, Hurley DL, Molly McMahon M, et al. Clinical

practice guidelines for the perioperative nutritional, metabolic, and nonsurgical support of the bariatric surgery patient--2013 update: cosponsored by American Association of Clinical Endocrinologists, the Obesity Society, and American Society for metabolic & bariatric surgery. Surg Obes Relat Dis. 2013;9:159–91. https://doi.org/10.1016/j.soard.2012.12.010.

20. Thorell A. Clinical nutrition university: nutritional support after bariatric surgery. E-SPEN. 2011;6:e96–100. https://doi.org/10.1016/j.eclnm.2011.01.002.
21. Shankar P, Boylan M, Sriram K. Micronutrient deficiencies after bariatric surgery. Nutrition. 2010;26:1031–7. https://doi.org/10.1016/j.nut.2009.12.003.
22. García-Ruiz-de-Gordejuela A, Madrazo-González Z, Casajoana-Badia A, Muñoz-Campaña A, Cuesta-González FJ, Pujol-Gebelli J. Evaluation of bariatric surgery patients at the emergency department of a tertiary referral hospital. Rev Esp Enferm Dig. 2015;107:23–8.

49 Mini Gastric Bypass: Why It Is Better than Gastric Bypass in India

Mohit Bhandari, Manoj Kumar Reddy, Winni Mathur, and Susmit Kosta

Mini gastric bypass is also known as single anastomosis gastric bypass. The procedure incorporates a long gastric tube of size 15–18 cm with a loop gastroenterostomy of size 4.5 cm. Essentially the procedure involves nonrestricted malabsorption. The limb lengths of biliopancreatic limb vary in different studies and centres. Most studies published have mentioned different limb lengths ranging from 150 cm to 300 cm [1].

Advantages of Mini Gastric Bypass

Mini gastric bypass is regarded as a safe, simple, reversible procedure. There is only one anastomosis and no mesenteric defect. It has shorter operative time. The procedure is safe and simple as the anastomosis is low lying and there is less tension on the anastomosis. In a gastric bypass, it is known that the anastomoses are close to the gastroesophageal junction and are in more tension than mini gastric bypass [2].

M. Bhandari (✉) · M. K. Reddy
W. Mathur · S. Kosta
Department of Surgery, Mohak Bariatrics and Robotics Surgical Center, Indore, India

Cons of Mini Gastric Bypass

There are concerns about a higher incidence of marginal ulcers, bile reflux, malignancies in long-term and excessive weight loss with protein-energy malnutrition of mini gastric bypass [3].

Reasons for Preference of Mini Gastric Bypass in India

The major reasons for preference of mini gastric bypass in India are as follows:

1. *Dietary habits*: Most Indians are vegetarians, and the diet consumed by most is full with carbohydrates and fats. This puts Indian subset of patients to do bulk eating and consuming huge quantity of fat. The protein in the diet is in very less proportion as compared to carbohydrates/fats. Mini gastric bypass having a wide anastomosis with propensity to cause fat malabsorption makes it a more durable and useful procedure for Indian patients.
2. *Severe type 2 diabetes*: India is now the world capital of diabetes. We have the highest number of individuals with type 2 diabetes across the world. The patients get diabetes at a lower BMI as compared to their Caucasian counterparts. The severity of diabetes is also high. The mini gastric bypass procedure is suitable as it has a long biliopancreatic limb which is more suitable for diabetics. The metabolic

J. Ettinger et al. (eds.), *Gastric Bypass*, https://doi.org/10.1007/978-3-030-28803-7_49

effects of a procedure in treatment of type 2 diabetes is dependent on BP limb.

3. *Technical ease*: Most surgeons in India are on the learning curve for bariatric, metabolic surgery. The country started with gastric banding in 2002 which later became unpopular due to weight regain and lack of compliance from patients. Then came the era of gastric bypass. Gastric bypass was a popular procedure in the country due to the strong metabolic effect until the advent of mini gastric bypass. The Roux-en-Y gastric bypass had many disadvantages. It was marred by excessive steep learning curve, two mesenteric defects and difficult anastomoses close to the gastroesophageal junction.

   In 2010, mini gastric bypass was introduced in India by Bhandari and Kular et al. The procedure had a long gastric tube that is easy to construct with a wide anastomosis. The proponents mentioned that there is no need to close internal hernia defects in mini gastric bypass as it did not have one and the reported incidence of Peterson's space hernia is very less. The anastomosis was simple to construct as it was close to the transverse colon. The procedure had some distinct advantages as it was safe, simple and effective. Now it has become the second most commonly performed procedure in the country [4].

4. *Better GQLI scoring*: Most studies conducted comparing sleeve, gastric bypass and mini gastric bypass mention better GQLI scoring with a mini bypass. The patients can eat with more ease, need not chew that much before they gulp the food and had forced compliance due to dumping effect forcing the patient to a Mediterranean diet.

   In India more than 10,000 mini gastric bypasses have been performed till date, and the results are better or equivalent to sleeve and gastric bypass. The reported incidence of resolution of type 2 diabetes is better with mini bypass due to a long BP limb.

Technique

1. *Patient position*:
   - Patient is placed in supine position. The reverse Trendelenburg position is used as per requirement during the procedure.
2. *Ports*:
   - Surgery is performed through six ports.
   - 10 mm midline port is placed approximately 15–18 cm below the xyphisternum (Camera port).
   - 12 mm port in between the right midclavicular and anterior axillary line, 6 cm above the level of midline port (right-hand working port).
   - 12 mm port in the left midclavicular line, at the level of midline port (for assistant).
   - 5 mm port 4–5 cm below the left subcostal region in between the left midclavicular and anterior axillary line.
   - 5 mm port 4 cm below the right subcostal region in between the right midclavicular and anterior axillary line.
   - 5 mm port in epigastric region for liver retraction.
3. Lesser omentum is dissected distal to the crow's foot (the junction between the antrum and body) near to lesser curvature of the stomach, creating a window for firing of the first staple.
4. The first staple (gold) is fired from the right-hand working port horizontally from the window created.
5. Further staples (blue) are fired cephalad towards the GE angle guided over 36 Fr bougie. Last staple is fired 1 cm away from GE angle. A gastric pouch of approximately 15 cm long and 3 cm wide is made, and gastrostomy is made with harmonic scalpel (Fig. 49.1).

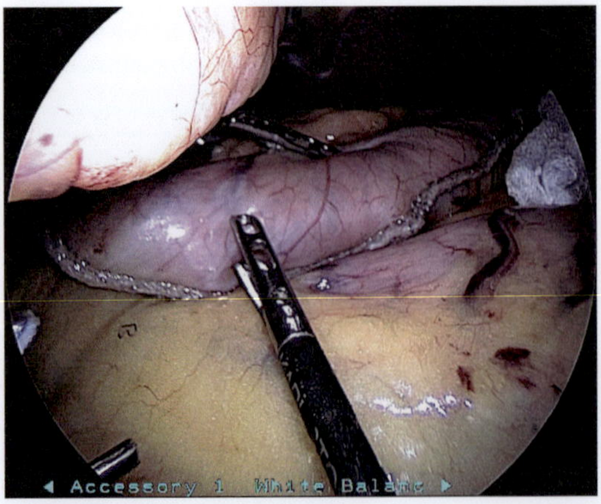

Fig. 49.1 Creating long pouch

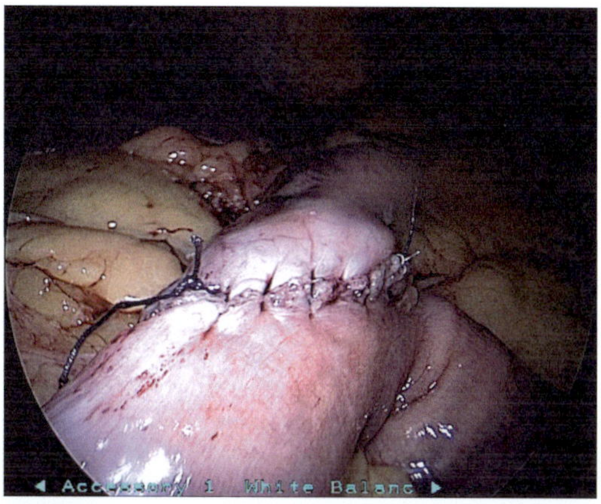

Fig. 49.2 Gastrojejunostomy

6. The omentum and transverse colon is retracted upwards and laterally to expose the ligament of Treitz. 180 cm of small bowel is measured for bypass.
7. Harmonic scalpel is used to create jejunostomy.
8. 3–4 cm stapled anastomosis is done with blue staple, and enterotomies are closed handsewn (Fig. 49.2).
9. No abdominal drains or Ryle's tube is used routinely.

Results/Complications

At our centre we did 3599 MGB from a total of 9445 bariatric procedures performed till date. We choose operation based on our algorithm. We perform MGB in patients with BMI greater than 40 and diabetic and have no GERD and hiatus hernia and are willing to come for regular follow-up. On the 6-year follow-up of our patients with follow-up rate of 72.7%, they had a %TWL and %EWL of 36.57% and 79.4%, respectively, with the lowest weight attained at 4 years. When compared to a study conducted by Kular and Rutledge, they had a 6-year weight loss post-MGB of 84%, whereas 7-year study of MGB had a 90% EWL. At 6 years diabetic resolution was seen in 86%, and resolution of hypertension was seen in 85%. Diabetes and hypertensive resolution of study conducted by Jammu was 95% and 85%, respectively, and 98% and 82%, respectively, in Kular's study. Early postoperative complications include staple line leak in one patient and staple line bleed in two patients of which one patient was managed conservatively with blood transfusion and one required exploration and staple suturing of pouch and remnant. Marginal ulcers were seen in four patients in which post-op endoscopy was done only in symptomatic patients. Reversal was done in one patient for recalcitrant marginal ulcer and in one patient for PCM [4, 5].

The incidence of nutrient, haemoglobin, albumin and protein deficiencies is higher at all times of follow-up; they are prone to iron and B12 deficiency because of the bypass of the duodenojejunal axis. In the incidence of anaemia, Hg < 11gm/dl was 12% in the OAGB at 6 years. Similar results have been reported by others after these operations [5–9]. Also, the incidence of hypoalbuminemia and hypoproteinaemia is significantly higher after OAGB/MGB. This is an issue of concern after OAGB/MGB, since in a subset of patients, the protein-caloric malnutrition becomes intractable, resulting in liver failure and need for surgical re-intervention and in some cases resulted in mortality [10, 11]. No patient in this series developed liver failure; however, two patients in the OAGB/MGB group had reoperations: one, a reversal because of excessive weight loss and hypoalbuminemia associated with an intractable marginal ulcer, and another, a revision operation because of hypoalbuminemia. Many needed intense nutritional support and counselling to control the mild cases of nutrient and protein-calorie malnutrition (PCM). The concern about PCM has made us and many other surgeons that perform the OAGB/MGB to modify the biliopancreatic limb length to 200 cm or less [12]. Patients with morbid obesity have lower QOL scores, and bariatric surgery improves QOL [13]. But new complaints like abdominal pain, nausea, vomiting, malodorous flatus, increased frequency of stools, etc. have been consistently reported by surgeons who perform either the MGB or OAGB [6, 14].

Obesity, particularly severe obesity, is such a burden to those afflicted that they are willing to accept certain outcomes which we may consider undesirable in exchange of the weight loss.

References

1. Chaim EA, Ramos AC, Cazzo E. Mini-gastric bypass: description of the technique and preliminary results. Arq Bras Cir Dig. 2017;30(4):264–6.
2. Noun R, Skaff J, Riachi E, Daher R, Antoun NA, Nasr M. One thousand consecutive mini-gastric bypass: short- and long-term outcome. Obes Surg. 2012;22(5):697–703.
3. Mahawar KK, Kumar P, Carr WR, et al. Current status of mini-gastric bypass. J Minim Access Surg. 2016;12(4):305–10.
4. Kular KS, Manchanda N, Rutledge R. A 6-year experience with 1,054 mini-gastric bypasses—first study from Indian subcontinent. Obes Surg. 2014;24:1430–5. https://doi.org/10.1007/s11695-014-1220-3.
5. Jammu GS, Sharma R. A 7-year clinical audit of 1107 cases comparing sleeve gastrectomy, Roux-en-Y gastric bypass, and mini-gastric bypass, to determine an effective and safe bariatric and metabolic procedure. Obes Surg. 2016;26:926–32.
6. Lee W-J, Ser K-H, Lee Y-C, Tsou J-J, Chen S-C, Chen J-C. Laparoscopic Roux-en-Y vs. mini-gastric bypass for the treatment of morbid obesity: a 10-year experience. Obes Surg. 2012;22:1827–34.
7. Johnson WH, Fernanadez AZ, Farrell TM, et al. Surgical revision of loop ("mini") gastric bypass procedure: multicenter review of complications and conversions to roux-en-Y gastric bypass. Surg Obes Relat Dis. 2007;3:37–41.
8. Magouliotis DE, Tasiopoulou VS, Svokos AA, Svokos KA, Sioka E, Zacharoulis D. One-anastomosis gastric bypass versus sleeve gastrectomy for morbid obesity: a systematic review and meta-analysis. Obes Surg. 2017;27(9):2479–87.
9. Bruzzi M, Rau C, Voron T, Guenzi M, Berger A, Chevallier JM. Single anastomosis or mini-gastric bypass: long-term results and quality of life after a 5-year follow-up. Surg Obes Relat Dis. 2015;11(2):321–6.
10. Milone M, Lupoli R, Maietta P, et al. Lipid profile changes in patients undergoing bariatric surgery: a comparative study between sleeve gastrectomy and mini-gastric bypass. Int J Surg. 2015;14:28–32.
11. Musella M, Susa A, Manno E, et al. Complications following the mini/one anastomosis gastric bypass (MGB/OAGB): a multi-institutional survey on 2678 patients with a mid-term (5 years) follow-up. Obes Surg. 2017;27(11):2956–67.
12. Mahawar KK, Jennings N, Brown J, Gupta A, Balupuri S, Small PK. "Mini" gastric bypass: systematic review of a controversial procedure. Obes Surg. 2013;23(11):1890–8.
13. Ballantyne GH. Measuring outcomes following bariatric surgery: weight loss parameters, improvement in co-morbid conditions, change in quality of life and patient satisfaction. Obes Surg. 2003;13:954–64.
14. Overs SE, Freeman RA, Zarshenas N, Walton KL, Jorgensen JO. Food tolerance and gastrointestinal quality of life following three bariatric procedures: adjustable gastric banding, Roux-en-Y gastric bypass, and sleeve gastrectomy. Obes Surg. 2012;22:536–43.

Can Bariatric Surgery Improve the Microvascular Complications of Type 2 Diabetes?

50

Loai A. Shakerdi, Carel W. le Roux, and Neil G. Docherty

Background

Obesity is now a critical global epidemic. In 2014, the WHO estimated that more than 1.9 billion adults were overweight and 600 million were obese. Overweight and obesity are affecting half of the population of most European countries. Overweight is defined as a BMI $\geq$ 25 kg/m^2 and obesity as a BMI $\geq$ 30 kg/m^2. Obesity increases the risk of type 2 diabetes mellitus (T2DM), and about 90% of type 2 diabetes is attributable to excess weight [1]. The number of patients with diabetes is predicted to rise from 171 million in 2000 to 366 million in 2030 [2], thus resulting in the prediction that diabetes will represent the seventh leading cause of death in 2030 [3]. The main characteristic of T2DM is an impaired β-cell sensitivity in tandem with increased insulin resistance. Insulin hypersecretion characterises the disease; however, its kinetic is not synchronised so as to optimise postprandial glycaemia. Hence, despite hyperinsulinaemia patients with T2DM exhibit reduced glucose tolerance and marked excursions in the postprandial period. Stimuli such as these are known to drive macrovascular and microvascular complications through the myriad pathways of glucotoxicity described hereafter.

The cumulative duration of exposure to risk factors such as glucotoxicity likely drives the incidence and progression of microvascular complications. Logic thus suggests that benefits in terms of end-organ damage should accrue following bariatric surgery given its capacity to arrest the key risk factors for microvascular end-organ damage.

Weight loss achieved through bariatric surgery is associated with prevention of diabetes, and in patients with pre-existing type 2 diabetes, it is associated with short-term remission and significant medium- to long-term improvement in the control of hyperglycaemia occurring in the context of a lowered medication burden. Other comorbidities such as essential hypertension are also more easily managed after surgery.

L. A. Shakerdi
Clinical Research Centre, St. Vincent's University Hospital, Dublin, Ireland

C. W. le Roux · N. G. Docherty (✉)
Diabetes Complications Research Centre, Conway Institute, School of Medicine, University College Dublin, Dublin, Ireland
e-mail: neil.docherty@ucd.ie

Glucotoxicity, Inflammation and Microvascular Complications of Diabetes

The exact mechanism of microvascular complications in patients with diabetes is not fully

J. Ettinger et al. (eds.), *Gastric Bypass*, https://doi.org/10.1007/978-3-030-28803-7_50

understood, but multiple factors are involved including metabolic, haemodynamic, inflammatory, genetic and immunological alterations.

Excess circulating glucose can bind to amino acids in the circulating or tissue proteins forming reversible glycation end products and eventually irreversible advanced glycation end products (AGEs), which accumulate in the tissues and contribute to the development of microvascular complications [4]. Chronic hyperglycaemia increases reactive oxygen species (ROS) and causes mitochondrial DNA damage. In the polyol pathway, glucose is reduced to sorbitol by aldose reductase (AR), which is then converted to fructose by sorbitol dehydrogenase (SDH). An overexpressed AR increases sorbitol content [5] and enhances oxidative stress [6]. The accumulation of sorbitol and fructose and its derivatives, such as fructose-6-phosphate and triose-phosphate, leads to the generation of oxidative stress and augments the production of AGEs [7]. Activation of the protein kinase C (PKC) pathway leads to increased vascular permeability, enhanced synthesis of extracellular matrix components and increased production of reactive oxygen species (ROS) and oxidative stress. Activation of ROS increases the production of AGEs and enhances glucose entry into the polyol pathway and PKC activation. In addition, ROS directly damage endothelial glycocalyx [8]. Hyperglycaemia contributes to the formation of unfolded or misfolded proteins within the endoplasmic reticulum (ER). Accumulation of dysfunctional proteins may cause ER stress in a response that contributes to the development of diabetic microvascular complications [9].

Mounting evidence supports the hypothesis that specific growth factors are involved in the development of microvascular complications of diabetes. Stressed and overloaded adipose tissue is an important source of inflammatory cytokines and growth factors such as tumour necrosis factor (TNF)-a and interleukin (IL)-6 [10] which characterise the systemic inflammatory milieu in T2DM. Vascular endothelial growth factor (VEGF) is a pro-angiogenic cytokine which is implicated in the development of nephropathy and retinopathy [11, 12].

Bariatric Surgery

The most commonly performed laparoscopic bariatric procedures are adjustable gastric banding (AGB), Roux-en-Y gastric bypass (RYGB) and vertical sleeve gastrectomy (VSG) [13]. Indications for bariatric surgery are a BMI > 40 kg/m^2 or BMI > 35 kg/m^2 with significant obesity-related comorbidities including T2DM (NIH,[1] ADA,[2] European, NICE[3] and NHMRC[4]).

Bariatric surgery can substantially improve the quality of life by reducing weight and reducing concomitant morbidities such as hypertension and dyslipidaemia and reducing the overall diabetes-related complications [14, 15]. The American Diabetes Association expert group defined remission of diabetes as an HbA_{1c} concentration in the normal range, fasting glucose concentration of 5·6 mmol/L or less without medical treatment for at least 1 year [16].

In a retrospective cohort study, Arterburn et al. identified 4434 adults with type 2 diabetes who had gastric bypass in the period from 1995 to 2008. Overall, 68.2% experienced an initial complete diabetes remission within 5 years after surgery. Among those, 35.1% redeveloped diabetes within 5 years [17]. In an unblinded randomised controlled trial that included 60 obese patients with recently diagnosed type 2 diabetes, it was found that 73% of patients achieved remission after 2 years of laparoscopic adjustable gastric banding [18]. A 3-year achievement of an American Diabetes Association composite treatment goal after 2 years of intensive lifestyle-medical management intervention, with and without Roux-en-Y gastric bypass, found no remission of diabetes in the medical management group at 36 months, whereas 17% of gastric bypass patients had full remission and 19% had partial remission [19]. A meta-analysis of randomised controlled trials, non-randomised

[1] *National Institutes of Health*

[2] *American Diabetes Association*

[3] National Institute for Clinical Excellence

[4] National Health and Medical Research Council

controlled clinical trials, cohort studies and case-control studies with follow-up for more than 2 years showed that 64.7% of patients achieved complete or partial remission of diabetes. The rate of diabetes recurrence ranged from 20.6% to 43.3% [20]. Several studies have demonstrated the long-term safety of bariatric surgery [14, 21, 22], with mortality rate ranges from 0.1% to 0.5%.

There is growing evidence suggesting that bariatric surgery can attenuate the development of microvascular complications of diabetes. Bariatric surgery was associated with a 65% reduction in major macrovascular and microvascular events in moderately and severely obese patients with T2DM [23]. The Swedish Obese Subjects (SOS) study was designed to investigate the overall mortality and the incidence of complications in two groups of obese patients; one group underwent bariatric surgery, whereas the other group received medical treatment. The study showed a marked (29%) long-term reduction in the overall mortality and complications, noticeably those associated with raised fasting insulins and patients with diabetes. The incidence of microvascular complications in type 2 diabetes mellitus was lower than that in patients managed with lifestyle interventions [21]. Schauer et al. evaluated 1160 patients who underwent LRYGBP (240 had IFG or T2DM) from July 1997 to May 2002. During this 5-year period, LRYGBP resulted in significant weight loss (60% of excess body weight loss) and resolution (83%) of T2DM [24].

Understanding the mechanism of weight loss associated with bariatric surgery, identifying the main factors contributing to improved comorbidities and reversing the progression of microvascular complication of diabetes have all been pursued in recent research studies. At least ten randomised controlled trials (RCTs) confirmed the superiority of surgery in achieving glycaemic control compared with conventional medical treatment [25, 26]. In most RCT studies, surgery resulted in a reduction in HbA1c by 2–3.5%, compared to 1–1.5% reduction by intensive medical therapy.

Bariatric Surgery and Diabetic Kidney Disease (DKD) (Table 50.1)

Microalbuminuria is the earliest laboratory marker of kidney damage associated with obesity and DKD and becomes manifest and progressive in 25–40% of patients. Microalbuminuria is defined as the presence of an abnormal levels of albumin in the urine (>30 mg/day or 20 μg/min; urinary albumin/creatinine ratio (ACR >3.0 mg/mmol). Albuminuria reflects pathological changes in the renal parenchyma characterised by cellular hypertrophy, thickening of the glomerular and tubular basement membranes and extracellular accumulation of matrix proteins. Loss of podocytes in glomeruli is an early pathological feature of DKD. Hypoadiponectinaemia is an established risk factor for these changes, and an adipose-renal axis acting via adiponectin is implicated in the health of the podocyte [27, 28].

Published case reports have demonstrated a remarkable resolution of diabetic nephropathy in obese patients following bariatric surgery. Up to 9 years of follow-up of 985 patients, undergoing bariatric surgery and 985 matched controls found that patients who underwent bariatric surgery had a 58% lower risk of an eGFR decline of ≥30% [29]. A retrospective evaluation of renal function in 32 obese patients with diabetes found a significant reduction in uACR after a mean follow-up of 1 year post RYGB [30]. In a prospective case-control study, RYGB surgery was superior to medical treatments for DKD [31]. An improvement in glomerular hyperfiltration was demonstrated in a prospective evaluation of a cohort of 19 obese patients with diabetes following RYGB [32]. Bariatric surgery significantly decreases urinary albumin excretion in DKD [33]. In a prospective case-control study of 70 obese surgical patients with type 2 diabetes, RYGB was superior to medical therapy for the treatments of DKD but not retinopathy or neuropathy. A 5-year retrospective follow-up of 52 obese subjects with T2D who underwent bariatric procedures (36 RYGB, 13 LAGB and 3 sleeve gastrectomy) reported a 58.3% remission of diabetic nephropathy [34].

Table 50.1 Summary of studies that analysed the effect of bariatric surgery on renal outcome in obese patients with T2DM

	Study design	No. of subjects	Follow-up	Intervention	Outcome
Izzedine et al. [47]	Case report	1	24 months	(RYGB)	Decreased proteinuria and serum creatinine levels
Perez et al. [48]	Case report	1	9 months	(RYGB)	Resolution of microalbuminuria
Agrawal et al. [30]	Retrospective	94 (32% T2DM)	12 months	(RYGB)	Significant reduction in albuminuria
DePaula, A. L. et al. [49]	Prospective	11	4–16 months	Ileal interposition into the proximal jejunum via a sleeve or diverted sleeve gastrectomy	Substantial improvement in microalbuminuria, macroalbuminuria and eGFR
Saliba et al. [32]	Prospective	35 (54% T2DM)	12 months	(RYGB)	Improved GFR
Navaneethan et al. [50]	Pilot	15	6	(RYGB, 9) (Other types, 6)	Reduction of albuminuria
Iaconelli et al. [35]	Case-control	22	10 years	(BPD versus medical care)	Improved GFR and remission of albuminuria
Heneghan, H. M. et al. [34]	Retrospective	52	5 years	GBP, SG, AGB	Diabetic nephropathy resolved in 58.3% at a mean follow-up of 66 months
Hou et al. [51]	Retrospective	233	12 months	RYGB, VSG and LAGB	Improvement in eGFR across grades of CKD and reduction in hyperfiltration
Stephenson et al. [52]	Retrospective analysis	23	3 years	LAGB	LAGB may improve or reverse renal damage
Jose et al. [53]	Retrospective observational study	25 (20% T2DM)	2–6 years	BPD	eGFR improved significantly a mean increase of 10.6 ± 15.45 at study end ($p = 0.048$)
Brethauer et al. [54]	Retrospective	217	5 years	RYGB, VSG and LAGB	Regression of diabetic nephropathy
Amor et al. [55]	Prospective	96	12 months	RYGB and VSG (observational)	Reduction and remission of albuminuria
Miras et al. [56]	Prospective case-control study	67	12–18 months	(RYGB)	ACR decreased significantly in the surgical group
Zakaria et al. [57]	Retrospective	20	13 years	LAGB	No unfavourable effect on kidney function and retinopathy

GBP gastric *bypass* procedure, *SG* sleeve gastrectomy, *BPD* biliopancreatic diversion, *AGB* adjustable gastric band, *LAGB* laparoscopic adjustable gastric banding

Renal complications were dramatically reduced in the surgical arm of biliopancreatic diversion in an unblinded, case-controlled trial with 10-years' follow-up, conducted from July 1998 through October 2009 [35]. Schauer et al. randomised 150 obese patients with uncontrolled type 2 diabetes to receive either intensive medical therapy alone or intensive medical therapy plus Roux-en-Y gastric bypass or sleeve gastrectomy. The primary end point was a glycated haemoglobin level of 6.0% or less. A notable outcome of this study was a 64% reduction in albuminuria after RYGB [36].

Bariatric surgery such as RYGB may however increase the risk of hyperoxaluria, supersaturation of calcium oxalate and subsequent nephrolithiasis. These side effects should be weighed against the overall benefits of these procedures.

Bariatric Surgery and Diabetic Retinopathy (DR) (Table 50.2)

Diabetic retinopathy (DR) is the most common microvascular complication of diabetes with a prevalence rate ranging from 10% to 50% depending on study population [37]. Depending on the presence or absence of abnormal new vessels, there are two main types of DR: proliferative retinopathy (PDR) and nonproliferative retinopathy (NPDR). The presence of red dots (microaneurysms and/or haemorrhages) and signs of vascular hypermeability such as hard and soft exudates and signs of capillary closure such as cotton-wool spots characterises NPDR. According to the international (AAO[5]) classification, NPDR is graded as mild, moderate and severe. The Royal College of Ophthalmologists classifies proliferative diabetic retinopathy (PDR) based on location and

[5]American Academy of Ophthalmology

Table 50.2 Summary of studies that analysed the effect of bariatric surgery on retinopathy outcome in obese patients with T2DM. *STDR* sight-threatening diabetic retinopathy

Study	No. of subjects	Follow-up	Outcome
DePaula, A. L. et al. [49]	11	4–16 months	Objective improvement in retinopathy was demonstrated in four patients (36.4%). Symptomatic improvement was observed in all 11 patients
Varadhan et al. [58]	22	6–12 months	9% development new DR 9% had progression of pre-existent retinopathy 59% had no DR before and after surgery 14% had stable DR through surgery 9% were noted to have regression of DR after surgery
Miras et al. [41]	67	12–18 months	1.5% progression of pre-existing DR 7.5% regression of pre-existing DR 91% no change
Abbatini et al. [59]	33	3 or 5 years	The Framingham risk score decreased significantly from 9.7% preoperatively to 4.7% postoperatively. No new diabetic retinopathy occurred during the whole period of observation
Johnson et al. [23]	15,951	20 months	Surgery vs. controls Diagnosis of blindness, <0.1% vs 0.3% Laser eye/retinal surgery required, 0.2% vs 0.6%
Thomas et al. [60]	38	12 months	Low incidence of new DR and progression of DR in those either without evidence of retinopathy or with minimal BDR prior to surgery with some subjects showing evidence of regression
Miras et al. [56]	Surgical: 56 Medical: 21	1 year	11% progression of pre-existing DR after bariatric surgery 11% regression of pre-existing DR after bariatric surgery 78% no change after bariatric surgery
Murphy et al. [61]	318	334 days	16% progression of pre-existing DR 11% regression of pre-existing DR 73% no change
Kim et al. [62]	20	12 months	All five patients with moderate nonproliferative DR or worse preoperatively had progression requiring intervention
Singh et al. [44]	150	2 years	There was no significant change in diabetic retinopathy scoring from baseline within and between each cohort
Banks et al. [43]	Surgical: 21 Medical: 24	2 years	DR showed significant progression for those in the control group ($p = 0.03$) but not in RYGB group ($p = 0.135$)
Zakaria et al. [57]	Surgical: 21 Medical: 24	13 years	No unfavourable effect on kidney function and retinopathy
Brynskov et al. [63]	56	1, 3, 6 and 12 months.	Diabetic retinopathy was clinically stable after bariatric surgery
Amin et al. [42]	Surgical: 152 Medical: 155	3 years	After bariatric surgery, patients with T2DM remain at risk for developing STDR. Surgery was associated with a lower progression to STDR or maculopathy compared with routine care

severity. There are two types according to location: the presence of new vessels on the disc (NVD) or within one disc diameter (DD) of the margin of the disc or new vessels elsewhere in the retina (NVE).

Neoangionesis, altered vascular permeability and inflammation are the main pathological drivers of diabetic retinopathy [38]. HbA1c and concomitant diabetic nephropathy are risk factors independently associated with progression of NPDR to PDR [39].

The postoperative probability of having diabetic retinopathy was associated with the extent of HbA1c reduction from presurgery HbA1c levels (Murphy, Jiang et al. 2015). An improved arteriole-to-venule ratio of retinal vessels was demonstrated after a median of 9 months following bariatric surgery of a 30-year-old patient with obesity WHO III [40]. A retrospective study analysed the outcome of bariatric surgery on 67 patients, reported a significant (17.8%) improvement in DR, compared with a worsening of 3.6% of cases [41]. A large, population-based, retrospective cohort study of adult obese patients with T2DM, conducted from 1996 to 2009, reported less ophthalmic manifestations in the bariatric surgery group as a secondary endpoint [23].

A retrospective cohort study investigated the impact of bariatric surgery on the progression to sight-threatening DR (STDR) in 152 patients with type 2 diabetes between January 2005 and December 2012. After bariatric surgery, patients with T2DM remain at risk for developing STDR, even those who did not have evidence of DR before surgery. However, surgery was associated with a lower progression to STDR or maculopathy compared with routine care [42].

A retrospective case-control study reported no significant differences in the progression or deterioration of DR in post RYGB compared with conservative medical treatment [31]. Similar findings were reported by Banks et al. [43]. The STAMPEDE trial did not demonstrate a significant difference in retinopathy outcomes following bariatric surgery compared to intensive medical therapy, but the study was likely underpowered as the majority of patients did not have retinopathy at baseline [44].

Bariatric Surgery and Diabetic Neuropathy (Table 50.3)

Diabetic polyneuropathy affects 30–50% of patients with diabetes mellitus. The pathogenesis

Table 50.3 Summary of studies that analysed the effect of bariatric surgery on the outcome of *neuropathy* in patients with T2D. *LRYGBP* laparoscopic Roux-en-Y gastric bypass

	Study design	No. of subjects	Follow-up	Intervention	Outcome
Philip R Schauer et al. [24]	Prospective follow-up	191 had IFG or T2DM	5 years	LRYGBP	Symptomatic improvement of diabetic neuropathy was reported by 50% of patients after surgery
DePaula, A. L. et al. [49]	Prospective cohort study	8	4–16 months	Ileal interposition into the proximal jejunum via a sleeve or diverted sleeve gastrectomy	Improvement in distal polyneuropathy occurred in 62.5%
Menezes, M. S. et al. [64]	Case report	3	1–4 months	(Restrictive method Roux-en-Y gastric bypass)	Three subjects developed, postoperatively, peripheral neuropathy
Muller-Stich et al. [46]	Prospective cohort study	20	6 months	RYGB	Symptomatic neuropathy was completely reversible in 67% of the patients
Miras et al. [56]	Prospective case-control study	54	12 months	RYGB	No clinically significant changes in any of the nerve conduction variables

IFG impaired fasting glucose

of diabetic DN is multifactorial. The main pathological manifestations are microangiopathy, segmental demyelination and Wallerian degeneration. Protein kinase C, polyol pathway, advanced glycation end products, reactive oxygen species and cytokines play a pivotal role in the pathogenesis of diabetic neuropathy.

A profound recovery from diabetes-associated comorbidities, such as nephropathy, peripheral neuropathy and retinopathy, was reported after sleeve gastrectomy [45]. However, there is not yet enough data to show the long-term impact of bariatric surgery on diabetic neuropathy. A single-armed prospective cohort study reported a significant improvement in *neuropathy* symptom *scores* (NSS) and *neuropathy* disability *scores* (NDS) early after laparoscopic RYGB in a group of obese patients with insulin-dependent T2DM. Symptomatic neuropathy was reversible in 67% of those patients [46].

Improved control of diabetes and amelioration of other risk factors following bariatric surgery may have beneficial effects on neuropathy. However, postoperative micronutrient deficiency specifically in B vitamins may detract from any potential benefits and nutritional status should this be managed in a specialised setting to optimise outcomes.

Conclusion

Intensive glycaemic control alone has been shown to be insufficient to prevent the incidence and the progression of microvascular complications of diabetes. Bariatric surgery is known to induce greater weight loss with a higher cure rate of obesity-related comorbidities. Identification of the precise mechanisms of postoperative weight loss and improved comorbidities could improve and optimise the surgical procedure, especially as many of the beneficial effects of surgery may be enhanced by adding medication such as metformin, angiotensin-converting enzyme inhibitors or statins. Understanding the role of the metabolic, hormonal, genetic and inflammatory factors involved in the aetiology and pathophysiology of obesity and diabetes remains a challenge. More RCTs are required to define the long-term impact of bariatric surgery on microvascular outcomes and to establish whether renal, retinal and neuropathic complications are impacted in similar or different fashions at follow-up. To date the best evidence base exists in relation to diabetic kidney disease. RCTs powered to compare surgery versus best medical approaches in terms of renal microvascular complications are currently underway, and results are eagerly anticipated.

References

1. Hossain P, Kawar B, El Nahas M. Obesity and diabetes in the developing world--a growing challenge. N Engl J Med. 2007;356(3):213–5.
2. Wild S, Roglic G, Green A, Sicree R, King H. Global prevalence of diabetes, estimates for the year 2000 and projections for 2030. Diabetes Care. 2004;27:1047–53.
3. Mathers CD, Loncar D. Projections of global mortality and burden of disease from 2002 to 2030. PLoS Med. 2006;3(11):e442.
4. Vlassara H. Protein glycation in the kidney: role in diabetes and aging. Kidney Int. 1996;49:1795–804.
5. Toth E, et al. Contribution of polyol pathway to arteriolar dysfunction in hyperglycemia. Role of oxidative stress, reduced NO, and enhanced PGH(2)/TXA(2) mediation. Am J Physiol Heart Circ Physiol. 2007;293(5):H3096–104.
6. Nyengaard JR, et al. Interactions between hyperglycemia and hypoxia: implications for diabetic retinopathy. Diabetes. 2004;53(11):2931–8.
7. Takagi Y, et al. Significance of fructose-induced protein oxidation and formation of advanced glycation end product. J Diabetes Complicat. 1995;9(2):87–91.
8. Dronavalli S, Duka I, Bakris GL. The pathogenesis of diabetic nephropathy. Nat Clin Pract Endocrinol Metab. 2008;4:444–4452.
9. Forbes JM, Cooper ME. Mechanisms of diabetic complications. Physiol Rev. 2013;93(1):137–88.
10. Leon CA, Raij L. Interaction of haemodynamic and metabolic pathways in the genesis of diabetic nephropathy. J Hypertens. 2005;23(11):1931–7.
11. Cha DR, et al. Role of vascular endothelial growth factor in diabetic nephropathy. Kidney Int Suppl. 2000;77:S104–12.
12. Matsuoka M, et al. Expression of pigment epithelium-derived factor and vascular endothelial growth factor in fibrovascular membranes from patients with proliferative diabetic retinopathy. Jpn J Ophthalmol. 2006;50(2):116–20.

13. Buchwald H, Oien DM. Metabolic/bariatric surgery worldwide 2008. Obes Surg. 2009;19(12):1605–11.
14. Adams TD, Gress R, Smith SC, et al. Long-term mortality after gastric bypass surgery. N Engl J Med. 2007;357:753–61.
15. Buchwald H, Avidor Y, Braunwald E, et al. Bariatric surgery: a systematic review and meta-analysis. JAMA. 2004;292:1724–37.
16. Buse JB, et al. How do we define cure of diabetes? Diabetes Care. 2009;32(11):2133–5.
17. Arterburn DE, et al. A multisite study of long-term remission and relapse of type 2 diabetes mellitus following gastric bypass. Obes Surg. 2013;23(1):93–102.
18. Dixon JB, O'Brien PE, Playfair J, et al. Adjustable gastric banding and conventional therapy for type 2 diabetes: a randomized controlled trial. JAMA. 2008;299:316–23.
19. Ikramuddin S, et al. Durability of addition of Roux-en-Y gastric bypass to lifestyle intervention and medical management in achieving primary treatment goals for uncontrolled type 2 diabetes in mild to moderate obesity: a randomized control trial. Diabetes Care. 2016;39(9):1510–8.
20. Yu J, et al. The long-term effects of bariatric surgery for type 2 diabetes: systematic review and meta-analysis of randomized and non-randomized evidence. Obes Surg. 2015;25(1):143–58.
21. Sjöström L. Review of the key results from the Swedish Obese Subjects (SOS) trial - a prospective controlled intervention study of bariatric surgery. J Intern Med. 2013;273(3):219–34.
22. Cohen RV, et al. Effects of gastric bypass surgery in patients with type 2 diabetes and only mild obesity. Diabetes Care. 2012;35(7):1420–8.
23. Johnson BL, et al. Bariatric surgery is associated with a reduction in major macrovascular and microvascular complications in moderately to severely obese patients with type 2 diabetes mellitus. J Am Coll Surg. 2013;216(4):545–56; discussion 556-8.
24. Schauer PR, et al. Effect of laparoscopic Roux-en Y gastric bypass on type 2 diabetes mellitus. Ann Surg. 2003;238(4):467–84; discussion 84-5.
25. Adams TD, et al. Clinical outcomes of metabolic surgery: microvascular and macrovascular complications. Diabetes Care. 2016;39(6):912–23.
26. Schauer PR, et al. Clinical outcomes of metabolic surgery: efficacy of glycemic control, weight loss, and remission of diabetes. Diabetes Care. 2016;39(6):902–11.
27. Iwashima Y, et al. Hypoadiponectinemia is an independent risk factor for hypertension. Hypertension. 2004;43(6):1318–23.
28. Sweiss N, Sharma K. Adiponectin effects on the kidney. Best Pract Res Clin Endocrinol Metab. 2014;28(1):71–9.
29. Chang AR, et al. Bariatric surgery is associated with improvement in kidney outcomes. Kidney Int. 2016;90(1):164–71.
30. Agrawal V, et al. The effect of weight loss after bariatric surgery on albuminuria. Clin Nephrol. 2008;70(3):194–202.
31. Alexander D, Miras LLC, Khalil N, Nicotra A, Vusirikala A, Baqai N, Graham C, Ravindra S, Lascaratos G, Oliver N, le Roux CW. Type 2 diabetes mellitus and microvascular complications 1 year after Roux-en-Y gastric bypass: a case–control study. Diabetologia. 2015;58:1443–7.
32. Saliba J, et al. Roux-en-Y gastric bypass reverses renal glomerular but not tubular abnormalities in excessively obese diabetics. Surgery. 2010;147(2):282–7.
33. Upala S, et al. Bariatric surgery reduces urinary albumin excretion in diabetic nephropathy: a systematic review and meta-analysis. Surg Obes Relat Dis. 2016;12(5):1037–44.
34. Heneghan HM, et al. Effects of bariatric surgery on diabetic nephropathy after 5 years of follow-up. Surg Obes Relat Dis. 2013;9(1):7–14.
35. Iaconelli A, et al. Effects of bilio-pancreatic diversion on diabetic complications: a 10-year follow-up. Diabetes Care. 2011;34(3):561–7.
36. Schauer PR, et al. Bariatric surgery versus intensive medical therapy for diabetes--3-year outcomes. N Engl J Med. 2014;370(21):2002–13.
37. Robinson R, et al. Update on animal models of diabetic retinopathy: from molecular approaches to mice and higher mammals. Dis Model Mech. 2012;5(4):444–56.
38. Fante RJ, Gardner TW, Sundstrom JM. Current and future management of diabetic retinopathy: a personalized evidence-based approach. Diabetes Manag (Lond). 2013;3(6):481–94.
39. Harris Nwanyanwu K, et al. Predicting development of proliferative diabetic retinopathy. Diabetes Care. 2013;36(6):1562–8.
40. Lammert A, et al. Improved arteriole-to-venule ratio of retinal vessels resulting from bariatric surgery. Obesity (Silver Spring). 2012;20(11):2262–7.
41. Miras AD, et al. Bariatric surgery does not exacerbate and may be beneficial for the microvascular complications of type 2 diabetes. Diabetes Care. 2012;35(12):e81.
42. Amin AM, et al. The impact of bariatric surgery on retinopathy in patients with type 2 diabetes: a retrospective cohort study. Surg Obes Relat Dis. 2016;12(3):606–12.
43. Banks J, et al. Roux-en-Y gastric bypass could slow progression of retinopathy in type 2 diabetes: a pilot study. Obes Surg. 2015;25(5):777–81.
44. Singh RP, et al. Effect of bariatric surgery versus intensive medical management on diabetic ophthalmic outcomes. Diabetes Care. 2015;38(3):e32–3.
45. DePaula AL, et al. Hormonal evaluation following laparoscopic treatment of type 2 diabetes mellitus patients with BMI 20-34. Surg Endosc. 2009;23(8):1724–32.
46. Muller-Stich BP, et al. Gastric bypass leads to improvement of diabetic neuropathy independent of

glucose normalization--results of a prospective cohort study (DiaSurg 1 study). Ann Surg. 2013;258(5):760–5; discussion 765-6.
47. Izzedine H, et al. Gastric bypass and resolution of proteinuria in an obese diabetic patient. Diabet Med. 2005;22(12):1761–2.
48. Perez G, et al. Resolution of early stage diabetic nephropathy in an obese diabetic patient after gastric bypass. Obes Surg. 2006;16(10):1388–91.
49. DePaula AL, et al. Laparoscopic treatment of type 2 diabetes mellitus for patients with a body mass index less than 35. Surg Endosc. 2008;22(3):706–16.
50. Navaneethan SD, et al. Urinary albumin excretion, HMW adiponectin, and insulin sensitivity in type 2 diabetic patients undergoing bariatric surgery. Obes Surg. 2010;20(3):308–15.
51. Hou CC, et al. Improved renal function 12 months after bariatric surgery. Surg Obes Relat Dis. 2013;9(2):202–6.
52. Stephenson DT, et al. Improvement in albuminuria in patients with type 2 diabetes after laparoscopic adjustable gastric banding. Diab Vasc Dis Res. 2013;10(6):514–9.
53. Jose B, et al. The effect of biliopancreatic diversion surgery on renal function--a retrospective study. Obes Surg. 2013;23(5):634–7.
54. Brethauer SA, et al. Can diabetes be surgically cured? Long-term metabolic effects of bariatric surgery in obese patients with type 2 diabetes mellitus. Ann Surg. 2013;258(4):628–36; discussion 636-7.
55. Amor A, et al. Weight loss independently predicts urinary albumin excretion normalization in morbidly obese type 2 diabetic patients undergoing bariatric surgery. Surg Endosc. 2013;27(6):2046–51.
56. Miras AD, et al. Type 2 diabetes mellitus and microvascular complications 1 year after Roux-en-Y gastric bypass: a case-control study. Diabetologia. 2015;58(7):1443–7.
57. Zakaria AS, et al. Effects of gastric banding on glucose tolerance, cardiovascular and renal function, and diabetic complications: a 13-year study of the morbidly obese. Surg Obes Relat Dis. 2016;12(3):587–95.
58. Varadhan L, et al. Bariatric surgery and diabetic retinopathy: a pilot analysis. Obes Surg. 2012;22(3):515–6.
59. Abbatini F, et al. Long-term remission of type 2 diabetes in morbidly obese patients after sleeve gastrectomy. Surg Obes Relat Dis. 2013;9(4):498–502.
60. Thomas RL, et al. Does bariatric surgery adversely impact on diabetic retinopathy in persons with morbid obesity and type 2 diabetes? A pilot study. J Diabetes Complicat. 2014;28(2):191–5.
61. Murphy R, et al. Progression of diabetic retinopathy after bariatric surgery. Diabet Med. 2015;32(9):1212–20.
62. Kim YJ, et al. Clinical course of diabetic retinopathy in Korean type 2 diabetes after bariatric surgery: a pilot study. Retina. 2015;35(5):935–43.
63. Brynskov T, et al. Monitoring of diabetic retinopathy in relation to bariatric surgery: a prospective observational study. Obes Surg. 2016;26(6):1279–86.
64. Menezes MS, Harada KO, Alvarez G. Painful peripheral polyneuropathy after bariatric surgery. Case reports. Rev Bras Anestesiol. 2008;58(3):252–9.

Index

A

ABCD score, 430
Abdominal pain, 14
  after gastric bypass, 235
    anastomotic stenosis, 239–240
    cholelithiasis, 240–241
    early intestinal obstruction, 237–238
    fistula, 236–237
    hernias in trocars site, 238
    incisional hernias, 241
    internal hernias, 241–242
    less frequent conditions post RYGB, 243
    marginal ulcer, 240
    portomesenteric thrombosis, 237
    remanescent gastric distension, 239
Abdominal ultrasound, 55–56
Abdominal wall, 189
Absorbable suture, mesenteric defect, 183
Acarbose, 309, 322
Accreditation Council for Graduate Medical Education (ACGME), 348
Adenosine triphosphate (ATP), 257, 322
Adipocytokines, 126–127
Adipokines, 13, 32, 34
Adiponectin, 125, 368
Adipose tissue, 369
  distribution, 128–129
  inflammation related to, 126
Adipose tissue macrophage (ATM), 126
Adjunctive therapy, 84
Adjustable gastric banding (AGB) surgery, 9, 273, 274
Advanced glycation end products (AGEs), 470
Adverse intraoperative events (AIEs), 187
Air leak test, gastrojejunostomy, 177–178
Airway evaluation
  handling of, 99
  in obese population, 99–102
Airway management, 103
  bariatric surgery, 222
  planning extubation, 106–107
  positioning, 103–104
  preoxygenation, 104–105
  simplified scoring system, 103
  unanticipated difficult airway, 105–106
Alcohol, pharmacokinetic changes of, 68
Alcohol use disorder (AUD), 218, 268
  American Society for Metabolic and Bariatric Surgery, 269–270
  bariatric surgery, 268–269
  DSM V diagnostic criteria, 268
Alimentary limb, 119, 198, 211, 251
Allopurinol, 261
American Academy of Sleep Medicine (AASM), 82
American Diabetes Association (ADA), 63
American Society for Metabolic and Bariatric Surgery (ASMBS), 230, 269–270, 276, 347, 348, 351, 355
American Society of Anesthesiologists (ASA), 99, 101
Aminoglycosides, 406
AMPK, 369
Anastomosis
  endoscopic measurement, 340–341
  endoscopic treatment, 339
  pouch, 338
  weight regain, 338
Anastomotic stenosis, 239–240
Anastomotic ulcer, 247, 251
Android obesity, 128
Anemia, 274–275
Anesthesia
  complications in bariatric surgery, 221, 224
    airway management, 222
    cardiovascular comorbidities, 223
    esophageal perforation, 224
    nerve injury, 221
    pharmacotherapy, 223
    venous thromboembolism, 223, 224
    ventilation, 222
Angle of His, 227–228
Anorexia nervosa (AN), 68, 287, 291
  crude mortality rate, 292
Antecolic alimentary loop, 197
Antecolic approach, mesenteric defect, 182
Antecolic Roux-en-Y loop, 197–199
Antecolic technique, 119
Anticipated difficult airway, 105
Antidepressants, binge eating, 288
Anti-incretin theory, 308

J. Ettinger et al. (eds.), *Gastric Bypass*, https://doi.org/10.1007/978-3-030-28803-7

Anti-obesity drugs, 161
Anxiety disorder (AD), 70, 217, 267
Apnea-hypopnea index (AHI), 81
Appetite regulation, 10
Appetite suppressors, 162
Argon plasma, 339, 341
Argon plasma coagulation (APC), 166, 333, 334
Arterial calcium-stimulation tests, 309
ASA Closed Claims 2005, 99
AspireAssist device, 26, 27
Asymptomatic gallbladder stone, 296
ATP-sensitive potassium channels (KATP channel), 322
Attention deficit hyperactivity disorder (ADHD), 216
AUD, *see* Alcohol use disorder (AUD)
Autonomic symptoms, hypoglycemia, 308
Awake fiberoptic intubation (AFI), 105

B

Balloon enteroscopy assisted ERCP (BEA-ERCP), 297, 299, 301
Banded gastric bypass
  results/complications, 134–136
  technique, 133–134
Banding, 163
Bardet-Biedl syndrome, 24
Bariatric endoscopy, role of, 329
Bariatric population, pyramid adaption, 282
Bariatric surgery (BS), 1, 27, 41, 47, 187, 215, 221, 454, 470
  age group, 68
  alcohol use disorder, 268–270
  analgesia, 459
  anesthetic complications in, 221, 224
    airway management, 222
    cardiovascular implication, 223
    esophageal perforation, 224
    nerve injury, 221
    pharmacotherapy, 223
    venous thromboembolism, 223–224
    ventilation, 222
  avoiding orogastric tubes/urinary catheters, 459
  behavioral changes, 68
  blood test after, 460
  complications, 403
  diabetes remission, 470
  and diabetic kidney disease, 471–472
  and diabetic neuropathy, 473–475
  and diabetic retinopathy, 471–474
  early ambulation, 459
  depressive disorders, 267–268
  eating behavior (*see* Eating disorder (ED))
  eating disorders, 68
  effectiveness of, 62
  endoscopic algorithm, 331
  enhanced recovery protocols, 459
  failure, 159–160
    causes and diagnosis, 160–161
    endoscopic revision, 165–166
    medical management, 161–162
    postoperative compliance, 160–161
    robotic revisional, 166–167
    surgical treatment, 162–165
  follow-up of, 67
  gastric pouch complication
    nasogastric tube, incidental transection, 228
    staple misfire, 227–228
    transection, 227
  gender, 68
  glucoregulatory effects, 454
  high levels of association, 68
  hypoglycemia, 307–311
    diagnosis, 308–309
    etiology, 308
    pathophysiology, 308
    treatment, 309–311
  indications, 470
  insufficient psychiatric anamnesis, 68
  intentional misinformation, 69
  laparoscopic access and safety, 224
    bowel injury, 226
    subcutaneous emphysema, 226–227
    vascular injury, 224–226
  leaks after, 331
  lung expansion protocols, 459
  mortality rate, 471
  obesity, 63, 215–216
    in anesthesia setting, 224 (*see also* Obesity)
  outcome of, 69–71
  pharmacokinetic changes of alcohol, 68
  postoperative diet, 459
  postoperative ICU admission, 460
  postoperative intra-abdominal infection, 403
    aminoglycosides doses, 406
    antibiotic treatment, 405–406
    ciprofloxacin, 406
    conservative treatment, 404
    enteral nutrition, 404, 405
    hemodynamic support, 404
    imaging methods, 404
    immunological support, 405
    intra-abdominal abscess, 407, 408
    metabolic support, 404–405
    methylene blue, oral administration of, 404
    parenteral nutrition, 405
    radiological findings, 404
    reoperation, indications of, 403–404
    secondary peritonitis, 407
    self-expandable esophageal stents, 404
    surgical repair, 407
    vancomycin doses, 406
  postoperative management
    multivitamin prescriptions, 461
    physical activity, 461
    proton pump inhibitors, 461
  postoperative mortality, 403
  postoperative period, 67
  prejudice, 215–216
  preoperative psychiatric evaluation, 217
  procedures, 117
  psychiatric complications, 67
  psychiatric disorders, 68–69, 217–218

recovery room, 231
restrictive fluid management, 459 (*see also* Roux-Y gastric bypass (RYGB))
STAMPEDE trial, 456
suicide cases, 270
Swedish Obese Subjects study, 412
T2DM, 375
on teenagers, 218
thromboprophylaxis, 459–460
training, 357
treatment for morbid obesity, 117
troublesome anastomosis, 228–231
weight loss after, 77
Bariatric Surgery Center of Excellence, 121
Bariatric surgical patient
cardiopulmonary function, 111–112
direct laryngoscopy, 113
injuries, 114–115
position during, 113–114
pre-oxygenation operating room table, 112
safe apnea period, 112–113
Trendelenburg position, 114
vocal cords during direct laryngoscopy, 113
Barrett's esophagus, 141
Behavioral interventions, binge eating, 288
Behavioral symptoms, 72
Beriberi, 71
Bile acids, 10–11, 365
T2DM, 385–387
Bile reflux, 118
Biliary lithiasis, 295
Biliopancreatic diversion (BPD) with/without duodenal switch (BPD/DS), 360, 376
vs. RYGB, 432–439
Biliopancreatic limb (BPL), 8, 149, 209
of jejunum, 119
omega side-to-side anastomosis, 149
Biliopancreatic loop, 211
Bilroth II reconstruction, 117
Binge eating disorder (BED), 42, 70, 216, 217, 287–292
diagnostic criteria, 287
features, 288
prevalence of, 288
treatment, 288, 289
Bioimpedance absorptiometry, 153
Bioliopancretic diversion with duodenal switch (BPD-DS), 165, 274, 276, 279, 283
Biotin deficiency, 279
Bipolar disorders (BD), 69, 216
Bipolar spectrum states, 68
Bleeding
extraluminal, 192
incidence, 191
intraluminal, 192–193
staple line, 192
BMI, *see* Body mass index (BMI)
BMI-CAD Collaboration Investigators, 32
Body mass index (BMI), 61, 102
prevalence of, 23
Bone mineral metabolism, 279
Bowel habits, 15
Bowel injury, laparoscopic bariatric surgery, 226
Bowel instrumental perforation, 190
Bowel obstruction, 182
BS, *see* Bariatric surgery (BS)
Bulimia nervosa (BN), 68, 287, 289
Bupropion, 26
Bypass Gastrico de Una Anastomosis (BAGUA), 139

C
Calcium antagonists, 322
Calorie malabsorption, 11
Cancer, obesity, 33–34
Carbohydrate addiction, 42
Cardiology, 56
Cardiopulmonary function, 111–112
Cardiovascular comorbidities, bariatric surgery, 223
Cardiovascular death, 33
Cardiovascular disease (CVD), 151
in diabetic patients, 412
obesity, 32–33
Catecholamines, 80
Centers for Medicare and Medicaid Services, 121
Central obesity, importance of, 127–128
Central sleep apnea (CSA), 79
Chenodeoxycholic acid (CDCA), 365
Cheyne-Stokes respiration, 79
Chiba needle, 301
Cholecystectomy, 296
Choledocholitiasis, 240, 296–304
Cholelithiasis, 55–56, 240–241, 295–296
Cholic acid, 13
Chronic obesity, 32
Chyme, dumping syndrome, 316
Ciprofloxacin, 406
Circular-stapled suture, 195, 196
Clavien-Dindo classification, 200
Closure of mesenteric defect, 181, 197, 200
antecolic/retrocolic approach, 182
laparoscopic grasper, 184
nonabsorbable *vs.* absorbable suture, 183
stapler technique, 183
Cognitive behavioral therapies (CBT)
binge eating, 288
bulimia nervosa, 289
Cognitive function, obesity, 36
Common bile duct (CBD), 296, 301, 303, 304
Compartmental syndrome, 257, 259, 262
Complete T2DM remission, 415
Comprehensive geriatric assessment, 153
Compression stocking, 223
Compressive maneuvers, 225
Compulsion change, 68
Computed tomography (CT), 243
gastric dilation, 199
gastrojejunostomy, 179
marginal ulcer, 250
metabolic bone disease, 280
rhabdomyolysis, 260–261
trocar puncture bleeding, 189
weight regain, 161

Continuous glucose monitoring (CGM), 309, 318–319
Continuous positive airway pressure (CPAP), 84
Contrast swallow study, gastrojejunostomy, 179
Cormack-Lehane classification, 102
Coronary artery disease (CAD), 32–33
Covidien stapler brand, 229
CPAP, 461
C-peptide, 309
C-reactive protein (CRP) level, 125, 460
Creatinine phosphokinase (CPK), 256, 257
  rhabdomyolysis, 259, 260
Crotch staple, 227
Crude mortality rate (CMR), anorexia nervosa, 292
Cyclic adenosine monophosphate (c-AMP), 385
Cytokines, 32, 126–127

D

DD, *see* Depressive disorders (DD)
Decompressive fasciotomy, 262
Deep venous thrombosis (DVT), 223, 224
Deleterious effects, 221
Delirium, 71
de novo lipogenesis (DNL), 422
Dental problems, 14
Deoxycholic acid (DCA), 365
Depression, obesity, 34
Depressive disorders (DD), 216, 217, 265
  bariatric surgery, 267–268
  pathophysiology of, 266–267
  prevalence of, 266
  treatment, 267
Depressive episode (DE), 265
  differential diagnosis, 266
  DSM V diagnostic criteria, 266
  treatment, 267
Diabetes
  comorbidities, 142
  obesity, 31–32
Diabetes remission, 470
Diabetes Surgery Study randomized clinical trial, 62
Diabetes Surgery Summit II (DSS-II), 64
Diabetic kidney disease (DKD), 471
Diabetic neuropathy, 473–475
Diabetic retinopathy (DR), 471–474
DiaRem scoring system, 415, 430
Diazoxide, 310
Difficult airway (DA), 99
  anticipated, 105
  obesity and, 101
  predictors of, 102–103
  unanticipated, 105–106
Difficult intubation predictive factors, 103
Difficult mask ventilation predictive factors, 102
Diffusion capacity, 76
Dilated gastric pouch, 163
Direct laryngoscopy (DL), 103, 113
Distal gastric bypass, 164–165
Diuretics, 261
Dormia basket, 302–304
Double-balloon endoscope, 299, 300
Double-contrast CT scan, gastrojejunostomy, 179
Doudenal switch (DS), 171
Dry hemostatic agents, 225
Dual energy X-ray absorptiometry (DEXA), 153
  metabolic bone disease, 279
Dumping symptom, incidence, 193
Dumping syndrome (DS), 15, 277, 307–310
  continuous glucose monitoring, 318–320
  defined, 316
  diagnosis, treatment algorithm, 325
  differential diagnosis, 321
  drug therapy, 322–324
  early dumping, 316–317
  homeostatic model assessment, 318–319
  late dumping, 317
  medical treatment, 324
  mixed meal tolerance test, 319–321
  oral glucose tolerance testing, 317–318
  pathophysiology treatment, 324
  scintigraphy, 321
  surgical therapy, 322–325
  symptoms of, 317
Duodenal-jejunal bypass (DJB), 382
Duodenal switch (DS), 273, 307
Dyslipidaemia resolution, 13
Dyslipidemia, 135

E

Eating disorders (ED), 216, 287
  anorexia nervosa, 291
  binge, 287–288
  bulimia nervosa, 289
  grazing, 290
  night eating syndrome, 289–290
  pagophagia, 290
  post-surgical eating avoidance disorder, 291–292
  prevalence, 287
Ectopic fat deposition, 32
ED, *see* Eating disorders (ED)
Electromyography (EMG), 80
  rhabdomyolysis, 261
Endocrine organ, 126
Endocrinology, 56
Endoscopic duodenal-jejunal liner sleeve (ELS), 382
Endoscopic gastric plication (EGP), 165–166
Endoscopic retrograde cholangiopancreatography (ERCP), 297, 298
  balloon enteroscopy assisted, 297, 299, 301
  laparoscopy-assisted transgastric, 298, 299
Endoscopic suturing methods, 341
Endoscopic vacuum therapy (EVT)
  RYGB, 331, 333
  weight regain, 333
Endoscopy
  gastrojejunostomy

intraoperative testing, 178
postoperative testing, 179
weight regain, 165–166
Endoscopy air leak test, 229
Energy expenditure (EE), 11
Entero-entero anastomosis (EEA), 148–149
Epidural anesthesia with general anesthesia, 223
Epworth sleepiness scale, 83
Escharotomy, 262
Escherichia coli, 368
Esophageal perforation, bariatric surgery, 224
Esophagogastric angle, 147
Esophagogastroduodenoscopy (EGD), 161
European Working Group on Sarcopenia in Older People (EWGSOP), 281
Excessive weight loss, 282–283
Expiratory reserve volume (ERV), 76, 111
predicted, 77
Extraluminal bleeding, soild organs, 192

F

Factitious disorder, 72
Faecalibacterium prausnitzii, 368
Farnesoid X receptor (FXR), 366
Fasting plasma glucose (FPG), 62
Fat free mass (FFM) loss, 280–281
Federal Council of Medicine, 152
Fellowship Council (FC), 347
Female infertility, 24
Ferrous sulphates, 275
FGF19, 363
FGF21, 363
Fibrin glue, 225
Fibroblast growth factor (FGF), 363
Fibromyalgia, 37
First Diabetes Surgery Summit (DSS-I), 63
Fistula, 173, 236–237
Folic acid deficiency, 14
Food intake
gut morphology, 8–9
hormonal, 9
mechanical factors, 8
neural responses, 9–10
weight loss, 7–11
Food preferences, 11
Fouchet tube, 208, 209
Framingham Offspring Cohort, 24
Functional clustering, of microbiota, 396
Functional MRI (fMRI), 11
Functional residual capacity (FRC), 75, 100, 111, 222

G

Gallstones, 15–16
risk of, 24
Gastric acid, 249
Gastric bypass (GB), 187
abdominal pain, 235–243
anastomotic stenosis, 239–240
cholelithiasis, 240–241
early intestinal obstruction, 237–238
fistula, 236–237
hernias in trocars site, 238
incisional hernias, 241
internal hernias, 241–242
less frequent conditions post RYGB, 243
marginal ulcer, 240
portomesenteric thrombosis, 237
remanescent gastric distension, 239
advent of, 99
behavioral changes, 42–43
biochemical testing, 42
complications and outcomes, 48–50
distal, 164–165
endoscopy, 44
laparoscopic method, 3, 117, 118
morbid obesity, 118
nutritional assessment, 42
patient selection, 41
postoperative weight loss, 47–48
preoperative weight loss, 43, 47, 50–51
procedures, 1, 3, 4
psychiatric evaluation, 43–44 (*see also* Roux-en-Y gastric bypass (RYGB))
results of, 159
step-by-step approach, 230
surgery, 117
teaching, 41–42
Gastric cancer, 141
Gastric contents aspiration, 100–101
Gastric dilation, 199
Gastric fistula, enteral nutrition in, 405
Gastric pouch, 119
and anastomosis revision, 163–164
bleeding, 230
complication during creation
nasogastric tube, incidental transection, 228
staple misfire, 227–228
transection, 227
construction, 146–148
position of, 210
preservation of neurovascular axis, 193
tube-related complications, 193–194
Gastric remnant distension, 16
Gastric restriction, laparoscopic restoration, 324
Gastric tube stenosis, 173
Gastric tube trapping, 193–194
Gastroenterostomy, 316
endoluminal revision of, 323
Gastroesophageal junction, 163
mini-gastric bypass, 137
Gastroesophageal reflux disease (GERD)
intractable, 172
Gastrogastric fistula, 161, 339
laparoscopic view, 161
treatment, 164
Gastrografhin swallow, 190

Gastrointestinal (GI) bleeding, postoperative, 230
Gastrointestinal operations, 412
Gastrointestinal surgery
  bile acids, 385–387
  gut microbial, 387
  lower intestinal hypothesis, 384–385
  starvation, 376
  stomach, 380
  upper intestinal hypothesis, 382
Gastrojejunal (GJ) anastomosis, 194–195, 338, 339
  leak at, 190
  stenosis, 195–196
Gastrojejunostomy (GJ), 119, 177, 212, 228
  intraoperative testing, 177
    advantages and disadvantages, 178
    endoscopy, 178
    methylene blue/air leak test, 177–178
  postoperative testing, 178–179
    contrast swallow study, 179
    double-contrast CT scan, 179
    endoscopy, 179
    methylene blue test, 179
  simplified gastric bypass, 147
Gastrostomy tube placement, 310, 311
Gastrotomy incision suture, 298
GE reflux disease (GERD), 138
Ghrelin, 9, 368, 380, 381
GIP receptors (GIPR), 381
GLP1, 366, 369
Glucacon like polypeptide 1 (GLP-1), 308, 384, 385
Glucagon like polypeptide 2 (GLP-2), 385
Glucagon-like peptide 1 (GLP-1), 277, 308, 310, 361
  analogs, 322
Glucose-dependent insulinotropic polypeptide (GIP), 363, 381
Glucose homeostasis, 380
Glycemic control, 411
  after RYGB
    signaling changes, 443
    weight-dependent mechanisms, 443–444
    weight-independent mechanisms, 443–445
G protein-coupled receptor, 366
Grazing, 287
  eating behavior, 290
Gut hormones, 308
Gut microbiota, 10
  after gastric bypass
    compositional alterations, 398
    functional changes, assessment of, 399–400
    metagenomics and back translation in rodents, 401
    phylogenetic comparison, 400
    pyrosequencing methods, 398
    shotgun sequencing of human faecal metagenome, 399
    UniFrac distance matrix analysis, 398
    white adipose tissue transcriptome, changes in, 398
  role in obesity and diabetes, 396–397
  structure and function of, 396
Gut morphology, 8–9

H

Hair loss, 14
  nutritional complications, 277–279
Handsewn anastomosis, 194
Hasson technique, 188
Health markers, 67
Health Professionals Follow-Up Study, 31
Helicobacter pylori (HP), 55, 141, 240, 249
Hemoglobin A1c (HbA1c), 360, 376
Hepaticojejunostomy, 301
Hernias
  incisional (*see* incisional hernias) (*see also specific hernias*)
  in trocars site, 238
Hiatal hernia (HH), 138
High calorie diet, 283
Home sleep apnea test (HSAT), 82, 83
Homeostatic model assessment (HOMA), 318
Homeostatic model assessment insulin resistance (HOMA-IR), 379
Hormonal disorder, 23
Hypercarbia, 80
Hypercortisolism, 23
Hyperglycemia, 411
Hyperinsulinemia, 35, 309, 311
Hyperinsulinemic hypoglycemia, 277, 307, 308, 316
  treatment, 309
Hyperuricemia, 260
Hypocalcaemia, 14, 262
Hypoglycemia, 277, 307–308
  diagnosis, 308–309
  etiology, 308
  pathophysiology, 308
  symptom, 307
  treatment, 309–311
Hypoglycemia-like symptoms, 307
Hypoglycemic agents, 460
Hypothyroidism, 23
Hypoventilation, 80
Hypovolemia, 261
Hypoxemia, 79
  perioperative, 100

I

ICU admission
  cardiac comorbidities, 460
  high-risk respiratory comorbidities, 460
Ileal transposition (IT), 385
Immunomodulation, 405
Incisional hernias, 241
Incretin effect, 361
Individualized metabolic surgery (IMS) score, 430
Indocyanine green (ICG) angiography, 231
Inflammation, related to adipose tissue, 126
Informed consent, 56–57
Initial haemostasis, rebleeding, 192
Insulin resistance, 126
Intensive medical diabetes and weight management (IMWM) program, 455
Interleukin 10 (IL-10), 125

Intermesenteric abscess, 190
Internal hernia, 120, 181–183, 197, 241–242
International Federation for the Surgery of Obesity and Metabolic Disorders (IFSO), 152, 337
Interstitial fluid glucose (IGF), 319
Intestinal gluconeogenesis, 365, 370
Intestinal glucose metabolism, 364
Intestinal intussusception, 243
Intestinal microbiota, 366–368
Intestinal obstruction, 237–238
Intra-abdominal abscess
  antibiotic treatment, 408
  percutaneous drainage, 407
  surgical drainage, 407
Intra-abdominal bleeding, 230
Intra-abdominal pressure, 115
Intractable gastroesophageal reflux disease (GERD), 172
Intra-ganglionic laminar endings (IGLEs), 10
Intragastric bougie, 207, 208
Intrahepatic triglyceride (IHTG), 37
Intraluminal bleeding, 192–193
Intraoperative bleeding, 191
Intraperitoneal bleeding, 192
Intrinsic PEEP (PEEPi), 100
Intubation laryngeal mask (ILMA), 105, 106
Iron deficiency, 14, 274, 278
Islets of Langerhans, 308
Isoperistaltic Billroth II reconstruction, 147

J

Jejunal loop
  alimentary position, 196–197
  antecolic Roux-en-Y loop, 197–199
  error in measurement, 196
  kinking of, 197
  Roux-en-o configuration, 196
Jejunojejunostomy, 173, 199–200
  alimentary limb, 198
Jejunojejunostomy mesentery, 181, 182
  See also Mesenteric defect closure
Jejunojenostomy, 119

K

Kidney stones, 15
Korsakoff psychosis, 275

L

Laparoscopic adjustable gastric band (LAGB), 280, 290, 376, 455
  vs. RYGB, 439
  T2DM, 379
Laparoscopic approach to Roux-en-Y gastric bypass (LRYGB), 118
Laparoscopic bariatric surgery, 224–227
  bowel injury, 226
  subcutaneous emphysema, 226–227
  vascular injury, 224–226
Laparoscopic bariatric surgery training
  bariatric privileges, 352
  bariatric trainees, 350
  credentialing, 351, 352
  curriculum guidelines, 348, 349
  leadership skills, 348
  LRYGB learning curve, 350, 351
  non-clinical endeavors, 348
  technical skills, 348
Laparoscopic cholecystectomy, 117, 296
Laparoscopic gastric bypass (LGBP), 187, 192, 205
  bleeding after, 191
  cardiology, 56
  cholelithiasis/abdominal ultrasound, 55–56
  endocrinology, 56
  GI evaluation, 54–55
  history, 53
  informed consent, 56–57
  intestinal time and anastomosis, 208–212
  intraoperative technical steps, 206–208
  laboratory testing, 54
  postoperative approaches, 212
  preoperative preparation, 205
  psychosocial and nutritional evaluation, 54
  pulmonary, 56
  surgical room checklist
    equipment and instrument, 206
    safe surgery, 206
    staff position, 206
  suture test, 212
Laparoscopic grasper, mesenteric defect, 184
Laparoscopic Roux-en-Y gastric bypass (LRYGBP), 3, 159–160, 188, 191, 193, 194, 227, 228, 350, 351, 416
  antecolic and antegastric route, 197
  bleeding after, 230
  early postoperative bleeding after, 230
  efficacy, 120
  intervention, 194
  linear stapled technique, 229
  laparoscopic operations, 120
  longterm follow-up, 120
  marginal ulceration (*see* Marginal ulcer (MU))
  multiple complications, 120
  nasogastric tube transection, 228
  perioperative risk factors, 121
  postoperative complication, 200
  quality of life, 121
  retrocolic and retrogastric route, 197
  technique description, 416–418
  tube-related complication, 194
  upper gastrointestinal hemorrhage after, 229
Laparoscopic simplified gastric bypass
  entero-entero anastomosis, 148–149
  gastric pouch construction, 146–148
  gastrojejunostomy, 147
  patient position and surgical team, 146
  Petersen space closure, 147–149
  pneumoperitoneum, 146
Laparoscopic sleeve gastrectomy (LSG), 137, 258, 275
  indications, 145
  to MGB, 140

Laparoscopy-assisted transgastric ERCP (LAT-ERCP), 298, 299, 301
Latex balloons, 299
L cells, 308
Lean tissue mass (LTM) loss, 280–281
Leptin, 9, 24
  hormone, 100
LGBP, *see* Laparoscopic gastric bypass (LGBP)
Linear-stapled suture, 195, 196
Linear stapler technique, 119
  anastomosis technique, 195
  laparoscopic Roux-en-Y gastric bypass, 229
Lipopolysaccharide (LPS), 397
Liraglutide, 26, 162
Lithiasis, 295
Lithocholic acid (LCA), 365
Liver, computed tomography, 50
L-lysine deficiency, 278
Longitudinal Assessement of Bariatric Surgery (LABS), 187, 191, 192, 230
Lönroth technique, 200
Look AHEAD trial, 25
Lorcaserin, 25
Loss of bone density, 15
Low-calorie diets (LCD), 50
Lower intestinal hypothesis, 384–385
LRYGB, *see* Laparoscopic Roux-en-Y gastric bypass (LRYGBP)
LSG, *see* Laparoscopic sleeve gastrectomy (LSG)
Lung volume
  severe obesity on, 77
  spirometric and subdivision of, 78
  subdivisions of, 76, 77

M

Macrophages, 127
Magnetic resonance imaging (MRI), rhabdomyolysis, 260–261
Major depressive disorder, 69
Malabsorptive jejunal bypass, 138
Male infertility, 24
Mallampati classification, 102
Mallampati score, 82, 222
Manual suture, 195, 196
Marginal ulcers (MU), 16, 240, 247, 248, 330
  anatomy, 248–249
  diagnosis, 250
  Helicobacter pylori, 249
  incidence, 247–248
  patient demographics, 249–250
  prevention, 250–251
  procedure type, 249
  surgical technique, 249
  symptomatology, 250
  treatment, 240, 250
Megaloblastic anemia, 276
Melanocortin receptor, mutation, 24
Melanocortin system, 13
Mental disorders, obesity, 215
Mesenteric defect, 197
Mesenteric defect closure, 181–184, 197, 200
  antecolic/retrocolic approach, 182
  laparoscopic grasper, 184
  nonabsorbable *vs.* absorbable suture, 183
  stapler technique, 183
Mesenteric irritation technique, 183
Mesocolic defect, 197
Metabolically healthy obese (MHO), 129
Metabolically obese normal weight (MONW), 129
Metabolically unhealthy normal weight (MUNW), 129
Metabolic and Bariatric Surgery Accreditation and Quality Improvement Program (MBSAQIP), 352, 357
Metabolic bone disease, 151, 172
  nutritional complications, 279–280
Metabolic surgery, 413, 455, 457
  blood test after, 460
  BMI, eligibility criteria, 413
  definition, 413
  DSS-2 guidelines, 414–415, 457
  eligibility criteria for, 414
  patient discharge, 461–462
  postoperative ICU admission, 460
  postoperative management, 459
    dyslipidemia, 461
    hypertension, 461
    obstructive sleep apnea, 461
    physical activity, 461
    proton pump inhibitors, 461
    type 2 diabetes, 460–461
  preoperative evaluation, 414
  randomized clinical trials, 455
  results, 413–416
  See also Bariatric surgery
Metabolic syndrome, 61, 125
Methylene blue, gastrojejunostomy
  intraoperative testing, 177–178
  postoperative testing, 179
Microalbuminuria, 471
Mini gastric bypass (MGB)
  advantages, 140, 465
  bariatric operations, 142
  comorbidities, 142
  complications, 467, 468
  components, 137
  disadvantages, 465
  follow-up, 467
  gastric cancer, 141
  harmonic scalpel, 467
  hypoalbuminemia, 138
  intake requirements, 141
  lap-band, 140
  lesser omentum dissection, 466
  LSG to, 140
  malabsorptive jejunal bypass, 138
  patient positioning, 466
  ports, 466
  pouch, 137
  preference in India, 465–466

rationale for, 140–141
staples, 466
weight loss after, 467
Mitochondrial dysfunction, 32
Mixed meal tolerance test (MMTT), 309, 319–321
Molecular microbiology, 395
Mood disorders (MD), 68, 216, 217
Morbid obesity, 23, 255, 453
associated complications, 24–25
genetic syndromes, 24
patient assessment, 23–24
rhabdomyolysis, 257–258
signs and symptoms, 23
systemic inflammation in, 125–126
treatment of, 25–27
very low-calorie diets, 25
Münchhausen syndrome, 72
Muscle biopsy, 261
Muscle weakness, 259
Muscular debridement, 262
Muscular injury, 255
Musculoskeletal disorders, obesity, 36–37
Myocytes, 255
Myoglobin, 256
Myonecrosis, 257

N

Naltrexone, 26
Nasogastric tube, incidental transection, 228
National Institute of Health (NIH), 152
Neck circumference (NC), 102
Nerve injury, bariatric surgery, 221
NES, *see* Night eating syndrome (NES)
Nesidioblastosis, 308–311
Neural responses, 9–10
Neurocognitive disorders, 218
Neuroglycopenia, 307
Neuro-paracrine actions, 364
Neuropathy, symptoms, 276
Neurovascular axis, preservation of, 193
Nifedipine, 310
Night eating syndrome (NES), 70, 287, 289–290
Nonabsorbable suture, mesenteric defect, 183
Nonalcoholic fatty liver disease (NAFLD), 24
obesity, 37
Noncommunicable diseases (NCDs), 359
Noninsulinoma pancreatogenous hypoglycemia, 308
Nonproliferative diabetic retinopathy (NPDR), 473
Nonsteroidal anti-inflammatory drugs (NSAIDs), 330
marginal ulcer, 249–251
Non-surgical "bariatric mimetic" approach, 401
Nutritional complications, 273
dumping syndrome, 277
excessive weight loss, 282–283
hair loss, 277–279
hypoglycemia, 277
lean tissue mass loss, 280–281
metabolic bone disease, 279–280
sarcopenia, 280–281
weight regain, 281–282
Nutritional deficiencies
anemia, 274–275
psychiatric disorders, 71
thiamine, 275–276
vitamin B_{12}, 276

O

Obesity, 23, 75, 215–216, 265, 454, 467, 469
airway evaluation in, 101–102
in anesthesia setting, 221–224
cancer, 33–34
cardiovascular disease (CVD), 32–33
cognitive function, 36
defined, 421
and depression, 34
diabetes, 31–32
and difficult airway (DA), 101
distribution of, 78
gas exchange in, 78–79
on male fertility, 35
minimally invasive surgery, 190
musculoskeletal disorders, 36–37
nonalcoholic fatty liver disease, 37, 38
non-physiologic position, 111
and perioperative hypoxemia, 100
perioperative management, 111
in physiologic changes, 78–79
prevalence, 255
pulmonary complications of, 75
and reproduction, 34–35
respiratory and airway changes in, 99–100
respiratory diseases, 35–36
and risk of gastric contents aspiration, 100–101 (*see also* Bariatric surgery (BS))
sexual function and, 35
on sleep, 79
treatment, 151, 152
vascular effects, 36
Obesity hypoventilation syndrome (OHS), 79–80
Obesity-induced type 2 diabetes mellitus, 453
Obesity Surgery Mortality Risk Score (OS-MRS), 152
Obsessive compulsive disorder, 70
Obstructive sleep apnea (OSA), 35, 79, 80
diagnosis and classification of, 82–84
evaluation for, 82
high risk of, 82
numerous screening tools, 82
pathogenesis of, 80
physical examination, 82
prevalence of, 100
probability of survival in patients, 81
severity of, 82
symptoms of, 82
treatment, 84
Octreotide (somatostatin), 310
Omega limb, 209
Omega loop, 199

Omental reinforcement, 228
One-anastomosis gastric bypass (OAGB), 139
  gastric pouch, 139
  intake requirements, 141
  rationale for, 140–141
Oral glucose tolerance test (OGTT), 317–318
  hyperglycemia, 309
Oral hypoglycemic agents, 460
Orlistat, 26, 162
Orogastric calibration tube, 194
Orogastric technique, 194
Orogastric tube,x methylene blue/air test through, 177–178
Osteoarthritis (OA), 37
Other specified feeding or eating disorders (OSFED), 287, 289
Overweight, defined, 469
Oxidative stress, 369

P
Pagophagia (Pica), 290
Palmer's point, 146, 226
Pancreatic resection, 310, 311
Partial pancreatectomy (PP), postprandial hypoglycemia, 308
Partial T2DM remission, 415
Pellagra, 71
Peptide YY (PYY), 362
Percutaneous transhepatic cholangiogram, 301, 302
Peripheral pulses, 262
Petersen's space, 181, 182, 197
  closure, 147–149, 210
  exposition, 210
Pharmacotherapy, bariatric surgery, 223
Phentermine, 25
Pica, 290
Pneumoperitoneum, 118
  laparoscopic simplified gastric bypass, 146
Polysomnogram (PSG), 82, 101
Portomesenteric thrombosis, 237
Positive end-expiratory pressure (PEEP), 114
Postoperative (PO) period
  epileptic fits, 72
  factitious disorder, 72
  immediate, 71
  late, 72
  mediate, 72
  Münchhausen syndrome, 72
  psychological/behavioral symptoms, 72
  psychopharmacological treatment in, 72
  simulation, 72
  somatization, 72
  surgical procedures, 71–72
Postpone surgery, 69
Postprandial hyperinsulinemic hypoglycemia, 307, 310
Postprandial hypoglycemia, 15, 308
  partial pancreatectomy, 308
  symptoms, 308
Postsurgical eating avoidance disorder (PSEAD), 68, 70, 291
Potassium channel activator, 322
Pouch
  endoscopic measurement, 340
  endoscopic treatment, 339
  weight regain, 338
Prader-Willi syndrome, 24, 218
Prejudice, 215–216
Preoxygenation, 104–105
Proglucagon-derived peptides (PGDPs), 384
Proinsulin, 309
Proliferative diabetic retinopathy (PDR), 473
Prolonged T2DM remission, 415
Proopiomelanocortin deficiency (POMC), 24
Prophylactic cholecystectomy, 55
Prophylactic surgery, 295
Prophylaxis, 100
Proton pump inhibitor (PPI), 141
  marginal ulcer, 250, 251
Psychiatric anamnesis, 68
Psychiatric disorders (PD), 215, 265, 267
  in bariatric surgery, 217–218
  identified during postoperative period, 68–69
  interference of, 69–71
  nutritional deficiencies, 71
  obesity, 215–216
  prevalence of, 67, 217
  suicide, 270
  weight loss, 71
Psychological symptoms, 72
Psychopharmacological treatment, 72
PubMed, 267
Pulmonary embolism (PE), 223
Pulmonary function tests, subdivisions, 75–77
Purse-string suture, 297, 298

Q
Quality of life (QoL), 265

R
Radiography, rhabdomyolysis, 260–261
Randomized controlled trials (RCT), 7, 47
Rapid eye movement (REM) sleep, 80
Reactive hypoglycemia, 307
Reduced resting energy expenditure (REE), 12
Refeeding, 276
Remanescent gastric distension, 239
Reproduction and obesity, 34–35
Residual volume (RV), 76, 100
Respiratory diseases and obesity, 35–36, 99–100
Respiratory function impairment, 25
Restorative Obesity Surgery Endoscopic (ROSE), 166
Retrocolic approach, mesenteric defect, 182
Retrocolic orientation, 119
Reverse Trendelenburg position, 112, 114, 118
Revisional surgery, 171
  indication, 172

Reward deficiency syndrome (RDS), 68
Rhabdomyolysis (RML), 255
  clinical features, 259
  clinical finding, 258–259
  complication, 259
  image examination, 260–261
  laboratory findings, 259–260
  in morbid obesity, 257
    incidence, 257
    prevention, 257–258
  pathophysiology, 255–257
  physical evaluation, 259–260
  postoperative, 255, 257
  research articles, 256
  risk factors, 259
  treatment, 261–262
Ring distal displacement, RYGB, 330–331
RML, *see* Rhabdomyolysis (RML)
Robotic bariatric surgeon
  credential vettings, 357–358
  intuitive surgical's curriculum, 356
  progression, surgical steps, 356–357
Robotic revisional bariatric surgery, 166–169
Roux-en-o configuration, 196
Roux-en-Y gastric bypass (RYGBP), 3, 4, 47, 93, 117, 145, 159, 177, 228, 273, 317, 319, 413, 421
  abdominal discomfort, 243–245
  anastomotic stricture, 329
  bariatric endoscopy, 329
  bile acids, 385
  clinical outcomes in randomized controlled trials
    vs. biliopancreatic diversion, 432–441
    vs. laparoscopic adjustable gastric banding, 439, 442
    vs. medical management, 432
    vs. sleeve gastrectomy, 432–438
  comorbidity improvement/resolution, 12
  complication rates, 13
  deficiency causes, 274
  diabetic kidney disease, 471
  DJB, 383
  in elderly patient, 151–153
    benefits, 153
    outcomes, 154
    postoperative complications, 155
    resolution of comorbidities, 155
    risks, 152
    surgical treatment, 153–154
  food impaction, 329
  hypoglycemia, 307–311
    diagnosis, 308–309
    etiology, 308
    pathophysiology, 308
    treatment, 309–311
  intragastric ring erosion, 330
  leaks after, 331–333
  marginal ulceration (*see* Marginal ulcer (MU))
  mesenteric defect closure, 183
  MGB, 140 (*see* Roux en Y gastric bypass (RYGB))
  ring distal displacement, 330–331
  sleeve gastrectomy, 171, 325, 347
    complication, 172, 173
    indications, 171, 172
    surgical technique, 173
  starvation, 376
  type 2 diabetes, 360
    adipose tissue effects, 369
    bile acid metabolism, 365
    caloric restriction, glycemia, 361
    fibroblast growth factor, 363
    gut hormones, 361
    intestinal glucose metabolism, 364
    intestinal lipid sensing, 364
    intestinal microbiota, 366–367
    islet cell dysfunction improvement, 368
  weight loss, 7–12
  weight regain, 333–334
Roux-en-Y gastrojejunostomy, 118
Roux-en-Y jejunojejunal anastomosis, 190
Roux-en-Y limb, 119, 120
Roux-en-Y loop, antecolic, 197–199
RYGBP, *see* Roux-en-Y gastric bypass (RYGBP)

S

Safe apnea period (SAP), 112–113
Sarcopenia, nutritional complications, 280–281
Schizophrenia, 70
Scintigraphy, dumping syndrome, 321
Self-expandable metallic stents (SEMS), 331
Septotomy, 332
Serum leptin, 81
Severe obesity, pathophysiology of T2D, 421–423
Sex hormone binding globulin (SHBG), 35
Sight-threatening diabetic retinopathy (STDR), 474
Silastic ring, 164
Simplified gastric bypass, 145–146
  laparoscopic
    entero-entero anastomosis, 148, 149
    gastric pouch construction, 146–148
    gastrojejunostomy, 147
    patient position and surgical team, 146
    Petersen space closure, 147–149
    pneumoperitoneum, 146
Simulation, 72
Single-anastomosis duodenoileal bypass (SADI), 171
Single-anastomosis duodeno-ileal bypass with sleeve gastrectomy (SADI-S), 140
Single anastomosis gastric bypass, *see* Mini gastric bypass
Single-balloon endoscope, 299
Single incision laparoscopic surgery (SILS), 120, 121
Sleep, obesity effect, 79
Sleep apnea, perioperative management, 85–86
Sleep disordered breathing (SDB), 79
  perioperative management of, 85–86
Sleeve gastrectomy (SG), 94, 181, 273, 274, 307, 347, 356, 376
  vs. Roux-en-Y gastric bypass, 171, 324, 325, 432–438
    complication, 172, 173
    indications, 171, 172
    surgical technique, 173

Small gastric curvature, 207
Snacking, 42
Society for Surgery of the Alimentary Tract (SSAT), 351
Society of American Gastrointestinal Endoscopic Surgeons (SAGES), 41, 351, 355
Sodium-glucose-cotransporter-1 (SGLT1), 364, 365
Soild organs
  extraluminal bleeding, 192
  injury, 188
Somatization, 72
Somatostatin analogs, 322
Spirometry, 76, 78
Splenectomy, incidence, 192
Staple line bleeding, 192
Stapler technique
  articulation, 208
  mesenteric defect, 183
  positioned for first shot, 208
Stapling gap suture closure, 210
Stenosis of gastrojejunal (GJ) anastomosis, 195–196
Stents, 331, 333
Stomal stenosis, 16
STOP-BANG questionnaire, 101
Stroke, 33
Subcostal trocar puncture, 189
Subcutaneous adipose tissue (SAT), 128
Subcutaneous emphysema, laparoscopic bariatric surgery, 226–227
Substance use disorders, 70
Sucralfate®, 250
Suicide, bariatric surgery and, 270
Superobesity, 49
  choice of procedure, 93–94
  clinical characteristics of, 91–92
  C-PAP treatment, 93
  definition, 91
  evaluation before bariatric/metabolic surgery, 92–93
  obesity-related comorbidities, 96
  postoperative care, 96
  preoperative evaluation, 92
  preoperative preparation of patients, 94–95
  preoperative work-up, 96
  special requirements for, 95
Supraceliac aortic clamping, 225
Supraglottic airway devices (SGD), 99
Supraglottic devices, 103
  emergence of, 105
Suture closure, of stapling gap, 210
Suture test, 212
Swedish Obesity Surgery Registry (SOReg), 187, 188
Swish Obesity Study (SOS), 281
Sympathetic fibres, 10
Systemic inflammation, in morbidly obese patient, 125–126

T

T2DM, *see* Type 2 diabetes mellitus (T2DM)
Technetium-99m pyrophosphate (99mTc-PYP) scintigraphy, rhabdomyolysis, 260–261
Teenagers, bariatric surgery, 218
Telogen effluvium, 278
Thiamine deficiency, 275–276
Thromboplastin, 256
Thrombosis, portomesenteric, 237
Tidal volumes (TV), 79
Tissue plasminogen, 256
Topicalization, 105
Topiramate, 25
  binge eating, 289
Total lung capacity (TLC), 76
Transoral outlet reduction (TORe), 166, 343
Transparetohepatic drainage, 241
Transumbilical gastric bypass (TUGB), 120
Transverse mesocolon elevation, 209
Treitz angle, 209
Trendelenburg position, 222
Trocar puncture
  access position, 206, 207
  bleeding, 189
  hernias, 238
  injuries, 188–189
  subcostal, 189
  wounds, 189
Trocars placement, laparoscopic simplified gastric bypass, 146
Type 2 diabetes (T2D), gastric bypass
  complications and long-term mortality, 430–432
  mechanisms of, 12–13, 359–360
  remission and relapse
    C-peptide measurement, 427
    glucagon-like peptide, 427
    long-term, 424–426
    predictors of, 427–430
    rates of, 423–427
    scoring systems, 430
  RYGB
    adipose tissue effects, 369
    bile acid metabolism, 365–366
    caloric restriction, glycemia, 361
    fibroblast growth factor, 363–364
    gut hormones, 361–363
    intestinal glucose metabolism, 364–365
    intestinal lipid sensing, 364
    intestinal microbiota, 366–368
    islet cell dysfunction improvement, 368
Type 2 diabetes mellitus (T2DM), 126, 159, 160, 411
  ADA criteria, 453
  Asiatic population, 61, 63
  bariatric surgery, 61–63 (*see* Bariatric surgery)
  body mass index, 61
  morbidity, 430
  mortalities, 431
  characteristic, 469
  deaths, 61
  Diabetes Surgery Study randomized clinical trial, 62
  gastrointestinal surgery
    bile acids, 385–387
    gut microbial, 387
    lower intestinal hypothesis, 384–385

starvation, 376–380
stomach, 380–382
upper intestinal hypothesis, 382–384
global prevalence of, 61
glucotoxicity, 469
glycaemic control, 61
LAGB, 379
laparoscopic sleeve gastrectomy, 456
lifestyle interventions and medication, 411
medical treatment, 64
metabolic abnormalities, 412
metabolic risk score, 64
microvascular complications, 469–471
night eating syndrome, 289–290
pathophysiology, 412
patient selection for metabolic surgery, 63, 64
prevalence, 421
prevention and treatment, 375
randomized trials, 62
remission, (*see* RYGB technique), 415
Roux-en-Y gastric bypass and, 62
surgical procedures, 62
treatment (*see* Metabolic surgery)

U
Ultracision®, 147
Ultrasound (US), rhabdomyolysis, 260–261
Uncoupling protein 1 (UCP1), 363
Upper gastrointestinal endoscopy, 161, 329
marginal ulcer, 330
Upper gastrointestinal hemorrhage (UGIH), 229
Upper gastrointestinal series (UGI), 54
Upper intestinal hypothesis, 382
Urinary myoglobin, 260
Ursodeoxycholic acid (UDCA), 296

V
Vagal afferent fibres, 10
Vagus nerve of Latarjet, 193
Vancomycin, 406
Vascular injury, laparoscopic bariatric surgery, 224–226
Venous thromboembolic events (VTE), 55
bariatric surgery, 223–224
Ventilation, bariatric surgery, 222
Veress technique, 188, 189
Vertical banding gastroplasty (VBG), 281
Very low-calorie diets (VLCD), 48, 50
Visceral fat area (VFA), 63
Visceral fat storage capacity, 128
Visceral injuries, 189–190
Vitamin B12 deficiency, 14, 71, 275, 276
Vitamin C, 275
Vitamin D deficiency, 14, 280
VTE, *see* Venous thromboembolism (VTE)

W
Wakeful stimuli, 80
Weight loss
daily energy intake, 8
failure in, 172
food intake, 7–11
postoperative, 47–48
preoperative, 43, 47, 50–51
psychiatric disorders, 71
Weight regain, 159, 310
causes and diagnosis, 160–161
endoscopic revision, 165–166
medical management, 161–162
nutritional complications, 281–282
postoperative compliance, 160–161
robotic revisional BS, 166–169
surgical treatment, 162–165
banding, 162, 163
BPD-DS, 165
conversion to distal gastric bypass, 164–165
gastric pouch and anastomosis revision, 163–164
gastrogastric fistula, 164
Weight regain after gastric bypass
abnormal anatomic, 342
anastomosis
endoscopic treatment, 339
measurement, 340–341
pouch, 338
endoscopic technique, 341–342
gastrojejunal anastomosis, 338
pouch measurement, 340
transoral outlet reduction, 343
Wernicke encephalopathy, 275
Wernicke-Korsakoff syndrome (WKS), 71, 292
Whipple's triad, 308
White adipose tissue (WAT), 127, 128
World Health Organization, 159

X
X-ray, marginal ulcer, 250

MIX
Papier aus verantwortungsvollen Quellen
Paper from responsible sources
FSC® C105338

If you have any concerns about our products,
you can contact us on
ProductSafety@springernature.com

In case Publisher is established outside the EU,
the EU authorized representative is:
Springer Nature Customer Service Center GmbH
Europaplatz 3, 69115 Heidelberg, Germany

Printed by Libri Plureos GmbH
in Hamburg, Germany